The Principles and Practice of
ULTRASONOGRAPHY
in OBSTETRICS
and GYNECOLOGY

fourth edition

The Principles and Practice of
ULTRASONOGRAPHY
in OBSTETRICS
and GYNECOLOGY
fourth edition

Edited by

Arthur C. Fleischer, MD
Professor of Radiology
Associate Professor of Obstetrics and Gynecology
Chief, Diagnostic Sonography
Department of Radiology and Radiologic Sciences
Vanderbilt University Medical Center
Nashville, Tennessee

Roberto Romero, MD
Associate Professor
Department of Obstetrics and Gynecology
Director of Perinatal Research
Yale University School of Medicine
New Haven, Connecticut

Frank A. Manning, MD
Chairman, Department of Obstetrics and Gynecology
University of Manitoba Faculty of Medicine
Women's Hospital
Winnipeg, Manitoba, Canada

Philippe Jeanty, MD
Associate Professor of Radiology
Assistant Professor of Obstetrics and Gynecology
Department of Radiology and Radiologic Sciences
Vanderbilt University Medical Center
Nashville, Tennessee

A. Everette James, Jr., ScM, JD, MD
Professor and Chairman
Department of Radiology and Radiologic Sciences
Vanderbilt University Medical Center
Nashville, Tennessee

APPLETON & LANGE
Norwalk, Connecticut/San Mateo, California

0-8385-7954-X

Notice: Our knowledge in clinical sciences is constantly changing. As new information becomes available, changes in treatment and in the use of drugs become necessary. The authors and the publisher of this volume have taken care to make certain that the doses of drugs and schedules of treatment are correct and compatible with the standards generally accepted at the time of publication. The reader is advised to consult carefully the instruction and information material included in the package insert of each drug or therapeutic agent before administration. This advice is especially important when using new or infrequently used drugs.

91 92 93 94 95 / 10 9 8 7 6 5 4 3 2 1

Prentice Hall International (UK) Limited, *London*
Prentice Hall of Australia Pty. Limited, *Sydney*
Prentice Hall Canada, Inc., *Toronto*
Prentice Hall Hispanoamericana, S.A., *Mexico*
Prentice Hall of India Private Limited, *New Delhi*
Prentice Hall of Japan, Inc., *Tokyo*
Simon & Schuster Asia Pte. Ltd., *Singapore*
Editora Prentice Hall do Brasil Ltda., *Rio de Janeiro*
Prentice Hall, *Englewood Cliffs, New Jersey*

Library of Congress Cataloging-in-Publication Data
The principles and practice of ultrasonography in obstetrics and gynecology/edited by Arthur C. Fleischer . . . [et al.].—4th ed.
    p.   cm.
ISBN 0–8385–7954–X
  1. Ultrasonics in obstetrics.   2. Generative organs. Female—Ultrasonic imaging.   3. Fleischer, Arthur C.
  [DNLM: 1. Genital Diseases, Female—diagnosis.   2. Pregnancy Complications—diagnosis.   3. Ultrasonic Diagnosis.]
RG527.5.U48U47   1991
618—dc20
DNLM/DLC
for Library of Congress   90–961
                                                                CIP

Designer: Janice Barsevich
Cover: Color Doppler sonogram of a 26-week pregnancy showing the umbilical cord, its paired arteries in blue, and vein in red. The back cover shows a transvaginal sonogram of an 8-week fetus.

PRINTED IN THE UNITED STATES OF AMERICA

To our children,
who we hope will continue to improve the quality of life
through refinements in technology.

CONTRIBUTORS

Apostolos P. Athanassiadis, MD
Postdoctoral Fellow
Department of Obstetrics and Gynecology
Yale University School of Medicine
New Haven, Connecticut

Cecilia Avila, MD
Postdoctoral Fellow
Department of Obstetrics and Gynecology
Yale University School of Medicine
New Haven, Connecticut

Giovanna Baccarani, MD
Department of Cardiovascular Diseases
Istituto delle Malattie Cardiovascolari
University of Bologna School of Medicine
Bologna, Italy

Beryl Benacerraf, MD
Clinical Associate Professor of Radiology and
    Obstetrics and Gynecology
Harvard Medical School
Brigham and Women's Hospital
Boston, Massachusetts

Frank H. Boehm, MD
Professor and Director
Division of Maternal/Fetal Medicine
Vanderbilt University Medical Center
Nashville, Tennessee

Luciano Bovicelli, MD
Section of Prenatal Pathophysiology
Department of Obstetrics and Gynecology
University of Bologna School of Medicine
Bologna, Italy

James D. Bowie, MD
Professor of Radiology
Chief, Section of Ultrasound
Assistant Professor Department of Obstetrics and
    Gynecology
Duke University Medical Center
Durham, North Carolina

Robert L. Bree, MD
Associate Professor of Radiology
Department of Radiology

University of Michigan Medical School
Chief, Radiology Services
Veterans Administration Medical Center
Ann Arbor, Michigan

Albert L. Bundy, MD, JD
Boston Ultrasound Consultants, P.C.
Brookline, Massachusetts

Peter S. Cartwright, MD
Assistant Professor
Department of Obstetrics and Gynecology
Vanderbilt University Medical Center
Nashville, Tennessee

James P. Crane, MD
Professor
Department of Obstetrics and Gynecology
    and Radiology
Washington University School of Medicine
St. Louis, Missouri

Jack Davies, MD
Emeritus Professor of Anatomy
Department of Cell Biology
Vanderbilt University Medical Center
Nashville, Tennessee

Peter J. Dempsey, MD
Radiologist
Doctors Hospital
Mobile, Alabama

Peter M. Doubilet, MD, PhD
Associate Professor of Radiology
Harvard Medical School
Director of Ultrasound
Brigham and Women's Hospital
Boston, Massachusetts

Stephen S. Entman, MD
Associate Professor and Vice Chairman
Department of Obstetrics and Gynecology
Vanderbilt University School of Medicine
Director, Division of Gynecology
Vanderbilt University Medical Center
Nashville, Tennessee

Calliope Fine, MD
Boston Ultrasound Consultants, P.C.
Brookline, Massachusetts

Arthur C. Fleischer, MD
Professor of Radiology
Associate Professor of Obstetrics and Gynecology
Chief, Diagnostic Sonography
Department of Radiology and Radiologic Sciences
Vanderbilt University Medical Center
Nashville, Tennessee

Sandro Gabrielli, MD
Section of Prenatal Pathophysiology
Department of Obstetrics and Gynecology
University of Bologna
Bologna, Italy

Kathleen A. Gadwood, MD
Clinical Assistant Professor
Michigan State University
Kalamazoo Center for Medical Studies
Kalamazoo, Michigan

William J. Garrett, MD
Professor of Obstetrics and Gynecology
Director of Department of Diagnostic Ultrasound
Royal Hospital for Women
Paddington, Sydney, Australia

Alan N. Gordon, MD
Assistant Professor of Obstetrics and Gynecology
Vanderbilt University Medical Center
Nashville, Tennessee

Lawrence P. Gordon, MD
Associate Professor of Pathology
State University of New York Health Science Center
    at Syracuse
Staff Pathologist
Crouse Irving Memorial Hospital
Syracuse, New York

David Graham, MD, FRCS(C)
Department of Obstetrics and Diagnostic Ultrasound
The Johns Hopkins Medical Institutions
Baltimore, Maryland

Dennis Gratton, RDMS
Educational Co-ordinator
Department of Ultrasound
Health Sciences Centre
Winnipeg, Manitoba, Canada

Christopher R. Harman, MD
Assistant Professor
University of Manitoba Faculty of Medicine
Director, Fetal Assessment Unit
Women's Hospital
Winnipeg, Manitoba, Canada

Carl Morse Herbert III, MD
Assistant Professor of Obstetrics and Gynecology
Acting Director
Division of Reproductive Endocrinology and Infertility
Vanderbilt University Medical Center
Nashville, Tennessee

Barbara S. Hertzberg, MD
Associate Professor
Department of Radiology
Section of Ultrasound
Duke University Medical Center
Durham, North Carolina

John C. Hobbins, MD
Professor, Deputy Chairman
Head, Section of Maternal/Fetal Medicine
Department of Obstetrics and Gynecology
Yale University School of Medicine
New Haven, Connecticut

Charles Hohler, MD (Deceased)
Director of Perinatology and Perinatal Ultrasound
Co-director, Division of Reproductive Medicine
St. Joseph's Hospital and Medical Center
Phoenix, Arizona

Mona Inati, MD
Genetics Associate
Department of Obstetrics and Gynecology
Yale University School of Medicine
New Haven, Connecticut

Valerie P. Jackson, MD
Professor of Radiology
Department of Radiology
Indiana University School of Medicine
Indianapolis, Indiana

A. Everette James, Jr., ScM, JD, MD
Professor and Chairman
Department of Radiology and Radiologic Sciences
Professor of Obstetrics and Gynecology
Professor of Medical Administration
Lecturer in Legal Medicine
Vanderbilt University Medical Center
Nashville, Tennessee

Everette James III, JD
Illinois Institute of Technology
Kent School of Law
Chicago, Illinois

Jeannette C. James, JD
Attorney at Law
Bass, Berry & Sims
Nashville, Tennessee

Philippe Jeanty, MD
Associate Professor of Radiology
Assistant Professor of Obstetrics and Gynecology
Department of Radiology and Radiologic Sciences
Vanderbilt University Medical Center
Nashville, Tennessee

Donna M. Kepple, RDMS
Chief Sonographer
Department of Radiology, Section of Ultrasound
Vanderbilt University Medical Center
Nashville, Tennessee

Faye C. Laing, MD
Professor of Radiology
University of California, San Francisco
Chief, Division of Ultrasound
San Francisco General Hospital
San Francisco, California

J. Patrick Lavery, MD
Clinical Professor
Department of Obstetrics and Gynecology
Michigan State University
Perinatologist
Bronson Methodist Hospital
Kalamazoo, Michigan

Clifford S. Levi, MD, FRCP(C)
Associate Professor
Department of Diagnostic Radiology
University of Manitoba Faculty of Medicine
Winnipeg, Manitoba, Canada

Daniel J. Lindsay, MD
Assistant Professor
Department of Radiology
University of Manitoba
Winnipeg, Manitoba, Canada

Edward A. Lyons, MD
Professor of Radiology
Professor of Obstetrics and Gynecology
University of Manitoba Faculty of Medicine

Acting Radiologist-in-Chief, Department of Radiology
Health Sciences Centre
Winnipeg, Manitoba, Canada

Frank A. Manning, MD
Chairman, Department of Obstetrics and Gynecology
University of Manitoba Faculty of Medicine
Women's Hospital
Winnipeg, Manitoba, Canada

Michael Moretti, MD
Associate Professor
Department of Obstetrics and Gynecology
University of Tennessee College of Medicine
Memphis, Tennessee

William D. O'Brien, Jr., PhD
Professor of Electrical and Computer Engineering
Professor of Bioengineering
Department of Electrical and Computer Engineering
Bioacoustics Research Laboratory
University of Illinois
Urbana, Illinois

Enrique Oyarzun, MD
Postdoctoral Fellow
Department of Obstetrics and Gynecology
Yale University School of Medicine
New Haven, Connecticut

David L. Page, MD
Professor of Pathology
Director of Anatomic Pathology
Department of Pathology
Vanderbilt University Medical Center
Nashville, Tennessee

Rebecca G. Pennell, MD
Clinical Assistant Professor of Radiology
Jefferson Medical College of Thomas Jefferson
   University
Philadelphia, Pennsylvania
Department of Radiology
Doylestown Hospital
Doylestown, Pennsylvania

Antonella Perolo, MD
Second Department of Obstetrics and Gynecology
Section of Prenatal Pathophysiology
University of Bologna School of Medicine
Bologna, Italy

Ferdinando M. Picchio, MD
Department of Cardiology
Istituto Malattie Cardiovascolari
University of Bologna School of Medicine
Bologna, Italy

Gianluigi Pilu, MD
Attending Physician
Section of Prenatal Pathophysiology
Second Department of Obstetrics and Gynecology
University of Bologna School of Medicine
Bologna, Italy

Ronald R. Price, PhD
Professor of Radiology and Radiologic Sciences
Associate Professor of Physics
Director, Division of Radiologic Sciences
Chief of Diagnostic Physics
Vanderbilt University Medical Center
Nashville, Tennessee

Marcos Pupkin, MD
Professor
Department of Obstetrics and Gynecology
University of Maryland School of Medicine
Baltimore, Maryland

Bhaskara K. Rao, MD
Assistant Professor of Radiology
Diagnostic Sonography
Vanderbilt University Medical Center
Nashville, Tennessee

Nicola Rizzo, MD
Section of Prenatal Pathophysiology
Department of Obstetrics and Gynecology
University of Bologna School of Medicine
Bologna, Italy

Roberto Romero, MD
Associate Professor
Department of Obstetrics and Gynecology
Director of Perinatal Research
Yale University School of Medicine
New Haven, Connecticut

Glynis A. Sacks, MD
Assistant Clinical Professor of Radiology
Vanderbilt University Medical Center
Nashville, Tennessee
Radiology Consultants
Nashville, Tennessee

Dinesh M. Shah, MD
Assistant Professor
Director, Obstetrics Diabetic Unit
Division of Maternal/Fetal Medicine
Department of Obstetrics and Gynecology
Vanderbilt University Medical Center
Nashville, Tennessee

Marina Sirtori, MD
Postdoctoral Fellow
Department of Obstetrics and Gynecology
Yale University School of Medicine
New Haven, Connecticut

Beverly A. Spirt, MD
Professor of Radiology
Chief, Department of Ultrasound
State University of New York Health Science Center
   at Syracuse
Syracuse, New York

Brian J. Trudinger, MD
Associate Professor
Department of Obstetrics and Gynaecology
University of Sydney at Westmead Hospital
Sydney, New South Wales, Australia

John R. Vallentine, MB, BS
The Australasian Medical Defense Union
Sydney, New South Wales, Australia

Anne Colston Wentz, MD
Professor of Obstetrics and Gynecology
Department of Obstetrics and Gynecology
Northwestern University Medical School
Head, Section of Reproductive Endocrinology and
   Infertility
Center for Assisted Reproduction
Northwestern Memorial Hospital
Chicago, Illinois

Alan C. Winfield, MD
Professor of Radiology
Department of Radiology and Radiologic Sciences
Vanderbilt University Medical Center
Nashville, Tennessee

Marvin C. Ziskin, MD
Professor of Radiology and Medical Physics
Department of Diagnostic Imaging
Temple University Medical School
Philadelphia, Pennsylvania

CONTENTS

PREFACE

Since the publication of the third edition, there have been several new developments in obstetric and gynecologic sonography. Foremost amongst these are the development and clinical application of transvaginal sonography, sonographically directed interventional procedures such as cordocentesis, and Doppler interrogation of uterine and uteroplacental circulation. These improvements have occurred along with better resolution conventional real-time imaging.

Because of the range and extent of new developments in this field, an almost complete revision of the prior edition was required. New chapters have been added concerning fetal blood sampling, the status of fetal interventional procedures, and early detection of ovarian carcinoma with sonography, to name a few. Many new illustrations have been included, such as line drawings to accompany transvaginal sonograms and numerous color prints depicting the use of color Doppler sonography.

We hope that this text will be of high educational value for medical imaging specialists, sonographers, and other health care related professionals who perform and interpret obstetric and gynecologic sonograms.

Arthur C. Fleischer, MD
Nashville, Tennessee
October, 1989

The Principles and Practice of
ULTRASONOGRAPHY
in OBSTETRICS
and GYNECOLOGY
fourth edition

1 Basic Physics of Ultrasound

Marvin C. Ziskin

THE NATURE OF SOUND

Sound is the propagation of energy by a mechanical wave through matter. A mechanical wave is a propagated vibration of particles in a medium. Sound requires a mass-containing medium to support its transmission and, therefore, cannot travel through a vacuum. In contrast, an electromagnetic wave sustains itself by the alternate exchange of energy between electric and magnetic fields and does not require matter for propagation. What the human ear perceives as sound is the pressure change on the eardrum caused by mechanical waves traveling through air.

The atomic and molecular structure of a medium will determine both the velocity and wave characteristics of any transmitted mechanical wave (sound). Let us consider the molecules (or structural units) of this medium represented by rigid spheres. The intermolecular forces are depicted by coiled springs between adjacent spheres (Fig. 1–1). A mechanical wave, such as sound, incident on this medium will cause a displacement of spheres so that they move back and forth in relation to one another. This longitudinal motion causes alternate crowding and uncrowding of adjacent spheres. The movement is periodic, with the distance between two bands of compression or rarefactions of the spheres determining the wavelength of the mechanical wave in the supporting medium (Fig. 1–2). Wavelengths ranging from 0.1 to 1.5 mm are utilized in medical applications. The wavelength is important because it determines the theoretical limit of resolution of the imaging system. Two structures closer than one wavelength apart will not be identified as separate entities in an ultrasound image.

The compressions and rarefactions of the spheres in our hypothetical medium plotted against time describe a sinusoidal curve like the one in the upper protion of Figure 1–2. Since pressure is proportional to molecular concentration, the local pressure is elevated in regions of compression and reduced in regions of rarefaction. Therefore, sinusoid also describes variations in pressure. The periodic change in pressure on the eardrum is called the frequency of sound. The human ear is capable of hearing frequencies of between 16 and 20,000 cycles per second. The unit of frequency is the Hertz, which is equal to one cycle per second, and is abbreviated Hz. One million Hertz equals one MegaHertz, abbreviated MHz. Ultrasound, by definition, is beyond the range of audible sound and therefore has a frequency greater than 20,000 Hz.

The Speed of Sound

The speed of sound through a medium is dependent on the density and compressibility of the medium. Materials with heavy molecules will tend to move more slowly than a light-molecular-weight material when there is any pressure change. Materials that are very compressible, such as gases, will have long excursions of individual molecules and will transmit pressure waves (sound) less rapidly. Therefore, increasing density or compressibility tends to decrease the speed of sound transmission. Some materials and their corresponding acoustic speeds are listed in Table 1–1. It is interesting to note that mercury is 13.6 times denser than water, but its speed is nearly the same. This occurs because mercury's compressibility is nearly 13.6 times less than that of water. Most liquids share this inverse proportionality between compressibility and density and, therefore, have similar acoustic speeds.

A fixed relationship between acoustic speed, wavelength and frequency exists as follows:

$$v = f\lambda \qquad [1]$$

where v is the speed of sound in conducting material (meters/second), f is the frequency (Hertz), and λ is the wavelength (meters). If the acoustic speed within any given material is constant, then as the frequency increases, the wavelength decreases. Thus, spatial resolution improves with increasing frequency.

Types of Waves

In the previous description, the vibratory motion of molecules is parallel to the direction of propagation. This is referred to as a longitudinal wave and is by far the predominant type of sound wave occurring within the body. A transverse sound wave is a wave in which the vibratory motion is perpendicular to the direction of propagation. Whereas solids, liquids, and gases can support longitudinal waves, only solids can support transverse waves. Surface or Rayleigh waves are waves in which the molecules move in an elliptic pattern. This type of wave occurs at the upper surface of a body of water.

With the exception of compact bone, the longitudinal waves are the only type observed within the body. In bone, both longitudinal and transverse waves can occur.

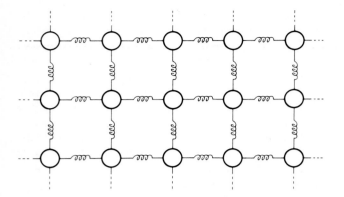

Fig. 1–1. Organization of matter. From the acoustic viewpoint, matter consists of an array of molecules connected to each of their immediate neighbors by elastic springs.

TABLE 1–1. ACOUSTIC SPEED IN VARIOUS TISSUES

Tissue or material	Acoustic speed (meters/sec)
Air	331
Fat	1,450
Water	1,495
Soft tissue (mean value)	1,540
Kidney	1,561
Muscle	1,585
Bone	4,080

Intensity of Sound

Intensity is the measure of the "strength" of a sound wave. Consider an imaginary plane positioned perpendicular to a sound wave. Power is then defined as the rate at which energy passes this plane. The unit of power is the watt. Intensity is defined as power per cross-sectional area and is expressed as watts per square centimeter (W/cm^2).

Table 1–2 lists intensities used in various medical applications. Note that intensities employed in most diagnostic applications are approximately 20 to 100 times less than those used in therapeutic applications. Some Doppler units, however, emit acoustic intensities approaching therapeutic levels. Because diagnostic intensities are so small, these are practically always given in units of milliwatts per square centimeter.

Sometimes, instead of absolute measurements, merely a comparison of two intensities is desired. This would normally imply a simple ratio of the two intensities. However, since such a ratio would range from zero to extremely large values, the logarithm of the ratio is used for comparison. Specifically, the intensity of a sound wave relative to some reference sound wave is expressed in decibel units (dB) as given by

$$dB = 10 \log_{10}(I/I_0) \qquad [2]$$

where I_0 is the intensity of the reference sound wave and I is the intensity of the sound wave being compared. Intensity and amplitude ratios are presented in Table 1–3.

Unless stated otherwise, whenever a sound intensity is expressed in decibel units, it is to be understood that the reference intensity is 10^{-16} W/cm^2, which is the lowest intensity perceptible to the human ear. Intensities of audible sound waves are most frequently expressed in decibel units. The greater the intensity, the greater the subjective sensation of loudness.

PRODUCTION OF SOUND

In the audible range, sound is usually produced mechanically by means of a loudspeaker, which consists of a paper cone or diaphragm connected to an electromag-

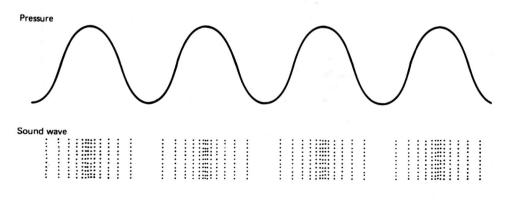

Fig. 1–2. Longitudinal sound wave and associated pressure wave.

TABLE 1–2. SOUND INTENSITIES EMPLOYED IN MEDICINE

Medical usage	Intensity* (W/cm²)
Surgical	> 10
Therapeutic	0.5–3.0
Diagnostic	
Pulse echo	0.001–0.1
Doppler	0.01–1.0

* Spatial-peak temporal-average intensity.

net. An electrical signal, whose voltage varies in accordance with the desired sound pattern, is applied to the electromagnet. This produces a corresponding motion of the diaphragm, which in turn produces a corresponding pressure variation in the air molecules in the vicinity of the diaphragm. This pressure variation propagates through the air and, on reaching the ear, is perceived as sound. However, because of their inertia, loudspeakers cannot vibrate rapidly enough to produce ultrasonic frequencies. Consequently, the generation of ultrasound had to await the discovery of piezoelectric crystals.

Most crystals do not possess the property of piezoelectricity. The most important natural crystal possessing this property is quartz. Although quartz has been used in ultrasonic generators for many years, it has now been replaced in medical devices almost entirely by synthetic ceramic crystals such as barium titanate and lead zirconate titanate (PZT), because these synthetic crystals possess better mechanical properties and are easier to fabricate than quartz.

The piezoelectric effect is the generation of an electric voltage when a crystal is compressed (Fig. 1–3). The voltage generated is proportional to the amount of compression. If the crystal is stretched, a voltage of the opposite polarity is generated. The reverse piezoelectric effect is the compression or expansion of a crystal induced by the application of a voltage (Fig. 1–4).

TABLE 1–3. DECIBEL UNITS AND CORRESPONDING INTENSITY AND AMPLITUDE RATIOS

dB	Intensity ratio	Amplitude ratio
60	1,000,000	1,000
50	100,000	320
40	10,000	100
30	1,000	32
20	100	10
10	10	3.2
0	1	1
−10	0.1	0.32
−20	0.01	0.1

Piezoelectric crystals are able to respond faithfully to applied electric signals at high frequencies to produce ultrasonic waves, and they likewise are able to convert accurately ultrasound waves into corresponding electric signals.

In medical application, these crystals are cut into thin wafers (less than 1 mm in thickness) and are mounted on a transducer probe.* The generation of sound waves is illustrated in Figure 1–5. The top row shows the transducer and the molecules in the surrounding medium at rest. In the next row, an electric voltage has been applied across the piezoelectric crystal. This induces an expansion of the crystal, which causes the molecules closest to the transducer to move toward the right. The resulting greater concentration of molecules is a condensation. The next row shows that, when the electric voltage is removed, the crystal returns to its initial shape whereas the condensation continues to move toward the right. The row next to the bottom shows the contraction of the crystal when an electric voltage of opposite polarity is applied. This results in a lesser concentration of molecules in the vicinity of the transducer. When the voltage is removed once more, the crystal returns to its original shape and the condensation and rarefaction continue moving toward the right. A repetitive alteration of the imposed electric voltage therefore generates a continuous sound wave. This is easily accomplished with present-day electronic circuitry.

Types of Transducers

Transducer probes come in a variety of shapes and sizes, each of which is designed for a particular application. Some of the more common types are cylindrical, flat, perivascular, aspiration, and multielement transducer arrays. The cylindrical or pencil-shaped transducer is designed for those examinations requiring scanning or searching for a particular structure. An example is the pencil-shaped Doppler transducer probe that is used to detect the fetal heart.

The flat transducer, in the shape of a disk, is useful for prolonged monitoring since it can be taped to the skin and need not be held throughout the examination period. It is particularly useful in fetal monitoring during labor.

The perivascular type is a cuff that is mounted around an exposed artery or vein at the time of surgery. Very small transducers can be made and mounted on catheter tips, which can then be inserted into blood ves-

---

* Technically speaking, a transducer is a device that converts one form of energy into another. In ultrasonics, the piezoelectric crystal is the actual transducer since it converts sonic energy into electric energy and vice versa. However, in common parlance, the combination of the crystal and its housing is usually referred to as the transducer.

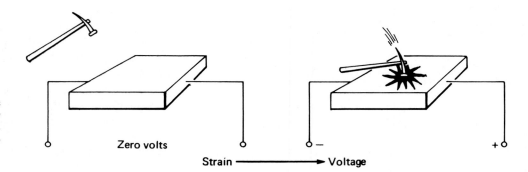

Fig. 1–3. The direct piezoelectric effect. (*Adapted from Goldberg B, et al. Diagnostic Uses of Ultrasound. New York, Grune & Stratton; 1975. By permission.*)

sels or the ureters, allowing close inspection of these structures.

The aspiration transducer is essentially a flat transducer with a central aperture through which a hypodermic needle can be inserted. This transducer allows simultaneous viewing of the needle tip location and surrounding anatomic structures and is useful for amniocentesis.

Various multielement transducer arrays are presently available. In these probes, as many as 64 or more individual piezoelectric crystals are mounted on a single unit. Excitation of these crystals in rapid sequence allows real-time viewing of moving internal structures and eliminates the need for manual scanning. "Real-time" connotes that one is able to see anatomic movements as they occur.

Sound Beams
Sound beams are classified as divergent, collimated, or focused (Fig. 1–6). The shape is determined by (1) the sound frequency, (2) the diameter of the transducer, and (3) the presence or absence of an acoustic lens. With a given transducer, the higher the frequency, the less the divergence of the beam. So that the sound beam may be sufficiently narrow to be useful in diagnostic applications, the frequency should be greater than 1 MHz. Obstetric applications usually employ ultrasonic frequencies ranging from 3 to 7 MHz. For collimated beams, the beam width is constant and is approximately equal to the transducer diameter.

A narrow, highly directional beam is required for good lateral resolution. The beam pattern of an unfocused transducer is determined by the wavelength and transducer diameter. A characteristic sound beam is depicted in Figure 1–7. There exists a parallel component, which is the Fresnel or near zone, and a diverging component called the Fraunhofer or far zone. The letter T designates the transition point between the Fresnel and Fraunhofer zones. The length of the Fresnel zone may be determined by the diameter of the transducer and the wavelength of the beam by the following relation:

$$T = r^2/\lambda \qquad [3]$$

where T is the length of Fresnel zone (cm), r is the radius of the transducer (cm), and λ is the wavelength (cm). The Fresnel zone is longest for a large transducer and for short wavelength (high frequency) ultrasound. Although both depth resolution and Fresnel zone length are increased with short wavelength (high frequency) ultrasound, the attenuation may become so high that deep structures cannot be imaged. Increasing the transducer size also has limitations, as large transducer diameters create wide beams with decreased lateral resolution.

To obtain the most resolution in examining deep, internal structures, focused beams are used. Focusing is achieved by means of an acoustic lens in fixed-focused transducers or by electronic switching techniques (dynamic focusing) in multielement transducer arrays. An acoustic lens is a thin piece of plastic whose center is thinner than its edges. This lens, placed on the front of

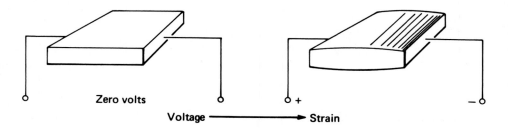

Fig. 1–4. The reverse piezoelectric effect. (*Adapted from Goldberg B, et al. Diagnostic Uses of Ultrasound. New York, Grune & Stratton; 1975. By permission.*)

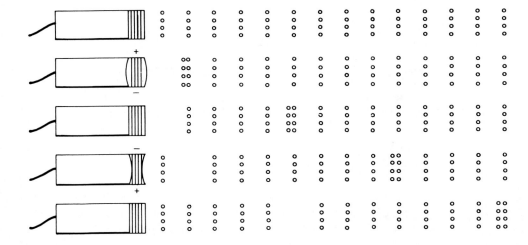

Fig. 1-5. Generation of ultrasound beam by transducer. Each row represents a successive instant in time. By imposing on oscillating electric signal, the transducer generates a continuous ultrasound beam.

the transducer probe, focuses the sound beam in the same manner as a glass lens focuses light. The focal length of a transducer is the distance from the transducer face to the focal point, which is the narrowest point in the sound beam. In dynamic focusing, the focal length can be varied continuously during scanning. A focal length of 9 to 13 cm is used for most obstetric and gynecologic examinations. For examination of more superficial structures, transducers with shorter focal length are preferred. In general, the narrowest part of the beam should occur at the depth where the greatest resolution is desired.

Modes of Operation

There are two modes of transducer operation: continuous and pulsed. In the continuous mode, a sustained electric oscillation is applied to the transducer crystal, and a continuous sound beam is produced. Because this crystal is dedicated to the generation of the sound beam, a second crystal is required to detect returning echoes. The second crystal is normally mounted on the same transducer probe. This mode of operation is used primarily in some Doppler units.

The pulsed mode of operation consists of emitting sound in very short pulses and bursts. Between pulses, the transducer is "silent" and able to detect returning echoes. Because the same crystal can act as both a sender and receiver of sound pulses, only one crystal is necessary in this mode of operation.

SOUND TRANSMISSION THROUGH TISSUE

Attenuation

The intensity of a sound beam constantly decreases as it travels through tissue. This decrease in intensity is called attenuation. It is due to three factors: (1) divergence of the sound beam, (2) absorption of sound energy by the tissue, and (3) deflection of sound out of the beam.

Divergence

As a sound beam diverges, its energy is spread over a larger cross-sectional area. Because intensity is proportional to energy per unit area, it decreases in proportion to the divergence of the beam.

Diverging

Collimated

Focused

Fig. 1-6. Beam patterns.

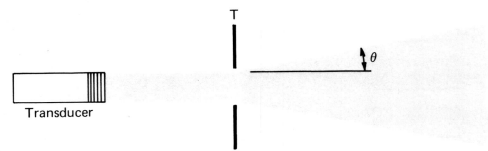

Fig. 1–7. Characteristic sound beam.

Absorption

Absorption is the transfer of energy from the sound beam to the tissue. The energy removed is used primarily in overcoming the internal frictional forces of the tissue and is ultimately degraded into heat production. The greater the sound frequency, the more rapidly the tissue molecules must move and the greater the energy expended in overcoming friction. Thus, absorption is proportional to frequency. At 1 MHz, approximately 50% of the energy is absorbed by the time sound travels 3 cm in soft tissue, and less than 1% of the original intensity remains after it has traveled 20 cm. At 10 MHz, with the absorption 10 times greater, 50% of the initial intensity remains at a 0.3-cm depth, and less than 1% at 2.0 cm. In order to detect deep abdominal structures, the frequency should be less than 5 MHz.

In addition to frequency, the amount of absorption depends on the viscosity of the tissue through which the sound travels. In general, the more rigid the tissue and the higher the collagen content, the greater the absorption. Bone absorbs approximately ten times more than most soft tissues, and these in turn absorb approximately 10 times more than body fluids such as blood and amniotic fluid.

Table 1–4 lists the absorption coefficients and the half-value layers of various tissues for a 1-MHz sound

TABLE 1–4. ABSORPTION COEFFICIENTS AND HALF-VALUE LAYERS OF VARIOUS TISSUES

Tissue or material	Absorption coefficient (dB/cm/MHz)	Half-value layer (cm)
Water	0.0022	1,360.00
Blood	0.15	20.38
Fat (subcutaneous)	0.61	4.95
Kidney	0.96	3.15
Uterus	1.04	2.89
Liver	1.22	2.45
Fat (peritoneal)	2.08	1.44
Bone	14.07	0.21

beam. The half-value layer is the distance the sound beam has penetrated into a tissue when its intensity has been reduced to one half of its initial value.

When sound encounters surfaces or boundaries between structures, a portion of the sound gets deflected out of the beam. Depending on the dimensions of the surface, the mechanism for the deflection will be that of scattering or reflection. Scattering occurs when the dimensions of the surface are as small as or smaller than the wavelength of the sound. The scattered sound leaves the surface in all directions, and is therefore frequently referred to as diffuse reflection. Because the scattered sound is emitted in all directions, the amount going in any one particular direction is very small and requires great amplification in order to be detected in B-scans.

Reflection

Whenever a sound beam reaches a large boundary between two tissues, some of the sound is reflected backward and the remainder is transmitted through the boundary (Fig. 1–8). This "mirror-like" type of reflection is called specular. The amounts of sound that are reflected and transmitted and the directions in which they travel are determined by certain properties of the two tissues and by the angle at which the incident sound beam strikes the boundary. This incident angle is labeled θ_i in Figure 1–8. As is true in the case of light, the direction of the transmitted beam is given by Snell's law:

$$\frac{\sin \theta_t}{\sin \theta_i} = \frac{v_2}{v_1} \qquad [4]$$

where v_1 is the speed of sound in tissue 1, v_2 is the speed of sound in tissue 2, and θ_t is as defined in Figure 1–8. The deviation of the direction of the transmitted beam from that of the incident beam is referred to as refraction.

The angle of reflection θ_r equals the angle of incidence. Therefore, in pulse echo techniques in which one uses the same transducer to both send pulses and receive echoes, the transducer should be positioned so that the sound beam is perpendicular to the boundary. This position will maximize the amount of echoes to return to the transducer and be detected.

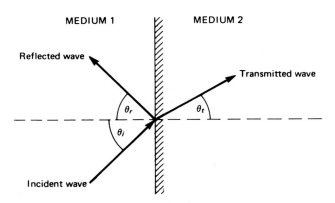

Fig. 1–8. Reflection and transmission of ultrasound at a boundary. (*Adapted from Goldberg B, et al. Diagnostic Uses of Ultrasound. New York, Grune & Stratton; 1975. By permission.*)

The amount of sound reflected is proportional to the difference in the acoustic impedances of the two tissues. Acoustic impedance is the resistance offered by a tissue to the passage of sound and is represented by the symbol Z. It can also be shown to equal the product of the density and the acoustic speed of the tissue:

$$Z = \rho v \qquad [5]$$

where ρ is the tissue density and v is the acoustic speed.

Table 1–5 lists the acoustic impedances for various tissues. Note that the acoustic impedance of air is extremely small compared to that of any other item in this list. Therefore, an air-tissue boundary presents such a large difference in acoustic impedances that virtually all of the sound incident on this boundary is reflected. This has several important consequences for diagnostic ultrasound.

The first consequence is that some coupling agent, such as mineral oil or Aquasonic, must be applied to the

TABLE 1–5. ACOUSTIC IMPEDANCES

Tissue or material	Acoustic impedance (rayl × 10⁻⁵)*
Air	0.0004
Fat	1.38
Water	1.48
Blood	1.61
Kidney	1.62
Soft tissue (mean value)	1.63
Liver	1.65
Muscle	1.70
Bone	7.80

* The rayl unit is equivalent to grams per square centimeter second.

surface of the skin so that no air exists between the transducer and the skin. The presence of air would cause all the sound to be reflected and prevent any penetration into the patient. The second consequence is that gas within the gastrointestinal tract also blocks any further penetration of a sound beam. Therefore, in order to examine any structure lying beneath a gas-containing intestinal loop, one must move the transducer to a different position to bypass the gas. This also applies to chest examination, where the first air-alveolar boundary effectively blocks any further penetration.

INSTRUMENTATION

Introduction

As mentioned previously, whenever sound enters the body, some of the sound is scattered and reflected backward and the remainder is transmitted through. Both the reflected echoes and the transmitted sound can be detected and analyzed to obtain medical information. This provides for three categories of ultrasonic techniques:

1. *Pulse-echo techniques*, which provide the location of anatomic structures by measuring the transit time for sound to reach the structure and return to the ultrasonic detector.
2. *Doppler techniques*, in which the frequencies of returning echoes are analyzed to determine the velocity of moving structures.
3. *Through-transmission techniques*, in which the sound completely traversing the body is analyzed for transit time, intensity, phase shift, and so forth.

Pulse-Echo Techniques

The purpose of a pulse-echo system is to transmit a short ultrasonic pulse and detect all returning echoes. As the transmitted pulse traverses the body, some of its energy is reflected backward at each tissue interface. The amplitude of each echo depends on the orientation of the reflecting surface and the difference in acoustic impedances of the tissues at the interface. Echoes detected by the transducer are displayed on an oscilloscope in either A-mode, B-mode, or B-scan presentations. As the transmitted pulse is approximately 1 microsecond in duration and the pulse repetition rate is typically 1,000 per second, the same transducer element is used for both transmitting and receiving,

The generation of each sound pulse is accomplished by applying a short electric impulse, called the excitation wave, to the transducer crystal (Fig. 1–9). This causes the crystal to "ring" at its natural frequency in a manner analogous to hitting a gong with a hammer. The natural

Fig. 1–9. Shock excitation. A short electric impulse is applied to the transducer crystal to produce the sound pulse. (*Adapted from Goldberg B, et al. Diagnostic Uses of Ultrasound. New York, Grune & Stratton; 1975. By permission.*)

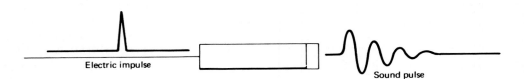

Electric impulse

Sound pulse

frequency is determined by the thickness of the crystal. So that the ringing not be too prolonged, damping is employed. This is accomplished by both electronic and mechanical means. In some instruments, a damping control is provided. This should be set so that approximately two complete cycles are contained in each pulse (Fig. 1–10). If overdamped, too little sound energy is transmitted and echoes are too weak to be detected. If underdamped, the pulse is so long that echoes from neighboring structures tend to overlap and thus resolution is decreased.

Returning echoes are converted by the transducer into an electric signal, the amplitude of which is directly proportional to the echo amplitude. The electric signal is processed and amplified in order to produce an adequate display on an oscilloscope (Fig. 1–11). An oscilloscope is frequently called a cathode ray tube (CRT). Depending on the manner in which the amplified signal is applied to the CRT, any one of several modes or displays can be obtained.

A-Mode. In the A-mode (amplitude modulation), echoes are displayed as vertical deflections along the CRT baseline, with the height of the deflection being proportional to the amplitude of the detected echo (Fig. 1–12). The distance between the transducer and the reflecting surface is indicated by the position of the deflection on the baseline. Using the value of 1,540 m/sec (the mean ve-

locity of sound through soft tissue), the baseline is calibrated so that depth measurements can be made to an accuracy of ±1 mm.

A time-compensated gain is customarily employed to compensate for the decreased amplitude of echoes arising from distant structures.

B-Mode. The B-mode (brightness modulation) differs from the A-mode in that echo information is applied to the Z-axis of the CRT instead of the vertical deflection circuit. Echoes appear as intensified points of illumination along the baseline. The B-mode is not useful by itself but is utilized in the creation of the M-mode and B-scan displays.

M-Mode. The M-mode (motion) display consists of the B-mode in which the baseline is continually raised. A timed photographic exposure records the movements of anatomic structure. This technique has been extremely valuable in studying dynamic changes in the heart. Much of this information, so easily obtained with ultrasound,

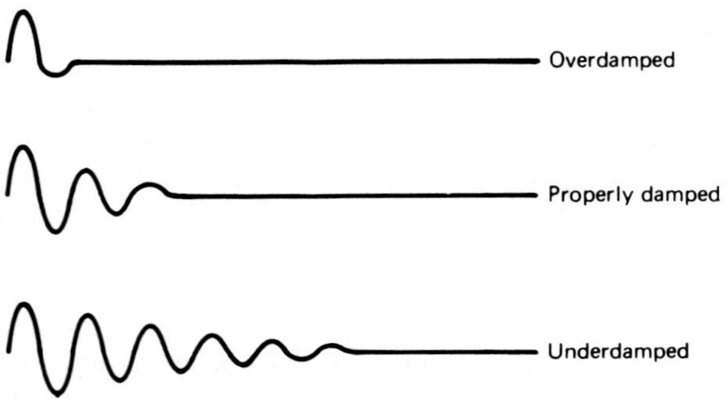

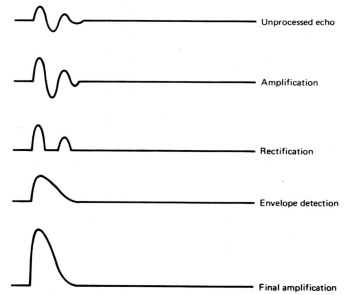

Unprocessed echo

Amplification

Rectification

Envelope detection

Final amplification

Fig. 1–11. Electronic processing of detected echoes. (*Adapted from Goldberg B, et al. Diagnostic Uses of Ultrasound. New York, Grune & Stratton; 1975. By permission.*)

Overdamped

Properly damped

Underdamped

Fig. 1–10. Effect of damping. (*Adapted from Goldberg B, et al. Diagnostic Uses of Ultrasound. New York, Grune & Stratton; 1975. By permission.*)

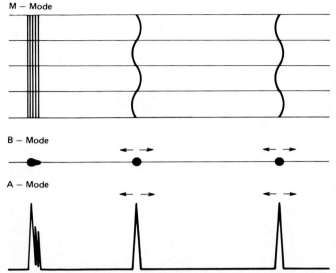

M — Mode

B — Mode

A — Mode

Fig. 1–12. Comparison of the A-mode, B-mode, and M-mode displays. The small arrows over the A-mode and B-mode displays signify that the indicated echoes move laterally upon direct observation of the CRT face. (*Adapted from Goldberg B, et al. Diagnostic Uses of Ultrasound. New York, Grune & Stratton; 1975. By permission.*)

cannot be attained with any other diagnostic technique. For example, the individual leaflets of cardiac valves are readily identified, and their excursions and velocities measured.

B-Scan. The B-scan provides a two-dimensional cross-sectional visualization of anatomic structures. This technique has become indispensable in many diagnostic applications. Of special value is its use in obstetrics, where it is desirable to keep x-ray examinations to a minimum. The B-scan is obtained by sweeping the ultrasound beam across the body and displaying the returning echoes in B-mode, but with the location and position of the oscilloscopic baseline accurately following that of the sound beam (Fig. 1–13). To accomplish this, accurate electronic sensing of the position and direction of the transducer and the sound beam must be maintained throughout the scanning procedure.

Scanning may be performed in any one of several ways: (1) mechanically moving the transducer with water bag coupling, (2) manually moving the transducer in contact with the skin, or (3) real-time imaging in which the transducer probe is held stationary against the skin and the ultrasound beam is made to sweep across the body. The first two scanning methods are called *static scanning*, and have for the most part been replaced by the third.

Figure 1–14 shows a B-scan examination being performed utilizing a hanging water bath. The transducer, within the water, is mechanically driven to produce high-quality, reproducible B-scans. Unfortunately, there are many mundane problems associated with this technique. The water has to be kept at a constant temperature and replenished frequently. The weight of the bag causes some discomfort to the patient, and in pregnant patients the pressure on the inferior vena cava may produce syncope. Furthermore, the bag has been known to rupture during an examination. Because of these problems, contact scanning has become the preferred technique for clinicians.

In contact static scanning, the transducer is mounted on a mechanical arm, which permits motion in one place. Positional sensors are mounted in each articulation of the arm, so that the position and orientation of the transducer can be accurately monitored. An acoustic coupling agent is applied to the skin surface and the transducer is manually moved across the skin (Fig. 1–15).

Real-Time Imaging. A standard B-scan takes approximately 20 seconds to complete. The photographic record

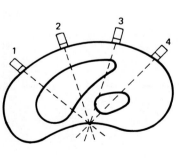

Patient

CRT Face

Fig. 1–13. Basic principle of the B-scan. The numbers 1 to 4 indicate different transducer placements in an abdominal examination and the corresponding B-scan on the CRT face. (*Adapted from Goldberg B, et al. Diagnostic Uses of Ultrasound. New York, Grune & Stratton; 1975. By permission.*)

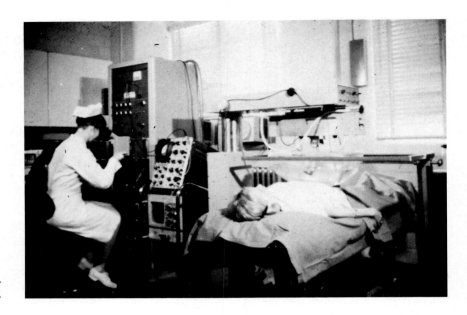

Fig. 1–14. B-scan ultrasound examination using a hanging water bath coupling techinque.

of such an examination does not provide any information concerning the motion of structures within the body. To study the dynamic action of moving structures, complete scans must be obtained much more rapidly than one per 20 seconds and, therefore, any manual scanning technique is precluded (Fig. 1–16).

By real time, we mean that the examination detects and displays motion as it occurs. Customarily, a frame rate of 15 per second or greater is considered adequate

for real-time imaging. Several different automated scanning techniques have been developed to provide real-time imaging. These techniques can be divided into mechanical scanners and multielement transducer arrays.

Mechanical Real-Time Scanners. Mechanical scanners physically move a transducer to scan the area being imaged. The movement of the transducer may be linear, pivoting, or rotational. Each is capable of producing scan

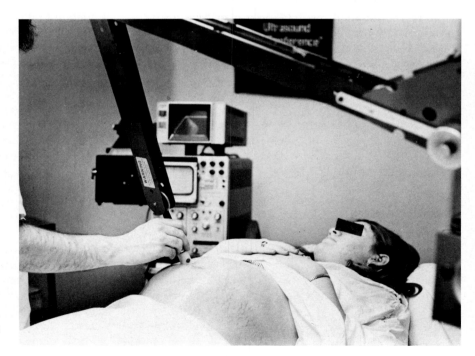

Fig. 1–15. Static B-scan ultrasound examination using contact scanning with a manually moved transducer.

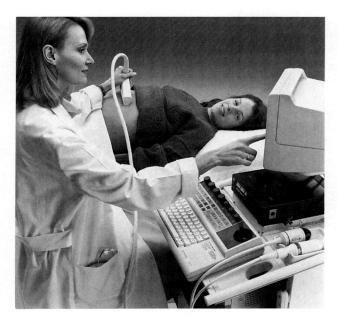

Fig. 1–16. Obstetrical sonography with a linear-array transducer. (*Courtesy of A.T.L., Inc.*)

rates of 30 frames per second in presently available instruments.

The linear mechanical scanner moves a single transducer back and forth parallel to the skin surface. The excursion of this motion may be several inches. Since the transducer is held fixed so that the sound beam is directed perpendicularly into the body, the resulting scan format is rectangular.

The pivoting mechanical scanner, sometimes called a *wobbler,* incorporates a mechanism for rocking the direction of the sound beam to produce a sector (pie-shaped) scan format. In some cases the transducer is rocked; in other cases, the transducer is held stationary and a pivoting acoustic mirror produces the scanning action.

The rotating mechanical scanner is simply a "side looking" transducer mounted on a rotating wheel. If contained within an acoustically transparent housing, this mechanism can scan an entire 360-degree field-of-view, such as that obtained in a commercially available rectal scanner. Much more commonly, however, the housing is designed to limit the egress of the sound beam to a sector ranging from 60 to 120 degrees. Sometimes two or more transducers may be mounted on the rotating wheel. In this way, it is no longer necessary to wait until the sole transducer rotates all the way back to the acoustic window in order to obtain echo information. Also, the transducer elements may be of differing frequencies or focal distances and thus may increase the amount of diagnostic information obtainable.

Multielement Transducer Arrays. This method of real-time imaging uses many piezoelectric crystals mounted on a single transducer probe, and electronically controls the excitation of these crystals so that an entire scan can be completed in a small fraction of a second. Because there are no moving parts, electronic switching is all that is required to produce frame rates of 60 per second or higher. In fact, the fundamental limitation to the speed of scanning is no longer the instrumentation but the speed of sound. That is, we can employ higher frame rates, but that will not allow sufficient time for sound to travel to deep structures and return prior to the emission of the next ultrasound pulse.

There are two methods of exciting the multielement arrays, multiplexing and phased array. In multiplexed systems, each crystal is excited and, following the necessary time for echoes to return to that crystal, the next crystal is excited, and so on until all the crystals have been excited. The total sequence constitutes a single frame. In presently available instruments, four or more crystals are excited at a time for improved beam shaping. The resulting scan pattern or anatomic window is rectangular in shape and has been particularly useful in obstetric applications.

In phased array systems, all of the crystals are excited as a single unit. However, there is a slight delay between each successive crystal, so that the sound pulse leaves the transducer at one end sooner than at the other end. This causes the direction of the emerging sound beam to deviate from the perpendicular. The amount of deviation is determined by the amount of delay. Rapid changing of the delay pattern can produce rapid beam steering. This electronic beam steering produces a sector type of scan, which has been particularly useful in cardiologic applications. Several of the most popular ultrasound scanners currently used in obstetrics are of the phased array type.

Gray Scale. Figure 1–17 shows a bistable B-scan of a fetal head in utero. Note that any point in the image is either white or black. There are no intermediate shades of gray. As a consequence, small echoes, such as those arising from the posterior uterine wall or from the vertically oriented side of the fetal head, are not displayed. This results in a discontinuous contour of anatomic boundaries. In many cases, it is quite difficult to decide which displayed echoes should go together to form an anatomic boundary and which neighboring echoes actually belong to separate structures. This confusion could be greatly reduced, if not totally eliminated, by the display of the smaller echoes. This is providing, of course, that the large echoes are not also increased to the point that they have completely "snowed" the image, making it totally white.

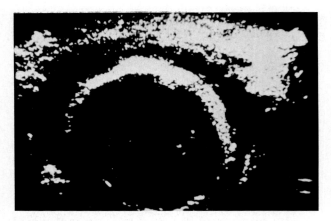

Fig. 1–17. Transverse B-scale of a pregnant abdomen. The large central ring of echoes represents the fetal head circumference. The large mass of dense echoes represents the anterior uterine wall and overlying skin. The echo-free area surrounding the fetal head is the amniotic fluid.

To gain better visualization of small echoes, gray scale capability has been added to B-scan systems. Gray scale refers to the number of distinguishable shades of gray, progressing from the blackest black to the whitest white in an image. The standard B-scan, as seen in Figure 1–17, has no shades of gray, only white or black. This is due to the imaging limitations of the storage CRT from which this B-scan was photographed. By bypassing the storage CRT and displaying the B-scan on a TV monitor, many shades of gray are obtained (Fig. 1–20). This is sufficient to provide the eye with an apparent continuously varying gray scale. Gray scale imaging is further enhanced by a nonlinear amplification of echo amplitudes. As seen in Figure 1–18, this results in the smaller echoes being more highly amplified than the large echoes. The resulting image is a significant improvement, as it displays the small echoes without total whitening by the large echoes.

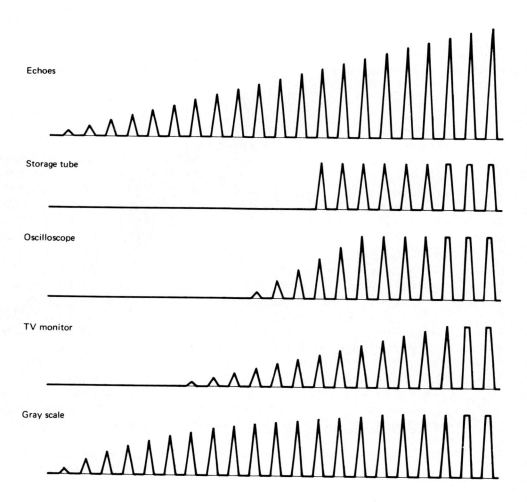

Fig. 1–18. Echo display amplitudes. The top row illustrates the range of echo amplitudes detected by the transducer. Echo amplitudes displayed on a storage CRT are either white or black with no intermediate shades of gray. A conventional oscilloscope and a TV monitor are able to display many shades of gray. Gray scale imaging incorporates nonlinear amplification of echoes, so that small echoes are rendered visible.

The value of an apparent, continuously varying gray scale can be seen in the interesting, although somewhat artificial, example illustrated in Figure 1–19. Close examination shows a 13 × 16 array of blocks. Each block possesses one of five shades of gray. The picture appears to be meaningless. However, if the distinct shades of gray are "smeared" so that the edges of each block appear intermediate in darkness, the picture will appear as though its gray scale were continuously varying. This is easily achieved by viewing the picture at a great distance, by squinting or, if one wears glasses, by removing them. By so doing, the intended pictorial information is easily recognized.

Figure 1–20 shows an example of the high quality B-scans that are obtainable using gray scale imaging. This technique clearly provides anatomic information sufficiently detailed for prenatal diagnoses. Further discussion of gray scale generation and perception will follow in Chapter 3.

Image Quality in Real Time. A sonogram is composed of a number of lines of echo information. The larger the number of lines, the greater the spatial resolution and the greater the amount of anatomic detail capable of being

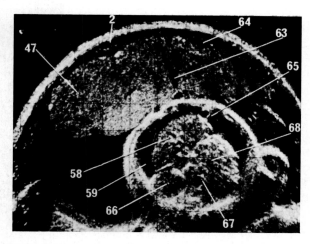

Fig. 1–20. Transverse B-scan with gray scale of fetus with hydrops *KEY:* 2, uterine muscle wall; 47, placenta; 58, liver; 59, ascites; 63, lobular divisions of placenta; 64, decidua basalis; 65, falciform ligament; 66, right kidney; 67, fetal aorta; 68, bowel. (*Reproduced with permission from Garrett W, et al. Gray scale echography in the diagnosis of hydrops due to fetal lung tumor. J Clin Ultrasound. 1975; 3:47.*)

displayed. However, the more lines required, the more time it takes to obtain a complete scan. This poses an important limitation for real-time imaging, where the time available for an individual scan frame is short (less than 1/15 of a second).

Each line of echo information requires an adequate time for sound to travel from the transducer to the deep-

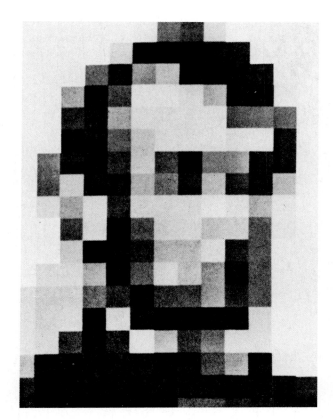

Fig. 1–19. Portrait of a famous man from history. See text for explanation.

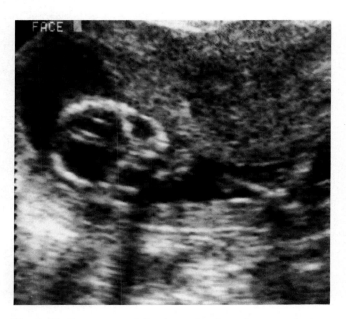

Fig. 1–21. Sonogram of the face of a fetus in coronal plane showing excellent image quality and anatomic detail.

est structures of interest and return to the transducer. Thirteen microseconds are required for each centimeter of depth. All of the above considerations can be related by:

$$\frac{\text{Frame}}{\text{rate}} \times \frac{\text{Lines per}}{\text{frame}} \times \frac{\text{Image}}{\text{depth}} = 77,000 \qquad [6]$$

This equation is of importance because it states an upper limit on the combination of desirable features in imaging: temporal resolution, spatial resolution, and field-of-view. For example, an instrument designed to provide a frame rate of 30 frames per second and 200 lines per frame will be limited to an image depth of 12.8 cm. To increase the depth of view, it would be necessary to decrease the frame rate or the number of lines. Fortunately for obstetric and gynecologic applications, those limitations are not so severe that they prevent excellent visualization of anatomic detail in real time.

Doppler Techniques

In accordance with the Doppler principle, echoes returning from moving structures are altered in frequency. The frequencies of echoes returning from structures moving toward the transducer are higher than the frequency originally transmitted by the transducer, whereas the frequencies of echoes returning from structures moving away are lower; those from stationary structures are unchanged. The amount of shift is directly proportional to the velocity of the moving structure. Under usual biologic conditions, the Doppler shift is between 0 and 2,000 Hz, and can be detected and applied to a loudspeaker to produce an audio signal. Alternately, this Doppler audio signal can be analyzed for its frequency content and displayed as a time-varying graph of blood velocity.

The primary use of Doppler techniques has been to detect and measure blood flow. Backscattered sound from the moving red blood cells provides the effective signal. The standard continuous-wave, nondirectional Doppler technique has been very useful in detecting fetal life (as early as 8 weeks of gestation), detecting nonpalpable arterial pulsations, and evaluating varicose veins.

Directional flow sensing has been provided by use of a single-sideband phasing technique. Pulsed Doppler systems can effectively separate signals from structures at various depths. Velocity profiles within blood vessels have been determined using this technique. The combination of pulsed Doppler and B-scan capabilities in duplex scanners provides both high resolution images of internal blood vessels and the simultaneous values of blood flow velocity within them. Measurements of umbilical blood flow have been used to obtain a physiologic overall assessment of fetal well-being. Recently, Doppler-shifted echoes have been color coded to provide a striking display of flow patterns superimposed on the gray-scale B-scan. This has been helpful in interpreting the complex bloodflow patterns existing within the body.

CONCLUSION

In the past several years, the advancement of ultrasonic instrumentation has been nothing less than spectacular. We are now beyond the point where just any image is acceptable. We have come to expect high-quality images with sufficient gray scale and resolution to provide reliable and accurate diagnostic information. Real-time imaging has provided us with dynamic views of anatomy never previously obtainable. Through-transmission techniques are still in their infancy. Other techniques, presently in the laboratory stage of development, also appear promising. Significant future progress is certain.

BIBLIOGRAPHY

Kremkau FK. *Diagnostic Ultrasound: Physical Principles and Exercises.* 3rd ed. Philadelphia: Saunders; 1989.

McDicken WN. *Diagnostic Ultrasonics, Principles and Use of Instruments.* New York: Wiley; 1981.

Wells PNT. *Biomedical Ultrasonics.* London: Academic; 1977.

Wells PNT, Ziskin MC. *New Techniques and Instrumentation in Ultrasonography.* New York: Churchill Livingstone; 1980.

2 Ultrasound Bioeffects Related to Obstetric Sonography

William D. O'Brien, Jr.

Ultrasound has had a profound influence on the practice of medicine, especially in obstetrics. It has been only three decades since some of the first ultrasonic devices were developed to provide an image of the fetus. The early studies with these devices showed a potential to provide high resolution information about the fetus, information that, if obtained by other techniques, could pose significant risks. Ultrasound did not appear to be associated with any known hazards. Diagnostic ultrasound also gained acceptance because it is convenient to use, comfortable for the patient, and not very expensive.

There continues to be a general belief in the medical community that ultrasound does not represent a risk to mother or fetus. But academic and government research scientists have continued to investigate and evaluate the risks. Many of these investigators (including this writer) have argued that the appropriate research has not been done to support a reliable assessment of the risks associated with human exposure to ultrasound. It could be properly argued, however, that there is always an insufficient data base to "prove" a modality totally safe.

The fact that there continues to be concern for the safety of ultrasound represents a continued interest by the clinical and basic science community in seeing that the use of this modality remains safe. Continued research will improve our data base and increase our confidence. And, if any risk is identified (which has not yet been the case), such information will then be disseminated to the clinical community so that appropriate risk-benefit decisions can be made.

It has been almost two decades since the first major efforts to assess the risk of ultrasonic energy were made.[1,2] Since then there have been numerous reviews and assessments.[3-24] Yet the basic status regarding risk assessment has remained unchanged during this time, viz, the studies necessary to support a reliable assessment of the risks associated with human exposure to ultrasound have not been undertaken. Therefore, rather than present another broad discussion of ultrasonic risk assessment, it seems to be much more reasonable to focus on one ultrasonically-induced biologic observation, namely, fetal weight reduction. Prior to a discussion of ultrasonically-induced fetal weight reduction, however, let us first consider an approach to risk assessment and then a review of general trends as they relate to diagnostic-level ultrasonic biologic effects. The effect of ultrasound on immunologic function and on sister chromatid exchange frequency will be considered as examples.

RISK ASSESSMENT APPROACH

With our current understanding of ultrasonically-induced biologic effects, it is difficult to argue against statements such as "diagnostic ultrasound is not harmful to the fetus." Experimental studies cannot be used to prove diagnostic ultrasound safe. Rather, what such studies will provide, if properly planned and executed, are data to aid in the overall assessment of risk associated with exposure to ultrasound. The term "safe" can imply the *complete* absence of an effect—that the procedure involves no risk. It simply is not possible, however, to prove that ultrasound, or for that matter any agent, produces no effect whatsoever at the levels employed diagnostically. The actual use of the word "safe" is also vague as it almost never refers to the absence of an effect and the term can also imply the *apparent* absence of an effect. A more useful and workable approach, therefore, is to examine the "risk" associated with ultrasonic exposure.

Some 35 years after the Curies discovered piezo-electricity in 1880,[25] the first use of ultrasonic energy was developed—underwater acoustic echoes were bounced off submerged objects.[26,27] During the course of this work, the first reported observation was made that ultrasonic energy had a lethal effect on small aquatic animals.[28] The first extensive investigation of the phenomenon confirmed that ultrasonic energy could kill small fishes and frogs within a minute or two.[29] In perhaps the first review paper of ultrasonically-induced biologic effects,[30] the physical, chemical, and biologic effects of ultrasound were evaluated. The effects on cells, isolated cells, bacteria, and tissues were summarized, with a view towards identifying the responsible mechanism. The ultrasonic exposure conditions in this early work were not well characterized, but the intensity levels were undoubtedly much higher than those currently in clinical use.

In the early pioneering studies where the ultrasonic exposure conditions were carefully controlled and specified, sciatic nerve paralysis was easily produced in the frog[31,32] and lesions were produced in central nervous system tissue.[33] In addition, high-intensity ultrasound was employed to produce lesions in adult cat and rat brain[33-38]; adult rat and neonatal mouse spinal cord[33,39,40]; adult frog muscle[41,42]; rabbit blood vessel[43]; rabbit kidney and testicle[44]; and rabbit ocular tissue.[45-47] The ultrasonic intensities were very much higher than those used in diagnostic ultrasound and, for the most part, these studies caused rather severe tissue damage. They have been extremely important in the elucidation of fundamental interaction processes. In terms of risk assessment, these studies support the view that the employed ultrasonic exposure conditions will more than likely not produce acute, gross irreversible damage.

These high-intensity studies further aided in recognizing the important fact that, at sufficient energy levels, ultrasound is capable of destroying biologic material. An approach, therefore, to the question of assessing the risk from ultrasound is as follows:

1. What biologic systems are most sensitive to ultrasound?
2. What exposure levels impose a significant risk on these systems?

This approach unfortunately has its difficulties. How does one determine significant risk? "Significant risk" usually means risk that is greater than some upper limit of acceptability. A benefit-versus-risk analysis is simple in principle but is not so easily implemented in practice.

An important consideration with respect to the evaluation of risk is an estimate of the extent of ultrasonic exposure that the patient receives. This may not give a good indication, however, as to the amount of ultrasonic energy that the patient population or a particular organ system receives because: (1) the number of examinations a patient receives is generally unknown, (2) multiple examinations may be performed with different types of equipment, and (3) the amount of ultrasonic energy that a patient receives varies from exam type to exam type and from examiner to examiner. Whereas no statistically-based survey is known to have documented the extent to which ultrasound has been used over the past 20 years, a number of indicators suggest that its use is increasing and that a large fraction of the human population will eventually be exposed, especially in utero.

In 1971, the US Food and Drug Administration's Bureau of Radiological Health surveyed 301 out of 6,306 short-term hospitals in the United States and found that 12% of the hospitals used diagnostic ultrasound.[48] The same Federal agency reported on the conduct of its 1974 hospital survey that 35% of the surveyed hospitals used

diagnostic ultrasound.[49,50] This represented an almost 200% increase in use between 1971 and 1974 (assuming that the surveys were identical), for an annualized increase of 43% during this time. The 1974 survey[49,50] further showed that an estimated 16% of the obstetric services in the United States used diagnostic ultrasound and that about one third of all US births for 1974 were delivered in these hospitals. Additionally, it was estimated that 470,000 pregnant women were exposed to diagnostic ultrasound in that year with about 35 to 40% of these women being examined more than once. In the more recent report of the National Council on Radiation Protection and Measurement,[12] it has been estimated that 40 to 60% of all ultrasonic imaging examinations are performed for obstetric purposes.

An examination of records in one US hospital setting[51] for two different years, 1975 and 1978, indicated that in 1975 11% of the lowest-risk pregnancy population was examined with ultrasound whereas 21% of that same risk population was examined in 1978. For the highest-risk pregnancy population, these percentages were 66 and 76 for 1975 and 1978, respectively. An evaluation of these data showed that the use of ultrasound in the lowest-risk pregnancy population was increasing at an annualized rate of about 25%, whereas for the highest-risk population it was increasing at a rate of about 5%. The rate of increase was greater in the lowest-risk population, which probably did not generally present with clinical problems. In the population that exhibited clinical problems, the use was much greater but the increase in use was not very high, owing perhaps to the fact that ultrasound was a relatively well-established diagnostic tool for this population of patients.

Sales growth information indicated that, in 1976 the ultrasonic industry's annual US dollar sales were around $30 million,[52] and for the following year about $40 million.[53] In the next four years, estimates of annual sales were 50, 79, 170, and 214 million dollars.[10] An increase from $30 million to $214 million from 1975 to 1980 represents an estimated average annual increase in sales of approximately 48%. In terms of the number of diagnostic devices, it was estimated that 3,500 systems had been sold in 1976 and approximately 12,400 in 1982,[54] for an annualized increase of about 24%.

The above data and reports represented the extent of use in the United States. Thus, in summary, if one were to estimate that about one half of all pregnant women are currently being examined with ultrasound and, additionally, that its usage is increasing at an annual rate of 10 to 25%, then virtually every fetus could be examined with ultrasound within a few years.

In countries other than the United States, no surveys or comparable data are available. In the United Kingdom, it was estimated that in the early 1970s the number of ultrasonic diagnostic examinations doubled every three years,[55] representing an annualized 26% increase. An international mail survey (which included the United States) suggested that, between 1963 and 1971, there was an average annual increase in the use of clinical ultrasound of approximately 10%.[56] In West Germany, official guidelines adopted in 1980 recommended the use of two ultrasound examinations during pregnancy[57] and, the Royal College of Obstetrics and Gynecology in the United Kingdom recommended that one screening ultrasonic examination be performed in every pregnancy.[13] A survey in Canada suggested that between 340,000 and 620,000 patients were examined with diagnostic ultrasound in 1977.[58]

Outside of the United States, therefore, there appears to be areas where screening is being recommended for all pregnancies. For the United States, at least one National Institutes of Health (NIH) document[13] has recommended against such screening. The bases for the NIH recommendations were in part that a theoretical risk could not be discounted and the utility of routine screening—as assessed through epidemiologic studies—could not be proved.

SOME GENERAL OBSERVATIONS

Experimental studies of ultrasonic biologic effects can be classified into morphologic or functional alterations.[59] Morphologic or tissue damage is usually permanent or irreversible. Such studies have been essential to the understanding of the mechanisms responsible for ultrasonically-induced alterations to biologic material. Ultrasound at high levels can cause damage to tissue by heating or by a phenomenon called *cavitation,* a general term used to describe the growth and subsequent dynamic behavior of gas bubbles produced in tissue by ultrasound. The action by ultrasound on these bubbles causes them to respond by producing large shearing forces within the bubble vicinity. These forces, in turn, can disrupt and destroy biologic tissues. Morphologic changes caused by both heating and cavitation have been identified and studied with very high ultrasonic intensities.

Biologic changes such as biochemical values, pH, function, activity, weight, and so forth, are termed functional alterations. These changes are not necessarily permanent. An example of a functional alteration is fetal weight change. There has been a large number of experimental studies that have evaluated the effect of ultrasonic exposure on the pregnant mouse. Some of the reports have shown the fetuses that were exposed in utero to be smaller at the time of birth than if they were not exposed.[60,61]

In general, much greater ultrasonic intensity levels are required to produce morphologic alterations as compared to functional alterations. The spatial peak, temporal average (SPTA) and spatial average, temporal average (SATA) intensity levels used in the fetal weight studies were much less than those used for studying morphologic alterations. Had these higher intensity levels been used to expose the mouse fetuses in utero, irreversible damage to the fetuses, and perhaps death, would have been the result.

Scientists and clinicians tend to question research findings of others whether they agree or disagree with them; such questioning is essential in science. It is interesting to observe, however, that the content of scientific conflict changes as the intensity level of ultrasound diminishes, especially with respect to ultrasonic bioeffect studies. Morphologic alterations are produced by quite high levels of ultrasonic energy. There is no conflict over whether or not the morphologic effect has occurred, but rather what caused the alteration (that is, heating, cavitation, or some other mechanism). These are the levels employed in the surgical application of ultrasound for which consistently well-defined, permanent biologic alterations can be produced. For example, three laboratories have independently confirmed that a highly focused ultrasonic beam can produce a lesion in mammalian (cat and rat) brain tissue.[35–38] Further, there is agreement that the effect has a threshold, and these investigators all agree as to the threshold. There is disagreement, however, as to what degree the effect is caused by a thermal mechanism or by cavitation.

At lower ultrasonic levels, usually within the therapeutic range, there are conflicting viewpoints as to whether or not and to what degree morphologic alterations have occurred. Most of the mouse fetal weight studies have been conducted at intensities in the therapeutic range (SATA intensities: 0.5–6 W/cm^2). There have been some 28 studies which have examined the effect of in utero ultrasonic exposure on fetal weight in either rats or mice.[16,19] Within these studies there is a number of perplexing and conflicting observations. For example, under the identical exposure and experimental conditions, in one strain of mouse statistically significant fetal weight reduction was determined, whereas in another strain of mouse, there was no change in the fetal weight. Both of these observations have been further confirmed in independent laboratories. Thus, under biologic conditions which are not understood, consistent and confirmed observations have been obtained for both positive effects and negative effects. (Additional comments about fetal weight studies will be made.)

For a third general category, at ultrasonic levels lower than those in the therapeutic range and sometimes into the diagnostic range (SATA intensities: 0.1–100 mW/cm^2), there are conflicting data as to whether or not a functional alteration occurred. This is aptly demonstrated in the numerous experimental studies that examined the effect of ultrasound on sister chromatid exchange (SCE) frequency (an indication of chromosome damage of which the biologic significance is unclear). Some of these studies have shown an effect when a diagnostic ultrasound device was used. However, some others have reported no change in SCE frequency[23] at diagnostic levels and at levels much higher than therapy. A study by Liebeskind and associates[62] appears to have received the greatest attention because it indicated an increase in human lymphocyte SCEs (a positive effect) from a diagnostic system. In another study by the same authors,[63] however, also with a diagnostic system, no change in SCEs was reported (a negative effect). In the latter study, two different types of cells were used. There have been two other positive observations[64,65] of increased SCEs, both with diagnostic levels of ultrasound. There have been at least ten other studies, however, some at diagnostic levels (both pulsed and continuous wave exposure conditions) and some at levels within or higher than therapeutic levels, which have reported no increase in SCEs. These 14 studies have been carefully and thoroughly reviewed by the American Institute of Ultrasound in Medicine Bioeffects Committee.[23] The committee's conclusion was that these studies do not suggest a hazard in diagnostic ultrasound.

One of the few studies in the early 1970s to show fetal weight reduction exposed rats in utero with diagnostic levels of pulsed ultrasound.[66] A positive finding was performed under a single exposure condition. An unsuccessful attempt to replicate the study by another group duplicated all experimental and animal protocols and, in addition, used ultrasonic exposure conditions equal to and higher than the original study.[67]

One of the more controversial studies in the early 1970s of prenatal ultrasonic exposure of pregnant mice was conducted with a commercial fetal Doppler device.[68,69] Whereas fetal abnormalities were observed in both the exposed and control groups, the differences were not significant. However, the rate of fetal death was increased significantly in the exposed group. The same researchers[69–71] found a statistically significant increase in fetal abnormalities in a different mouse strain. In both of these studies, pregnant mice were given an initial dose of sodium nembutal that was effective for about one hour, after which the animals awoke and struggled in their harness for 4 hours; the ultrasound exposure duration was 5 hours. Edmonds[72] drew attention to errors in the statistical analyses, the conclusions drawn, and the effective ultrasound power (about 280 mW). He concluded that the reported effects were related to a combination of prolonged binding of the mice and ultrasonic hyperthermia.

A significant reduction in the frequency of mitotic cells in surgically-simulated rat liver from diagnostic level, continuous wave ultrasound (SATA intensity: 60 mW/cm^2) was reported.[73] However, this observation was not able to be confirmed under virtually the identical research protocol, even when the SATA ultrasonic intensity ranged from 60 mW/cm^2 up to 16 W/cm^2.[74]

These are a few of the many studies reporting ultrasonically-induced biologic effects at intensity levels below 100 mW/cm^2 for which attempts at replication failed. There are also many more studies for which no attempt has been made to replicate the original finding because, in general, research funding does not support this type of activity.

FETAL WEIGHT STUDIES

Over the past decade, experimental observations have suggested that subtle effects occur in rodent embryos and fetuses when they are exposed to ultrasound in utero. The balance of this chapter selectively examines ultrasonically-induced fetal weight reduction in experimental animals. In choosing this topic, an attempt has been made to approach the assessment of risk from ultrasound for this single biologic endpoint. It is not known whether or not this biologic system is very sensitive (in a chemical and physical sense) to ultrasonic energy but, clearly, it is sensitive in an emotional and political sense. It behooves us, therefore, to understand the experimental data that show that ultrasonic energy does influence fetal weight when the system is exposed to ultrasound in utero.

One of the earliest studies that suggested in utero ultrasonic irradiation affected prenatal growth and development was reported in experimental animals about 12 years ago.[60] Timemated mice received continuous wave (1 MHz) ultrasound on the eighth day of gestation under well-controlled and documented exposure conditions.[75] The fetuses were weighed on the eighteenth day of gestation, and a statistically significant weight reduction of up to 17.5% relative to controls was observed. Two hundred seventy-two litters (2,866 fetuses) were examined in seven separate ultrasound groups, including a sham group. The SATA intensity ranged from 0.5 to 5.5 W/cm^2, and the exposure time ranged from 10 to 300 seconds (Table 2–1).

A detailed account of the initial finding[60] and an extension of the data analysis[61] showed that a dose-effect response was observed. Here the dose-effect response of the exposure condition versus fetal weight was developed by defining the dose parameter I^2t, where I is the exposure intensity (W/cm^2) and t is the exposure time (seconds) as listed in Table 2–1 for each of the six exposure conditions.

There is a basis for the I^2t dose parameter in the ultrasonic literature and in the literature of the other energy forms. Threshold ultrasonic dosages for structural

TABLE 2–1. SUMMARY OF CF₁ MOUSE FETAL WEIGHT STUDY

I (W/cm^2)	t (sec)	I^2t	Percentage weight change (against sham)
0.5	300	75	− 5.3
2.0	20	80	− 6.1
3.0	10	90	− 6.1
0.7	300	147	− 8.8
3.0	20	180	− 7.9
5.5	10	303	−17.5

The mice were ultrasonically exposed (continuous wave at 1 MHz) in utero on day eight of gestation and the fetuses were examined on the eighteenth day of gestation.
I = SATA intensity; t = exposure time.
Data from O'Brien WD Jr.[60,61]

TABLE 2–2. SUMMARY OF LAF₁/J MOUSE FETAL WEIGHT STUDY

I (W/cm^2)	t (sec)	I^2t	Percentage weight change (against sham)
25.6	20	13,100	− 5.4
35.3	20	24,900	− 0
45.0	20	40,500	− 0
50.8	20	51,600	−18.8

The mice were ultrasonically exposed (pulsed, SPTA intensity = 1,936 W/cm^2, 1 MHz, pulsed repetition frequency = 1 kHz) in utero on the eighth day of gestation and the fetuses were weighed on the eighteenth day of gestation.
I = SPTA intensity; t = exposure time.
Data from Fry FJ, et al.[83]

changes in the adult mammalian central nervous system results in a mathematical dependency between the ultrasonic intensity, I, and the exposure duration, t,[35,37,76–78] which is described by the product of I^2 and t equaling a constant value. In other words, if I equals 20 W/cm^2 (I^2 = 400) and t equals 0.5 seconds for the threshold of an ultrasonically-induced change, then I^2t equals 200. The same biologic threshold would occur under the ultrasonic exposure conditions in which I equals 10 W/cm^2 (I^2 = 100) and t equals 2.0 seconds; that is, I^2t = 200 again.

A similar type of I^2t dependency has been observed for ultrasonically-induced hind limb paralysis of neonatal mice,[37,79] threshold focal lesions in cat liver,[80] as well as focal lesions in rabbit liver, kidney, and testis.[44] In comparison to other forms of energy, a similar dose dependency has been observed for mammary neoplasms at low ionizing radiation doses wherein two x-ray secondary particles (produced by a single neutron) are required to elicit the effect.[81] In photochemical and photobiologic studies at high energy concentrations, biophotonic excitation (two photons required to produce the effect) has been observed.[82]

What does an I^2t type of dependency for a biologic effect mean? Basically, it means that two energy events are required to produce the biologic effect. However, there is not enough fundamental information available at this time to speculate on whether or not the reduced fetal weight observations reported herein can be explained by this dosimetric model. The numerical representation in such a model nevertheless begins to provide a basis for extrapolating biologic effect observations. (Such an extrapolation will be done shortly in terms of assessing the potential for ultrasonically-induced fetal weight reduction in humans based on the mouse data.) Thus, the following fetal weight observations will be presented in terms of the I^2t dependency.

The observation that ultrasonic exposure in utero can cause weight reduction in mouse fetuses has been confirmed by two other research groups using two different strains of mice.[83,84] For the data listed in Table 2–2,[83] relatively high level, pulsed ultrasound conditions were employed. Here the mice were exposed to ultrasound on the eighth day of gestation and the fetuses were individually weighed on the eighteenth day of gestation. A statistically significant 18.8% weight reduction was observed for SPTA intensities above 50 W/cm^2 (SPTA intensity of 1,936 W/cm^2 and exposure time of 20 seconds) when irradiated on day eight of gestation. At and below a SPTA intensity of 45 W/cm^2, no statistically significant change in the fetal weight was observed.

The data listed in Table 2–3[84] show mean fetal weight reductions that range up to 25% relative to the sham under continuous wave (2 MHz) exposure conditions at

TABLE 2–3. SUMMARY OF CFW SWISS WEBSTER MOUSE FETAL WEIGHT STUDY

I (W/cm^2)	t (sec)	I^2t	Percentage weight change (against sham) Day 0	Day 7	Day 12
1	80	80	− 2.7	+ 5.1	− 3.9
1	100	100	+ 1.6	+ 3.9	− 5.6
1	120	120	− 0.4	− 0.4	− 5.3
1	140	140	+ 2.9	− 8.7	−13.3
1	160	160	− 1.8	−11.2	−22.2
1	180	180	−19.1	−11.0	−11.3
1	200	200	−25.1	−11.5	−18.4

The mice were ultrasonically exposed (continuous wave of 2 MHz) in utero on days 0, 7 OR 12 of gestation and the fetuses were weighed on the seventeenth day of gestation.
I = SATA intensity, t = exposure time.
Data from Stolzenberg SC, et al.[84]

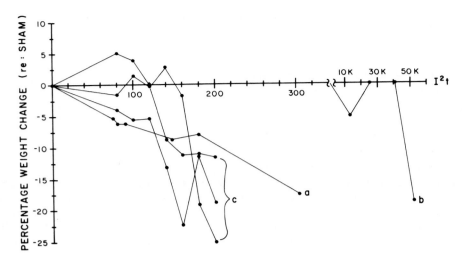

Fig. 2–1. Summary of fetal weight studies in terms of the dose effect parameter I^2t. Curves a, b, and c represent data from Tables 2–1, 2–2, and 2–3, respectively.

a SATA intensity of 1 W/cm^2 for exposure times up to 200 seconds at gestation ages of 0, 7, and 12. The fetuses were individually weighed on the seventeenth day of gestation. These results compare most directly with the previous finding[60,61] in which similar mean fetal weight reductions were observed.

Figure 2–1 graphically summarizes in a unified way the three published studies[61,83,84] that reported statistically significant effects of fetal weight reduction from in utero exposure to ultrasound. Here the data from Tables 2–1, 2–2, and 2–3 are represented by the percentage weight change (against sham) as a function of the calculated dose parameter I^2t. All three studies graphically show that as the value of I^2t increases, the fetal weight (against sham) decreases.

DOSE-EFFECT APPROACH

Experimental studies consist of exposing the specimen to ultrasound, and evaluating whether or not there have been any biologic changes that can be attributed directly to the exposure. The choice of exposure quantity and the type of biologic effect are critical elements of the experimental protocol. Exposure quantity variables include, but are not limited to, the following: pulsed or continuous wave conditions; frequency; power; SATA intensity; SPTA intensity; spacial peak, pulse average (SPPA) intensity (if pulsed); peak pressure values; unfocused or focused fields; and exposure duration. If a diagnostic machine is the exposure source for the experiment, then its output quantities generally do not vary. Only exposure duration could be varied with a diagnostic system because most of the other output quantities are fixed within the system. On the other hand, when specially designed exposure systems are used, virtually every exposure

quantity is under the investigator's control. It is essential to have control over all exposure quantities because only then can dose-effect studies be properly planned and conducted.

What is meant by dose? It is quite difficult to determine the exposure time that the human fetal heart, for example, is undergoing during an examination, especially when the ultrasonic beam is rapidly scanning from the transducer assembly and the transducer assembly is also being moved. Under such conditions the ultrasonic dose is quite difficult to quantify. Further, it is not known which of the various ultrasonic intensity quantities are relevant in terms of the dose determination. Consider the fact that the very high SPPA intensity acts for only a millionth of a second, and this action repeats itself every thousandth of a second, whereas the very much lower SATA intensity acts for quite a long period of time. Dose for the former could be much lower than that for the latter.

Dose-effect studies are still important for two reasons: (1) they provide the capability to extrapolate the amount or kind of effect at the doses used experimentally to the dose generated by diagnostic systems (note it is easier to determine what is generated than what a tissue receives), and (2) they provide the fundamental basis from which the biophysic mechanisms causing the effect can be evaluated (ie, was it due to heating, cavitation, or some other cause). To obtain measurable and highly repeatable biologic effects in experimental studies, the dose conditions are higher than those used diagnostically. The dose is varied over this higher range and the effect is evaluated. In this way, extrapolation to diagnostic dose levels is placed on a scientific basis. Let us consider two examples. In one case, the effect might be proportional in such a way that, when extrapolated, it does not go to zero (or to a normal level) until the dose goes to zero.

This would be considered a no-threshold effect. In another case, the experimental study could yield an effect which goes to zero (or a normal level) at some non-zero dose. This would be an example of a threshold effect. In the first case, the degree of the effect would have to be evaluated when extrapolated to diagnostic levels. In the latter, the evaluation would depend on where the threshold occurred.

Consider the mouse dose-effect fetal weight data shown in Figure 2–1. If we were to apply this dose-effect curve to a clinical exposure condition for purposes of assessing risk, we would first examine the upper value of the dose parameter I^2t for static pulse echo scanners.[14] For a single pulse, the SPPA intensity could be 500 W/cm^2 and the exposure time (here the pulse duration) about 1 microsecond, yielding an I^2t around 0.25. For the time average case, the SPTA intensity could be 200 mW/cm^2 and the exposure time (here the length of the exam for maximum effect) is about 30 minutes, yielding an I^2t around 72. Of course, this latter case would require examining the same tissue volume for the entire length of time. This might not be the situation with static pulse echo scanner but is quite possible for a Doppler fetal monitor wherein the spatial peak intensity is about 75 mW/cm^2. For an exposure time of 1 hour, the I^2t dose parameter calculates at about 20. The point made is that, one is in a better position to examine what might be the effect under clinical conditions with a dose-effect model. The model would have to be validated for such applicability, of course. There is a long way to go with respect to ultrasound.

Acknowledgments

The author gratefully acknowledges the partial support by a grant from the National Institutes of Health's National Cancer Institute (CA 36029) and the National Institute of Child Health and Health Development (HD 19805).

REFERENCES

1. Reid JM, Sikov MR, eds. *Interaction of ultrasound and biological tissues workshop proceedings.* Washington, D.C.: US Government Printing Office; DHEW Publication (FDA) 73–8008 BRH-DBE.

2. O'Brien WD, Shore ML, Fred RK, et al. On the assessment of risk of ultrasound. In: deKlerk J, ed. *1972 Ultrasonics Symposium Proceedings.* New York: 1972; 486–490. IEEE Cat. No. 72 CHO 708–8 SU.

3. Ulrick WD. Ultrasound dosage for nontherapeutic use on human beings—extrapolation from a literature survey. *IEEE Trans Biomed Eng.* 1974: BME-21:48.

4. Wells PNT. The possibility of harmful biological effects in ultrasonic diagnosis. In: Reneman RS, ed. *Cardiovascular Applications of Ultrasound.* New York: Elsevier; 1974; 1–17.

5. Hazzard DG, Litz ML, eds. *Symposium on biological effects and characterization of ultrasound sources proceedings.* Washington, D.C.: US Government Printing Office; 1977. DHEW Publication (FDA) 78–8084.

6. O'Brien WD Jr. Safety of ultrasound. In: deVlieger M, et al, eds. *Clinical Handbook of Ultrasound.* New York: Wiley, 1978; 99–108.

7. Repacholi MH, Benwell DA, eds. *Ultrasound short course transactions.* Canada: Radiation Protection Bureau, Health Protection Branch, National Health and Welfare; 1979.

8. Repacholi MH. *Ultrasound: Characteristics and biological action.* Ottawa, Canada: National Research Council of Canada; 1981. Publication NRCC 19244.

9. Dunn F, Frizzell LA. Bioeffects of ultrasound. In: Lehmann JF, ed. *Therapeutic Heat and Cold.* Baltimore: Williams & Wilkins; 1982; 386–403.

10. Stewart HF, Stratmeyer ME. *An overview of ultrasound: Theory, measurement, medical applications, and biological effects.* Washington, D.C.: US Government Printing Office; 1982. HHS Publication FDA 82–8190.

11. Environmental Health Criteria 22. Geneva, Switzerland: World Health Organization; 1982.

12. *Biological Effects of Ultrasound: Mechanisms and Clinical Implications.* Washington, D.C.: National Council on Radiation Protection and Measurement Document 74; 1984.

13. *The Use of Diagnostic Ultrasound Imaging in Pregnancy.* National Institute of Child Health and Human Development. NIH Consensus Development Conference process. Washington, DC: US Government Printing Office; 1984.

14. AIUM/NEMA Safety Standard for Diagnostic Ultrasound Equipment. AIUM/NEMA Standards Publication UL1–1981. Bethesda, MD: American Institute of Ultrasound in Medicine, or Washington, D.C.: National Electrical Manufacturers Association. *J Ultrasound Med.* 1983; 2–52.

15. AIUM Bioeffects Committee. Safety considerations for diagnostic ultrasound. Bethesda, MD: American Institute of Ultrasound in Medicine; 1984. AIUM publication 316.

16. O'Brien WD Jr. Safety of ultrasound with selected emphasis for obstetrics, In: Raymond HW, Zwiebel WJ, eds. *Seminars in Ultrasound,* 5. Orlando, FL: Grune & Stratton; 1984; 105–120.

17. O'Brien WD Jr. Ultrasonic bioeffects: A view of experimental studies. *Birth.* Fall, 1984; 11:143–157.

18. Nyborg WL. Optimization of exposure conditions for medical ultrasound. *Ultrasound Med Biol.* 1985; 11:246–260.

19. O'Brien WD Jr, Withrow TJ. An approach to ultrasonic risk assessment and an analysis of selected experimental studies. In: Sanders RC, James AE Jr, eds. *Principles and practices of Ultrasound in Obstetrics and Gynecology.* Norwalk, CT: Appleton-Century-Crofts; 1985; 15–22.

20. O'Brien WD Jr. Biological effects of ultrasound: Rationale for the measurement of selected ultrasonic output quantities. *Echocardiography—A Review of Cardiovascular Ultrasound.* 1986; 3:165–179.

21. Sikov MR. Effect of ultrasound on development: I: Introduction and studies in inframammalian species. *J Ultrasound Med.* 1986; 5:577–583.

22. Sikov MR. Effect of ultrasound on development: II: Studies in mammalian species and overview. *J Ultrasound Med.* 1986; 5:651–661.

23. Goss SA. Sister chromatid exchange and ultrasound. *J Ultrasound Med.* 1984; 3:463–470.

24. AIUM Bioeffects Committee. *AIUM safety report.* Bethesda, MD: American Institute of Ultrasound in Medicine; 1988.

25. Cady WG. *Piezoelectricity,* 1. New York: Dover; 1946.

26. Urick RJ. *Principles of Underwater Sound for Engineers.* New York: MacGraw-Hill; 1967.

27. Van Went JM. *Ultrasonic and Ultrashort Waves in Medicine.* New York: Elsevier; 1954.

28. Graber P. Biological actions of ultrasonic waves. In: Lawrence JH, Tobias CA, eds. *Advances in Biological Physics,* 3. New York: Academic; 1953: 191–246.

29. Wood RW, Loomis AL. The physical and biological effects of high-frequency sound-waves of great intensity. *Philos Mag.* 1927; 4:417.

30. Harvey EN. Biological aspects of ultrasonic waves: A general survey. *Biol Bull.* 1930; 59:306.

31. Fry WJ, Wulff VJ, Tucker D, et al. Physical factors involved in ultrasonically induced changes in living systems: I: Identification of non-temperature effects. *J Acoust Soc Am.* 1950; 22:867.

32. Fry WJ, Tucker D, Fry FJ, et al. Physical factors involved in ultrasonically induced changes in living systems: II: Amplitude duration relations and the effect of hydrostatic pressure for nerve tissue. *J Acoust Soc Am.* 1951; 23:365.

33. Fry WJ. Intense ultrasound in investigation of the central nervous system. *Adv Biol Med Phys.* 1958; 6:281.

34. Hueter TF, Ballantine HT Jr, Cotter WC. Production of lesions in the central nervous system with focused ultrasound. A study of dosage factors. *J Acoust Soc Am.* 1956; 28:192.

35. Fry FJ, Kossoff G, Eggleton RC, Dunn F. Threshold ultrasonic dosages for structural changes in the mammalian brain. *J Acoust Soc Am.* 1970; 48:1413.

36. Pond JB. The role of heat in the production of ultrasonic focal lesions. *J Acoust Soc Am.* 1970; 47:1607.

37. Dunn F, Fry FJ. Ultrasonic threshold dosages for the mammalian central nervous system. *IEEE Trans Biomed Eng.* 1971:BME-18:253.

38. Robinson TC, Lele PP. An analysis of lesion development in the brain and in plastics by high-intensity focused ultrasound at low-megahertz frequencies. *J Acoust Soc Am.* 1972; 51:1333.

39. Dunn F. Physical mechanisms of the action of intense ultrasound on tissue. *Am J Phys Med.* 1958; 37:148.

40. Taylor KJW, Pond J. The effects of ultrasound on varying frequencies on rat liver. *J Path.* 1969; 100:287.

41. Eggleton RC, Kelly E, Fry FJ, et al. Morphology of ultrasonically irradiated skeletal muscle. In: Kelly E, ed. *Ultrasonic Energy.* Urbana, IL: University of Illinois Press; 1965:117.

42. Ravitz MJ, Schnitzler RM. Morphological changes induced in the frog semitendinosus muscle fiber by localized ultrasound. *Exptl Cell Res.* 1970; 60:78.

43. Fallon JT, Stephens WF. Effect of ultrasound on arteries. *Arch Path.* 1972; 94:380.

44. Frizzell LA, Linke CA, Carstensen EL, et al. Thresholds for focal ultrasonic lesions in rabbit kidney, liver and testicle. *IEEE Trans Biomed Eng.* 1977; BME-24:393.

45. Coleman DJ, Lizzi F, Burt W, et al. Ultrasonically induced cataract. *Am J Ophthal.* 1971; 71:1284.

46. Sokollu A. Destructive effect of ultrasound on ocular tissue. In: Reid JM, Sikov M, eds. *Interaction of Ultrasound and Biological Tissue.* Washington, D.C.: US Government Printing Office; 1972. DHEW Publication (FDA) 73–8008:129.

47. Lizzi FL, Parker AJ, Coleman, DJ. Experimental cataract production by high frequency ultrasound. *Ann Ophthal.* 1978; 10:934.

48. Landau E. Are there ultrasonic dangers for the unborn? *Prac Radiol.* 1973; 1:27.

49. Roney PL, Albrecht RM. Hospital survey of obstetric ultrasound. Presented at Ad Hoc Review Panel on Ultrasound Bioeffect and Measurement meeting; April 9–10, 1976; Bureau of Radiological Health, FDA.

50. Roney PL, Albrecht RM. Hospital survey of obstetric ultrasound—United States 1974. In: Hazzard DG, Litz ML, eds. *Symposium on Biological Effects and Characterization of Ultrasound Sources Proceedings.* Washington, D.C.: US Government Printing Office; 1977. HEW Publication (FDA) 78–8048:29–30.

51. Read JL, Stern RS, Thibodeau LA, et al. Variations in antenatal testing over time and between clinic settings. *J Am Med Assoc.* 1983; 249:1605–1609.

52. Smith SW. *Diagnostic ultrasound: A review of clinical applications and the state of the art of commercial and experimental systems.* Washington, D.C.: US Government Printing Office; 1976. HEW Publication (FDA) 76–8055.

53. Smith SW. Diagnostic equipment and its use. Presented at Eighth Annual National Conference on Radiation Control; Springfield, IL, May 1–7, 1976.

54. Emmitt RB. Dynamic 40 percent increase in ultrasound sales. *Diagn Imaging.* 1979; 1:10.

55. Wells, PNT. What is the future of ultrasonics? *Ultrasonics.* 1973; 11:16.

56. Ziskin MC. Survey of patient exposure to diagnostic. In: Reid JM, Sikov MR, eds. *Interaction of Ultrasound and Biological Tissues.* Washington, D.C.: US Government Printing Office, 1972. DHEW Publication (FDA) 78–8008.

57. Mutterschaftsrichlinien. Beilage 4–80 zum Brundesanzeiger 22 von 1 Feb 1980. (Guidelines for Maternity Care. February 1, 1980; suppl: 4–80 to Federal Bulletin 22.

58. Benwell DA. Use of diagnostic ultrasound devices in Canada. *Ultrasound Med Biol.* 1981; 7:145–154.

59. Sarvazyan AP. Some general problems of biological action of ultrasound. *IEEE Trans Sonics and Ultrasonics.* 1983; SU-30:2–12.

60. O'Brien WD Jr. Ultrasonically induced fetal weight reduction in mice. In: White D, Barnes R, eds. *Ultrasound in Medicine.* New York: Plenum; 1976; 531–532.

61. O'Brien WD Jr. Dose-dependent effect of ultrasound on fetal weight in mice. *J Ultrasound Med.* 1983; 2:1.

62. Liebeskind D, Bases R, Mendex F, et al. Sister chromatid exchanges in human lymphocytes after exposure to diagnostic ultrasound. *Science.* 1979; 205:1273.

63. Liebeskind D, Bases R, Elequin F, et al. Diagnostic ultrasound: Effects on the DNA and growth patterns of animal cells. *Radiology.* 1979; 131:177.

64. Haupt M, Martin AO, Simpson JL, et al. Ultrasonic induction of sister chromatid exchanges in human lymphocytes. *Hum Genet.* 1981; 59:221.

65. Ehlinger CA, Katayama KP, Roesler MR, et al. Diagnostic ultrasound increases sister chromatid exchange. Preliminary report. *Wisconsin Med J.* 1981; 80:21–23.

66. Pizzarello DJ, Vivino A, Maden B, et al. Effect of pulsed low-power ultrasound on growing tissues. *Exp Cell Biol.* 1978; 46:179–191.

67. Carstensen EL, Gates AH. The effects of pulsed ultrasound on the fetus. *J Ultrasound Med.* 1984; 3:145–147.

68. Shoji R, Momma E, Shimizu T, et al. An experimental study on the effect of low-intensity ultrasound on developing mouse embryos. *J Faculty Science* (Hokkaido University, Series VI). 1971; 18:51–56.

69. Shoji R, Momma T, Shimizu T, Matsuda S. Experimental studies on the effect of ultrasound on mouse embryos. *Teratology.* 1972; 6:119.

70. Shoji R, Murakami U, Shimizu T. Influence of low-intensity ultrasonic irradiation on prenatal development of two inbred mouse strains. *Teratology.* 1975; 12:227–232.

71. Shimizu T, Shoji R. *Experimental safety-study on mice exposed to low-intensity ultrasound.* Second Congress on Ultrasonics in Medicine; June, 1973; Rotterdam, The Netherlands.

72. Edmonds PD. Further skeptical comment of reported adverse effects of alleged low-intensity ultrasound. *Proceeding of 1980 AIUN Conference.* New Orleans: 1980; 50.

73. Kremkau FW, Witkofski RL. Mitotic reduction in rat liver exposed to ultrasound. *J Clin Ultrasound.* 1974; 2:123–126.

74. Miller MW, Kaufman GE, Cataldo FL, Carstensen EL. Absence of mitotic reduction in regenerating rat livers exposed to ultrasound. *J Clin Ultrasound.* 1976; 4:169–172.

75. O'Brien WD Jr, Christman DL, Yarrow S. Ultrasonic biological effect exposure system. In: deKlerk J, ed. *1974 Ultrasonic Symposium Proceedings.* New York: 1974; 57–64. IEEE Catalog No. 74 CHO 896-ISU.

76. Dunn F, Lohnes JE, Fry FJ. Frequency dependence of threshold ultrasonic dosages for irreversible structural changes in mammalian brain. *J Acoust Soc Am.* 1975; 58:512.

77. Johnston RL, Dunn F. Influence of subarachnoid structures on transmeningeal ultrasonic propagation. *J Acoust Soc Am.* 1976; 60:1225.

78. Johnston RL, Dunn F. Ultrasonic absorbed dose, dose rate, and produced lesion volume. *Ultrasonics.* 1976; 14:153.

79. Fry WJ, Dunn F. Ultrasonic irradiation of the central nervous system at high sound levels. *J Acoust Soc Am.* 1956; 28:129.

80. Chan SK, Frizzell LA. Ultrasonic thresholds for structural changes in the mammalian liver. In: deKlerk J, McAvoy BR, eds. *1977 Ultrasonic Symposium Proceedings.* New York: 1977; 153–156. IEEE Catalog No. 77 CH2364-ISU.

81. Rossi HH, Kellerer AM. Radiation carcinogenesis at low doses. *Science.* 1972; 175:200.

82. Wang SY. Introductory concepts for photochemistry of nucleic acids. In: Wang SY, ed. *Photochemistry and Photobiology of Nucleic Acids,* 1. New York: Academic; 1976; 1–21.

83. Fry FJ, Erdmann WA, Johnson LK, et al. Ultrasonic toxicity study. *Ultrasound Med Biol.* 1978; 3:351.

84. Stolzenberg SC, Torbit CA, Edmonds PD, et al. Effects of ultrasound on the mouse exposed at different stages of gestation: Acute study. *Radiation Environmental Biophysics* 1980; 17:245.

3 Sonographic Instrumentation

Ronald R. Price • Arthur C. Fleischer

Recent improvements in sonographic (ultrasound) instrumentation have primarily been the result of more complete integration of high-speed digital electronics. Special purpose microcomputers are now being used to steer and dynamically focus array transducers, allowing greater flexibility and control over image formation and producing images with both higher spatial and intensity resolution. Recent developments in real-time color Doppler systems have also been the product of high-speed special-purpose microprocessors. Selection of a satisfactory scanner from the wide variety of equipment available today can often be puzzling and time consuming. It is difficult to obtain an unbiased opinion. While there are no definite guidelines, some general considerations are presented here. Discussion will largely be restricted to those aspects of ultrasound imaging technology applicable to general abdominal and obstetric and gynecologic imaging.

In general, it is important to understand the principles of ultrasound and to have a fundamental knowledge of how the image is formed. In addition, the patient population to be scanned must be analyzed since it will largely determine the variety of examinations to be performed and the type of equipment needed.

The focus of this chapter will be to review each of the various categories of real-time scanners, to describe the relative advantages and disadvantages of each and to discuss recent advances in each design. In addition, the features of the various types of transducer/probes relative to their clinical use will be emphasized.

SCANNER COMPONENTS

Real-time instruments rapidly sweep the ultrasound beam through a sector or rectangular area by either mechanical or electronic means. Frame rates greater than 15 frames per second are required to produce flicker-free images and to observe moving structures. Because real-time probes are usually not attached to a scanning arm, the sonographer has great flexibility in selecting the image plane orientation.

Ultrasound scanning systems typically consist of the following:

1. A mechanical or electronic means of moving the ultrasound beam through an image plane.
2. An electronic signal processing unit with controls for varying the transducer power output, overall receiver gain, and other operational parameters such as time-gain compensation (TGC).
3. A gray scale display unit equipped with controls for varying the image brightness and contrast.
4. A device for permanently recording the images—Polaroid, multi-image format camera, or videotape.

Modern instruments should also have a keyboard for superimposing on the recorded image the patient identification, exam date, and study information.

TRANSDUCER DESIGNS

Transducers are characterized by their frequency, size (effective aperture in the case of arrays), and degree of focusing. Typically, the range of frequency for diagnostic ultrasound imaging is 3.5 to 10.0 MHz. The degree of focusing is either short (1 to 4 cm), medium (4 to 8 cm) or long (6 to 12 cm). Focusing is achieved internally by the crystal shape, externally by an acoustic lens, electronically by selective pulsing of individual elements of an array, or by a combination of these three methods. The length of the zone available for focusing (Fresnel zone) is governed by the effective transducer aperture and its operating frequency. In selecting a transducer which has the optimum combination of frequency, aperture size and focal zone for a particular type of examination, the following general points should be considered:

1. Increasing transducer frequency generally results in enhanced axial resolution, but at the expense of reduced tissue penetration. The highest frequency consistent with adequate tissue penetration should be used.
2. For a selected transducer frequency, decreasing the transducer aperture improves lateral resolution in the near field. However, the length of the Fresnel zone (useful working range of the transducer) is reduced; lateral resolution beyond this zone (the Fraunhaufer zone) is degraded because of beam divergence. Decreasing the transducer aperture also decreases its sensitivity. It is important to note that many new array systems provide the capability of "dynamic aperture," which means that the effective aperture size can be varied by utilizing smaller or larger subunit-transducers depending upon the depth of focus chosen.

3. Larger aperture transducers are more suited to lower frequencies so that good lateral resolution is preserved at depth; smaller apertures are better suited to higher frequency transducers to provide improved lateral resolution over the shorter range.
4. Focused transducers provide improved lateral resolution and sensitivity at the depth of the focal zone, which is limited by the length of the Fresnel zone. The choice of focal zone, therefore, depends on the depth of structures to be resolved.

ALTERNATIVES IN SCANNER DESIGN

The evolution of the real-time scanners has led to a development of a variety of types of real-time scanner designs and configurations. It is generally true that no single design provides maximum performance of all image parameters, but rather optimizes some image parameters at the expense of others. Examples of these are the trade-off of axial resolution obtained from higher frequencies with depth-of-penetration, good lateral resolution at a specific depth resulting from a large aperture transducer with decreased lateral resolution at other depths, the convenience of fully electronic scanners against less expensive mechanical scanners, and the large echo dynamic range of mechanically driven single-element transducers against the more rapid multielement arrays which may have a more limited echo dynamic range. Real-time scanners can be grouped according to how they form the beam (focusing), and how the beam is steered (scanned) to form the image. In each case (focusing and steering), the task may be accomplished either mechanically or electronically. Mechanical focusing is the name frequently given to the use of acoustic lenses. Single-element transducers use mechanical means exclusively for beam focusing, whereas multielement arrays utilize pulse timing to bring about a convergent beam in the plane of the array, and use mechanical means to converge the beam in the "slice-thickness" direction (perpendicular to the array axis). Beam steering can be accomplished either by mechanically moving the transducer (or alternatively an acoustic mirror), or by electronic steering by means of pulse-timing sequences in multielement systems. Hybrid systems are also available which utilize a combination of array focusing and mechanical steering.

As noted above, new advances in real-time ultrasonic imaging are largely the result of the more complete integration of high-speed dedicated digital electronics (computers) into imaging systems. The term "computed sonography" is now being used to emphasize this increased dependence of the ultrasound image formation on the digital computer.

Single-Element, Mechanically Steered Scanners

Most single-element, mechanically steered scanners produce a sector (pie-shaped) format image. The sector opening angles may range from 30 degrees to 120 degrees (most are around 90 degrees). The ultrasonic beam may be steered by moving the transducer itself or by reflecting the beam from an oscillating "acoustic mirror." Because of the difficulty of maintaining adequate skin contact with either the moving transducer or moving mirror, most mechanically steered scanners utilize a fluid-filled case with an acoustically transparent window to contain the moving parts. In this manner, skin contact is made with the acoustic window case rather than directly with the moving components. This configuration insures adequate acoustic coupling even at relatively large steering angles.

Mechanically steered scanners have two main advantages relative to electronically steered scanners:

1. The use of a single-element transducer requires less sophisticated electronics and generally allows for a more simple transducer head design.
2. Image artifacts due to side lobes and grating lobes (unique to electronically steered beams) are less.

The disadvantages of mechanically steered arrays are:

1. The beam focus and beam pattern are fixed for a given transducer. To change the focus, one must change the entire transducer head.
2. The image framing rate depends on how rapidly the transducer is oscillated. The framing rate is governed by the line density needed to produce an image of diagnostic quality and by the depth of the field-of-view. The velocity of ultrasound in tissue is the ultimate factor governing the oscillation rate of the transducer. The framing rate thus may become quite low when large fields-of-view are chosen that require large excursions of the transducer element.
3. Field-of-view and image frame rates are in competition in sector format images when the total number of scan lines per image is kept constant. Thus, large opening angles are needed for large field sizes, and small opening angles are required for high resolution. In other words, the sector angle must decrease if higher line density is desired. This problem is not unique to mechanical scanners, however, and will be discussed again in regard to electronically steered scanners.

Although many variations on the mechanical oscillating transducer design have been designed and built, the most common design is a transducer which oscillates

TRANSDUCER (SERVO-SECTOR)

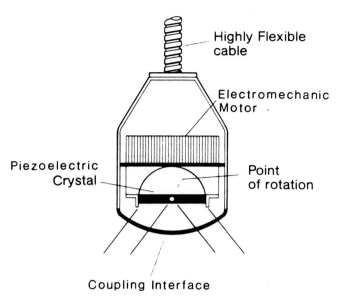

Fig. 3–1. Mechanical sector real-time scanner of the oscillating single-element fixed-focus design.

about a single fixed point and yields a sector-shaped image format (Fig. 3–1).

When a single element "wobbler" transducer is placed in contact with the skin surface, it is rocked from side to side in a small arc by means of an electrical motor. Each individual line of the B-mode image is produced and displayed as a radius of a circle with the transducer at the center.

Beam formation in mechanical scanners is achieved through mechanical focusing, using either shaped transducer (internal focus) or an acoustic lens which is attached to the transducer surface (external focus) (Fig. 3–2). One of the disadvantages of this design is that in order to change the focal zone, one must physically replace the transducer and, consequently, the focal zone cannot be conveniently changed during scanning. Electronically focused scanners achieve focusing by delayed pulse sequences, allowing the focal zone to be changed without physically altering the scanner.

An alternative approach to beam steering in a mechanical scanner is to keep the transducer stationary and to utilize an oscillating acoustic mirror to move the beam in a sector format (Fig. 3–3). This design requires that the mirror and transducer also be contained within a fluid-filled housing so that the moving mirror does not make direct contact with the patient.

The oscillating mirror design offers an advantage over the oscillating transducer design by eliminating the

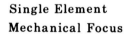

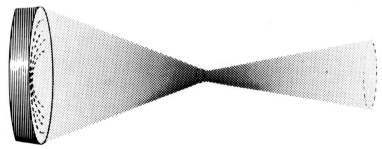

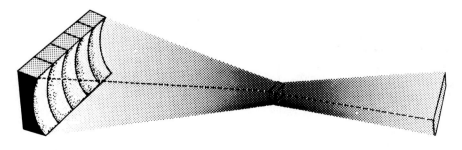

Fig. 3–2. Single-element scanners require curved transducer crystals or an attached acoustic lens to achieve focusing (*top*). Single-element transducers are thus focused to a specific depth (fixed focus). Array focusing is achieved by altering the times at which each sub-element is pulsed, thus allowing multiple focal depths (*bottom*).

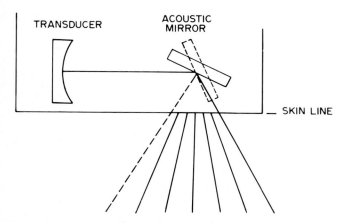

TRANSDUCER

ACOUSTIC
MIRROR

— SKIN LINE

Fig. 3–3. A mechanical sector scanner using an oscillating acoustic mirror for beam steering. Focal depth is determined by the mechanical focus of the transducer and is not affected by the presence of the mirror. Oscillating mirrors are also used to steer annular arrays in some systems.

need to move an electrically active component (the transducer). In addition, the mirror is usually lighter and can be moved more easily and rapidly. The lighter mirror results in the need for a smaller motor, which results in a more compact and lighter transducer probe.

A plane mirror only changes the direction of the beam and does not affect the beam focus. Thus, the focal characteristics are entirely determined by the transducer and its mechanical construction. The angle at which the beam is reflected from the mirror surface is equal to the angle of beam incidence analogous to light reflection—with essentially no energy loss in the reflection process. The fluid-path length, by necessity, will be slightly longer (approximately 1 cm) than scanners that use an oscillating transducer without a mirror, thus making the image field-of-view more trapezoidal in format. This is not necessarily a disadvantage, however, since the additional offset of the skin-line usually results in the better lateral resolution by moving the skin-line away from the transducer face and closer to the focal zone of the transducer. Scanners

2-Element Oscillating   **3-Element Rotating Wheel**

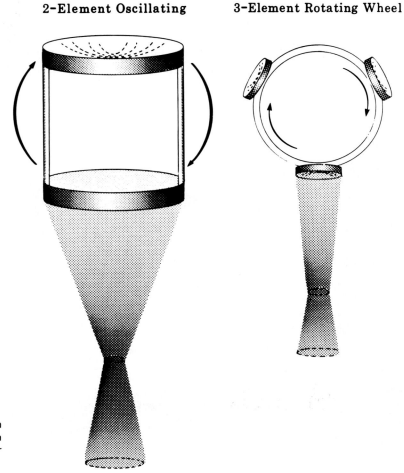

Fig. 3–4. Rotating-wheel mechanical scanners with multiple elements provide more rapid frame rates than single-element scanners and may also produce wider fields-of-view.

of this design operate typically at 15 to 30 frames per second.

Another common design for mechanical scanners is the rotating wheel, which consists of multiple (usually three) transducers mounted on a wheel which is rotated by an external motor (Fig. 3–4). The wheel is rotated in the same direction, making the mechanical assembly much simpler. The wheel and transducer are housed in a fluid-filled case with an acoustic window at the lower surface, which makes contact with the patient. As the transducers rotate, the output is switched from one transducer to the next in sequence, depending on which transducer has rotated in front of the acoustic window. This design allows for rapid framing without flicker—typically 30 frames per second. The design produces a sector-shaped field-of-view and allows a wide-opening angle of 90 degrees or more.

Electronically Steered Scanners

Included in this category are linear phased arrays, multielement linear sequenced arrays and multielement annular arrays. Through the proper phasing of the transmit-receive timing of the transducer elements which are used to fabricate the arrays, a composite ultrasonic beam can be created. In this manner, the beam can be focused and steered electronically. Fundamental to electronic focusing is the fact that each element of the array generates an ultrasonic wave, which has a definite phase relationship with the waves from the other elements. The ultrasonic waves generated by each element can be superimposed in a precise manner to create the effect of a single wave front.

Multielement linear sequenced arrays sequentially pulse subunits of transducers so as to produce a wave front which moves normal to the transducer face, thus yielding a rectangular field. On the other hand, linear phased arrays pulse all of the available transducers for each line, and thus must steer as well as focus (Fig. 3–5A). An interesting and valuable variation on this general field-geometry is the field shape produced by "radial" or "convex" linear array transducers (Fig. 3–5B). Radial arrays operate in much the same way that conventional linear sequenced arrays operate but, rather than being aligned in a straight line, the transducer sub-elements are aligned along an arc. The advantages of this design are several: by launching the ultrasound wave perpendicular to the transducer face as well as the skin, better transmission is achieved; beam steering is achieved geometrically rather than by pulse timing, eliminating increased grating-lobe artifacts seen in phased arrays at large steering-angles; there is increased field-of-view at depth unlike with conventional sequenced arrays which produce rectangular fields-of-view.

The transducer array is usually composed of many (typically 128 to 256) small piezoelectric crystals (M) arranged in a row (Fig. 3–6). Since the field from a single

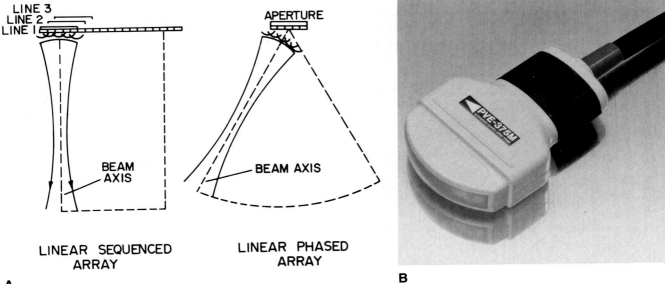

A

Fig. 3–5. A. Traditional linear-sequenced arrays (*left*) produce rectangular fields-of-view and use both transmit and receive array focusing. Phased linear arrays (*right*) are steered to produce a sector-shaped field-of-view and also to use both transmit and receive focusing. **B.** Radial or convex linear arrays provide increased field-of-view with depth without electronic scanning, thus reducing grating-lobe artifacts that accompany traditional phased arrays when large steering angles are used.

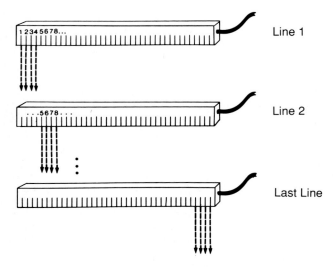

Fig. 3–6. Linear sequenced arrays scan the beam by sequentially pulsing transducer subgroups along the length of the array; thus only a small portion of the crystals is used to form any one line.

activated first and the inner transducers are delayed in time, with the central transducer having the greater delay to yield a wave axis perpendicular to the plane of the transducer. By varying the order of the delay, the wave can be focused at a specified depth and the wave axis can be scanned through a sector of 60 to 90 degrees. Properly selected delays can produce steering and focusing simultaneously. One distinction between linear sequenced arrays and linear phased arrays is that, in the phased array, every element is used to form the beam for each line. In the linear sequenced array, only a small subset of the transducers is used to create a given line.

The phased annular array scanner represents a hybrid system and possesses characteristics of both mechanical and electronic designs. The transducer is comprised of a series of independent transducers; each element has the shape of an annular ring and multiple elements are arranged in concentric rings about a central transducer element (Fig. 3–8).

Beam formation and focusing are achieved electronically by proper phasing of the transducer elements.

small crystal element diverges very rapidly, several elements (**N**) are driven simultaneously, and electronic focusing is utilized. In the subgroup of **N** crystals, the outer crystals may be pulsed first with the inner crystals delayed. In this circumstance, the field from the **N** elements will be focused at a depth that depends on the magnitude (time interval) of the delays. By changing the magnitudes of the delays, the focal zone can be chosen for a specific depth. The elements may also be designed so as to be sensitive to the returning waves in a manner determined by the same delay factors used in transmission, thus constituting a focusing effect on the returning signals. A signal scan line in the real-time image is formed in this manner. The next adjacent scan line is generated by utilizing another group of **N** crystals formed by shifting from the previous **N** crystals, one crystal position along the transducer array. The same transmit-receive pattern is then repeated for this set of **N** crystals and, subsequently, for all other sets of **N** crystals along the array in a cyclic manner. Focusing in the plane of the transducer elements improves lateral resolution as well as sensitivity by increasing the amount of energy in the focal zone (constructive interference). Focusing in the plane perpendicular to the scan lines determines the slice thickness, and is accomplished by the use of mechanically focused elements (double focusing, see Fig. 3–2).

The linear phased array is frequently termed an electronic-sector scanner since the resulting field is pie-shaped, with the field diverging as the distance from the transducers is increased. How this field shape is created is illustrated in Figure 3–7. The outside transducers are

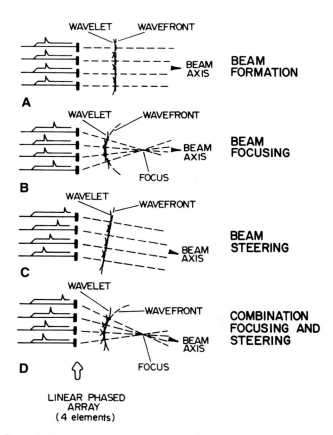

Fig. 3–7. Phased arrays are capable of electronic beam formation (**A**), beam focusing (**B**), beam steering (**C**), or any combination of focusing and steering (**D**) allowing dynamic focusing and steering.

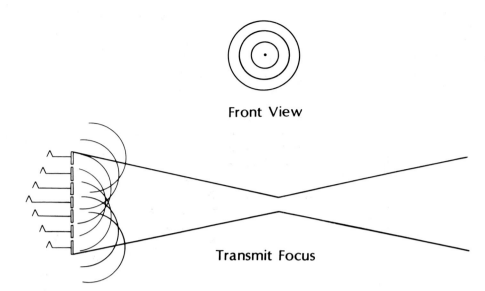

Front View

Transmit Focus

Fig. 3–8. Phased annular arrays are also capable of dynamic focusing and offer the added advantage that the beam is focused in two dimensions, unlike linear arrays that are only capable of electronic focusing in the plane of the array. For linear arrays, focusing in the slice-thickness direction must be accomplished mechanically. Annular arrays, however, must be steered mechanically.

An advantage of this design is readily recognized in that focusing is achieved in two dimensions similar to that with a single focused element; but, unlike mechanical focusing, the focal zone can be changed without physically changing the transducer. Beam steering, on the other hand, must be achieved mechanically. The beam is swept through a trapezoidal field-of-view with an oscillating mirror, or the transducer itself may be oscillated. As with other mechanically steered scanners, the transducers, the mirrors, or both, are contained within a fluid-filled housing.

In the oscillating mirror design, the transducer may be quite large, typically 10 cm or more. A large transducer aperture can be used to achieve a long focal zone, which may be appropriately positioned in the area of interest by choosing the fluid-path length properly. As the fluid-path length is usually longer than the maximum depth of view in the patient, no reverberation artifacts resulting from echoes reflected back and forth between the patient's skin and the transducer face will be seen in the images. Because of the exceedingly long path length, however, the pulse repetition rate must be reduced relative to hand-held scanners. Typical frame rates are at 12 frames/second (128-line resolution) and high resolution images at 1 frame/second.

Commercially available annular-array scanners offer a variable focal zone option that allows the user to specify one of several focal zones. The systems also operate in a survey scan mode, in which the transducers are cyclically scanned through the available focal zones while the operator observes the images. Once a particular depth of interest is specified, the operator terminates the survey scan and selects the appropriate focal zone for optimum visualization.

DISPLAY AND STORAGE OF REAL-TIME IMAGES

The number of gray shades displayed in the ultrasound image depends on the characteristics of *scan converter* that translates the pressure change received by the transducer to electrical impulses.

Most instruments for B-mode imaging use *digital* scan converters (Fig. 3–9). In these systems, the analog voltage levels—which correspond to the returning echo amplitudes for each line of the image—are digitized by an analog-to-digital converter. The generated array of numbers is then stored in a digital memory. The digital memory is divided into a number of picture elements or *pixels*. Typically, each pixel element depicts 1 × 1 mm of the image. The size of the memory can be described by the number of pixel elements, such as 512 × 512. Each pixel represents a region in the body whose size is equal to the image field-of-view divided by the number of pixels. For example, a 25-cm field-of-view imaged with a 512- × 512-pixel matrix would yield pixel sizes of approximately 0.5 mm × 0.5 mm. The memory can then be interrogated and the image displayed on a video monitor. The brightness of the TV signal representing each picture element is controlled by the value stored in the corresponding digital word. The number of shades of gray available is determined by the size of the digital word used to store the information for each picture element. The size of the word is measured in terms of the number of bits, and frequently referred to as the *depth* of the memory. Three-bit words provide the capacity for displaying eight shades of gray, four bits provide 16 shades of gray, and five bits provide 32 shades of gray. Most digital memories used for real-time scanners are at least

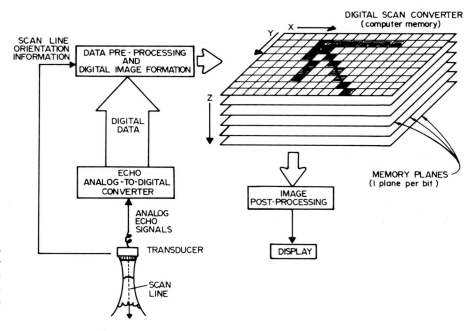

Fig. 3–9. Block diagram of a digital ultrasound system. Echo signals detected by the transducer are digitized and then stored in a computer memory (digital scan converter), which is then read out to a video monitor.

512 × 512 by 6 to 8 bits deep (64 to 256 shades of gray).

The discreteness of both the spatial domain and the gray-scale shades provides an image that is not as "smooth" as the analog image. The appearance of the image will be different, and the margin between picture elements (pixels) will be more definite than with analog displays. However, as the number of pixels increases and these become smaller, it becomes difficult to distinguish between the two types of images. Images are frequently processed by linear interpolation to produce more esthetically pleasing images. Interpolation "fills in" between picture elements without altering the original image data. However, the digital system is more stable, does not drift, and is less sensitive to heat. This eliminates long start-up time and allows one to institute predigital and postdigital image processing.

The two most common methods for permanent archiving of ultrasound images are multi-image format film and video tape. Multiformat film imagers have become the recording device of choice not only for ultrasound but also for computed tomography, nuclear medicine, and magnetic resonance imaging. Due to the transportability of most ultrasound systems, multiformat cameras are usually chosen in the "compact" design. In most applications, the 9 on 1 format on 8" × 10" film is adequate size for viewing and measurements. If larger recorded images are desired, the 6 on 1 format is also readily available.

Videotape recorders have also become very popular storage devices because of their ability to allow a real-time study to be recorded just as it was performed—often with superimposed audio from the operator for

further study and clarification on orientation, and other descriptive findings.

Video recorders using one-half inch VHS standard videotape are relatively inexpensive and store several hours of video on a single tape with acceptable resolution. These units generally include slow/fast motion playback modes, still-frame replay mode, and automatic search capabilities. Care should be taken to recognize that in most units when still-frame imaging is used the number of displayed lines will be reduced to approximately one half of the real-time display resolution.

COMPUTED ULTRASOUND

In addition to the use of digital scan converters, which have now become commonplace in current real-time systems, several manufacturers have extended the use of digital technology by replacing many of the traditional analog portions of the system's pulsing and receiving hardware. In the past, it has been appreciated that digital components provide flexibility through software programmability that analog systems cannot. However, the price and speed of digital systems has only recently been such that the replacement of analog circuits could be considered. High-speed parallel processors, under program control, driving multielement array transducers have made it possible to dynamically vary pulsing and receiving signal-processing steps. This is unlike analog circuits that must be physically changed each time a change in signal processing is made.

As described previously, a beam can be formed and

steered by pulse timing of transducer arrays. The beam will have a focal depth that depends on the values of the time delays between the pulsing of the outer transducer elements relative to the center elements. Once a beam is launched from the transducer, there is no further control that can be gained over the transmitted beam. In the case of transmit focus, the digital flexibility primarily benefits by allowing one to choose the focal zone before each scan without having to physically change the transducers. This is an important practical benefit but does not change the resultant image quality relative to analog systems.

The most significant improvement in image quality that has resulted directly from the use of the digital system has been benefits derived from the dynamic signal processing on the returning echoes. This is often referred to as *receive focusing* or *dynamic focusing*. Even though the transmitted beam can have only a single focal zone, it is possible to selectively "listen" to the returning echoes. Because returning echoes from different depths arrive at different times, reflections from nearby are detected first, followed by reflections from deeper sites. Accepting only those echoes which have the proper pattern of arrival times assures that the returning signals are in focus for each depth (Fig. 3–10). This is the essence of dynamic focusing. In order to accomplish dynamic focusing, it is essential that the system have almost complete control over the pulsing and receiving of each individual transducer element. It is this fact that requires the power of high-speed parallel processing. Conventional multielement scanners sum the received signal with equal weightings from the various elements to produce the echo signal. In the parallel-processed systems, the gain of each element is controlled separately. This dynamically variable gain capability is referred to as *dynamic apodization*. Dynamic variations in the individual gains can be used to discard echoes from off-axis sites to minimize side-lobe and grating-lobe artifacts. The same technique can also be used to effectively change the size of the aperture during the scan, depending on whether or not one is scanning in the near- or far-field.

INTRALUMINAL TRANSDUCER/PROBES

Recent advances in transducer designs have afforded development of transducers that can be mounted on probes to be placed in various lumen within the body. Specifically, the two major types of intraluminal probes that have gained recent clinical application include transducer/probes (for imaging of the uterus, early pregnancy, and the adnexa), and transrectal transducer/probes (for imaging of the cervix and parametrium).

Because of the proximity of the organ of interest to the transducer, both transvaginal and transrectal probes can use high frequency transducers—usually 5 or 7.5 MHz. In general, the use of these probes can contribute to increased diagnostic specificity through the improved resolution afforded by proximity of the transducer to the area of interest, and by the higher transducer frequencies that can be used.

As illustrated in the chapters on early obstetrical sonography and gynecologic infertility sonography, transvaginal transducer/probes significantly enhance the sonographic evaluation of the uterus and adnexa. At present, there are between 10 and 15 different types of commercially available probes (Table 3–1). The major types of transvaginal probes include those that use a single-element mechanical oscillating transducer, those with a curved linear array, those that use an eletronically phased steering of multiple-transducer elements, and those that are a single-element transducer that rotates (Figs. 3–11A and B).

In general, the field-of-view of most transvaginal probes is approximately 10 cm, with the focal range varying from 2 to 7 cm—depending on the type and design of the transducers. The sector of the field-of-view is typically 90 to 100 degrees with some rotating-wheel designs going as high as 240 degrees. The design of the actual probe housing ranges from a straight shaft, with a transducer mounted on the end, to some in which the trans-

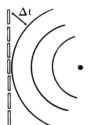

Echoes from Distant Reflectors

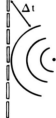

Echoes from Near Reflectors

Fig. 3–10. Receive focus is carried out in real-time by means of high-speed digital processors capable of monitoring the response received by each individual transducer element. By using predetermined time-delay patterns, the system can distinguish echoes which come from different depths by the relative time delays ($\triangle t$) observed by the array elements.

TABLE 3–1. TRANSVAGINAL TRANSDUCERS

Manufacturer	Freq. (MHz)	Focal range (mm)	Field-of-view	Type	Insertion length (cm)	Diameter (cm)
Acuson	5.0	15–40	90°	Phased-array Sector	16.0	0.8 max.
ADR Ultrasound	3.0 5.0	40–60 30–60	90° 90°	Mechanical Sector	16/0	1.9–2.5
Ausonics	7.5	20–40	90°	Mechanical Sector	17.0	1.2–2.5
Bruel & Kjaer Instruments	7.5	10–60	115°	Mechanical Sector	7.2	2.1–3.8
Cone Instruments	5.0 7.0	30–70 20–50	112° or 240°	Mechanical Sector	15.0	1.2–2.6
Corometrics Medical Systems	5.0	15–45	60°	Curvilinear (convex)	14.0	1.6–2.0
Diasonics	7.5	20–40	100°	Mechanical Sector	20.2	1.5–1.7
Elscint	6.5	20–60	30°–105°	Mechanical Sector	16.1	2.6 max.
General Electric Medical Systems	5.0	25–80	90°	Phased-array Sector	19.2	1.0–2.5
Philips Ultrasound International	5.0 7.5	30–70 20–65	90°	Mechanical Sector	15.0	2.3–3.3
Picker International	3.5 5.0 7.5	20–40 (approx.)	100° (approx.)	Mechanical Sector	23.0 (approx.)	2.0 max. (approx.)
Pie Medical USA	5.0	Sector: 40–120 Linear: 40–80	Sector: 110° Linear: 5 cm	Mechanical Sector or Linear	Sector: 15 Linear: 19	Sector: 3.5 Linear: 1.2–2.0
Siemens Medical Systems	7.0	20–70	220°	Mechanical Sector	14.0	1.0–2.0
Toshiba Medical Systems	5.0	50 (auto-focus point)	86°	Curvilinear (convex)	20.0	2.2–2.7

ducer's face is inclined relative to the handle. Needle guides are available on several transvaginal transducer/probes and attach onto the shaft.

When selecting a type of transvaginal transducer probe to be used, one should keep in mind that they vary according to the size of the actual imaging surface or "footprint," the size of the shaft, and angle of the handle. Handles that assist the operator in determining probe orientation are preferred. Probes with the smallest shaft size may be preferred in virgins or young girls and in older women with atrophic vaginas.

Transrectal probes are used extensively for evaluation of the prostate in men (Figs. 3–12A and B). These probes usually contain one or more than one array of transducers. For imaging in the sagittal plane, a series of linear-array elements with electronic or phased-array focusing is usually used. For those probes that have two elements, the axial view is usually obtained by a single-element mechanically oscillated transducer, curved linear array, or phased-array transducer array.

Static-scanner biopsy probes have been largely replaced by real-time transducers with biopsy guide attachments. A unique advantage is the ability to select the needle path on a real-time, two-dimensional image and then to directly observe the needle penetrating the organ, tumor, or fluid collection.

DOPPLER SCANNERS

Doppler scanners have evolved from the relatively simple continuous wave (CW) units, which yielded an audible frequency to the users' earphones, to current pulsed-Doppler systems that are now capable of yielding color-coded flow images in real-time. This evolution has been made possible in large part by the advent of relatively inexpensive high-speed parallel-processing computers. The basic interaction of the Doppler effect has not changed over the years, but rather the ability to rapidly process and analyze the returning echo data.

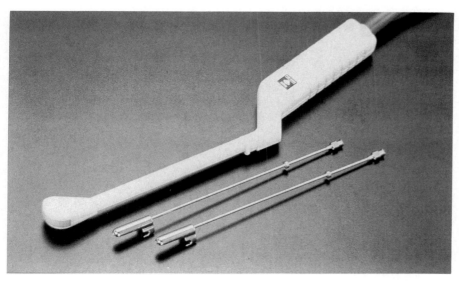

A

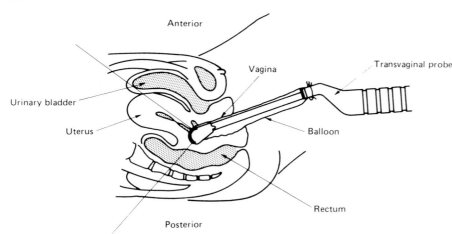

Anterior

Vagina

Transvaginal probe

Urinary bladder

Uterus

Balloon

Rectum

Posterior

Fig. 3–11A. Transvaginal probe of the curved linear array design shown with needle guide attachments. **B.** Diagram of curved linear array transvaginal probe, illustrating approximate field-of-view. (*Courtesy of Toshiba, Inc.*)

B

The general effect of sound that passes through the body is to be either absorbed (a decrease in beam intensity of about 1 dB/cm/MHz), or to be reflected. Sound is reflected at each point along the beam where the relative acoustical impedance changes. If this reflecting interface is stationary, the frequency of the reflected wave will be identical to the incident beam. If the interface is moving, the reflected echo frequency will be shifted up or down (relative to the incident wave) by an amount proportional to the velocity along the beam direction. This shift Δf is the Doppler shift and is given by the following equation:

$$\Delta f = \frac{2\,V f_o}{c} \cos\theta \qquad [1]$$

where Δf is the Doppler shift frequency (Hz), V is the velocity of the moving interface (cm/sec), f_o is the frequency of the incident sound (Hz), c is the velocity of

sound in tissue (cm/sec), and θ is the angle in degrees between the sound beam direction and the direction of the moving interface.

Their actual received frequency (fr) from the moving interface would thus be:

$$fr = f_o + \Delta f \qquad [2]$$

When the impinging ultrasound beam passes through a blood vessel, scattering of the sound wave occurs. In this process, small amounts of sound energy are absorbed by each red cell and re-radiated in all directions. If the red blood cell is moving with respect to the source, the backscattered energy returning to the receiving transducer will be shifted in frequency; the magnitude and direction of this shift is proportional to the velocity of the respective cell. If the ultrasound beam is considered to fill the entire lumen of a blood vessel,

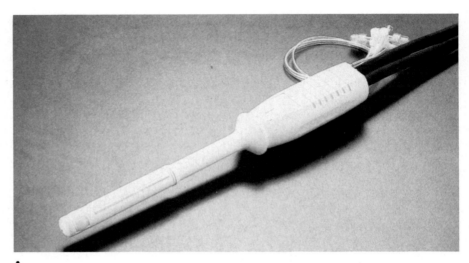

A

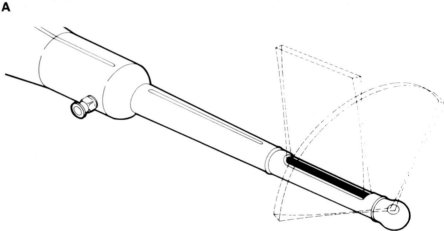

Fig. 3–12A. Transrectal probe with bi-
planar capability (both linear and sector
scanners incorporated into a single
probe). **B.** Diagram of field-of-view and
scan plane orientations for the biplane
dual-transducer transrectal probe. (*Courtesy of Toshiba and A.T.L., Inc.*)

B

then the backscattered signal will consist of all the Doppler shifts produced by the red cells moving through the
ultrasonic beam. Because there will always be a range
of velocities present, from zero at the vessel wall to a
peak value near the center of the vessel lumen, a spectrum of Doppler shift frequencies will always be present.
The frequency spectrum is derived from the application
of a mathematical operation called a Fourier transformation to the returning echo wave train. This spectrum
can become quite complex with pulsating blood flow and
vessel wall motion, especially when blood flow disturbances due to anatomical defects are present. Vessel wall
irregularity, ulcerated plaques, narrowed or partially occluded vessels, or such other abnormalities as stenotic
heart valves cause velocity variation readily detected by
differences in the frequency spectrum of the Doppler
signal.

A number of imaging schemes have been devised
to give the user other information on vessel anatomy in
addition to blood flow. The simplest of these uses a CW
Doppler transducer fixed to a mechanical arm. As the
transducer moves back and forth over a vessel of interest,
an image is produced on a storage oscilloscope corresponding to each site of inquiry. A serious deficiency of
this simple CW Doppler instrument is depth resolution.

The most practical way to add depth resolution to
a Doppler instrument is to pulse the source and add a
range gate to the receiver. Such pulsed Doppler devices
are similar to a pulse echo instrument in that bursts of
ultrasound are emitted at a regular repetition rate into
the body tissue. A new pulse will not be transmitted until
echoes from the previous pulse have ceased or significantly diminished. The depth of a pulse can be determined by noting the time of its flight to an interface and
return. Relatively short bursts of approximately 0.5 to
1.0 second duration can be used to give high axial resolution for detection of the location and separation of
interfaces within 1 mm or less.

The principle for the pulsed Doppler is actually quite
different from that employed with a pulse echo instrument. To determine simultaneously the Doppler spectrum of a reflected wave from many depths in real-time

requires extremely fast parallel processes to carry out the many Fourier transformations. To display these multidimensional data (flow magnitude, direction, and location), color-coded images are often used. In the image, color is used to encode direction and hue is used to encode relative magnitude.

A disadvantage of pulsed Doppler scanners is their inability to accurately determine rapid flow; this may present aliased results in which a high-flow location is actually presented as a low-flow location. The maximum flow that can be measured by a pulsed Doppler system is determined by the pulse repetition (PRF) of the system. Specifically, the detected Doppler shift frequency ($\triangle f$) cannot be greater than PRF/2. To increase PRF to allow estimates of rapid flow unfortunately limits the field-of-view to very superficial structures and also adds the potential for range ambiguity errors. (Range ambiguity errors occur when echoes from previous lines are received as echoes from the current line.) Fortunately, flow aliasing can often be recognized and will not generally lead to mistaken diagnoses.

QUALITY CONTROL

The purpose of a quality assurance program is to ensure that the diagnostic quality of all ultrasonic images is maintained at the maximum attainable level. Part of this program must include monitoring procedures that will ensure the proper and consistent operation of all equip-

ment. Equipment acceptance tests must be performed on delivery of new equipment and repeated whenever major equipment repairs are made. Quality assurance tests should be performed on a routine basis to detect deviations from the baseline acceptance tests. Quality assurance is a joint responsibility of physician, technologist, and the service support personnel.

There are numerous test objects and instruments that are now available for assessing the performance of ultrasonic equipment. A number of documents are also available that contain detailed protocols for establishing a quality assurance program. Probably the single most versatile and complete test object that can be used in these studies is the American Institute of Ultrasound in Medicine (AIUM) Standard 100-mm Test Object (Fig. 3–13A). The standard AIUM test object is filled with a relatively non-attenuating medium. Phantoms with a similar configuration, but filled with an attenuating "tissue-equivalent" material, are also commercially available. These tissue-equivalent phantoms provide system beam-parameter measurements in a more patient-like environment.

A minimal quality assurance program should include routine monitoring of the performance of the gray scale photography, image system sensitivity, axial resolution, and the accuracy and linearity of distance markers. In addition to evaluation of the gray scale system, the AIUM test object may be used to assess each of the other system parameters. The minimal quality assurance program provides relative parameter values. Relative values are use-

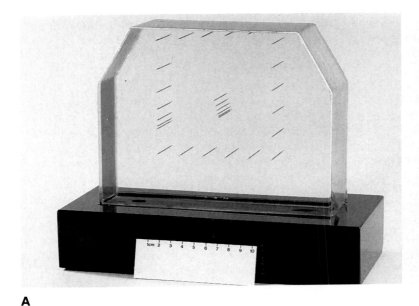

A

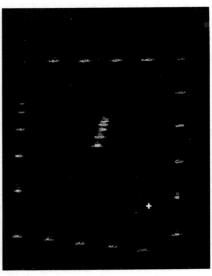

B

Fig. 3–13A. Photograph of the AIUM Standard 100-mm Test Object. **B.** Scan image of the AIUM phantom illustrating axial-resolution wire-set (*center*), dead-zone wire-set (*top*), and distance markers (*vertical and horizontal*).

ful for detecting early changes in image system characteristics. Absolute measurements of system parameters are more difficult and may require additional test objects and equipment.

Of equal importance to the actual performance testing is the documentation of the test results. These recorded data are essential for accurate monitoring of equipment performance, and are useful to both the equipment service personnel and the equipment manufacturer. It is also an incumbent possibility that this will be required by government regulatory and certifying agencies in the near future.

The initial camera settings and scan converter output controls depend largely on individual points of reference. Once a baseline has been established, a daily evaluation should be made to ensure that the same range of echo amplitudes can be seen as was present on previous test exposures.

Most systems now generate gray scale bars displayed to one side or at the bottom of the image. This bar should be examined daily for consistency of step distribution and display. The comparison can be made either by visual inspection or with the aid of a densitometer, which is more quantitative.

A simple test for system sensitivity stability can be performed with the aid of the AIUM phantom. After carefully positioning the transducer directly above the reference wires, which are spaced 2 cm apart (making sure the transducer face is flat against the phantom surface), the system gain (attenuation or output) settings should be adjusted to display a one-division echo from the most distant wire. These gain settings should not change on subsequent recordings. Similarly, the minimum gain settings required to yield a discernable echo in the B-mode image should not change with time. By this method the stability of the instrumentation over time can be determined.

A single image of the AIUM phantom will provide data on axial resolution as well as the accuracy and linearity of the distance markers. Axial resolution is assessed from the minimum resolvable spacing in the set of diagonal wires at the center of the phantom (Fig. 3–13B). Within this set, wire spacings range from 5 mm to 1 mm. Most imaging systems should exhibit the ability to resolve 2-mm wire spacings, and this value should remain constant over time.

The accuracy and linearity of the system-generated distance markers can be evaluated by direct measurement of the distances of the vertical and horizontal wires from a B-mode image. The distance between the uppermost and bottom wires in the 2-cm spaced group is

actually 10 cm, and this distance—as estimated by the markers—should not differ by more than 2 mm.

SUMMARY

This chapter has discussed and illustrated the pivotal and clinically pertinent principles involved in sonographic imaging.

BIBLIOGRAPHY

Physics

Christensen EE, Curry T, Dowdey J. *Introduction to the Physics of Diagnostic Radiology*, 3rd ed. Philadelphia: Lea & Febiger; 1984.

Kremkau FW. *Diagnostic Ultrasound Principles, Instrumentation and Exercises*, 2nd ed. New York: Grune & Stratton; 1984.

Powis R, Powis W. *A Thinker's Guide to Ultrasonic Imaging*. Baltimore: Urban & Schwarzenberg; 1984.

Price RR, Jones T. Fleischer AC, James AE. Ultrasound basic principles. In: Coulam GM, et al, *The Physical Basis of Medical Imaging*. New York: Appleton-Century-Crofts; 1981; 155.

Doppler

Merritt, CRB. Imaging blood flow with Doppler. *Diagnostic Imaging*. November 1986; 146.

Taylor KJW. Going to the depths with duplex Doppler. *Diagnostic Imaging*. October 1987; 106.

Taylor, KJW, Morse SS, Rigsby CM, et al. Vascular complications in renal allografts. Detection with duplex Doppler ultrasound. *Radiology*. 1987; 62:31–38.

Zagzebski, JA. Physics and instrumentation of Doppler ultrasonography. *Seminar Ultrasound*. 1981; 11:246.

Intraluminal Probes

Berneschek G, Tatru G, Janisch H. Rectal sonography—A major advance in the diagnosis of recurrence of cervical malignancies. *Radiology*. 1985; 155:557.

Platt LD. New look in ultrasound: The vaginal probe. *Contemporary Obstet Gynecol*. October 1987; 99–105.

Quality Assurance

Goldstein A. *Quality Assurance in Diagnostic Ultrasound: A Manual for the Clinical User*. Washington, DC: US Government Printing Office; 1980. HHS Publication FDA 81–8139.

Goldstein A, Madrazo BL. Slice-thickness artifacts in gray-scale ultrasound. *Journal of Clinical Ultrasound*. 1981; 9:365–375.

4 Sonography in Early Intrauterine Pregnancy Emphasizing Transvaginal Scanning

Arthur C. Fleischer • Rebecca G. Pennell •
Glynis A. Sacks • Donna M. Kepple • Jack Davies

Conventional transabdominal sonography is an established modality for the evaluation of early pregnancy. Besides establishing that the pregnancy is indeed within the uterus, sonography is frequently used to evaluate whether or not the embryo/fetus is alive—particularly in those pregnant patients who experience bleeding and pain. The recent availability of transvaginal sonography has greatly improved the evaluation of both normal and abnormal early intrauterine pregnancy. In general, this technique allows earlier and more definitive diagnoses than the conventional transabdominal techniques.

This chapter discusses the role of sonography in evaluation of first trimester pregnancy that is within the uterus. The next chapter is devoted to sonographic evaluation of ectopic pregnancy.

CLINICAL INDICATIONS

Sonography has several clinical indications in the first trimester of pregnancy. The majority of these involves the establishment of the location of the pregnancy and detection of embryonic/fetal life. Others concern establishing the cause of the bleeding and the severity of the disorder.

Approximately 20% to 50% of patients may experience bleeding in the first few weeks of pregnancy.[1] This bleeding has been attributed to the anchoring of the choriodecidua as it burrows into the decidualized endometrium. This bleeding is usually limited and not associated with cramping. On the other hand, 20% to 30% of patients with bleeding will progress to a threatened abortion.[1] This condition is probably related to extension of retrochorionic hemorrhage to involve more of the implantation site. The size of the retrochorionic hemorrhage can be correlated to clinical outcome.[2]

Sonography has a major role in evaluation of patients with suspected ectopic pregnancy. Most importantly, sonography can accurately establish that the pregnancy is intrauterine, virtually excluding the possibility it is ectopic. This can be accomplished best by transvaginal

scanning that can document an intrauterine pregnancy as early as four to five postmenstrual weeks.[3,7]

Thus, the major indications for sonography in the first trimester include:

1. Establishment of intrauterine pregnancy, particularly when ectopic pregnancy is suspected.
2. Evaluation of complicated early pregnancy such as retrochorionic hemorrhage, incomplete abortion, anembryonic pregnancy, or completed abortion.
3. Detection of embryonic/fetal life.
4. Precise localization of IUDs associated with early pregnancy.

INSTRUMENTATION AND SCANNING TECHNIQUE

In most cases, transvaginal scanning is the method of choice over transabdominal scanning for evaluation of first trimester pregnancies. This is primarily due to its improved resolution of the intrauterine contents and better patient acceptance.[3] Because of the theoretic potential for ascending infection, transvaginal sonography should not be used when there is active bleeding and a dilated external cervical os. Transabdominal sonography still is an accurate means for confirmation of location and viability of pregnancies greater than eight to ten weeks, and can be used solely or in conjunction with transvaginal sonography.

The technique for transvaginal scanning begins with covering the transducer probe with a condom and placing some ultrasonic lubricant within the condom. Then the transducer/probe is inserted through the introitus and into the midvagina. When placed within the vagina, the transducer can be manipulated in semicoronal and sagittal planes for delineation of the uterus and the adnexa in long and short axes. A slightly distended bladder may assist in placing a very anteflexed uterus to a more neutral or horizontal position. However, greater degrees of bladder filling may displace the uterus away from the focal zone of the transducer, making detailed examination of the embryo and choriodecidua difficult.

On a routine first trimester transvaginal sonogram, certain structures should be clearly documented. These landmarks can be correlated to a specific range of beta-hCG values.[14,15] These include the position and regularity of the choriodecidua of the gestational sac, the presence or absence of a yolk sac and/or embryo/fetus, and evaluation of the adnexa and cul-de-sac. When an embryo is identified, its crown rump length should be measured accurately. If an embryo cannot be delineated, gestational sac dimensions are useful alternative parameters for measurement to determine gestational duration. For this measurement, the three inner-to-inner dimensions (long, short, and anterior–posterior) are obtained and then averaged. Prior to depicting an embryo, the sonographic documentation of a yolk sac within the gestational sac is a reliable means to confirm that the pregnancy is indeed intrauterine.[13]

Although transvaginal scanning is usually sufficient in early pregnancy, occasionally structures that are superior to the uterus and outside the field of view of transvaginal probe may be difficult to image. For these, a routine transabdominal scan with a fully distended bladder may be helpful. In some patients who are hesitant to have a transvaginal scan, transabdominal scanning remains an accurate means for evaluating most complications that occur in early pregnancy.

Normal First Trimester Pregnancy

This discussion of normal development is divided into considerations of 4 to 6 weeks, 7 to 8 weeks, and 9 to 11 weeks.

During the embryonic period, all of the main viscera are formed. In the fetal period, these formed structures grow and complete their functional development. This distinction is somewhat arbitrary and is based on terminology used in embryology. The terms used by embryologic texts, specifically gestational age, vary in meaning from those used clinically. Embryologic texts typically describe development in terms of the time from conception (gestational age), whereas menstrual age is used in a clinical setting because it dates from a recordable event. Although there is usually a two-week interval between the time of fertilization and last day of menses, this can vary by plus or minus eight days. The events described in this chapter are classified by their menstrual dates.

Four to Six Weeks

The midembryonic period of development can generally be defined from the fourth to sixth menstrual weeks (Figs. 4–1 and 4–2). The embryonic anatomy present in early embryonic development is generally below the resolution of most currently available systems. Variations in the time

of ovulation (up to 12 days) and implantation (up to three days) may influence what is depicted on a transvaginal scan in this early stage of pregnancy.

Using transvaginal sonography, one of the first signs of intrauterine pregnancy is a hypoechoic complex within the thickened decidualized endometrium. This complex measures only a few millimeters. The gestational sac can be seen as early as four weeks and three days but should be routinely detected by transvaginal sonography after five weeks.[8] Within the sac, a few-millimeter double sac structure—representing the developing primary yolk sac and extraembryonic coelom (double bleb)—can be seen surrounded by the echogenic layer of choriodecidua at five weeks.[10] The embryo (which is not visible at this stage) is termed a trilaminar embryo since, microscopically, three distinct layers (endoderm, mesoderm, and ectoderm) are present.

Because transvaginal scanning is a relatively new clinical modality, additional experience with this technique is needed before absolute standards for sac sizes relative to yolk sac/embryo visualization are established. Using data collected from patients undergoing in vitro fertilization, one study has indicated that a gestational sac can be seen routinely between four and five weeks' menstrual age.[8] Our experience in following one in vitro fertilization patient indicated that an intrauterine sac could be seen at 18 days postconception. In general, a yolk sac can usually be demonstrated within the gestational sac by transvaginal scanning when the sac is approximately 1 cm in size; an embryo is usually seen in sacs that average 1.5 cm.[9] Similarly, preliminary experience has suggested that the beta-hCG level at which early gestational sacs are seen by transvaginal sonography is in the range of 500 to 800 mIU units (the second international standard). This is significantly lower than the level reported with transabdominal sonography (1,800 to 3,000 mIU units).[9] The gestational sac itself grows approximately 1 to 2 mm in size each day at this time, and can usually be delineated within the thickened decidua vera.

During the middle of the fifth postmenstrual week (three and one half weeks' gestational age), the embryo measures between 2 and 5 mm and is located adjacent to the relatively prominent secondary yolk sac—which appears as a rounded hypoechoic structure between 3 and 4 mm in size. The embryo/yolk sac complex lies adjacent to the edge of the gestational sac and has been described as forming a "double bleb," representing the amniotic sac–embryo/yolk sac complex.[10] By the end of the first half of the embryonic period, the choriodecidua forms the boundaries of the gestational sac—which appears as an echogenic ring of tissue. At four weeks' menstrual age, the gestational sac measures only 3 to 5 mm in diameter and grows to approximately 1 cm at five weeks.

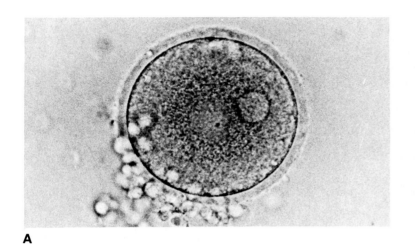

A

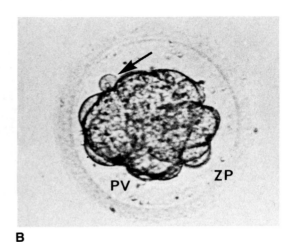

B

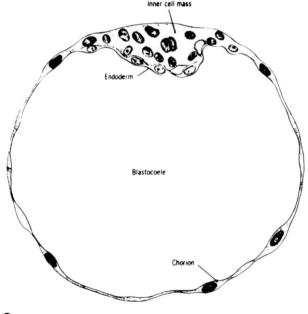

C

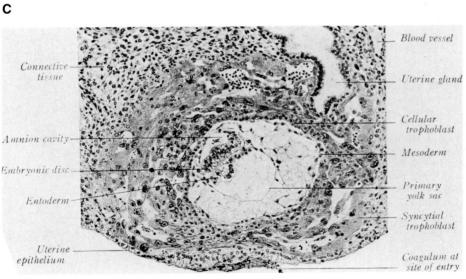

D

Fig. 4–1. Diagrammatic representation of embryonic/early fetal development. **A.** Human oocyte in process of fertilization (×420). **B.** A preimplantation baboon embryo (similar to the human) as the morula is transforming into a blastocyst. Arrow, column segmentation cavity; PV, perivitelline space; ZP, zona pellucida. **C.** Line drawing of blastocyst showing early inner cell mass and trophoblast. (*Reprinted with permission from Davies J: Human Developmental Anatomy, New York, Ronald, 1963.*) **D.** Section of 11-day human embryo showing cellular and syncytial trophoblast. (*Reprinted with permission from Arey B: Developmental Anatomy, Philadelphia, Saunders, 1962.*) (*Figure continued.*)

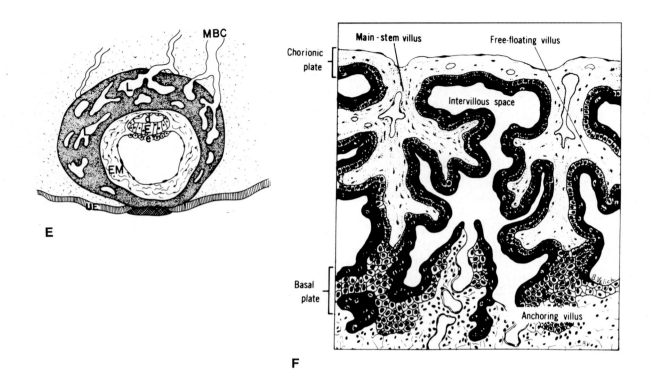

E

F

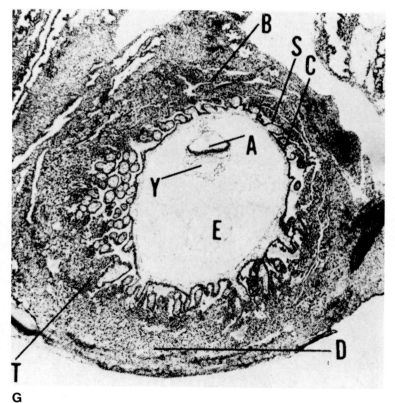

Fig. 4–1. (*continued*). The first stages of embryonic development, **E.** 12-day implanted embryo; a, amnion and amniotic cavity; E, embryonic ectoderm; e, embryonic entoderm; EM, extraembryonic mesenchyme; L, maternal blood lacuna in the trophoblast; Ue, uterine epithelium; MBC, maternal blood circulation. (*Redrawn by Panigel: In Grasse (ed), Traité de Zoologie, Masson, 1976. Reprinted with permission from Hertig and Rock and from Starck.*) **F.** Cross section of early human placenta that demonstrates portions of the villous tree and stem villi anchored to the decidua basalis. (*Reprinted with permission from Davies J: Human Developmental Anatomy, New York, Ronald, 1963.*) **G.** Cross section through an early (16 day) gestational sac. B, decidual basalis; D, decidual capsularis; T, cytotrophoblast; C, chorion, S, secondary villus; A, amnion, Y, yolk sac; E, exocoelomic cavity. (*Reprinted with permission from Gruenwald P: The Placenta, 1st ed, Baltimore, University Park, 1975.*)   (*Figure continued.*)

G

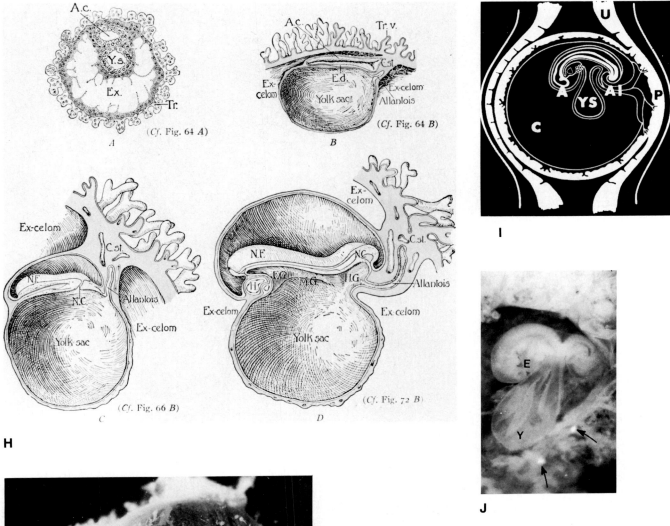

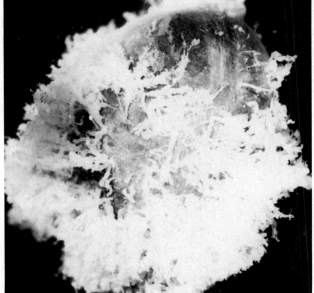

Fig. 4–1. (continued). H. Diagrams showing progressive growth (A through D) of the amniotic sac, yolk sac, and embryo. (*Reprinted with permission from Arey B: Developmental Anatomy, Philadelphia, Saunders, 1962, p 89.*) **I.** Diagram of **J** showing 10-mm human embryo with its membranes and surrounding villous trophoblast. C, amniotic cavity; P, placenta; U, uterus; YS, yolk sac; **J.** 10-mm embryo, E; yolk sac, Y; and the chorionic villi (*arrows*). **K.** The external surface of a human chorionic sac showing both the chorion frondosum and chorion laeve areas. (*Figure continued.*)

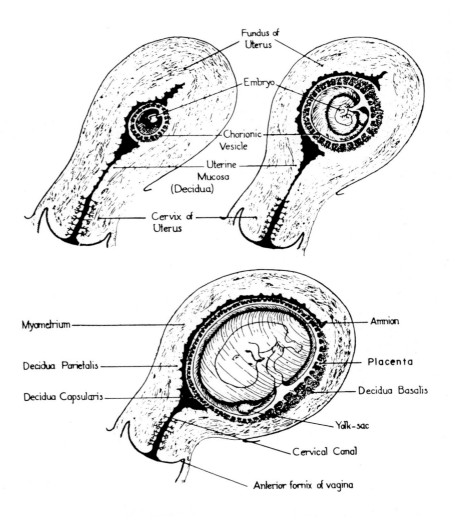

Fig. 4–1. (continued). L. Diagrams in cross section of uterus at 6, 8, and 10 weeks' menstrual age showing embryonic membranes and their development.

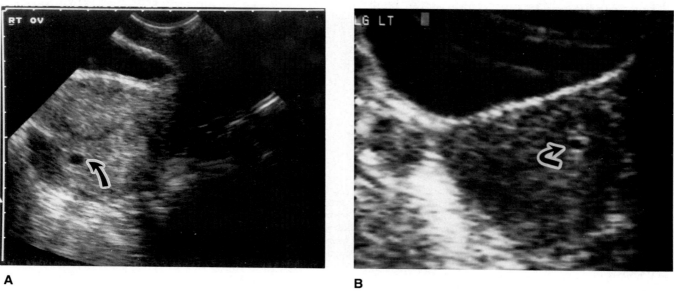

Fig. 4–2. Normal 5-week intrauterine pregnancy (IUP). **A.** Transvaginal (TV) sonogram of 4-week, 6-day pregnancy demonstrating 5-mm anechoic sac (*arrow*) within decidua. **B.** Transabdominal (TA) sonogram of 5-week IUP (*arrow*) as depicted on magnified transverse scan.   (*Figure continued.*)

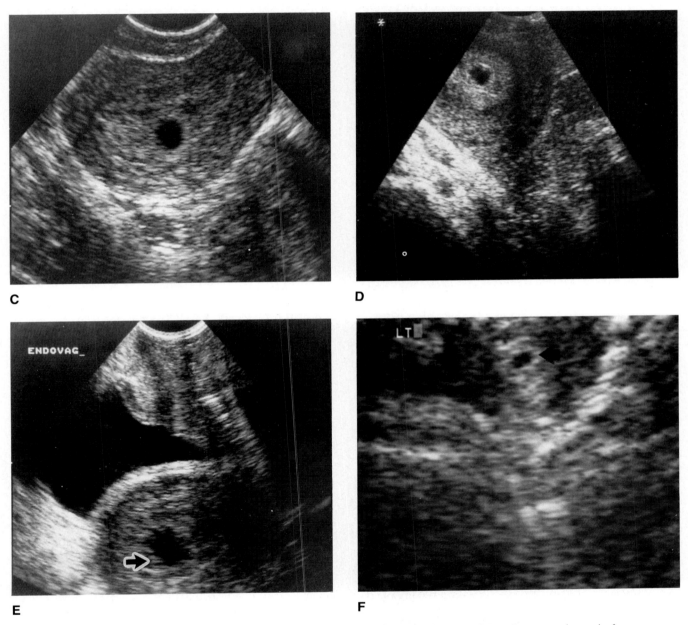

Fig. 4–2. (*continued*). Normal 5-week intrauterine pregnancy (IUP). **C.** TV scan of 7- to 8-mm sac (*arrow*) of 5-week IUP. **D.** TV sonogram US of 5-week IUP appearing as anechoic area within the thickened decidualized endometrium. **E.** TV scan of 5-week 6-day intrauterine pregnancy in a retroflexed uterus, demonstrating a embryo/yolk sac complex (*arrowhead*). **F.** Magnified transverse TA scan of 5- to 6-week IUP showing concentric layers of decidua (*arrow*) and a "double bleb."

During the early embryonic period the embryo may be barely visible on transvaginal sonography. Although many of the structures are present, they cannot be resolved sonographically. The neural tube is closed in its mid portion but open at its rostral and caudal ends. Brachial arches form and the somites develop as rounded surface elevations. Forty-two or forty-four somites form; these paired structures eventually give rise to the axial skeleton and associated musculature.

Seven to Eight Weeks

During the latter half of the embryonic period, sonographic scanning can depict a gestational sac, developing embryo and its heart beat, surrounding membranes, and choriodecidua. During this period, organogenesis of the major body viscera occurs (Figs. 4–3 to 4–6).

On both transvaginal and transabdominal sonography, heart pulsations can be depicted during this period of gestation. Transvaginal sonography is most precise in depicting early heart pulsation after six postmenstrual weeks, when the developing embryo forms from two enfolding fusiform tubes and begins contractile activity.

During the seventh postmenstrual week (fifth week gestational age), the developing embryo grows from 6 to 11 mm in crown rump length. During this phase of development, the head growth is extensive—resulting primarily from rapid development of the brain. A cystic area can be identified in the brain representing the rhombencephalon.[11] The yolk sac is relatively large (5 to 10 mm) and floats within the gestational sac between the chorion and amnion, attached to the developing umbilical cord.

During the eighth postmenstrual week of embryonic development (six weeks' gestational age), the embryo grows from 14 to 21 mm in length. The head remains a large and prominent structure and is bent over the heart prominence. The yolk sac becomes progressively smaller, and the intestines enter the extraembryonic celom beginning the normal process of umbilical herniation. By the end of the ninth postmenstrual week (seventh week of gestational age), the embryo has attained human features.[4] The head, body, and extremities can be identified sonographically. The intestine is still within the proximal portion of the umbilical cord. Occasionally, this physiologic umbilical herniation of bowel is particularly well depicted with transvaginal scanning. Because this process of physiologic herniation of bowel into the umbilical cord is normal, abnormalities of the ventral wall should be suspected only if the bowel remains outside of the abdomen at 12 weeks or beyond.

Another structure that can be depicted in the late embryonic period is the amniotic membrane.[5] The amniotic cavity forms from an area deep in the trilaminar embryo, and the amniotic membrane can be seen on a fully floating linear interface in the outer portion of the amniotic cavity. The amnion approximates with the chorion only late in the first trimester of pregnancy (14 to 18 weeks).[12] At six to eight weeks, the membrane can be seen as a thin rounded structure that encircles the embryo/fetus on transvaginal sonography. Prior to this, the amniotic membrane may appear as a linear echogenic interface projected within the gestational sac in proximity to the embryo.

Besides depiction of the embryo/fetus, the choriodecidua is seen as it begins to thicken at the implantation site during the late embryonic and early fetal period. The anatomic and functional fusing of decidua basalis and chorion frondosum forms the future placenta.

Nine to Eleven Weeks

After nine weeks, the fetus is clearly depicted both with transabdominal and transvaginal scanning. The fetus begins to move into trunk and extremities and can be seen to do an occasional somersault within the uterus. The fetal brain has relatively large lateral ventricles that are mostly filled with choroid plexus (Figs. 4–5 to 4–8).

COMPLICATED EARLY INTRAUTERINE PREGNANCY

As stated previously, it is not unusual for the pregnant patient to experience painless spotting in the first few weeks of pregnancy. This probably is related to trophoblastic implantation within the decidualized endometrium. As the gestational sac develops, small (2 to 5 mm) hypoechoic areas may be seen immediately beneath the echogenic choriodecidua that probably represent an area of blood pools or lacunae (Fig. 4–8).

Patients who present with extensive bleeding may have retrochorionic hemorrhage. In this disorder, there is more extensive bleeding behind the chorion—appearing as a hypoechoic area surrounding the gestational sac. Using the formula for a prolate ellipse volume (cc): length (cm) × width (cm) × height (cm) × 0.5, the relative size of the retrochorionic hemorrhage can be quantified in relation to the size of the gestational sac itself. It has been shown that the relative size of the retrochorionic hemorrhage has some implications as to whether or not the pregnancy will progress.[3] When the area of the retrochorionic hemorrhage is less than one fourth of the gestational sac or less than 60 mL, it is likely that the pregnancy will progress.[3]

In spontaneous incomplete abortions, there is usually passage of the fetus or embryo with retained choriodecidua. This tissue typically appears as echogenic material within the uterine lumen. The choriodecidua is irregular and the gestational sac itself appears "deflated."

In cases of blighted ovum or anembryonic pregnancy, there is failed or abnormal development of the

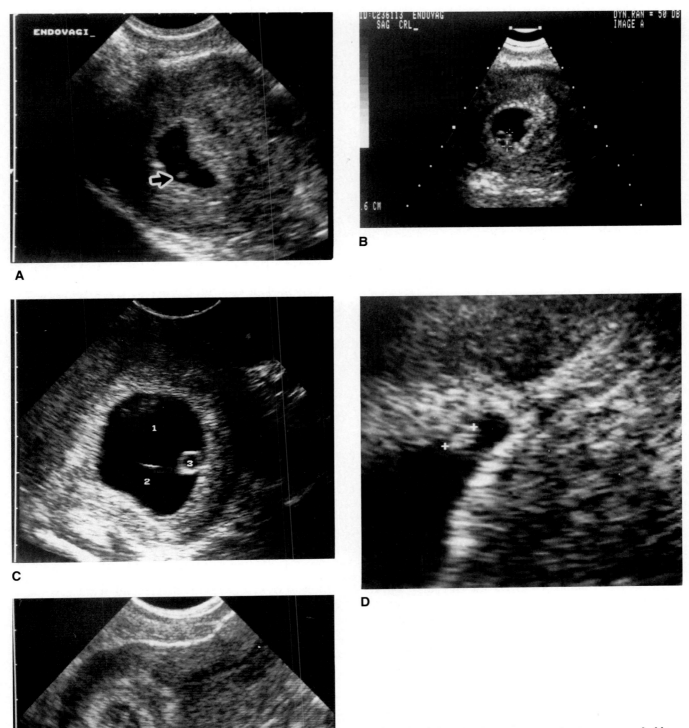

Fig. 4–3. Normal 6- to 7-week intrauterine pregnancy. **A.** Magnified TV sonogram of 3-mm embryo/yolk sac (*arrow*). Compare to Figure 4–1H. **B.** TV sonogram of 6-week IUP with 6-mm embryo (between xs) adjacent to the yolk sac. **C.** Magnified TV scan of 6-week IUP demonstrating embryo within embryonic cavity (1), extra embryonic celom (2), and yolk sac (3). **D.** Magnified TV sonogram of 6-mm embryo located in an edge of the gestational sac. **E.** TV scan of 6-week IUP demonstrating embryo/yolk sac complex and decidua capsularis and vera. Compare to Figure 4–1L.

embryo and its associated umbilical cord and body stalk. Thus, even though a gestational sac may appear normally formed, no embryo or, on occasion, no yolk sac will be identified within the uterus. Anembryonic pregnancy is usually a reflection of a chromosomally aberrant conceptus.

Embryonic demise can be documented by transvaginal sonography when there is lack of heart motion in an embryo that measures over 6 mm in length. In some cases of failed embryonic development, amorphous internal debris can be present within the sac—probably representing strands of blood or sloughed decidual tissues.

In completed miscarriages, there is close apposition of relatively thin and regular endometrial interfaces. Although one might argue that ectopic pregnancies may demonstrate this appearance, correlation with beta-hCG values may be helpful in confirming a completed miscarriage. In completed miscarriage, serial beta-hCG values will typically fall precipitously whereas in ectopic pregnancy this value slowly decreases or plateaus.[6]

OTHER APPLICATIONS

It is important in some patients with intrauterine contraceptive devices and complicated pregnancies to confirm the presence of an IUD and establish its location relative to the gestational sac in developing choriodecidua. Clearly, IUDs that are implanted superior to the gestational sac are more difficult to extract than those that are inferior. The amount of retrochorionic hemorrhage associated with an IUD can also be quantified using transvaginal sonography.

Transvaginal sonography may also be helpful in evaluation of first trimester pregnancies complicated by trophoblastic disease. Although large hydropic villi may not be present in trophoblastic disease at this stage, the abnormal tissue can be diagnosed as well as its relative amount. However, trophoblastic tissue frequently has the sonographic appearance of retained choriodecidua. This disorder is discussed in detail in Chapter 31.

SUMMARY

The recent development of transvaginal sonography as providing a means to evaluate complicated early intrauterine pregnancy has been discussed in this chapter. Transvaginal sonography primarily has a role in diagnosis of early intrauterine pregnancy in patients suspected of ectopic pregnancy, and of detecting embryonic or fetal life in those patients with extensive bleeding, cramping, or both in the first trimester.

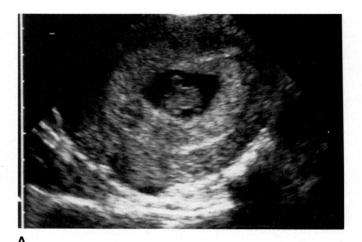

A

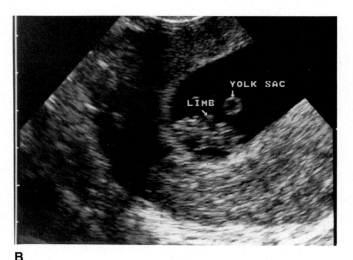

B

C

Fig. 4–4. Normal embryo at 7 to 8 weeks. **A.** TV sonogram of 8-mm embryo with a yolk sac adjacent to embryo. **B.** 10-mm embryo demonstrating limb and yolk sac. **C.** TV scan of 8-week embryo in coronal plane, demonstrating early ossification of clavicle (*arrow*).

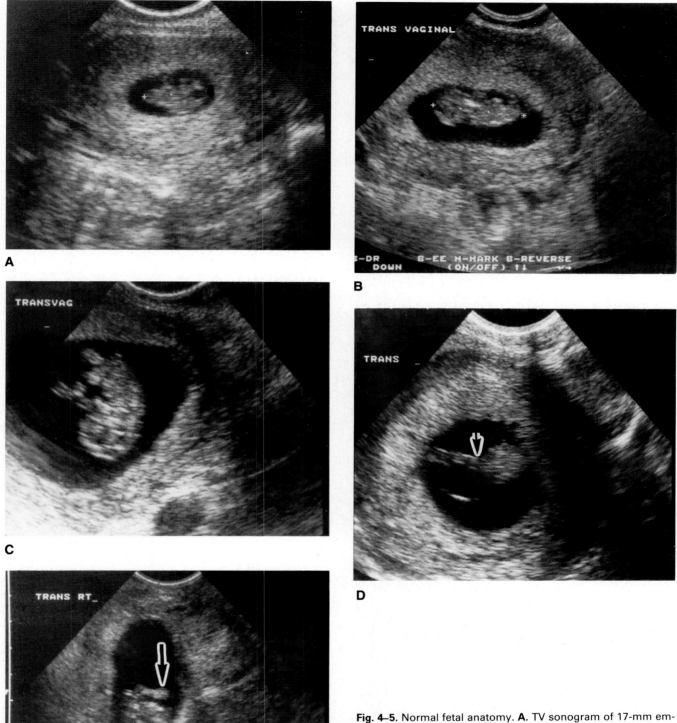

Fig. 4–5. Normal fetal anatomy. **A.** TV sonogram of 17-mm embryo demonstrating prominent cystic area of brain corresponding to rhombencephalon. **B.** TV scan of 28-mm fetus. **C.** TV scan of 10-week fetus demonstrating arms and legs. **D.** Transverse of same fetus showing umbilical cord insertion within some physiologic herniation of bow into base of umbilical cord. **E.** TV sonogram showing hands on or near face of 11-week fetus.   (*Figure continued.*)

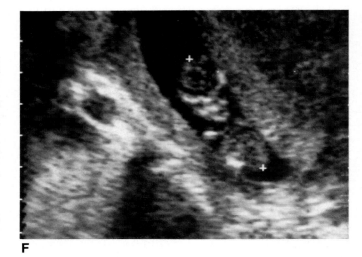

F

Fig. 4–5. (*continued*). Normal fetal anatomy. F. TA scan of 11-week fetus (between +s).

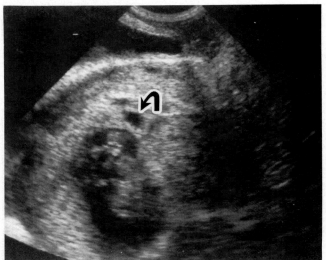

A

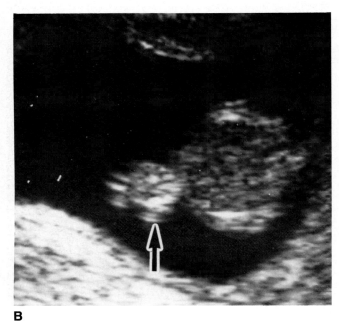

B

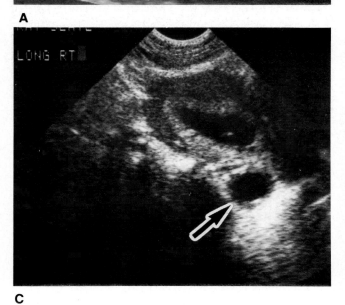

C

Fig. 4–6. Other normal features. A. Hypoechoic lacunae around decidual basalis of 10-week IUP. B. Magnified TV sonogram of 11-week fetus with bowel herniated into base of cord. C. TA scan of corpus luteum cyst of pregnancy. D. TA scan showing unoccupied lumen (*curved arrow*) at 6 weeks. (*Figure continued.*)

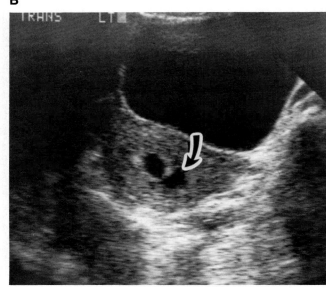

D

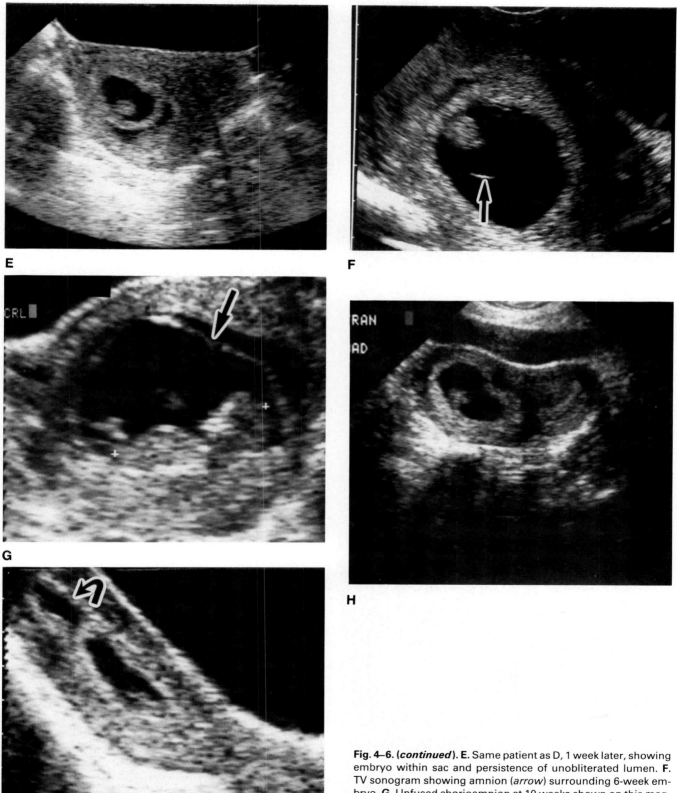

E

F

G

H

I

Fig. 4–6. (*continued*). E. Same patient as D, 1 week later, showing embryo within sac and persistence of unobliterated lumen. F. TV sonogram showing amnion (*arrow*) surrounding 6-week embryo. G. Unfused chorioamnion at 10 weeks shown on this magnified TA scan. H. Transabdominal sonogram of 6-week IUP within the right cornu of a bicornuate uterus. I. TA scan showing prominent retrochorionic blood pool (*curved arrow*).

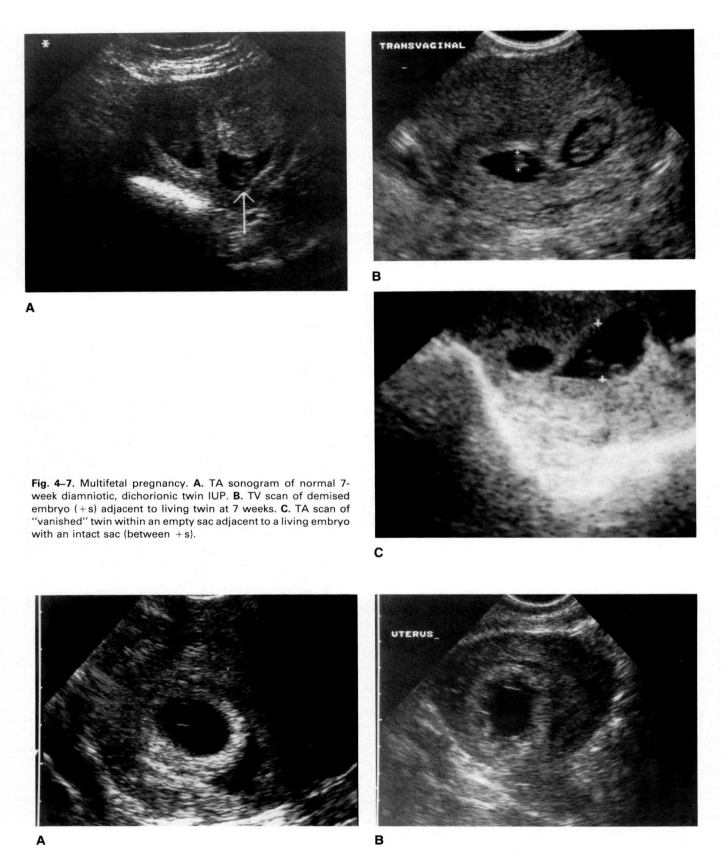

Fig. 4–7. Multifetal pregnancy. **A.** TA sonogram of normal 7-week diamniotic, dichorionic twin IUP. **B.** TV scan of demised embryo (+s) adjacent to living twin at 7 weeks. **C.** TA scan of "vanished" twin within an empty sac adjacent to a living embryo with an intact sac (between +s).

Fig. 4–8. Complicated early pregnancy. **A.** TV sonogram of anembryonic pregnancy. **B.** Semi-axial TV scan of incomplete abortion with irregular choriodecidua and deflated sac. (*Figure continued.*)

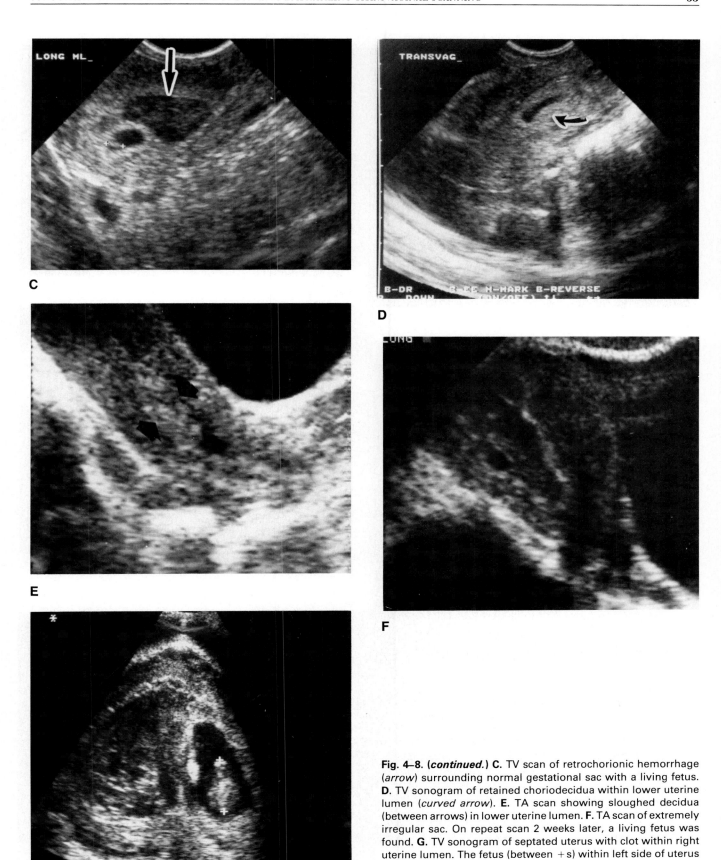

Fig. 4–8. (*continued.*) C. TV scan of retrochorionic hemorrhage (*arrow*) surrounding normal gestational sac with a living fetus. **D.** TV sonogram of retained choriodecidua within lower uterine lumen (*curved arrow*). **E.** TA scan showing sloughed decidua (between arrows) in lower uterine lumen. **F.** TA scan of extremely irregular sac. On repeat scan 2 weeks later, a living fetus was found. **G.** TV sonogram of septated uterus with clot within right uterine lumen. The fetus (between + s) within left side of uterus was living. (*Figure continued.*)

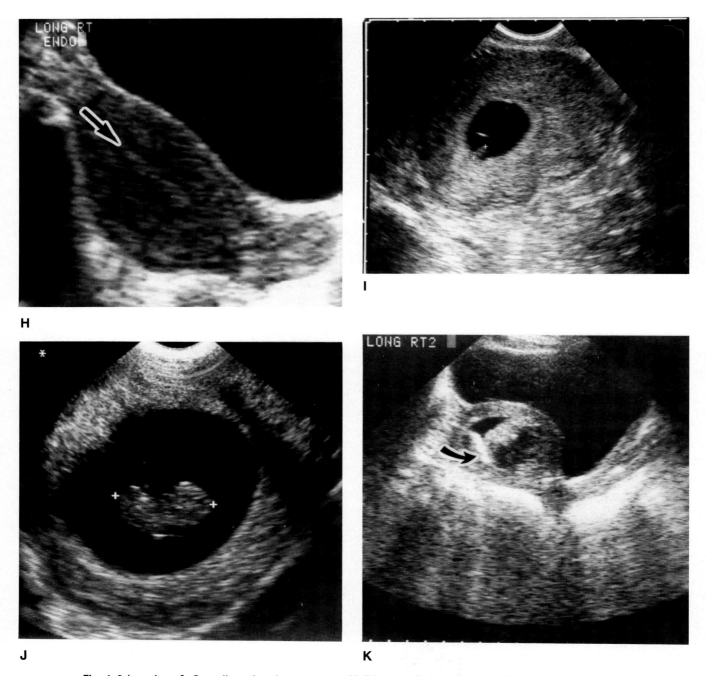

Fig. 4–8 (*continued*). Complicated early pregnancy. **H.** TA scan of completed abortion. Note thinness and regularity of endometrial interfaces (*arrow*). **I.** TV sonogram of embryonic demise at 6 weeks. No heart activity was detected. **J.** TV scan of fetal demise at 9 weeks. No heart motion was detected. **K.** TA scan showing retrochorionic hemorrhage surrounding an IUD (*curved arrow*). The deflated sac is seen inferior to the IUD.

REFERENCES

1. Pritchard L, MacDonald PC, Gant NF, eds. *Williams Obstetrics,* 16th ed. Norwalk, Conn: Appleton-Century-Crofts; 1985.
2. Sauerbrei EE, Pham DH. Placental abruption and sub-chorionic hemorrhage in the first half of pregnancy: US appearance and clinical outcome. *Radiology.* 1986; 160: 109–112.
3. Pennell RG, Baltarowich OH, Kurtz AB, et al. Complicated first-trimester pregnancies: Evaluation with endovaginal US versus transabdominal technique. *Radiology.* 1987; 165:79–83.

4. Moore K. *The Developing Human*. Philadelphia: Saunders; 1987.

5. Jeanty P. Sonographic appearance of normal amnion. *J Ultrasound Med*. 1982; 1:243.

6. Steier JA, Bergsjo P, Myking OL. Human chorionic gonadotrophin in maternal plasma after induced abortion, spontaneous abortion, and removed ectopic pregnancy. *Obstet Gynecol*. 1984; 64:391.

7. Timor-Tritsch IE, Rottem S, Thaler I. Review of transvaginal ultrasonography: A description with clinical application. *Ultrasound Quarterly*. 1988; 6(1):1–34.

8. de Crespigny L, Cooper D, McKenna M. Early detection of intrauterine pregnancy with ultrasound. *J Ultrasound Med*. 1988; 7:7–10.

9. Timor-Tritsch IE, Rottem S. *Transvaginal Sonography*. New York, Elsevier; 1988; 98.

10. Yeh HC, Rabinowitz JG. Amniotic sac development: ultrasound features of early pregnancy—the double bleb sign. *Radiology*. 1988; 166:97–103.

11. Cyr D, Mack L, Nyberg D, et al. Fetal rhombencephalon: normal US findings. *Radiology*. 1988; 166:691–692.

12. Torpin R. Fetal malformations caused by amnion rupture during gestation. In: Torpin R, ed. *The Human Placenta*. Springfield, Ill: Thomas: 1968; 1–76.

13. Nyberg DA, Mack LA, Harvey D, Wang K. Value of the yolk sac in evaluating early pregnancies. *J Ultrasound Med*. 1988; 7:129–135.

14. Batzer FR, Weiner S, Corson SL. Landmarks during the first forty-two days of gestation demonstrated by the B subunit of human chorionic gonadotrophin and ultrasound. *Am J Obstet Gynecol*. 1983; 146:973.

15. Nyberg DA, Filly RA, Mahony BS, et al. Early gestation: Correlation of hCG levels and sonographic identification. *AJR*. 1985; 144:951.

5 Sonography of Ectopic Pregnancy with Transabdominal and Transvaginal Scanning

Arthur C. Fleischer • *Peter S. Cartwright* • *Rebecca G. Pennell* • *Glynis A. Sacks*

Recent improvements in the sonographic depiction of uterine and adnexal structures with transvaginal sonography and refinements in radioimmunoassay (RIA) of the beta subunit of human chorionic gonadotropin (β-hCG) have markedly enhanced the sonologist's ability to diagnose ectopic pregnancy. Although the sonographic findings in ectopic pregnancy can be subtle, a definitive diagnosis of this entity is possible in most cases when sonographic findings are combined with results of a single or serial β-hCG assay. Most importantly, sonography is useful in evaluation of patients with suspected ectopic pregnancy to verify the presence or absence of an intrauterine pregnancy.

The possibility that a tube containing an ectopic pregnancy can be "salvaged" by linear salpingostomy with subsequent resuture is closely related to the stage at which the ectopic pregnancy is detected. Once the tube has ruptured, it usually cannot be salvaged. It is therefore most desirable to diagnose an ectopic pregnancy as early as possible.

The use of transvaginal sonography (TV US) has greatly enhanced the sonographic evaluation of patients with suspected ectopic pregnancy. Specifically, the presence or absence of an intrauterine gestation can be documented approximately 1 week earlier with TV US than with transabdominal sonography (TA US). In addition, adnexal masses created by ectopic pregnancies can more frequently be detected by transvaginal sonography.

With these modalities and laboratory tests, a very high degree of accuracy (over 90%) is now possible in establishing the presence or excluding the possibility of ectopic pregnancy.[1]

If left unrecognized, an ectopic pregnancy can result in significant maternal morbidity and mortality. Ectopic pregnancy is currently responsible for 4% to 10% of all maternal deaths.[2,3] Even though the diagnosis of ectopic pregnancy is often considered in women who present with lower abdominal pain and amenorrhea, it is missed by the initial examining physician in up to 70% of cases.[4]

Expeditious and accurate diagnosis of patients who are suspected of having ectopic pregnancy is therefore important so proper management can be instituted. If it is recognized early, before tubal rupture, it may be possible to surgically remove the gestational sac by linear salpingotomy—thereby preserving the tube and future chances of achieving pregnancy. Since salpingectomy is frequently required for advanced ectopic pregnancies, a history of the disorder can be a contributing factor to female infertility. Once a patient has had an ectopic pregnancy, there is a significant chance (about one in four) of recurrence.[4]

INCIDENCE

Several epidemiologic studies have shown that the incidence of ectopic pregnancies is increasing, which may be a reflection of the increased prevalence of salpingitis.[5,6] For example, the age-adjusted incidence of ectopic pregnancy rose from 55.5 to 84.2 per 100,000 women in northern California from 1972 to 1978.[5] Nationwide, the number of ectopic pregnancies has ranged from 17,800 in 1970 to 42,000 in 1978.[6] The death rate, however, decreased by 75% during this period. The incidence of ectopic pregnancies is greatest in patients with salpingitis, previous tubal surgery, or IUD use.[24,25]

PATHOGENESIS

The term ectopic pregnancy refers to an implantation of the conceptus outside the endometrial cavity. Ninety-five percent of ectopic pregnancies are tubal, and the majority of these occur in the ampullary or isthmic portions of the oviduct. The remaining 5% occur in the abdomen, ovary, cervix, and the retroperitoneal space.

In ectopic tubal pregnancy, the conceptus implants beneath the epithelium of the Fallopian tube to form a fluid-filled gestational sac—lined with trophoblastic tissue—in the wall of the tube. Since the Fallopian tube has only two thin layers of muscle, the trophoblastic cells that burrow deep into the tubal epithelium distend it and can eventually cause rupture. The gestational sac within the tube of a ruptured ectopic pregnancy is usually surrounded by fluid or blood due to erosion of adjacent vessels. In the vast majority of cases, the separation of the decidua from the wall of the tube causes death of the embryo. In rare cases, the embryo may survive an attempt at abortion by reimplantation within the abdomen and reestablishment of the blood supply from the omentum or the mesentery.

Mild uterine enlargement and decidualization of the endometrium are usually present with an ectopic pregnancy and can occasionally be detected clinically. If dilatation and curettage (D&C) is performed on a patient with an ectopic pregnancy, only decidua without chorionic villi will be obtained.

Recent studies have indicated that up to one third of all ectopic embryos have an abnormal karyotype, a factor which contributes to their demise and resultant deficient decidual support.[2] Because the ectopic implanted embryo frequently dies before the sixth week of gestation, decidualization may be interrupted and faulty.[7] Other contributing factors may include endocrine dysfunction, current IUD use, and previous tubal surgery.[24,25]

Another possible etiology of recurrent ectopic pregnancies is the transperitoneal migration of the fertilized egg into the contralateral tube. Predictably, this would result in delayed and faulty implantation of the trophoblasts into the tubal wall. As the relative contribution of those factors to the development of ectopic pregnancy are better understood, measures which can prevent ectopic pregnancy may be determined.

CLINICAL ASPECTS

Proposed explanations for development of ectopic pregnancy include delayed ovulation or delayed transit of the fertilized zygote secondary to Fallopian tube malfunction, ovulation from the contralateral ovary with delayed passage of the zygote through the tube, obstruction of zygote passage secondary to adhesions from pelvic inflammatory disease, and abnormal angulation of the tube relative to the uterine cornu.[2]

Prior to the use of antibiotics for pelvic inflammatory disease, tubal inflammation resulted in a much higher incidence of complete tubal closure and subsequent sterility. The recent two- to three-fold increased incidence of ectopic gestations among previously pregnant patients has been attributed paradoxically to the use of antibiotics

for treatment of tubal inflammation.[8] Antibiotics have reduced the incidence of sterility but have resulted in more women with open, but malfunctioning, tubes. The result is an increased incidence of ectopic pregnancy among patients with previous tubal infection. In addition to patients who have a history of pelvic inflammatory disease, patients who have undergone tubal surgery, have a history of infertility, and those who used IUDs have an increased chance of developing an ectopic pregnancy.[24] Ectopic pregnancy is a double-edged sword because it results in both a nonviable pregnancy and ability to render the patient infertile.[25] Again, once a patient has had an ectopic pregnancy, there is a one in four chance of recurrence.[4]

In the United States, the incidence of ectopic pregnancy is currently between 1 in 100 and 1 in 400 pregnancies, but in some populations it is as high as 1 in 32 live births.[2,4] Clinically, however, ectopic pregnancy should be considered in the differential diagnosis of any patient presenting with lower abdominal pain. This is because the sometimes massive intraperitoneal bleeding associated with rupture of an ectopic pregnancy is such a serious complication. An analogy can be made between ectopic pregnancy now and the great masquerade of pulmonary tuberculosis in the 1930s; its clinical symptoms at presentation vary so much in type and severity.[2] In fact, clinicians are now taught to "think ectopic" for any woman of childbearing age who presents with lower abdominal pain.

The most common presenting symptoms of ectopic pregnancy are pelvic pain—which may be mild and intermittent, or persistent and severe—and abnormal vaginal bleeding. The clinical symptomatology and routine laboratory findings in ectopic pregnancy are usually not diagnostic by themselves. Abnormal vaginal bleeding is seen in approximately three quarters of patients with such pregnancies and can be confused with other causes of first trimester bleeding (such as threatened or spontaneous abortion). However, there is no bleeding or menstrual history that is inconsistent with an ectopic gestation. Statistically, vaginal bleeding is more commonly associated with other first trimester conditions (such as threatened spontaneous abortion, cervical polyp, or infection) than with ectopic pregnancy. Diffuse abdominal pain may be present, as may rebound tenderness from peritoneal irritation resulting from free intraperitoneal bleeding.

The presence of an adnexal mass is not specific for the diagnosis of ectopic pregnancy because a mass can occur in many other conditions (such as corpus luteum cyst, dermoid cyst, or leiomyomata). In our experience, a palpable adnexal mass is noted in less than one third of cases and does not predict whether or not the gestation has ruptured.[9] Although uncommon, the presence of a palpable adnexal mass (that is, separate from both ovaries and uterine fundus) is highly suggestive of an ectopic pregnancy.

In an emergency setting, culdocentesis (the transvaginal aspiration of fluid from the posterior cul-de-sac) remains an alternative diagnostic aid for evaluating patients suspected of having an ectopic gestation. The aspiration of nonclotting blood indicates the presence of a hemoperitoneum. However, this finding is not diagnostic of an ectopic pregnancy; it also may result from a hemorrhagic corpus luteum, complete or incomplete abortion, ovulation, or previous attempts at culdocentesis. In our experience, 70% of patients with an ectopic pregnancy who underwent this procedure had positive taps; this was one of the key factors resulting in the patient's admission to the hospital.[10] In only 56% of these patients, however, was the tube ruptured; intact tubal pregnancy may produce several liters of hemoperitoneum by bleeding through the fimbriated end of the tube. A negative culdocentesis usually excludes a ruptured tube.

The clinical course of an ectopic pregnancy is related to its site of implantation. The ampullary portion of the tube is the most common location for ectopic implantation. As in other sites, the ectopic pregnancy can expand the tube until it ruptures. Complete or partial tubal abortion may also occur, with the contents of the sac extruded through the fimbriated end of the tube into the peritoneal cavity. If the fimbriated end of the tube is occluded, hematosalpinx will result. Ectopic pregnancies that occur in the narrow isthmic portion of the tube usually distend it eccentrically and, because of the tube's small diameter, rupture early in the pregnancy.

Ectopic pregnancy in the interstitial portion of the tube is uncommon (3% to 4% of all ectopic pregnancies) but potentially has the most serious complications. Because of its location within the muscular portion of the uterus near the major uterine vessels, the pregnancy can survive until three to four months' gestation. Massive bleeding from the uterine arteries and veins can then result.

Chronic ectopic pregnancies may occur, resulting in hematoma formation in the cul-de-sac.[11] Such patients usually present with recurrent, intermittent low-grade fever associated with a palpable solid mass. On physical examination, there is usually a firm pelvic mass located in the midline and difficult to separate from the uterus. Culdocentesis may be negative because the blood in the cul-de-sac is clotted. In very rare cases, the embryo and products of conception will undergo dehydration in situ with formation of a lithopedian pregnancy.

Other rare sites of implantation include intra-abdominal, ovarian, cervical, and extraperitoneal. True advanced abdominal ectopic pregnancies may be difficult to differentiate from normal intrauterine pregnancy; the

uterus must be defined separately from the amniotic sac and its contents.[12] Abdominal pregnancies are thought to be the result of reimplantation of an aborted fetus after is passes out the fimbriated end of the tube and reimplants on the mesentery or omentum. These pregnancies can progress to term without symptoms, and first present because of difficulty during the initial stages of labor. Extraperitoneal ectopic pregnancies are quite rare and are probably the result of tubal rupture with expulsion of the fetus between the leaves of the broad ligament. The rupture occurs between the fimbriated end of the tube (where it is not covered by peritoneum) and the site where the two folds of the broad ligament are loosely opposed. The tubal contents may empty into the soft tissue and mesosalpinx and implant in that region.

BETA-hCG ASSAY

To properly evaluate a patient in whom an ectopic pregnancy is suspected, it is absolutely imperative to correlate the sonographic findings with a pregnancy test. In addition, it is extremely important for the sonologist to be aware of the type and relative sensitivity of the pregnancy test that is used.

The recently developed enzyme-linked immunoassay (ELISA) β-hCG urine pregnancy tests are a dramatic improvement over the sensitivity of non-qualitative tests generally available as office tests. The β-hCG assay is accurate in determining the presence or absence of pregnancy. However, the blood β-hCG assay that detects a quantitated level is most helpful in those cases in which diagnosis of early intrauterine or ectopic pregnancy, or its viability, is in question. Serial quantitated β-hCGs are therefore indicated in some cases and enhance accuracy by allowing specific correlation of certain sonographic landmarks (such as detection of embryo/yolk sac and size of gestational sac) to a particular level of β-hCG.

The RIA for serum beta subunit of human chorionic gonadotropin (β-hCG) is now widely available, and allows the diagnosis of pregnancy as early as 10 days after conception ($3\frac{1}{2}$ weeks' menstrual age). The development of monoclonal antibodies and the ELISA has also allowed the urine pregnancy tests to improve markedly. These newer urine tests assay for the whole hCG molecule and are exquisitely sensitive and specific, routinely detecting a normal pregnancy about 8 to 14 days after conception or $3\frac{1}{2}$ weeks after the last menstrual period.

The newer ELISA urine tests also markedly improve our ability to detect the presence of hCG in patients with an ectopic pregnancy.[13] The older agglutination inhibition assays are relatively insensitive and nonspecific, with negative results in over half of the patients with an ectopic pregnancy.[14] This is due mainly to the decreased amount

TABLE 5-1. TV US AND EMBRYOLOGIC MILESTONES

Menstrual Week	Chorionic Sac Mean Dimension (mm)[a]	Embryo Length (mm)[a]	Mean β-hCG mIU/mL[b,c]
4	inner: 1.5 outer: 2.8	.5	28
5	8–15	1.5–3	300
6	15–40	4–8	3,000
7	40–100	9–16	50,000

[a] Data from Davies J. *Hum Dev Anat.* New York, NY: Ronald Press; 1962.
[b] Data from Cartwright P. *Obstet Gynecol.* 1984.
[c] Second International Standard.[13]

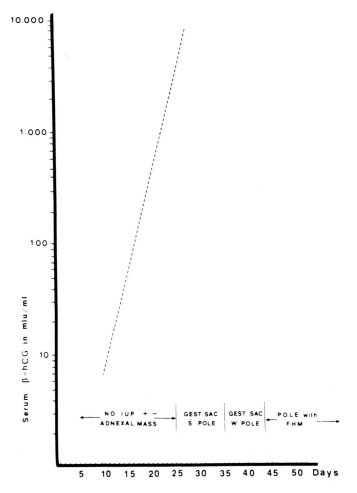

Fig. 5-1. β-hCG and TA US milestones.[13]

of hCG elaborated by most ectopic gestations.[13,14] Conversely, the newer ELISA urine tests are positive in about 99% of patients with a symptomatic ectopic gestation and may be easily performed within a few minutes. These tests, however, are only qualitative. The serum β-hCG RIA is exquisitely sensitive and offers a means to quantitate the patient's level of β-hCG. This assay is also highly specific and does not cross-react with luteinizing hormone or other nonspecific proteins.

Recently, there has been much controversy and confusion regarding comparison of β-hCG assays that use different standards. Whereas most centers use an assay compared to the Second International Standard, some use the International Reference Preparation which is reported in values approximately double that of the Second International Standard. It is important, therefore, for the obstetrician and sonologist to be aware of these differences and to be familiar with the particular assay their institutions use.

The ability to quantitate serum levels of β-hCG allows the clinician to estimate the gestational age of a pregnancy, assuming it is normal. The β-hCG value can then be correlated with the presence or absence of certain sonographically apparent developmental "milestones" (Table 5-1). Transabdominal and transvaginal sonographic features that are expected at the various β-hCG levels are summarized in Figure 5-1. Correlating the serum level of β-hCG with sonographic findings enables the clinician to evaluate the normalcy of the pregnancy in question.

A "discriminatory" hCG zone has been defined for discerning normal (viable) intrauterine pregnancies from ectopic pregnancies by means of TA US.[15,16] This zone lies between 1,800 and 3,600 mIU/mL of the Second International Standard or 3,600 and 6,500 mIU/mL of the International Reference Preparation (about twice the Second International Standard). The absence of an intrauterine gestational sac in conjunction with an hCG value above this discriminatory level signifies the pres-

ence of ectopic pregnancy in the majority of cases. The absence of an intrauterine gestational sac associated with hCG value below the discriminatory zone can either be associated with an early intrauterine pregnancy or an ectopic pregnancy. It has, therefore, been suggested that, if the initial sonographic features cannot distinguish between an intrauterine and extrauterine pregnancy, the sonographic examination should be repeated when the value would be expected to be 3,600 mIU/mL. For example, if a nondiagnostic sonogram is obtained in a patient whose beta subunit assay is 2,000 mIU/mL, repeat examination in two days should be able to discriminate between an intrauterine and ectopic pregnancy because at that time an intrauterine pregnancy should exhibit a well-defined gestational sac.

The amount of β-hCG produced with an ectopic pregnancy is usually less than with a viable intrauterine pregnancy of the same gestational age.[13] This may be the result of less extensive trophoblastic proliferation in ec-

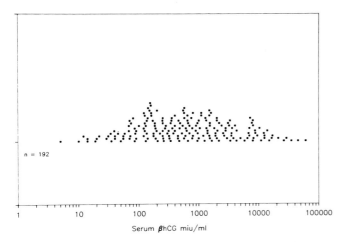

Fig. 5–2. β-hCG at time of presentation in 192 surgically proven ectopic pregnancies.[13]

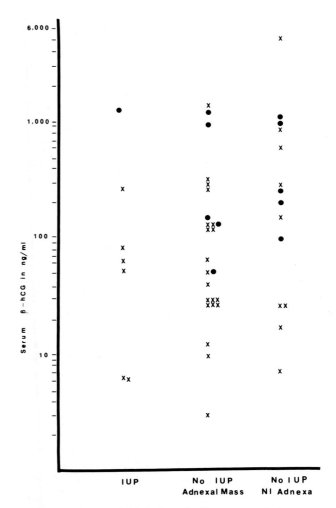

Fig. 5–4. β-hCG, US (TA) findings in 46 proven ectopic pregnancies.[13]

topic pregnancy, or of a difference in implantation in the tube and endometrium. This fact is useful, however, only if the date of conception is known. The serum β-hCG level for 192 women with a proven ectopic pregnancy at the time of their initial clinical presentation is shown in Figure 5–2. It is clear that an accurate assay, sensitive to 5 mIU/mL of the Second International Standard, must be used. The majority of these patients presented with serum β-hCG level below the discriminatory zone.

The level of serum β-hCG tends to be proportional to the size of a tubal pregnancy (Fig. 5–3). Ruptured tubal pregnancies tend to be associated with a higher level than unruptured. The range of serum β-hCG levels for any given situation is so broad, however, that this observation is of little clinical relevance.

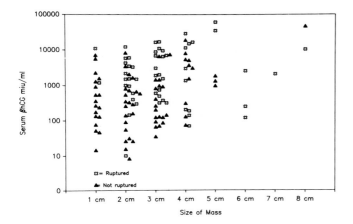

Fig. 5–3. β-hCG versus size of mass.

Figure 5–4 presents data collected at our institution with TA US, and correlates sonographic findings with serum β-hCG levels for 46 patients with ectopic pregnancies.[13] It has been observed that patients with levels above the discriminatory zone had an "empty" uterus (no decidual changes) by sonographic scanning, whereas six patients had pseudogestational sacs and levels below this zone.

In our experience and that of others, a normal gestational sac can only rarely be discerned by TA US when hCG levels are below 1,800 mIU/mL.[16] At this point, the lack of uterine changes makes an early intrauterine pregnancy look like an ectopic pregnancy. The presence of an adnexal mass in a patient with a β-hCG of less than 2,000 mIU/mL (even with fluid in the cul-de-sac) is still compatible with a viable intrauterine pregnancy and a hemorrhagic corpus luteum. Using a transvaginal probe, a normal intrauterine gestational sac is often visualized when serum levels are about 800 mIU/mL of the Second International Standard.[17,26] Although knowledge of the hCG level at the time of sonographic evaluation is likely to help distinguish a pseudogestational sac from a viable gestation, most patients still present with serum hCG levels so low that a normal gestation would not be seen by sonography. In this case, waiting to repeat sonography in one week may delay the diagnosis. One might postulate that rupture could occur in this interim. However, most pseudogestational sacs associated with ectopic pregnancy are smaller and more irregular than those expected for an intrauterine pregnancy at a particular stage.

Serial determinations of β-hCG levels have proven useful for patients in whom sonographic findings are non-diagnostic. Figure 5–5 shows the β-hCG progression in 25 clinically stable patients with ectopic gestation.[13] The first known value is arbitrarily placed on the standard line, and subsequent values plotted accordingly. It is apparent that most patients had levels that plateaued or fell during the period of preoperative evaluation. This plateau or fall is diagnostic of nonviability if it occurs while levels are below 3,000 mIU/mL, and after at least 48 hours. It does not distinguish the nonviable intra-uterine gestation from the ectopic, but it does allow one to make appropriate management decisions. It is also apparent from Figure 5–5 that some ectopic pregnancies produce early rises in β-hCG levels that are identical to normal gestations. This rise quickly falls off, however, and is found only while β-hCG levels are low and the pregnancy is very early. By plotting serial β-hCG values on the standard line, one can evaluate gestational viability while levels are below the discriminatory zone without knowing the menstrual history or calculating doubling times. Patients showing a plateau or fall while levels are 3,000 mIU/mL or less have a nonviable gestation and intervention is warranted. Those having an abnormal rise, but no plateau or fall, may still have a viable gestation.

SONOGRAPHIC EVALUATION

The use of TV US has greatly enhanced the sonographic evaluation of patients with suspected ectopic pregnancy.[18,26] In particular, the presence or absence of an intrauterine gestation can be documented or excluded at an earlier stage (approximately 1 week earlier) than with transabdominal sonography. In addition, adnexal masses and reliable collections of intraperitoneal fluid created by ectopic pregnancies can more frequently be detected by transvaginal sonography. The use of trans-abdominal and transvaginal sonography with highly sen-

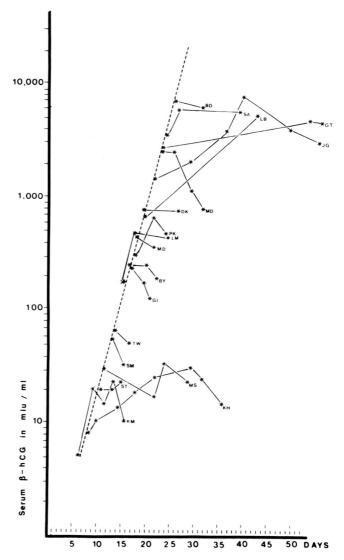

Fig. 5–5. Serial β-hCG in 19 clinically stable patients.[13]

sitive pregnancy tests has markedly enhanced the ability to detect ectopic pregnancies over techniques and tests available in the recent past. A very high degree of ac-curacy now exists in ability to establish the presence or exclude the possibility of ectopic pregnancy.[19,26]

Transvaginal sonography plays a major role in eval-uation of patients with suspected ectopic pregnancy. Most importantly, vaginal transducer/probes allow ac-curate and definitive inclusion or exclusion of an intra-uterine pregnancy by demonstration of an intrauterine gestational sac. Secondly, TV US can be used to dem-onstrate an extrauterine gestational sac, corpus luteum, or both. Transabdominal sonography can be used to eval-uate these parameters but is, in general, less accurate or definitive. Since the field-of-view of TV US is limited,

TA US can be helpful in identification of intraperitoneal fluid associated with ectopic pregnancy hemorrhage, rupture, or both.

SCANNING TECHNIQUE

On both TA US and TV US, sonographic examinations should begin by delineation of the uterus in its long axis. One should carefully evaluate the endometrial interfaces for the presence or absence of a gestational sac or decidual thickening. Once the uterus is adequately evaluated, the adnexal region should be carefully examined. If possible, both ovaries should be identified since some ectopic pregnancies are associated with coexisting corpus luteum. On a transverse transvaginal scan, the relative position of the proximal segment of tube can be approximated by recognition of several anatomic landmarks. These include delineation of the round ligament as it courses directly anterior to the tube near the uterine fundus, and location of the interstitial portion of the tube by its proximity to the endometrium (which invaginates into the uterine outline on a transverse scan).

SONOGRAPHIC FINDINGS

The sonographic findings that are encountered in a patient with ectopic pregnancy vary according to the stage of pregnancy in which the patient is examined, and whether or not rupture has occurred. In addition, they depend on what type of transducer/probe is used. The following discussion is organized into uterine, adnexal, and peritoneal sonographic findings.

Uterine

In most ectopic pregnancies, the uterus demonstrates a thickened endometrial interface due to the decidualization of the endometrium (Fig. 5–6). Particularly with TV scans, the increased fluid content of the decidualized endometrium can be appreciated due to enhanced through-transmission distal to this layer. In more advanced ectopic pregnancies, fluid or blood may be present within the decidualized endometrium simulating the appearance of an early gestational sac. In some cases, prior to sloughing of the decidua, a hypoechoic interface beneath the decidua can be seen that represents hemorrhage between the necrotic decidua and inner myometrium. In contradistinction to normal intrauterine pregnancies, where the gestational sac is spherical and well-defined, the pseudogestational sac created by sloughing decidua and found in some advanced ectopic pregnancies is more irregular and angulated. For a more detailed discussion of the sonographic changes that occur within the uterus in early intrauterine pregnancy refer to Chapter 41.

Adnexal

Typically, ectopic pregnancies occur as rounded masses, varying from 1 cm to 3 cm in size, which are located in the parauterine region. Masses that result from an ectopic pregnancy typically consist of a central hypoechoic area surrounded by an echogenic rim of trophoblastic tissue and muscle layer. An embryo can rarely be identified within the gestational sac of an ectopic pregnancy; a yolk sac may occasionally be present. In general, a corpus luteum appears as a hypoechoic structure surrounded by a rim of ovarian tissue. Usually, the corpus luteum is more centrally located within the ovarian structure than the more concentric halo representing the rim of trophoblastic tissue and muscle of an ectopic pregnancy.

Transvaginal sonography is particularly helpful in identification of adnexal masses resulting from ectopic gestations (Fig. 5–7). In our study, TV US was able to identify adnexal masses in the 1- to 3-cm range that had β-hCGs between 800 and 1,000 mIU/mL.[26]

Peritoneal

Along with evaluation of the uterus and adnexa, sonography can detect intraperitoneal fluid that may be associated with hemorrhage, rupture, or both of an ectopic pregnancy (Fig. 5–8). The presence of intraperitoneal fluid does not always correlate with the presence of rupture as there may be hemorrhage out of the fimbriated ends of tubes in patients with unruptured ectopic pregnancies. Large amounts of intraperitoneal fluid, such as that seen when this fluid extends into the hepatorenal pouch, is usually associated with rupture of ectopic pregnancy.

RARE TYPES OF ECTOPIC PREGNANCY

Although the majority of ectopic pregnancies (95%) occurs within the tube, there are some rare types that can occur within the uterine cornu, cervix, ovary, and peritoneal (abdominal) spaces (Fig. 5–9). Rarely, a patient can present after tubal rupture with a chronic ectopic pregnancy.

Transvaginal sonography is helpful in diagnosing interstitial ectopic pregnancies. One should be aware that the normal intrauterine pregnancy may have a very eccentrically located gestational sac early in development (at approximately 5 to 7 weeks). However, in interstitial ectopic pregnancies, the gestational sac can be identified outside the decidualized endometrium. It may sometimes be difficult to distinguish a cornual ectopic pregnancy that is very eccentrically located within the uterus from one located within the isthmic portion of the tube.

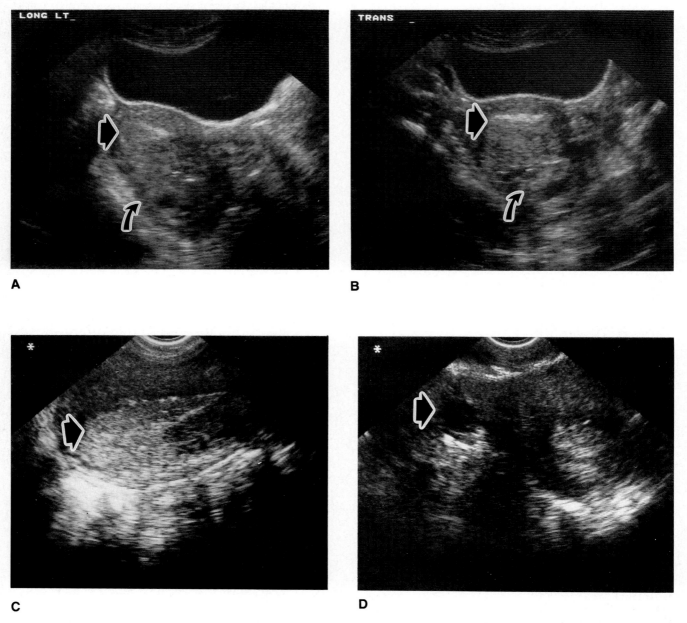

Fig. 5–6. Ectopic pregnancy: uterine US findings. **A.** Longitudinal TA sonogram of unruptured ectopic pregnancy appearing as a complex retrouterine mass posterior to uterus (*curved arrow*). Uterus contains thickened, decidualized endometrium (*arrow*). **B.** Transverse TA US of *A* showing thickened endometrium (*arrow*) and left adnexal ectopic gestation (*curved arrow*). **C.** TV US of unruptured ectopic pregnancy. Long axis of uterus shows thickened decidualized endometrium (*arrow*). **D.** Semiaxial TV US of *C* showing right adnexal mass (*arrow*), which represents an unruptured ectopic pregnancy. A yolk sac is present within gestational sac. (*Figure continued.*)

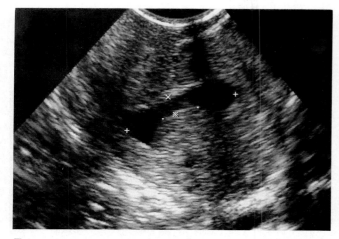

E

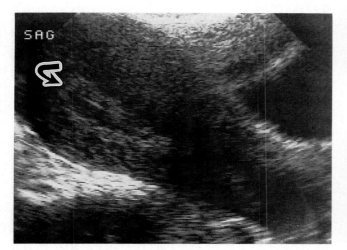

G

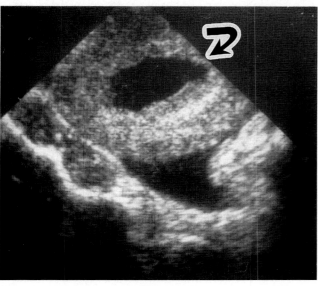

I

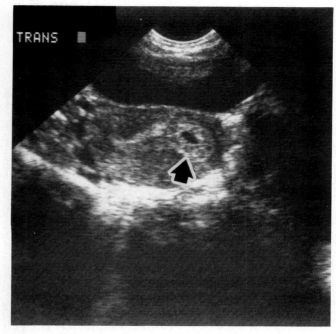

F

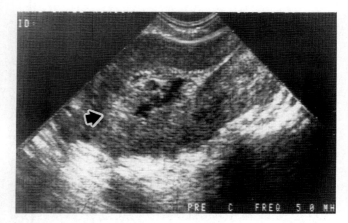

H

Fig. 5–6 (*continued*). E. TV US of pseudogestational sac in patient with proven ectopic pregnancy. The irregular sac (between +s) was mistaken for deformed intrauterine sac. **F.** Transverse TA US of a 6-week intrauterine pregnancy showing typically eccentric location of gestational sac (*arrow*) within uterine lumen. **G.** TA US showing irregularly thickened decidualized endometrium (*curved arrow*). **H.** TV US of patient in **G,** more clearly showing irregular decidualized endometrium (*arrow*) of proven ectopic pregnancy. **I.** TV US of decidual cast (*curved arrow*) with blood-distended uterine lumen. Intraperitoneal fluid was also present in cul-de-sac.

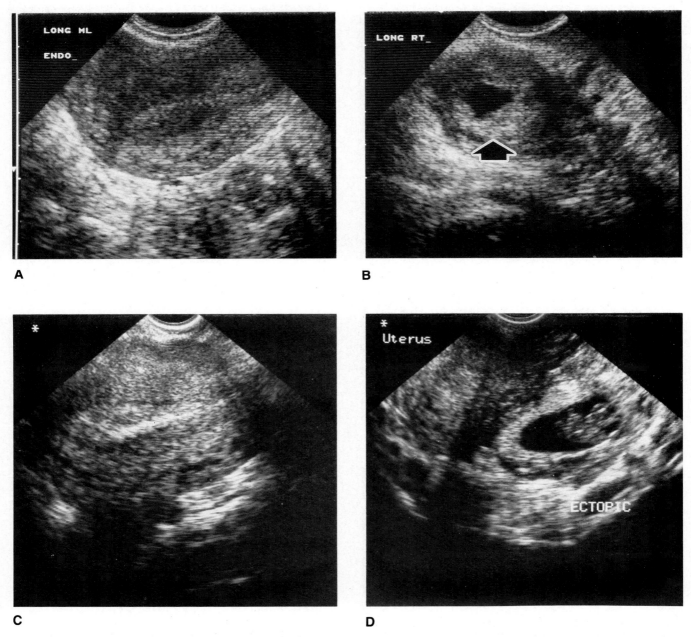

A

B

C

D

Fig. 5–7. Ectopic pregnancy: adnexal findings. **A.** TV sonogram showing lack of gestational sac within uterus. **B.** TV US of patient in **A,** showing distended tube containing irregular gestational sac (*arrow*). **C.** TV sonogram of uterus in long axis and **D.** left adnexa in advanced (8-week) unruptured ectopic pregnancy. Fetus demonstrated heart activity. (*Figure continued.*)

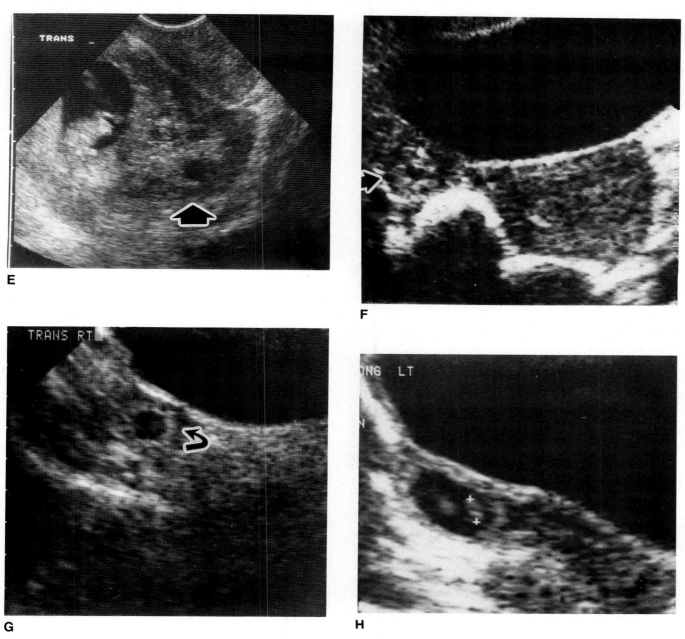

Fig. 5–7 (*continued*). Adnexal findings. **E.** TV sonogram of advanced (9-week) ruptured ectopic pregnancy. There is clotted blood (*arrow*) within cul-de-sac adjacent to ectopic gestation secondary to rupture of this ectopic pregnancy. Pregnancy had intraluminal fluid as depicted in **E. F.** Magnified transverse TA US of unruptured right-tubal pregnancy (*arrow*). (*Courtesy of Gary Thieme, MD.*) **G.** Transverse TA US of ectopic gestation with embryo within sac (*arrow*). **H.** Magnified longitudinal TA US of 7-week ectopic pregnancy showing embryo (between +s). (*Courtesy of Philippe Jeanty, MD, PhD.*) (*Figure continued.*)

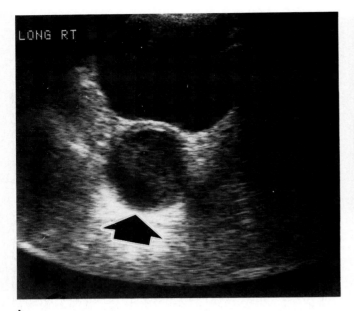

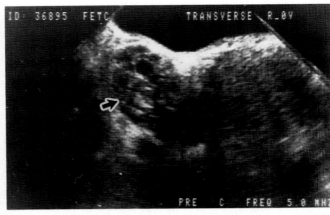

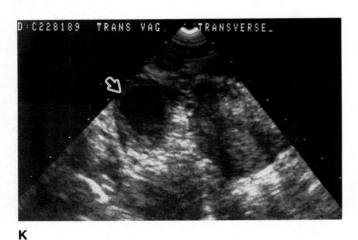

Fig. 5–7 (continued). Adnexal findings. **I.** TA US of hematosalpinx (*arrow*) secondary to ruptured ectopic pregnancy. **J.** TV US of hematosalpinx (*arrow*) secondary to ruptured ectopic pregnancy. **K.** TV US of hemorrhagic corpus luteum (*arrow*) that simulated an ovarian ectopic pregnancy.

Another condition that can be confused with an interstitial ectopic pregnancy is an early intrauterine pregnancy in a bicornuate uterus. Transvaginal sonography is particularly helpful in establishing the presence of two endometrial lumina in patients with a bicornuate uterus.

Cervical ectopic pregnancies appear as gestational sacs that are abnormally low within the uterus. These can be mimicked by nonviable pregnancies that are in the process of aborting.

Abdominal pregnancies result from abortion or tubal rupture with subsequent fixation of the decidua onto bowel, omentum, or mesentery. These types of ectopic pregnancy may be difficult to recognize because the uterine wall surrounding some intrauterine pregnancies is so thin. Clues to this disorder include abnormal fetal lie, oligohydramnios, and intraperitoneal fluid. To confirm an intra-abdominal pregnancy, one should endeavor to delineate the uterus as a separate structure from the fetus and placenta. In some cases, magnetic resonance imaging can be useful in assessing whether or not the pregnancy is within the uterus by demonstrating its relationship to the cervix and myometrium of the uterus.

Chronic ectopic pregnancies result from rupture of the tube with subsequent hematoma formation. The hematoma may also incite an inflammatory reaction with development of adhesions. These masses typically appear as rounded solid structures. They can be surrounded by a hydrosalpinx or pyosalpinx. In some cases of chronic ectopic pregnancy, the trophoblasts will be necrotic and the β-hCG low or absent.

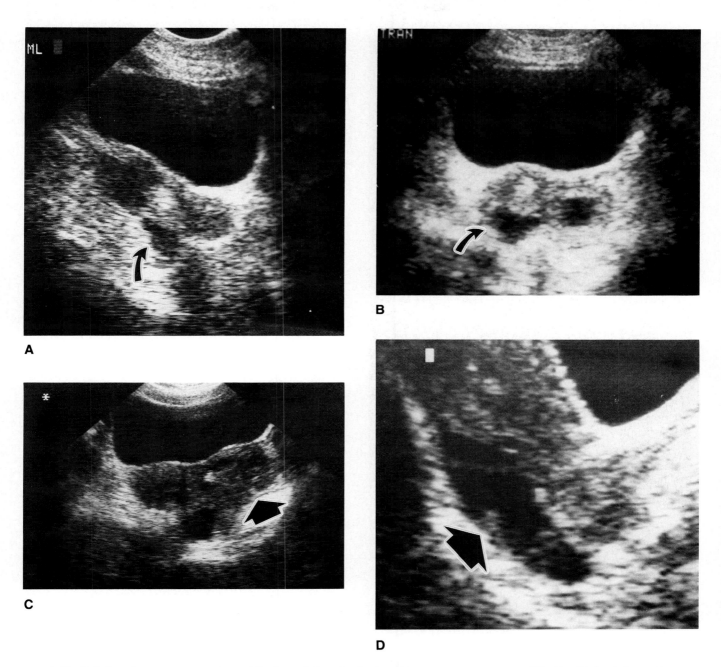

Fig. 5–8. Ectopic pregnancy: peritoneal findings. **A.** Longitudinal and **B.** transverse sonogram of "leaking" left tubal ectopic pregnancy with unclotted cul-de-sac hemorrhage (*curved arrow*). **C.** Transverse TA US of clotted hemorrhage secondary to chronic ruptured ectopic pregnancy. Transverse TA US of intraperitoneal hemorrhage associated with ruptured abdominal pregnancy. **D.** Magnified longitudinal TA US showing partially clotted cul-de-sac hemorrhage (*arrow*) secondary to ruptured ectopic pregnancy. (*Figure continued.*)

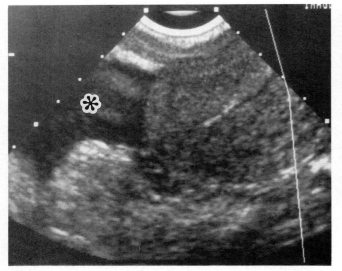

E

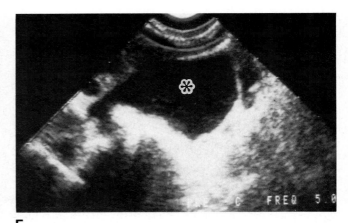

F

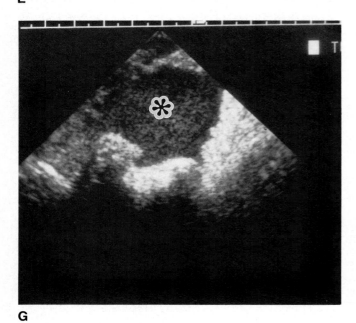

G

Fig. 5–8 (continued). Peritoneal findings. **E.** TV US long axis showing clotted blood (∗) superior to fundus. **F.** TV US showing intraperitoneal free blood (∗). Low-level echoes were within this partially clotted blood collection in cul-de-sac. **G.** TV US of free blood (∗) in cul-de-sac secondary to ruptured ectopic pregnancy. TA US low-level echoes probably were from clotted portions of intraperitoneal blood collection.

Although sonographic documentation of an intrauterine pregnancy virtually excludes the possibility of an ectopic pregnancy, one should not totally disregard the possibility of the latter, particularly in a patient who has undergone ovulation induction.[20] The incidence of combined intrauterine and extrauterine pregnancy is low and has been reported to be between 1 in 2,000 to 1 in 30,000 deliveries.[21]

Ectopic pregnancy can coexist with other adnexal masses. For example, we have examined patients in whom an ectopic pregnancy was found coexisting with a dermoid cyst, ovarian cystadenoma, and fibroids.

Whether or not the presence of these masses contributed to the chance of developing an ectopic pregnancy is only speculative. However, the presence of these masses may alter the angle and course of the tube.

OTHER ADNEXAL MASSES

Transvaginal sonography is particularly helpful in distinguishing corpus luteum that occurs within the ovary from ectopic pregnancies (Fig. 5–10). In general, a corpus luteum appears as a hypoechoic area within the ovary.

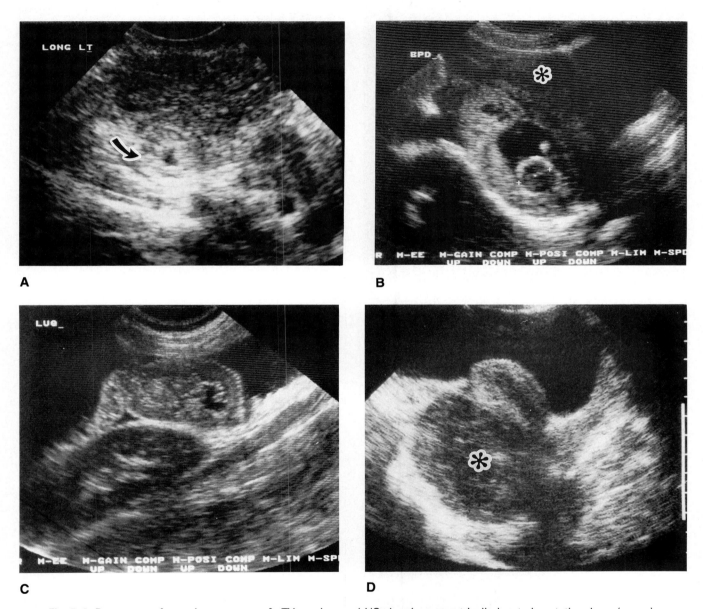

Fig. 5–9. Rare types of ectopic pregnancy. **A.** TV semicoronal US showing eccentrically located gestational sac (*arrow*) that was found at surgery to represent cornual ectopic pregnancy. **B.** Longitudinal TA US showing 12-week fetus outside uterus (∗). **C.** Same patient as B, showing large amount of intraperitoneal fluid surrounding bowel in this ruptured abdominal ectopic pregnancy. **D.** Longitudinal TA US showing solid retrouterine mass (∗) that represented chronic ectopic pregnancy. The β-hCG was negative. (*Figure continued.*)

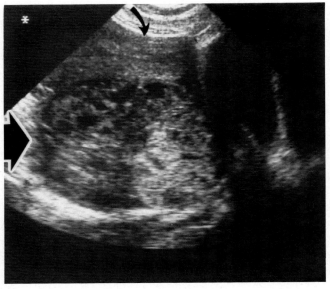

E

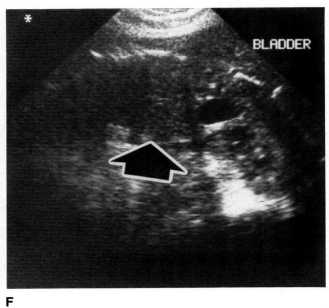

F

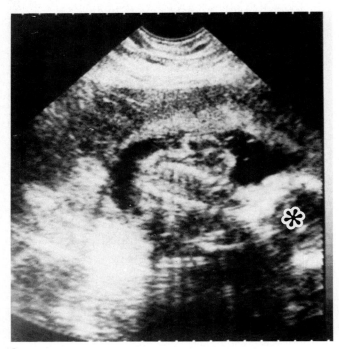

G

Fig. 5–9 (*continued*). Rare types of ectopic pregnancy. **E.** Longitudinal TA US showing hydropic placenta (*big arrow*) posterior to non-gravid uterus (*curved arrow*). **F.** Fetus in **E** was in right upper quadrant. **G.** Transverse TA US of 24-week fetus found to be surrounded by ovarian tissue. Fetal head (∗) and cervical spine are shown. (*Figure continued.*)

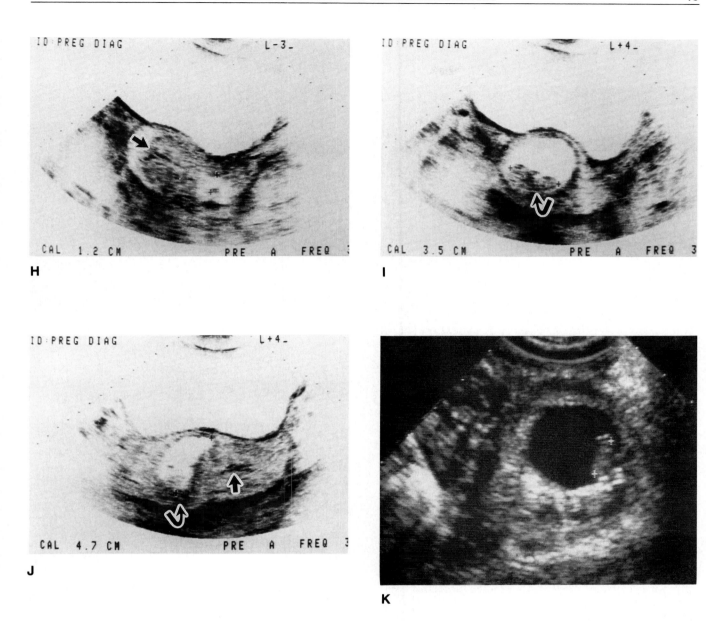

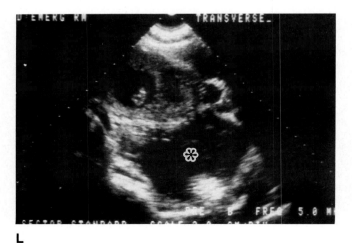

Fig. 5–9 (continued). Rare types of ectopic pregnancy. **H.** and **I.** Longitudinal and transverse; **J.** TA US (black-on-white format) showing an interstitial ectopic pregnancy at 8 weeks. The endometrial lumen (*straight arrow*) is nondistended by the interstitial ectopic gestational sac (*curved arrow*). (*Courtesy of Grady Stewart, MD.*) **K.** TV US of left ovarian ectopic pregnancy. An embryo can be identified within the left ovary. **L.** Transverse TA US of IUP and ruptured ectopic pregnancy appearing as localized collection of blood in cul-de-sac (∗).

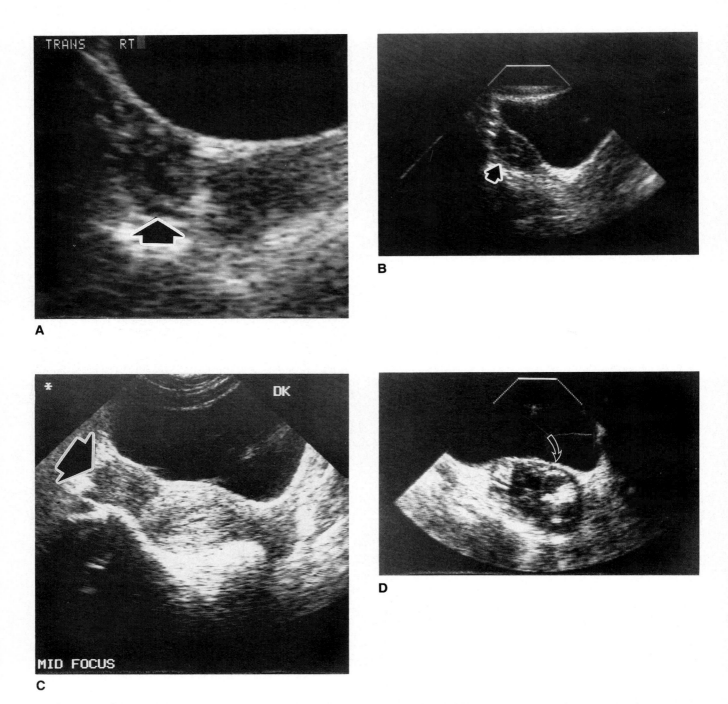

Fig. 5–10. Other adnexal masses and conditions. **A.** Magnified transverse TA US of corpus luteum (*arrow*) within right ovary having similar appearance to ectopic pregnancy. Hypoechoic center is surrounded by echogenic rim of tissue. **B.** Longitudinal TA US of group of endometriomas (*arrow*) that appear similar to ectopic pregnancy. **C.** Longitudinal TA US of pedunculated fibroid (*arrow*) adjacent to uterine fundus, simulating appearance of ectopic pregnancy. Patient's pregnancy test was positive even though intrauterine gestation could not be depicted with TA US. **D.** Transverse TA sonogram of patient with unruptured ectopic pregnancy adjacent to dermoid cyst. (*Figure continued.*)

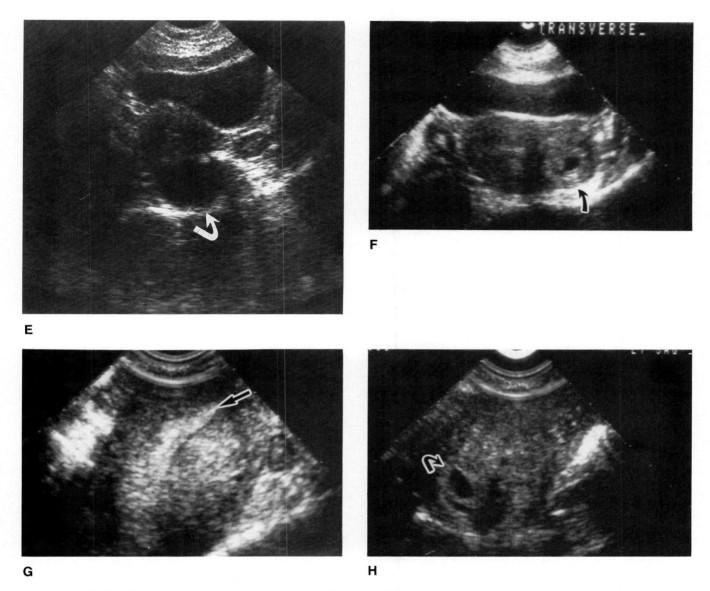

Fig. 5–10 (continued). Other adnexal masses and conditions. **E.** Transverse TA sonogram of patient with cystic adnexal mass and positive pregnancy test. At surgery, ectopic pregnancy was found next to a cystadenoma of left ovary. **F.** Transverse TA sonogram showing eccentrically located gestational sac (*curved arrow*). **G.** TV sonogram showing thickened endometrium (*arrow*) of nongravid horn of a bicornuate uterus. **H.** Left horn contained gestational sac (*curved arrow*).

Corpora lutea typically tend to be eccentrically located within the ovary, although this is not an absolute criterion for their recognition. A hydrosalpinx can be differentiated from an ectopic pregnancy by delineation of its shape and orientation. It may be difficult in some cases of tubo-ovarian abscess and ectopic pregnancy to determine which mass actually represents the ectopic pregnancy.

MEDICO-LEGAL CONSIDERATIONS

For medico-legal purposes, the sonologist should be aware that in up to 20% of proven ectopic pregnancies the sonographic appearance of uterus and adnexa were normal with TA US.[22] It therefore may be advisable in some cases where sonographic findings are inconclusive to incorporate a statement in the official report such as the following: "Although the possibility of an ectopic pregnancy is unlikely, it cannot be totally excluded."[23]

SUMMARY

In conclusion, it is believed that the use of TA US, TV US, or both, with sensitive pregnancy tests can result in a high degree of accuracy in the detection or exclusion of an extrauterine pregnancy. In most cases, it is important to correlate sonographic findings with the β-hCG level. With TV US, most normal intrauterine pregnancies will demonstrate a gestational sac at a level of 800 to 1,000 mIU/mL (Second International Standard).[17] In other words, if an intrauterine gestational sac cannot be identified when the β-hCG is above this value, an ectopic pregnancy should be considered.[26] It is anticipated that earlier diagnosis of ectopic pregnancy will result in better clinical outcome because it may improve the chance for successful surgical treatment.

REFERENCES

1. Weckstein LN, Boucher AR, Tucker H, Gibson D, Rettenmaier MA. Accurate diagnosis of early ectopic pregnancy. *Obstet Gynecol.* 1985;65:393–397.
2. Laing F. Ectopic pregnancy. In: Ferrucci J, ed. *Diagnostic Imaging.* Philadelphia: Lippincott; 1988:1.
3. Tancer M, Delke L, Veridiano N. A fifteen year experience with ectopic pregnancy. *Surg Gynecol Obstet.* 1981;152:179.
4. Breen J. A 21-year survey of 654 ectopic pregnancies. *Am J Obstet Gynecol.* 1970;106:1004.
5. Shiono P, Harlap S, Pellegrin F. Ectopic pregnancies: Rising incidence rates in Northern California. *Am J Public Health.* 1982;72:173.
6. Rubin G, Peterson H, Dorfman S, et al. Ectopic pregnancy in the United States 1970 through 1978. *JAMA.* 1983;249:1725.
7. Laing F, Jeffrey R. Ultrasound evaluation of ectopic pregnancy. *Radiol Clin North Am.* 1982;20:383.
8. Kleiner G, Roberts T. Current factors and causation of tubal pregnancy: A prospective clinical pathologic study. *Am J Obstet Gynecol.* 1967;99:21.
9. Ackerman R, Deutsch S, Krumholtz B. Levels of human chorionic gonadotropin in unruptured and ruptured ectopic pregnancy. *Obstet Gynecol.* 1982;60:13.
10. Cartwright P, Vaughn W, Tuttle D. Culdocentesis and ectopic pregnancy. *J Reprod Med.* 1984;29:88.
11. Bedi DG, Fagan CJ, Nocera RM. Chronic ectopic pregnancy. *J Ultrasound Med.* 1984;3:347–352.
12. Stanley R, Horger J, Fagan C, Andriole J, Fleischer A. Sonographic findings in abdominal pregnancies. *AJR.* 1986;147:1043.
13. Cartwright P, DiPietro D. Ectopic pregnancy: Change in serum hCG concentrations. *Obstet Gynecol.* 1984;63:76.
14. Schwartz R, DiPietro D. Beta hCG is a diagnostic aid for suspected ectopic pregnancy. *Obstet Gynecol.* 1980; 56:197.
15. Kadar N, DeVore G, Romero R. Discriminatory hCG zone: Its use in sonographic evaluation for ectopic pregnancy. *Obstet Gynecol.* 1981;58:156.
16. Nyberg DA, Filly RA, Laing FC, Mack LA, Zarutskie PW. Ectopic pregnancy: Diagnosis by sonography correlated with quantitative hCG levels. *J Ultrasound Med.* 1987;6:145–150.
17. Rottem S, Timor-Tritsch IE. Think ectopic. In: Timor-Tritsch IE, Rottem S, eds. *Transvaginal Sonography.* New York: Elsevier; 1988:125–141.
18. Nyberg DA, Mack LA, Jeffrey RB, Laing FC. Endovaginal sonographic evaluation of ectopic pregnancy: A prospective study. *AJR.* 1987;149:1181–1186.
19. Filly RA. Ectopic pregnancy: The role of sonography. *Radiology.* 1987;162:661–668.
20. Yaghoobian J, Pinck RL, Ramanathan K, Ibarra J. Sonographic demonstration of simultaneous intrauterine and extrauterine gestation. *J Ultrasound Med.* 1986;5:309–312.
21. Hann LE, Bachmann DL, McArdle CR. Coexistent intrauterine and ectopic pregnancy: A reevaluation. *Radiology.* 1984;152:151.
22. Mahony BS, Filly RA, Nyberg DA, et al. Sonographic evaluation of ectopic pregnancy. *J Ultrasound Med.* 1985;4:221.
23. James AE Jr, Fleischer A, Sacks G, et al. Ectopic pregnancy: The paradigm of a sonographic "missed lesion." *Clinics in Diagnostic Ultrasound.* 1986;26:99.
24. Marchbanks PA, Annegers JF, Coulam CB, Strathy JH, Kurland LT. Risk factors for ectopic pregnancy: A population-based study. *JAMA.* 1988;259:1823–1827.
25. Taylor RN. Ectopic pregnancy and reproductive technology. *JAMA.* 1988;259:1862–1864.
26. Fleischer A, Herbert C, Hill G, Cartwright P, Sacks G, Jeanty P. Ectopic pregnancy: Features of transvaginal sonography. *Radiology.* 1990;174:375–378.

6 Sonographic Depiction of Normal Fetal Anatomy

Philippe Jeanty

To many, anatomy is a subject that brings back nightmares of medical school. It is probably one of the most difficult subjects to learn because it does not lend itself to simplification by reasoning and can only be memorized. This dislike probably still affects a large number of those who perform obstetrical ultrasound examinations; so it is likely that few readers will have rushed to this particular chapter after glancing at the book's table of contents.

Yet there are many reasons to learn more about anatomy as it relates to ultrasound. To be able to identify the correct planes of scanning was formerly one of the most important. Now, with an improved level of competence of those performing obstetric ultrasound examinations, this knowledge is more prevalent.

Most of all, it is vital to be able to distinguish normal structures from pathologic ones. Despite the fact that not everyone is willing to diagnose congenital malformations, one would not want to refer a patient for a high-resolution or level II scan to verify a finding that turns out to be a perfectly normal structure. Earlier, it was reported, for example, that fetal ears had been confused with encephalocele. Callen demonstrated that what was previously thought to represent artifactual ascites were actually abdominal muscles of the fetus. In intracranial anatomy, multiple errors were made; for example, the cavum septum pellucidum was confused with the third ventricle, the insula was confused with the Sylvian fissure, and some deep cerebral veins were confused with the roof of the lateral ventricle. Our understanding of sonographic findings has considerably increased over the years.

Among all the subjects that can be imaged by ultrasound, the fetus is by far the most challenging. Numerous tiny fetal structures can test whether or not the equipment is able to image small structures or differentiate them from adjacent ones by differences in echogenicity. When dealing with such small anatomical details a better understanding of the anatomy and fetal anatomy becomes necessary.

To allow the reader to compare the importance of anatomical knowledge to resolution in computerized sonography, we have elected to use some images provided by low- or medium-cost machines, as well as some by old and discontinued machines. Many of these machines provide outstanding resolution. As a general rule, the limiting factor in detection of anatomy and anomalies does not lie in the equipment but in the user's knowledge of anatomy, and his or her perception of what is normal and abnormal.

ANATOMY

Early Gestations

The most important advance in the high-resolution evaluation of the early fetus has come through more widespread use and improved resolution of transvaginal transducers. Fetal structures are easier to recognize, especially in obese patients (Fig. 6–1). See Chapter 4.

Head

Eyes. The different components of the eye that can be observed with ultrasound are the globe, including the vitreous body, the lens, and the anterior chamber. In early gestation, what probably corresponds to the interface of the conjunctival sac (Fig. 6–2) can also be seen. In the retro-orbital region, one can recognize the external (Fig. 6–3) and internal rectus muscle, as well as the superior oblique. The optic nerve (Fig. 6–4) and the ophthalmic artery are also discernible. An equatorial section obtained in a fetus facing toward the transducer best demonstrates these structures. The vitreous body, lens, and anterior chamber can be seen in most circumstances. The conjunctival sac is formed by closure of the eyelids in front of the globe at about the eighth week of menstrual age. It reopens at about the seventh month. The lateral (or external) rectus muscle is seen as a thin hypoechoic line, close to the orbital surface of the zygomatic bone (see Fig. 6–1). The latter appears brightly echogenic (due to acoustic enhancement behind the vitreous body) with distal shadowing. The internal (or medial) rectus muscle can be seen along the orbital plate of the ethmoid bone. When the plane of section is slightly asynclinal, one can image some of the other extraocular muscles. The easiest to demonstrate is the superior oblique muscle, which is slightly more medial and superior to the medial rectus

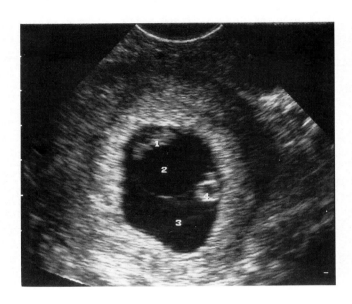

Fig. 6–1. The transvaginal approach allows extremely high resolution of the early gestational sac. This illustration demonstrates embryo (1) in the amniotic cavity (2). The yolk sac (4) is in the extraembryonic coelom (3). The membrane between amniotic cavity and extraembryonic coelom is the amnion. (*Reprinted with permission from Jeanty P, Daniel TL. Fetal anatomy in ultrasonography. In: Hobbins JC, Benacerraf BR, eds.* Clinics in Diagnostic Ultrasound, *25. New York: Churchill Livingstone; 1989.*)

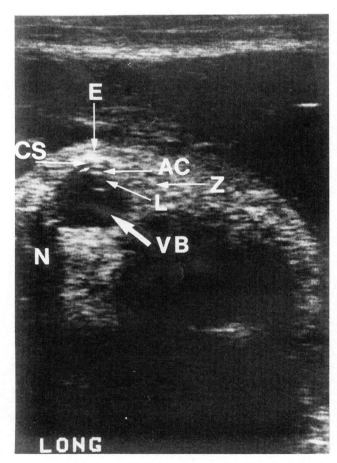

Fig. 6–2. Scan of fetal eye. The fetus is facing the top left of image and nose is at left border of image. One can recognize the vitreous body (VB) inside the globe, the lens between (L), anterior chamber between (AC), conjunctival sac between (CS), and the eyelid between (E). The zygomatic bone is at right side of orbit. (*Reprinted with permission from Jeanty P, Romero R, Hobbins JC. Fetal facial anatomy.* J Ultrasound Med. *1986;5:607.*)

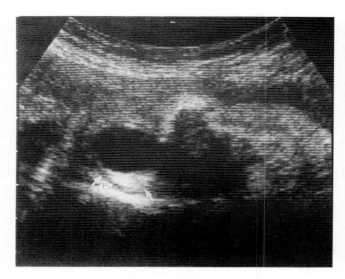

Fig. 6–3. The lateral rectus muscle (*arrow*) and also the superior rectus muscle directly behind the globe.

muscle. When the section is obtained high in the orbit, the complex of the superior rectus muscle and the levator palpebrae superioris is seen. Identification of the extraocular muscle is greatly facilitated by fetal eye movements. The pulling action of the muscles is then clearly differentiated from the passive "tail waving" movement of the optic nerve.

The optic nerve is easily recognized in the equatorial section (see Fig. 6–4), as a hypoechoic structure exiting the globe opposite to the lens. Its contours are more fuzzy than those of the muscles, and its medial course in the conus region helps distinguish it from muscle. The

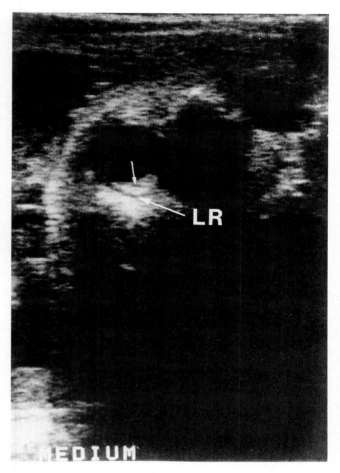

Fig. 6–5. Scan demonstrates lateral rectus muscle and also ophthalmic artery (*small arrow*). The ophthalmic artery has some better defined walls than the optic nerve or rectus muscle. (*Reprinted with permission from Jeanty P, Romero R, Hobbins JC. Vascular anatomy of the fetus. J Ultrasound Med. 1984;3:113.*)

pulsation of the ophthalmic artery can also be recognized (Fig. 6–5). The ophthalmic artery has a "rail" shape appearance (two bright echos surrounding a lucency), instead of the homogenous gray of the optic nerve and rectus muscles.

Ears. The helix, scaphoid fossa, triangular fossa, concha, antihelix, tragus, antitragus, intertragic incisure, and lobule can be seen (Fig. 6–6). The internal auditory canal, as well as the middle and inner ear, are concealed in the petrouse bone and its acoustic shadow.

Nose and Lips. The tip of the nose, the alae nasi, and the columna are seen above the upper lip (Fig. 6–7). The observation of the fetal nose would be of poor clinical interest if it were not for the diagnosis of cleft lip. In cleft lip, the nonunion of the maxillary process with the

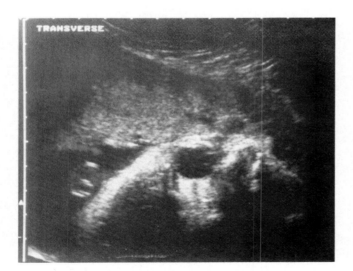

Fig. 6–4. Optic nerve originating at back of the eye.

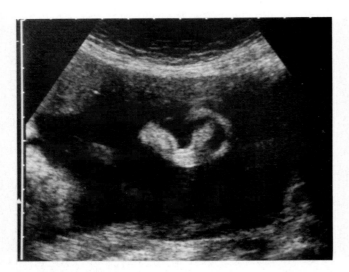

Fig. 6–6. Fetal ear. One can recognize the helix, scaphoid fossa, triangular fossa, concha, antihelix, tragus, antitragus, intertragic incisure, and the lobule. (*Reprinted with permission from Jeanty P, Daniel TL. Fetal anatomy in ultrasonography. In: Hobbins JC, Benacerraf BR, eds. Clinics in Diagnostic Ultrasound, 25. New York: Churchill Livingstone; 1989.*)

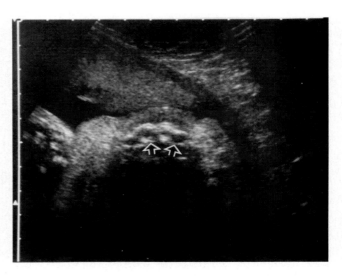

Fig. 6–8. Cheeks are visible on both sides of the upper teeth (*arrows*). (*Reprinted with permission from Jeanty P, Daniel TL. Fetal anatomy in ultrasonography. In: Hobbins JC, Benacerraf BR, eds. Clinics in Diagnostic Ultrasound, 25. New York: Churchill Livingstone; 1989.*)

fronto-nasal process leaves a groove that extends from the nostril to the mouth. Since cleft lip is a common malformation, and since the section demonstrating the nose and upper lip is easy to obtain, some degree of familiarity with the normal anatomy of the region is worthwhile knowing.

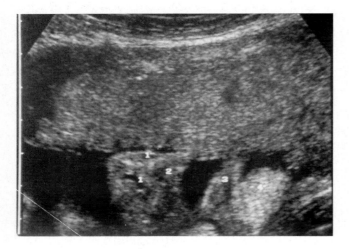

Fig. 6–7. Nose and lips. Tangential scan to the most anterior portion of the mouth demonstrates the tip of the nose on left portion of figure, two nostrils (1), upper lip (2), lower lip (3), and chin (4). (*Reprinted with permission from Jeanty P, Daniel TL. Fetal anatomy in ultrasonography. In: Hobbins JC, Benacerraf BR, eds. Clinics in Diagnostic Ultrasound, 25. New York: Churchill Livingstone; 1989.*)

Cheeks. In a transverse section of the cheek, one can recognize from medial to lateral the tongue, buccinator muscle, and Bichat's fat pad (the corpus adiposum buccae) (Fig. 6–8). More posteriorly, the ascending branch of the mandible is seen medial and anterior to the masseter muscle.

Teeth. The teeth bud is included in the dental sac, which is a rounded hypoechoic area (Fig. 6–9). The low echogenicity is probably due to the loose mesenchyma of the stellate reticulum which surrounds the dental papilla. The bright echo that surrounds the teeth buds probably corresponds to the interface between the stellate reticulum and the gum plus the adjacent interfaces produced by the gingival and glossal sulci. Teeth buds for the incisor, the canine, and the premolar are usually recognized. They start calcifying between the fourth and fifth gestational month. In a fetus with a cleft lip, the failure to recognize the upper row of teeth buds is suggestive of a concomitant cleft palate. More posteriorly, the jugular vein and the carotid artery are seen anterior and lateral to the cartilaginous portion of the vertebral body.

Tongue, Epiglottis, and Larynx. The tongue can be seen both during movements and at rest. The median sulcus is occasionally visible. At the root of the tongue, the epiglottis and the vestibulum of the larynx are seen (Fig. 6–10). The epiglottis is visible both in transverse scans of the base of the head and in coronal sections of the

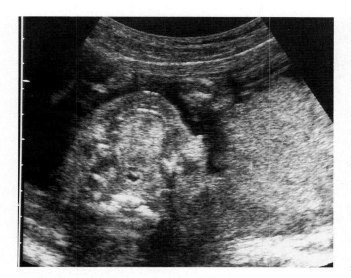

Fig. 6–9. The tongue in a coronal section of the mouth. (*Reprinted with permission from Jeanty P, Daniel TL. Fetal anatomy in ultrasonography. In: Hobbins JC, Benacerraf BR, eds.* Clinics in Diagnostic Ultrasound, *25. New York: Churchill Livingstone; 1989.*)

neck. The vestibulum of the larynx should not be confused with the foramen magnum, which is more posterior. In a coronal section of the neck, the vocal cords are seen slightly below the larynx in the trachea.

Intracranial Anatomy. Intracranial anatomy as imaged by ultrasound is now fairly well delineated. The anatomy varies between early gestation and late gestation. In early gestation, most of the intracranial structure is a large hypoechoic mass that is symmetrically located on either side of the midline. This echogenic mass represents the choroid plexus. The hypoechoic structure around this mass represents the cortical mantle and not the cerebral spinal fluid as previously thought. The hypoechoic temporal lobe is thought to be related to the relatively sparse myelination of the cervical cortex with fetuses up to 28 to 30 gestational weeks.

As growth progresses, the relative size of the choroid plexus is less important and cortical mantle is more visible. One can also observe the inward incurvation of the convexity and the level of the insula; both the frontal and occipital opercula can also be seen. In the second half of the gestation, in a typical scan one can observe the two sutures (the coronal and lambdoidal suture). At that time, one can recognize in the brain the cortical mantle and the lateral ventricle containing the choroid plexus, which is echogenic (Fig. 6–11). In the midline area one can see the cavum septum pellucidum (from the anterior aspect going to the back of the head), the two thalami, and in their midst the fourth ventricle. The posterior fossa demonstrates the lateral lobes of the cerebellum as well as the vermis. The cisterna magna is usually visible as a large hypoechoic space. while angling the transducer in the sagittal plane, one can observe the entrance of the spinal cord into the posterior fossa.

Spine

The vertebral body of the fetal spine is not completely ossified. There are typically three ossification centers that are recognizable by ultrasound. One is the ossification center of the vertical body and the other two are ossification centers of the posterior lamina. Identification of the latter two ossification centers has been quite important in the diagnosis of neural tube defects.

In a normal fetus, the three ossification centers should be at the corners of a triangle whose tip is pointing toward the center of the fetus. In fetuses with spina bifida, there will be some splitting between the two ossification centers of the posterior lamina, and their distance will be increased. Other findings, of course, will be the absence of skin covering the vertebrae over the defect and a bulging thin membrane representing the meninges. In a normal fetus, the vertebral body and posterior lamina ossification centers can be imaged in a plane in which they are aligned to resemble what has been nicknamed "the railroad tract image." In that type of image, the

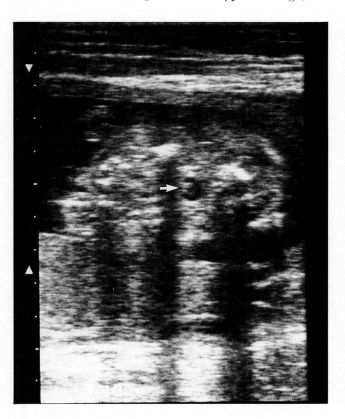

Fig. 6–10. Scan through the neck demonstrates larynx and epiglottis in its middle.

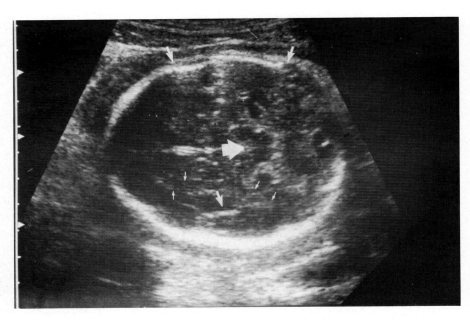

Fig. 6–11. In cranial anatomy: the thalami (*large arrow*), choroid plexus (*small arrow*), cortical mantle, insula (*medium arrow*), and sutures (*top arrows*).

external echoes are generated by the posterior lamina and the middle echoes are created by the vertebral ossification center. More important than the three lines is a section that demonstrates only two lines, which present the posterior lamina alone without the vertebral body ossification center. Often, when the vertebral body ossification center is included in the scan, the section is too anterior to correctly demonstrate a spinal defect.

One should be aware that an oblique section going through a posterior lamina and a vertebral body ossification center will also demonstrate a two-line image. That image is inadequate to distinguish spinal defects because it does not pass by the spinal defect. These two-line images are recognizable because on one side of the spine there is a small amount of fetal tissue whereas while on the other side of the spine (the side toward the vertebral body) there is a large amount of fetal tissue corresponding to the entire chest or abdomen of the fetus, depending on the level of the scan. Another congenital malformation that can be distinguished in the coronal section is the absence of a portion of vertebral body such as occurs in VATER assocation (with congenital scoliosis). This is discussed in the section on neural tube defect.

Neck

The common carotids are roughly parallel and slightly posterior to the trachea in the neck. The jugular vein can be seen lateral to the carotid artery. The carotids have sharply defined walls, and their pulsation can be recorded. The jugular veins are closer to the skin than the carotid and are larger. The trachea is recognizable by its larger diameter. The vertebral arteries can be demonstrated along the cervical spine. They can be dis-

tinguished from the carotids by their more posterior course (Figs. 6–12 and 6–13). The course of the vertebral artery in the vertebral canal can be seen because the canal is only cartilaginous (Fig. 6–14).

Chest

Rib Cage. The fetal ribs are easily identifiable. Very rarely, one can observe bifid ribs. The scapula is also visible, as is the clavicle.

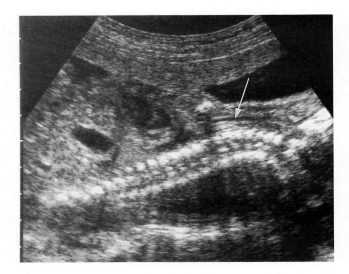

Fig. 6–12. Carotid artery (*arrow*) seen in the middle of the neck. (*Reprinted with permission from Jeanty P, Daniel TL. Fetal anatomy in ultrasonography. In: Hobbins JC, Benacerraf BR, eds. Clinics in Diagnostic Ultrasound, 25. New York: Churchill Livingstone; 1989.*)

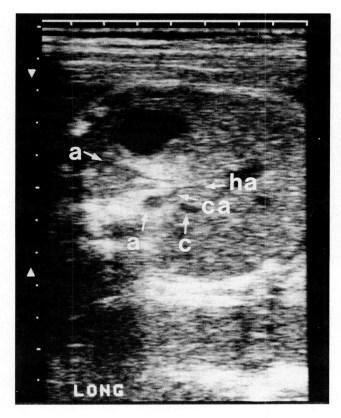

Fig. 6–24. Transverse section through the abdomen demonstrates stomach on the top portion of image and the spine at bottom left. In front of the spine, one can recognize the aorta and, to its right, the inferior vena cava (c). Originating from the aorta (a) is the celiac axis (ca). The hepatic artery going to the right side (ha) can be seen as well as the splenic artery (a) entering the spleen directly behind the stomach at the left side of image. (*Reprinted with permission from Jeanty P, Daniel TL. Fetal anatomy in ultrasonography. In: Hobbins JC, Benacerraf BR, eds.* Clinics in Diagnostic Ultrasound, *25. New York: Churchill Livingstone; 1989.*)

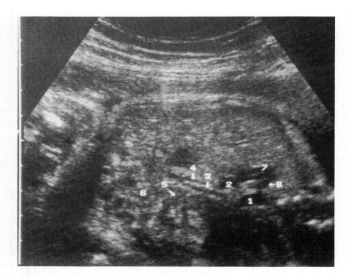

Fig. 6–25. Transverse and oblique section in the fetus demonstrates the origin of the superior mesenteric artery. The aorta (1) is in front of the vertebral body, which is on the right side of image. Above the aorta, one can recognize the vena cava (2) adjacent to the more medial portion of the right adrenal (7). Behind the adrenal one can see the crux of diaphragm (8). Coming out ouf the aorta, one can recognize the superior mesenteric artery (3). Alongside the superior mesenteric artery and to its right, and slightly larger, one can also observe the superior mesenteric vein. (5) shows smaller branches of division of the superior mesenteric artery. 6 represents bowel. (*Reprinted with permission from Jeanty P, Daniel TL. Fetal anatomy in ultrasonography. In: Hobbins JC, Benacerraf BR, eds.* Clinics in Diagnostic Ultrasound, *25. New York: Churchill Livingstone; 1989.*)

the liver and divides into the right and the left portal vein (Fig. 6–29). This division of the main portal vein is the landmark used to obtain the abdominal perimeter. The right portal vein divides into an anterior and a posterior branch. The left portal vein receives the umbilical portion of the umbilical vein.

Stomach. The stomach is visible on the left side of the abdomen. At the level of the stomach, the pylorus and duodenal bulb can be seen. Behind the stomach one can see the spleen on the external side of the fetus and the tail of the pancreas on the posterior. The pancreas is usually hyperechoic, not only because of the acoustic enhancement of the beam behind the stomach, but also because of the natural echogenicity of the pancreas. The

spleen is of homogenous density and can be recognized by its relationship between the diaphragm (which is hypoechogenic and posterosuperior to the spleen) and the stomach (which is more medial and inferior). The rest of the gastrointestinal and genitourinary anatomy is described at length in chapters concerning anomalies of these organ systems, and need not be repeated here.

The liver occupies two thirds of the abdomen in a section that goes through the portal vein. The anatomy of the intrahepatic vessels has been described above.

Small Bowel. Some authors have attempted to correlate the echogenicity of the small bowel with the lung maturity. This has not been universally accepted. Occasionally, small bowel may appear hyperechogenic due to intraluminal meconium and mucus, and may be confused with a mass.

The transverse colon is also visible as a hypoechoic structure just below the liver. Its position is not only transverse but oblique from the posterior right side of the abdomen to anterior left.

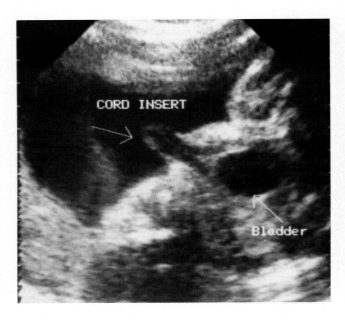

Fig. 6–26. The abdominal portions of both umbilical arteries are visible alongside the bladder; they also move toward the umbilicus and perforate the abdominal wall at this level.

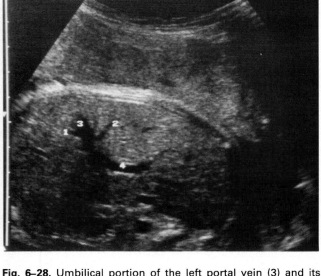

Fig. 6–28. Umbilical portion of the left portal vein (3) and its junction with the left portal vein (4) is visible. Vena advehentes (1,2) can be recognized. The ductus venosus (dv) can be seen connecting the portal system and the inferior vena cava (ivc). On the right side of the portal vein, one can recognize the right anterior portal vein (rapv). See the right posterior vein (rppv). (*Reprinted with permission from Jeanty P, Daniel TL. Fetal anatomy in ultrasonography. In: Hobbins JC, Benacerraf BR, eds. Clinics in Diagnostic Ultrasound, 25. New York: Churchill Livingstone; 1989.*)

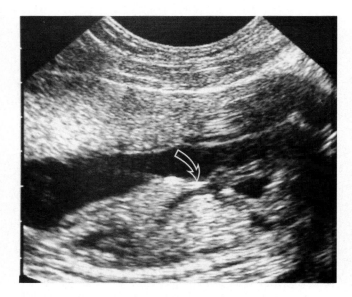

Fig. 6–27. The sharp cephalic bend of the umbilical vein (*arrow*) below and in the liver is visible in this sagittal section of the fetus. (*Reprinted with permission from Jeanty P, Daniel TL. Fetal anatomy in ultrasonography. In: Hobbins JC, Benacerraf BR, eds. Clinics in Diagnostic Ultrasound, 25. New York: Churchill Livingstone; 1989.*)

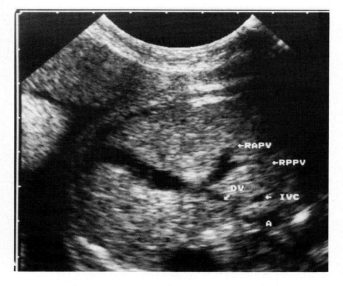

Fig. 6–29. The blood flows either to the ductus venosus or to the portal system. (*Reprinted with permission from Jeanty P, Daniel TL. Fetal anatomy in ultrasonography. In: Hobbins JC, Benacerraf BR, eds. Clinics in Diagnostic Ultrasound, 25. New York: Churchill Livingstone; 1989.*)

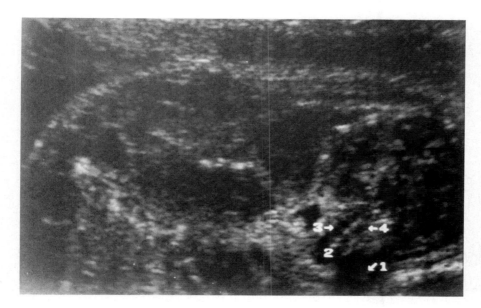

Fig. 6–30. The renal vessels can occasionally be seen. Here, the kidney is on the right side of image, and the renal vein (3) and renal artery (4) are recognizable.

Genitourinary (GU) Anatomy

The kidneys are visible from 14 weeks on; however, they are not always distinguishable. They become more obvious at about 20 weeks. Initially, they are hypoechoic but the renal anatomy becomes progressively more obvious and the echogenicity becomes mixed. The pyramids remain hypoechoic and the cortex is slightly echogenic. Occasionally, the arcuate arteries are visible. The main renal vessels (main artery and vein, Fig. 6–30) can sometimes be recognized.

The renal pelvis forms a group of mildly echogenic interfaces. The pelvis can be slightly (5 to 7 mm) distended when there is diuresis.

Nondistended ureters are usually not visible.

The bladder is visible at the midline as a fluid structure in the pelvis. It is typically bordered on both sides by the abdominal portion of the iliac vein. This important landmark allows one to differentiate the bladder from other cystic structures that might exist in the pelvis—such as distended loop of bowel or hydrometrocolpus. The umbilical arteries can be seen in some 16- to 20-week fetuses as a tubular structure, extending from the dome of the bladder to the base of the umbilical cord.

Limbs

Chinn has shown that the cartilaginous portion of the long bones (Fig. 6–31), as well as the cartilaginous bone of the wrist, could be demonstrated (Fig. 6–32). He also demonstrated the tendons of the hands. Birnholtz (personal communication) has shown that the fingernails (Fig. 6–33) could be imaged. Further, one can also image the palmar skin creases, a subject of potential interest in the noninvasive diagnosis of Trisomy 21 (Fig. 6–34).

Imaging Individual Limb Bones. Imaging of the limb bones is best done in a systematic fashion to avoid mislabeling limb segments. The preferred technique for recognizing each bone varies with different authors. Some have recommended identifying the spine first, and then turning the transducer 70 degrees to identify the femur. This approach requires demonstrating a longitudinal section of the spine and assumes that all fetuses have their

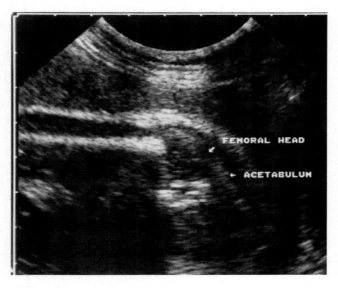

Fig. 6–31. The acetabulum and femoral head of this fetus can readily be observed. (*Reprinted with permission from Jeanty P, Daniel TL. Fetal anatomy in ultrasonography. In: Hobbins JC, Benacerraf BR, eds. Clinics in Diagnostic Ultrasound, 25. New York: Churchill Livingstone; 1989.*)

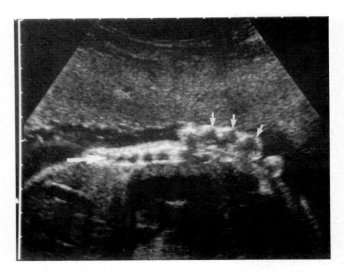

Fig. 6–32. Section passing through the anterior chest of the fetus. One hand (*arrows*) is lying on the sternum; the chondrocostal cartilage can be seen on the left side of picture. The section through the cartilaginous of the fingers is seen on the right side. (*Reprinted with permission from Jeanty P, Daniel TL. Fetal anatomy in ultrasonography. In: Hobbins JC, Benacerraf BR, eds.* Clinics in Diagnostic Ultrasound, *25. New York: Churchill Livingstone; 1989.*)

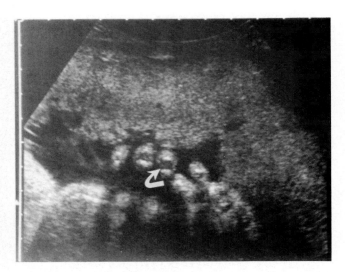

Fig. 6–33. Fingernails. (*Reprinted with permission from Jeanty P, Daniel TL. Fetal anatomy in ultrasonography. In: Hobbins JC, Benacerraf BR, eds.* Clinics in Diagnostic Ultrasound, *25. New York: Churchill Livingstone; 1989.*)

legs at a 70-degree angle from the spine. The technique that we recommend for identifying all long bones, including the femur, is based on the spatial orientation of the fetus from an easily recognizable landmark, such as the heart.

The Upper Extremity. To find the bones of the arm, identify the scapula (which is close to the heart and appears as a large echogenic area external to the rib cage). Then, follow the scapula to demonstrate a more external echo that corresponds to the humerus. This "bull's-eye" image represents the echogenic humerus surrounded by the hypoechogenic muscles of the arm, enclosed in the hyperechogenic subcutaneous and cutaneous tissues. Few movements are usually necessary to go from the scapula to the humerus, and the most common error is to make large sweeps, thereby losing the target. Once the humerus has been identified (usually in a transverse section), the principal movement that should be performed to image the whole length of the humerus is to rotate the transducer around an imaginary line perpendicular to the patient's skin. Rocking, tilting, or otherwise moving the transducer is generally not advised. If the section of the humerus that is displayed increases in length as a result of the movement, the movement should be continued in the same direction. Otherwise, rotation in the opposite direction is suggested.

A general problem that beginners encounter at this stage is "losing" the bone, usually because of imperceptible translations of the transducer on the slippery maternal abdomen. Once the humerus has been measured, one can identify the distal end and proceed to the elbow in order to image the ulna and the radius. The same rotational procedure is used to image the length of the radius or ulna. The distal ends of the two bones occasionally appear fused, and their individual participation can be difficult to assess. The ulna can be differentiated from the radius because the olecranon is closer to the surface of the flexed elbow than is the radius. The ulna, therefore, appears a few millimeters longer than the radius.

The Lower Extremity. The procedure to image the bones of the lower extremity is basically the same as that used in the upper extremity but, of course, the landmarks are different. Once the fetal heart has been identified, sweep down the trunk to image the fetal bladder. A bright echo in close proximity to the bladder is the ilium. Once it is located, the next most external and caudal echo corresponds to the femur. Again, careful rotation of the transducer around the femoral section will display the femoral length. The tibia and fibula are slightly easier to demonstrate than the radius and ulna because the latitude of movements permitted by the knee joint is smaller than that which occurs at the elbow. The tibia is the thicker of the two leg bones and lies medial to the fibula.

The fetal feet are more difficult to observe than the hand because they are usually closely apposed to the

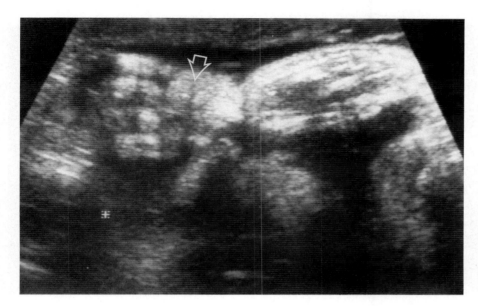

Fig. 6–34. Simian crease in the hand of a fetus with trisomy 21. (*Reprinted with permission from Jeanty P, Daniel TL. Fetal anatomy in ultrasonography. In: Hobbins JC, Benacerraf BR, eds.* Clinics in Diagnostic Ultrasound, *25. New York: Churchill Livingstone; 1989.*)

uterine wall (or to the placenta) and therefore lack the contrast provided by the amniotic fluid. There are more ossification centers in the foot than in the hand; at birth, the calcaneus, the talus, and the cuboid are usually calcified, and these can be imaged in the late stages of pregnancy. The metatarsal and the phalanges are also easily recognizable.

Measuring the Long Bones. Various authors have produced nomograms of fetal bone growth (usually the femur). They have used the same landmarks: the major trochanter and the distal end of the femoral shaft. The head of the femur has never been included in the measurement because it is not adequately ossified for visualization during much of the pregnancy. For the other long bone, the same rules are applied; only the shaft of the bone is included in the measurement, and the distal or proximal epiphysis is not measured.

An important criterion for the definition of an adequate plane for measurement is that the acoustic shadow should be sufficiently well-defined to conceal all posterior structures. The intersection of the shadow with the bone often provides the best position for placement of measurement calipers. Exceptions to this rule are the acoustic shadows produced by the head of the femur and spurious acoustic shadows that originate from adjacent structures (such as the ilium or bones of the contralateral limb). As a general rule, it is better to measure the bones proximal to the transducer than the distal bones.

SUMMARY

This survey of fetal anatomy is not intended to demonstrate the entire extent of the current state of the art, but only to highlight the fact that a large number of very small fetal structures can indeed be seen with today's ultrasound equipment.

The anatomic structures that should be routinely evaluated and documented have been specified in a joint statement issued by the American Institute of Ultrasound in Medicine and the American College of Radiology. The reader is encouraged to be familiar with the items specified in this list.

REFERENCES

Arey LB. *Developmental Anatomy.* Philadelphia: Saunders; 1974.

Birnholz JC. The development of fetal eye movement patterns. *Science.* 1981;213:679–681.

Chinn DH, Bolding DB, Callen PW, et al: Ultrasonographic identification of fetal lower extremity epiphyseal ossification centers. *Radiology.* 1983;147:815–818.

Chinn DH, Bolding DB, Callen PW, et al. Ultrasonographic identification of fetal lower extremity epiphyseal ossification centers. *Radiology.* 1983;147:815–818.

Fink IJ, Chinn DH, Callen PW. A potential pitfall in the ultrasonographic diagnosis of fetal encephalocele. *J Ultrasound Med.* 1983;2:313–314.

Hamilton WJ, Mossman HW. *Human Embryology.* Baltimore: Williams & Wilkins; 1972;274–276.

Hashimoto BE, Filly RA, Callen PW. Fetal Pseudoascites: Further anatomic observations. *J Ultrasound Med.* 1986;5:151–152.

Hertzberg BS, Bowie JD, Burger PC, et al. The three lines: Origin of sonographic landmarks in the fetal head. *AJR.* 1987;149:1009–1012.

Jeanty P, Chervenak F, Romero R, Michiels M, Hobbins JC. The sylvian fissure: A commonly mislabelled cranial landmark. *J Ultrasound Med.* 1984;3:15–18.

Jeffrey RB, Laing FC. High-resolution realtime sonography of fetal cardiovascular anatomy. *J Ultrasound Med.* 1982;1:249–251.

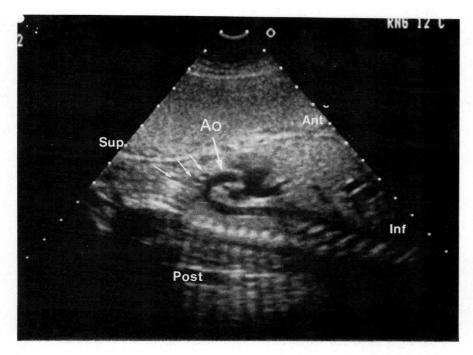

Fig. 8–6. Aortic arch (Ao) viewed from the anterior thoracic wall. Head and neck vessels are indicated by small arrows. (*Reproduced with permission from Romero R, et al.* Prenatal Diagnosis of Congenital Anomalies. *Norwalk, Conn: Appleton & Lange, 1987.*)

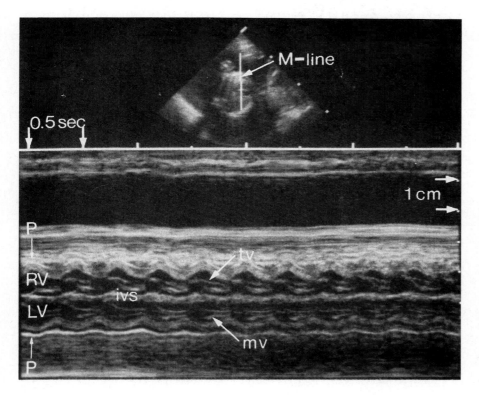

Fig. 8–7. With ultrasound equipment that has the option of real-time directed M-mode, the position of the cursor (M-line) can easily be selected during real-time examination. M-mode echocardiogram of the ventricular cavities (RV, LV) at the level of the atrioventricular valves (tv, mv) is shown. Undulations of free ventricular walls and interventricular septum (ivs) reflect systole and dyastole. P = pericardium. (*Reproduced with permission from Romero R, et al.* Prenatal Diagnosis of Congenital Anomalies. *Norwalk, Conn: Appleton & Lange; 1987.*)

size of the ventricular chambers and great vessels.[14,16,17] Measurement of ventricular chambers and determination of contractility have been suggested as a mean for assessment of cardiac function[16] although the clinical value of such evaluation is still undetermined. At present, M-mode ultrasound is particularly valuable in identification and differential diagnosis of fetal dysrhythmias.[18-21]

Pulsed Doppler ultrasound evaluation has recently been applied to the study of the heart function in the human fetus.[22-30] Adequate recordings of velocity waveforms of blood flow through the atrioventricular valves, great vessels, and inferior vena cava can be obtained in almost all cases starting at 18 to 20 weeks (Fig. 8–8). Several authors have pointed out remarkable differences between in utero and postnatal Doppler studies. The higher velocity in flow at the ventricular inlet that is dependent on atrial contraction, when compared to passive venous filling, has been interpreted as a sign of the

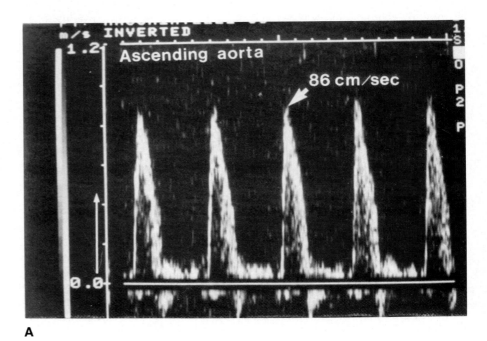

A

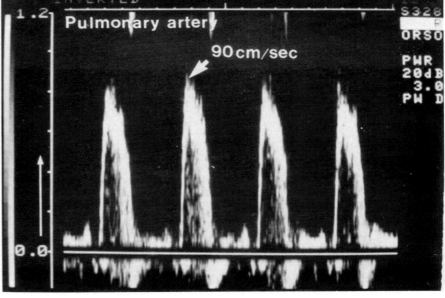

B

Fig. 8–8. Doppler velocity waveforms of the ascending aorta (**A**), pulmonary artery (**B**), ductus arteriosus (**C**), left ventricle (**D**), and inferior vena cava close to the right atrium (**E**). Correction of Doppler shift for the angle of incidence allows estimation of blood velocity. Waveforms of blood flow within the ascending aorta and pulmonary artery are similar, with maximal velocities usually less than, or close to, 1 m/sec in normal fetuses. The waveform in the ductus arteriosus differs from the pulmonary artery and ascending aorta because of the presence of significant blood velocities in diastole (*curved arrows*) that probably reflect low impedance. (*Figure continued.*)

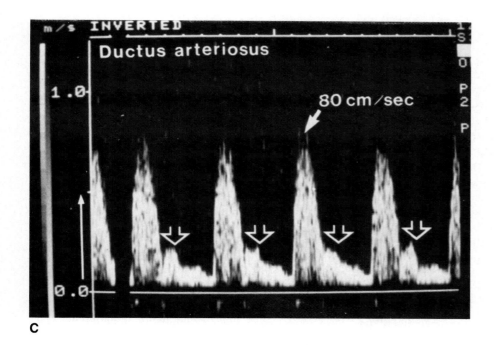

C

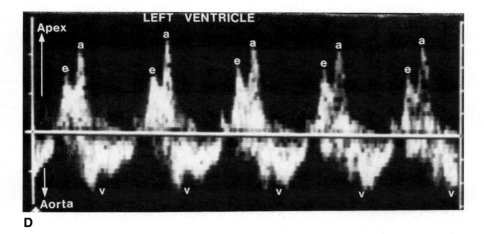

D

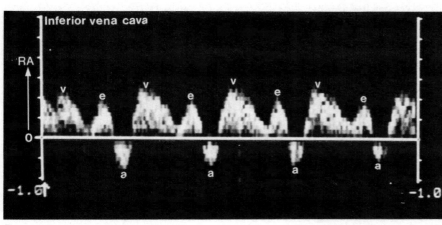

E

Fig. 8–8 (continued). Doppler velocity waveforms. In (**D**), the sampling volume is positioned within the left ventricle apical to the mitral valve. Both ventricular inflow and outflow are recorded. Diastolic filling is characterized by blood moving toward the apex of the heart in a biphasic velocity waveform. The e peak corresponds to passive venous filling and the a peak to atrial systole. The waveform with opposite direction (v) corresponds to blood flow moving toward the aorta in systole. The higher velocity recorded in blood flow, dependent on atrial contraction when compared to passive filling, has been interpreted as a sign of physiologic "stiffness" of the fetal myocardium. Evaluation of this Doppler sonogram allows correlation of atrial and ventricular systole and inference of the sequence of excitation. A pulsatile waveform is recorded within the inferior vena cava in proximity of the right atrium (**E**). Blood flows toward the right atrium during ventricular systole (v) and passive diastolic filling (e). Flow in the opposite direction is recorded during atrial systole (a). This tracing (**D**), similarly to **E**, allows inference of atrioventricular sequence of excitation.

physiologic "stiffness" of the fetal myocardium.[24] Pulsed Doppler ultrasound, in combination with two-dimensional and M-mode sonography, has proved useful in evaluation of both fetal dysrhythmias and structural anomalies. In this regard, Doppler is valuable in documenting atrioventricular valve insufficiency (Fig. 8–9). It has been recently demonstrated that the association of structural heart disease, hydrops, and atrioventricular valve insufficiency carries a very poor prognosis.[23] It has also been found that, in normal fetuses, the peak velocity in both ascending aorta and pulmonary artery is less than 1 m/sec.[26] This observation is relevant for the prenatal diagnosis of pulmonic and aortic stenosis, which are associated with poststenotic turbulence.

However, the use of Doppler in the fetus is still an area of ongoing research. Sophisticated analyses of cardiac function are appearing with increasing frequency.

CARDIAC STRUCTURAL ANOMALIES

Atrial and Ventricular Septal Defects

Atrial septal defects (ASD), which cover a wide range of severity, are commonly divided into primum and secundum types. *Primum* ASD is the simplest form of atrioventricular defect. The most severe form is the complete atrioventricular canal. Atrioventricular canal is found in more than 50% of infants with trisomy 21.[31] *Secundum* ASD may be a part of the Holt-Oram syndrome with autosomal dominant transmission.

Due to the presence of the foramen ovalis valve, it is usually difficult to properly assess the integrity of the septum secundum in the fetus. It is also questionable if isolated, small defects in this area can be recognized in utero. We have never identified secundum ASD prior to birth. Conversely, primum ASD is easily seen. The complete atrioventricular canal is identified by the association of an ASD with a ventricular septal defect and a common atrioventricular valve. The insertion of the two atrioventricular valves at the same level of the ventricular septum is a useful echocardiographic sign of this anomaly (Fig. 8–10).

Atrial septal defects do not cause impairment of cardiac function in utero as does a large right-to-left shunt at the level of the atria in the fetus. Most affected infants are asymptomatic even in the neonatal period. In the complete form of atrioventricular canal, the common atrioventricular valve may be incompetent and systolic blood regurgitation from the ventricles to the atria may give rise to congestive heart failure.[32] Pulsed Doppler ultrasound allows identification of the regurgitant jet.[23]

Ventricular septal defects (VSD) are probably the most common congenital cardiac defects. The echocardiographic diagnosis depends on the demonstration of a dropout of echoes in the ventricular septum (Fig. 8–11). Obviously, VSDs smaller than 1- to 2-mm will fall beyond the resolution ability of current ultrasound equipment and will escape detection. There is no evidence that VSDs are responsible for hemodynamic compromise in utero. Even a large interventricular communication gives probable rise only to small bidirectional shunts in the fetus—

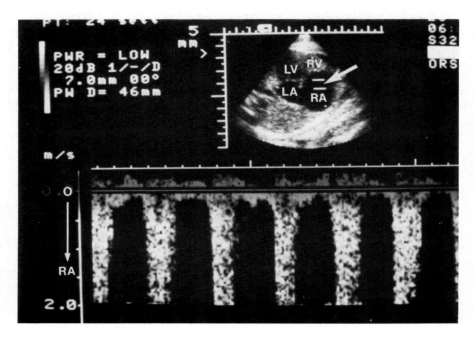

Fig. 8–9. In this fetus with Ebstein anomaly of the tricuspid valve, sampling volume (*arrow*) is positioned within the right atrium (RA) close to the tricuspid valve. A systolic regurgitant jet with velocity exceeding 2 m/sec is recorded. This finding is consistent with insufficiency of the tricuspid valve. The fetus had nonimmune hydrops. LV = left ventricle; RV = right ventricle; LA = left atrium.

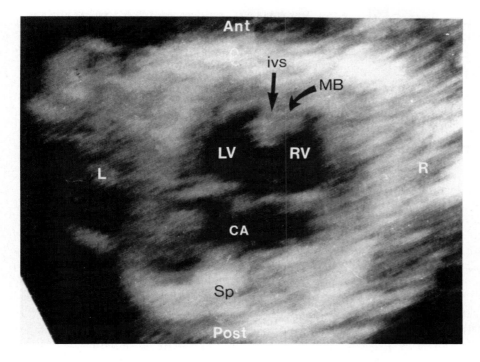

Fig. 8–10. Four-chamber view of the fetal heart reveals a large defect of the interventricular septum (ivs), a common atrioventricular valve, and absence of the atrial septum. This is complete atrioventricular canal with a common atrium (CA). LV = left ventricle; RV = right ventricle; MB = moderator band; Sp = spine. (*Reproduced with permission from Romero R, et al. Prenatal Diagnosis of Congenital Anomalies. Norwalk, Conn: Appleton & Lange; 1987.*)

as during intrauterine life the right and left ventricular pressures are believed to be equal.[33] The vast majority of infants with such anomolies are not symptomatic in the neonatal period.[34]

Pulmonary Stenosis

The most common form of pulmonary stenosis is the valvular type, due to the fusion of the pulmonary leaflets.

Hemodynamics is altered in proportion to the degree of the stenosis. The work of the right ventricle is increased, as well as the pressure, leading to hypertrophy of the ventricular walls. In the most severe cases, right-ventricular overload results in congestive heart failure.

Postnatal diagnosis of pulmonary stenosis depends on a cross-sectional demonstration of doming of the pulmonary cusps, and poststenotic turbulence detected by

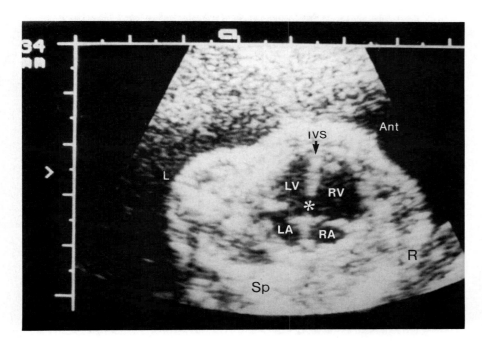

Fig. 8–11. Four-chamber view of the fetal heart demonstrating perimembranous ventricular septal defect (*). LV = left ventricle; RV = right ventricle; LA = left atrium; RA = right atrium; Sp = spine.

Doppler ultrasound.[35] M-mode examination is an unreliable tool. Prenatal diagnosis is probably difficult, because only a few very severe cases have been described. These were mainly cases with enlargement of the right ventricle, poststenotic enlargement, or hypoplasia of the pulmonary artery (Fig. 8–12). Recently, we have been able to demonstrate abnormally high velocities in the main pulmonary trunk in two fetuses with tetralogy of Fallot and infundibular pulmonic stenosis (Fig. 8–13).

Aortic Stenosis

Aortic stenosis is commonly divided into supravalvular, valvular, and subaortic forms. The subaortic forms include a fixed type (which is the consequence of a fibrous or fibromuscular obstruction) and a dynamic type (which is due to a thickened ventricular septum obstructing the outflow tract of the left ventricle). The latter is also known as asymmetric septal hypertrophy or idiopathic hypertrophic subaortic stenosis. In the most severe cases, the association of left-ventricular pressure overload and subendocardial ischemia (due to decrease in coronary perfusion) may lead to early intrauterine impairment of cardiac function.[36] Insufficiency of the mitral valve and systolic regurgitation may ensue. Intrauterine hemodynamic disturbance following aortic stenosis is indirectly attested by the very high incidence of intrauterine growth retardation in infants affected by this anomaly.[37] Neither supravalvular nor subaortic stenosis are usually clinically manifested in newborns.

The same considerations previously reported for the prenatal echocardiographic diagnosis of pulmonic stenosis apply to aortic stenosis. Severe cases of this condition have been described frequently in the current literature.[36,38] Pulsed Doppler ultrasound is valuable in assessing the presence of mitral valve insufficiency.[23]

Asymmetric septal hypertrophy has been identified in a fetus.[39] The only reported case, however, is probably an exception. There is evidence indicating that this anomaly usually has an evolutive course and is not apparent in the neonatal period.[40] We are not aware of any case of supravalvular aortic stenosis detected in utero.

Tetralogy of Fallot

Tetralogy of Fallot has the following features: a ventricular septal defect, usually in the perimembranous area; infundibular pulmonic stenosis; aortic valve overriding the ventricular septum; and hypertrophy of the right ventricle. Both pathologic studies in infants and echocardiographic studies in live fetuses seem to agree in documenting a late onset of right ventricular hypertrophy.[11,41]

In the most severe cases, the infundibulum of the right ventricle and the pulmonary artery may be atretic and the anomaly is commonly referred to as pulmonary atresia with VSD. Associated defects, including atrial septal defects and bicuspid or absent pulmonary valve, are frequently seen. The main factor affecting hemodynamics is the degree of hypoplasia of the right-ventricular outflow tract; this causes both a decrease in pulmonary blood flow and a right-to-left shunt at the level of the

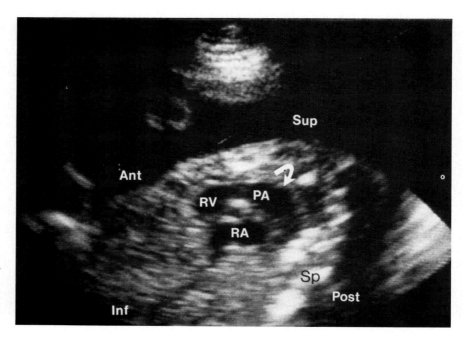

Fig. 8–12. Curved arrow indicates enlargement of main pulmonary artery (PA). Moderate pulmonic stenosis was found at birth. RA = right atrium; RV = ventricle; Sp = spine.

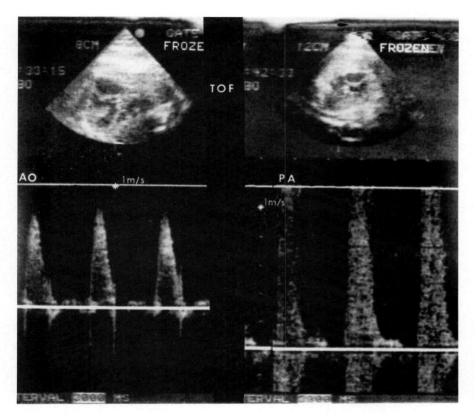

Fig. 8–13. Doppler velocity waveforms of blood flow within the ascending aorta (Ao) and pulmonary artery (PA) in a fetus with tetralogy of Fallot. Maximal velocities in the pulmonary artery that exceed 1 m/sec and cause an alias are consistent with pulmonic stenosis.

ascending aorta with decreased oxygen saturation. However, tetralogy of Fallot does not seem to cause hemodynamic compromise in utero. Even in the case of very tight infundibular stenosis or pulmonary atresia, the combined output of both ventricles is directed toward the aorta, and the pulmonary vascular bed is supplied by reverse flow through the ductus arteriosus. This concept is supported by the observation of normal intrauterine fetal growth in affected fetuses.[37] Congestive heart failure is very rarely seen in neonates and it usually occurs only in those with absent pulmonary valves.

Echocardiographic diagnosis of tetralogy of Fallot can be made by demonstrating the aorta overriding the ventricular septum (Fig. 8–14).[11,32] Caution is recommended as artifacts are seen rather frequently. In our experience, all fetuses with tetralogy of Fallot have an enlargement of the ascending aorta that is striking on real-time examination and should raise the index of suspicion. The study of the right-ventricular outflow tract and pulmonary artery provides important clinical information by allowing assessment of the degree of infundibular stenosis. Doppler ultrasound is valuable in assessing the presence of blood flow in the pulmonary artery (see Fig. 8–13). Enlargement of the right ventricle, main pulmonary trunk, and pulmonary artery suggest absence of the pulmonary valve.[32]

Transposition of the Great Arteries

Transposition of the great arteries (TGA) is commonly subdivided into two forms: complete TGA and corrected TGA. In complete TGA, the aorta arises from the morphologic right ventricle, and the pulmonary artery from the left ventricle, in the presence of a normal atrioventricular connection. Associated cardiac anomalies are frequently found. According to Becker and Anderson,[6] three main varieties can be distinguished: transposition with intact ventricular septum, with or without pulmonic stenosis; transposition with VSD; and transposition with VSD and pulmonic stenosis. Other anomalies commonly found include abnormalities of the atrioventricular valves, underdevelopment of either the right or left ventricle, and coarctation of the aorta.

Corrected transposition of the great arteries is associated with an atrioventricular and a ventriculo-arterial discordance. The right atrium is connected to the left ventricle which is connected to the pulmonic aorta; the left atrium is connected to the right ventricle which is connected to the ascending aorta.

Fetal echocardiography allows identification of abnormalities of the ventriculo-arterial connection. In both complete and corrected transposition, the two great vessels arise parallel from the base of the heart. With careful scanning, the aorta and pulmonic artery can be identified,

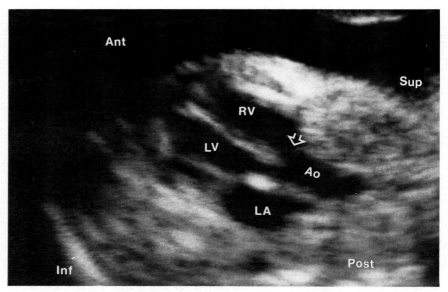

A

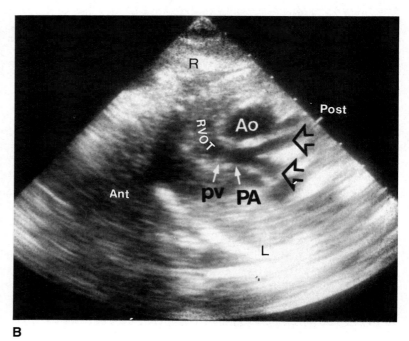

B

Fig. 8-14. **A.** Long-axis view of the left ventricle demonstrating the aorta (Ao) (*arrow*) overriding a ventricular septum defect by almost 50%. This is tetralogy of Fallot. (*Reproduced with permission from Bovicelli L, Baccarani G, Picchio FM, Pilu G. Ecocardiografia Fetale. La Diagnosi ed il Trattamento Prenatale delle Cardiopatie Congenite. Milan: Masson; 1985.*) **B.** Short-axis view of the great vessels in a fetus with tetralogy of Fallot demonstrates obvious disproportion between the size of the ascending aorta and main pulmonary artery. The outflow tract of the right ventricle (RVOT) is narrow. Findings are consistent with severe infundibular stenosis of the pulmonary artery. Right and left pulmonary arteries are indicated by open arrows. LA = left atrium; LV = left ventricle; ivs = interventricular septum; pv = pulmonary valve.

and their relationship with each ventricle assessed (Fig. 8-15). Differential diagnosis between complete and corrected transposition depends on identification of the morphologic right and left ventricles by visualization of the moderator band, papillary muscles, and insertion of atrioventricular valves. The atrioventricular connection can be further recognized by demonstration of the systemic and pulmonary venous return.

Fetuses with uncomplicated complete transposition should not undergo hemodynamic compromise in utero. Survival after birth depends on the persistence of fetal circulation. In corrected transposition, discordance between atrioventricular and ventriculo-arterial connection cancel one another; and, ideally, there should not be any hemodynamic imbalance. Corrected transposition may indeed be occasionally found at autopsy. However, im-

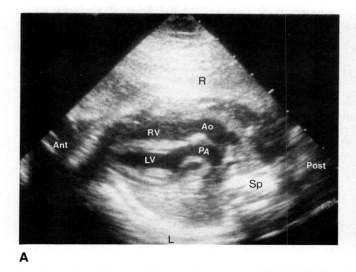

A

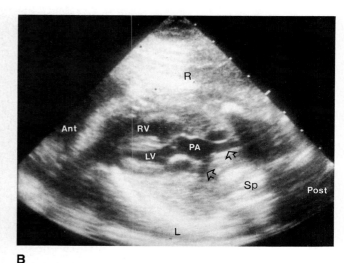

B

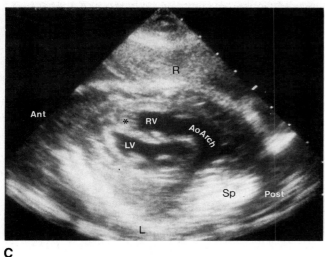

C

Fig. 8–15. Transposition of the great arteries. **A.** Two vessels (Ao, PA) are seen arising parallel from the base of the heart. **B.** The vessel connected to the left ventricle (LV) can be positively identified as the main pulmonary trunk by following its course to bifurcation into the right and left pulmonary artery (*open arrows*). **C.** The vessel arising from the right ventricle (RV) can be identified as the ascending aorta by following its long upward course to the aortic arch (AoArch). Visualization of the moderator band (*) identifies the anterior ventricle as the right one.

portant associated cardiac anomalies are found in the vast majority of cases (VSDs, pulmonic stenosis, abnormalities of the atrioventricular valves, and atrioventricular block).

Double Outlet Right Ventricle
In double outlet right ventricle (DORV) most of the aorta and pulmonary artery arise from the right ventricle (Fig. 8–16). The relation between the two great vessels may vary. A defect of the ventricular septum is almost always associated with DORV, as well as with other anomalies (atrial septal defects, pulmonary stenosis, and abnormalities of the atrioventricular valves). By definition, the term DORV includes those cases of tetralogy of Fallot in which the aorta arises predominantly from the right ventricle. Prenatal diagnosis of DORV has been reported.[42] However, differentiation from other conotrun-

cal anomalies, such as transposition of the great vessels and tetralogy of Fallot, is notoriously difficult.[43]

Hypoplastic Left Heart Syndrome
Hypoplastic left heart syndrome (HLHS) is characterized by a very small left ventricle with mitral or aortic atresia, or both. Blood flow to the head and neck vessels and coronary artery is supplied in a retrograde manner via the ductus arteriosus. Hypoplastic left heart syndrome is frequently associated with intrauterine heart failure. The prognosis is always extremely poor. Untreated infants usually die in the very first days of life. Palliative procedures have been proposed and long-term survivors have been reported. Recently, cardiac transplantation in the neonatal period has also been attempted.

Echocardiographic diagnosis of HLHS in the fetus

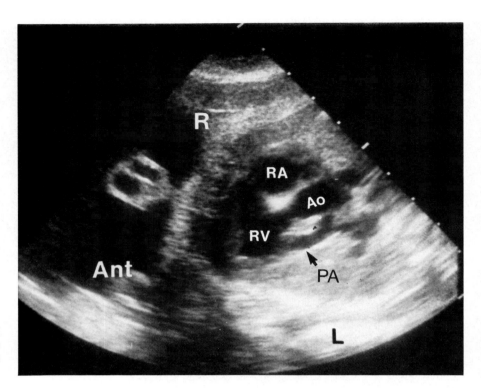

Fig. 8–16. Both large aorta (Ao) and a small stenotic pulmonary artery (PA) are seen arising from the right ventricle (RV). This is double-outlet right ventricle.

depends on the demonstration of a diminutive left ventricle.[44,45] The ascending aorta is severely hypoplastic. The right ventricle, right atrium, and pulmonary artery are usually enlarged (Fig. 8–17). With the use of pulsed Doppler ultrasound, it should be possible to demonstrate retrograde blood flow in the ascending aorta and a regurgitant jet in those cases with tricuspid insufficiency. In most cases, the ultrasound appearance is striking and the diagnosis an easy one.

Pulmonary Atresia with Intact Ventricular Septum

Pulmonary atresia with intact ventricular septum (PA:IVS) in infants is usually associated with a hypoplastic right ventricle (Fig. 8–18). Fetuses with an enlarged right ventricle and atrium have been described with unusual frequency (Fig. 8–19).[46] Although prenatal series report a small number, it is possible that the discrepancy with pediatric literature is due to the very high perinatal loss that is found in dilated cases. Enlargement of the ventricle and atrium are probably the consequence of tricuspid insufficiency. Prenatal diagnosis of PA:IVS relies on demonstration of a small pulmonary artery with an atretic pulmonary valve. We have recently been able to confirm real-time two-dimensional diagnosis of pulmo-

nary atresia by using Doppler ultrasound to show the absence of blood flow within the main pulmonary trunk and reverse flow through the ductus arteriosus.

Univentricular Heart

According to Becker and Anderson,[6] the term univentricular heart defines a group of anomalies unified by the presence of an atrioventricular junction that is entirely connected to only one chamber in the ventricular mass. Based on this definition (which we find very suitable for fetal echocardiographic studies), the univentricular heart includes cases in which two atrial chambers are connected (by either two distinct atrioventricular valves or by a common one) to a main ventricular chamber (classic "double-inlet single ventricle"). The term also includes cases in which, because of absence of one atrioventricular connection (tricuspid or mitral atresia), one of the ventricular chambers is either rudimentary or absent. The main ventricular chamber may be either of left or right type and, in some cases, of indeterminate type. A rudimentary ventricular chamber lacking atrioventricular connection is a frequent, but not constant, finding. Antenatal echocardiographic diagnosis is usually easy. An example of a double-inlet single ventricle heart is shown in Fig. 8–20. The hemodynamics may vary greatly from case to case, depending on the type of ventriculo-arterial

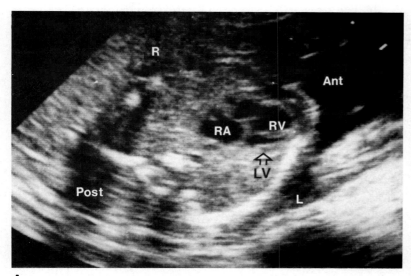

A

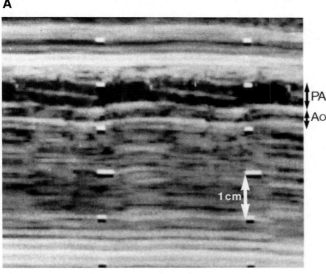

B

Fig. 8–17. **A.** In this four-chamber view of a fetal heart, the left ventricle (LV) cannot be visualized. Only a solid mass of thickened myocardium is seen. The right atrium and ventricle (RA and RV) are enlarged. **B.** M-mode echocardiogram in the same case, comparing the pulmonary artery (PA) and ascending aorta (Ao). The ascending aorta is hypoplastic, and no aortic valve movement could be detected by either real-time or M-mode sonography. Findings are consistent with hypoplastic left heart.

connection and the sum of associated cardiac anomalies frequently seen.

Cardiomyopathies

Congenital cardiomyopathies include a heterogeneous group of myocardial disorders commonly subdivided into nonobstructive and obstructive forms. The etiologies of *nonobstructive forms* include inborn errors of metabolism, muscular dystrophies, and infections. *Obstructive forms* include hypertrophic cardiomyopathy of infants of diabetic mothers and asymmetric septal hypertrophy (previously considered). Hypertrophic cardiomyopathy is found in 30% to 50% of infants of diabetic mothers, even if it clinically manifests in a much smaller proportion.[47] The etiology of this condition is controversial, but it is commonly accepted to represent the final consequence of fetal hyperglycemia and hyperinsulinemia.

Cardiomyopathies of both obstructive and nonobstructive types share (as a consequence of pump failure and/or valvular regurgitation, or as a result of obstruction to ventricular outflow) a more-or-less marked tendency toward congestive heart failure. The onset and extent of symptoms are extremely variable from case to case. While most newborns are asymptomatic, cases associated with intrauterine heart failure have been described.[11,48]

Echocardiographic diagnosis of nonobstructive forms relies on demonstration of cardiomegaly and poor contractility of ventricular chambers (Fig. 8–21).[48] In obstructive forms, thickening of the interventricular septum has been reported (Fig. 8–22).[39,49]

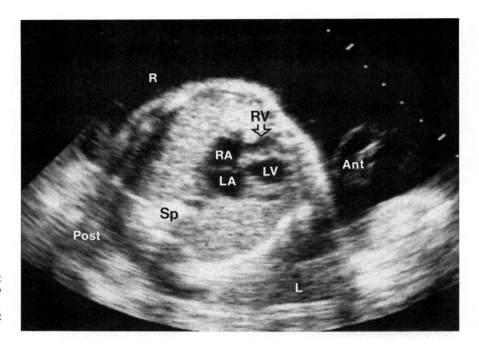

Fig. 8–18. Pulmonary atresia with intact ventricular septum. Four-chamber view reveals small right ventricle (RV). LV = left ventricle; RA = right atrium; LA = left atrium.

Coarctation of the Aorta

The pathogenesis of coarctation of the aorta is controversial. Three hypotheses have been suggested. According to these different views, coarctation may be (1) a true malformation arising from an embryogenetic abnormality; (2) the consequence of aberrant ductal tissue in the aortic wall resulting in narrowing of the isthmus at time of closure of the ductus (the so-called Skodaic theory); or (3) the anatomic result of an intrauterine hemodynamic perturbance caused by an intracardiac anomaly diverting blood flow from the aorta into the pulmonary artery and ductus arteriosus. There is clinical as well as pathologic evidence supporting at least the last two hypotheses.

A discrete shelf between the isthmus and the de-

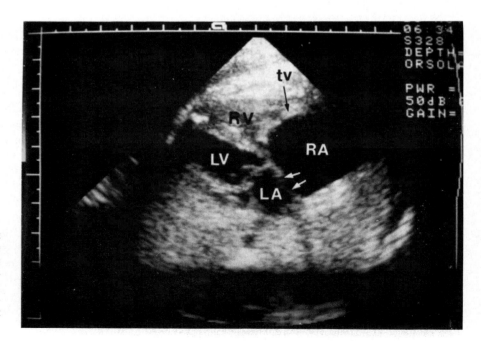

Fig. 8–19. Pulmonary atresia with intact ventricular septum. The right ventricle (RV) and particularly the right atrium (RA) are enlarged. The interatrial septum (*arrows*) bulges toward the left atrium (LA). Doppler echocardiography revealed tricuspid valve (tv) insufficiency. LV = left ventricle.

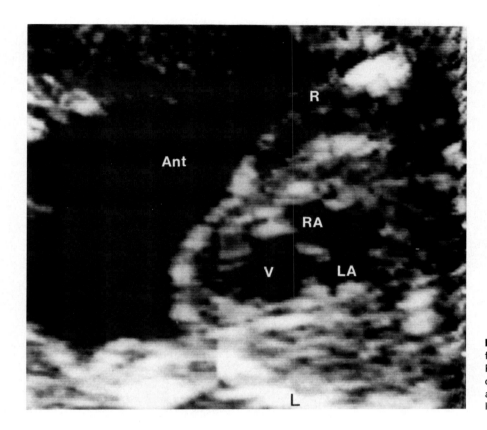

Fig. 8–20. This four-chamber view of the fetal heart reveals that the two atria (LA, RA) are connected to a single ventricular chamber (V). There are two separate atrioventricular valves. This is double-inlet single ventricule heart.

scending aorta is the most common finding at anatomic dissection. Tubular hypoplasia of a segment of the aortic arch is seen less frequently. Coarctation may be a postnatal event, and this limits prenatal diagnosis in many cases. However, this anomaly has been described in the fetus although only in late pregnancy.[50] In one case seen in our laboratory, echocardiography was negative at 20 weeks. At 30 weeks, enlargement of the right ventricle was found and the aortic isthmus appeared severely narrowed (Fig. 8–23). As the blood flow through the isthmus

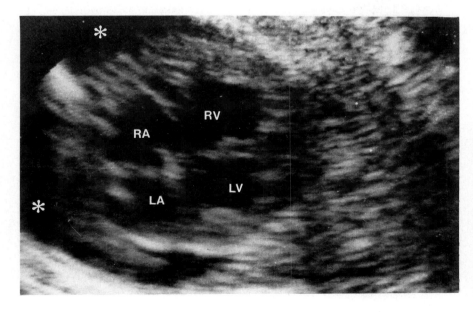

Fig. 8–21. Non-obstructive cardiomyopathy (primary endocardial fibroelastosis) in a third-trimester fetus with nonimmune hydrops. There is obvious cardiomegaly, and poor contractility of ventricular walls was noted on real-time examination. A large layer of pleural effusion is seen in this view (*). RV and LV = right and left ventricle; RA and LA = right and left atrium. (*Reproduced with permission from Bovicelli L, et al. Prenatal diagnosis of endocardial fibroelastosis.* Prenat Diagn. *1984;4:67.*)

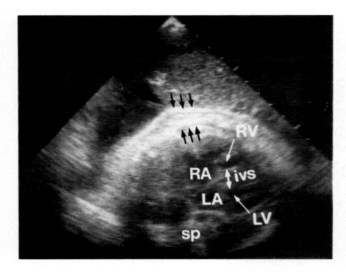

Fig. 8–22. Hypertrophic cardiomyopathy in fetus of an insulin-dependent diabetic mother. There is a disproportionate increase in the thickness of the interventricular septum (IVS) that measures 14 mm. An unusually large layer of subcutaneous fat tissue is seen at the level of the thoracic wall (*black arrows*), suggesting severe macrosomia. LV and RV = left and right ventricle; RA and LA = right and left atrium. (*Reproduced with permission from Romero R, et al.* Prenatal Diagnosis of Congenital Anomalies, *Norwalk, Conn: Appleton & Lange; 1987.*)

is minimal during intrauterine life (the descending aorta being mainly supplied via the ductus arteriosus), isolated coarctation is not expected to significantly alter hemodynamics. However, cases with tubular hypoplasia of the aortic arch may result in a greater hemodynamic burden; this could explain the dilatation of the right heart that has been documented with echocardiography prior to birth.

FETAL DYSRHYTHMIAS

Irregular patterns of fetal heart rhythms are a frequent finding. Brief periods of tachycardia, bradycardia, and ectopic beats also are commonly seen. In the vast majority of cases they have no clinical significance. The electrical instability of the fetal heart has not yet been clearly explained. Catecholamine release or accessory pathways have been suggested as playing a role. Although realizing that differentiating clearly between physiologic variations and pathologic alterations is not possible in many cases, a distinction must be attempted for practical clinical purposes. According to the pragmatic approach suggested by Allan and associates,[18] sustained bradycardia of less than 100 beats per minute, sustained tachycardia of more than 200 beats per minute, and irregular beats occurring more than one in ten must be considered abnormal and require further investigation.

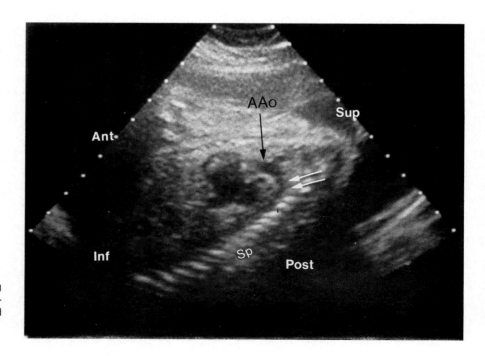

Fig. 8–23. In this 30-week fetus, narrowing of the aortic isthmus is seen (*white arrows*). Severe coarctation was confirmed at birth. AAo = ascending aorta; Sp = spine.

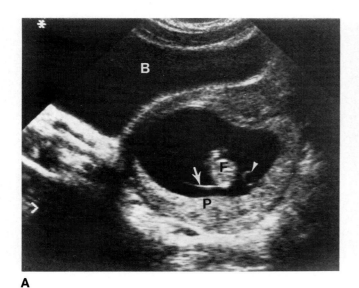

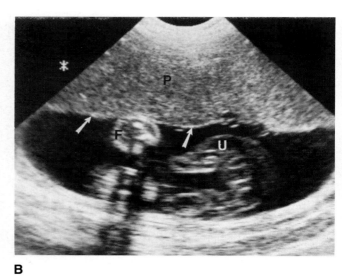

Fig. 9–2. (Left.) **A.** Transverse sector scan at 10.8 weeks shows the amniotic membrane (*arrow*) separate from the posterior placenta (P). The yolk sac (*arrowhead*) is seen between the amnion and placenta. F = fetus; B = maternal bladder. **B.** Transverse sector scan at 27 weeks shows clearly-defined chorionic plate (*arrows*). U = umbilical cord.

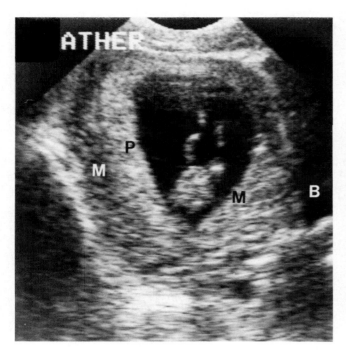

Fig. 9–3. Sagittal sector scan at 11.5 weeks clearly shows posterior placenta (P). Retroplacental myometrium (M) appears relatively hypoechoic while the myometrium (M) on inferior aspect of uterus appears more echogenic. B = maternal bladder.

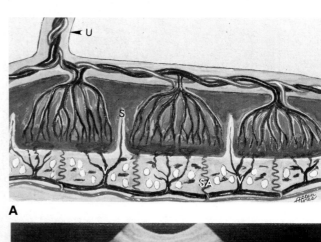

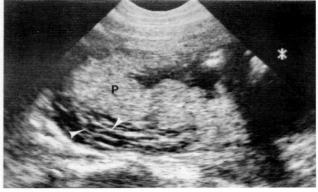

Fig. 9–4. A. Diagram of placental circulation. U = umbilical cord; SA = spiral arterioles; V = draining veins; S = septum. (*Reprinted with permission from* Semin Ultrasound. *Grune & Stratton; 1980; 1:293.*) **B.** Sector scan at 20 weeks demonstrating venous drainage of placenta (*arrowheads*). P = placenta.

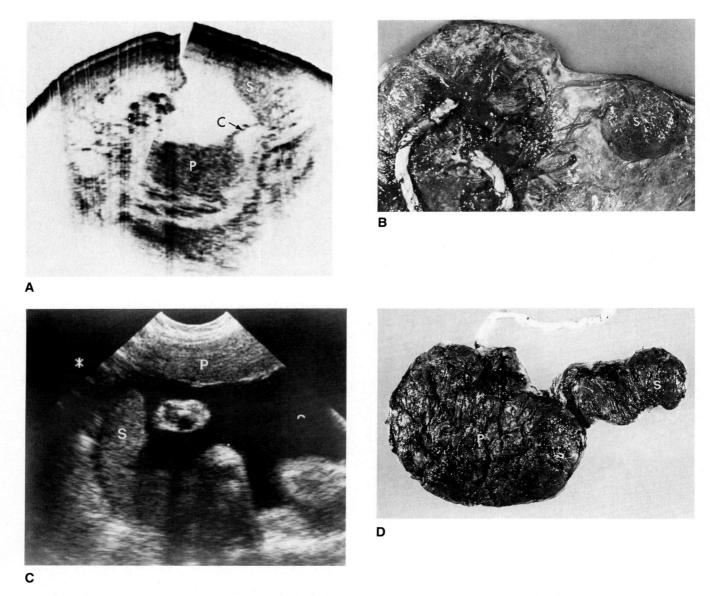

Fig. 9–5. A. Transverse sonogram at 28 weeks demonstrates posterior placenta (P) with left succenturiate lobe (S). C = elevated membranes over a sonolucent space representing a submembranous hematoma, confirmed at delivery. **B.** Gross examination of placenta shows succenturiate lobe (S). (*Reprinted with permission from* J Clin Ultrasound. *1981; 9:139.*) **C.** Sector scan at 33 weeks demonstrates anterior placenta (P), with posterior succenturiate lobe (S). **D.** Maternal surface of gross specimen shows succenturiate lobe (S) separate from main body of placenta (P).

are present.[1,11–13] These consist of separate masses of chorionic villi connected to the main placenta by vessels within the membrane. A succenturiate lobe may also be continuous with the placenta via a bridge of chorionic tissue. Succenturiate lobes may be demonstrated by sonography (Fig. 9–5). It is important to diagnose a succenturiate lobe antenatally because of the following complications: it may be retained in utero, resulting in

postpartum hemorrhage; it may overlie the internal cervical os; or, the vessels that connect it to the main placental mass may traverse the internal os (vasa previa) and rupture during labor, resulting in fetal blood loss.

A placenta in which the fetal membranes do not extend to its edge, so that the chorionic plate is smaller than the basal plate, is called placenta extrachorialis. The attachment of the fetal membranes to the chorionic plate

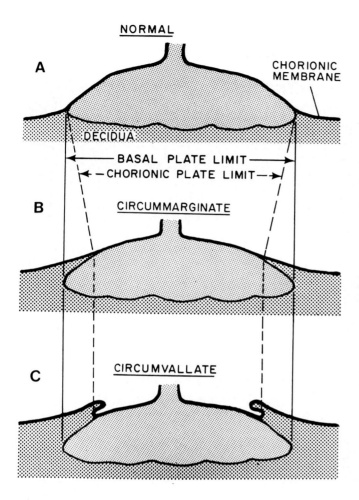

Fig. 9–6. Cross-sectional diagram comparing extrachorial placentas with normal placenta. **A.** Normal placenta, showing transition of membranous to villous chorion at placental edge. **B.** Circummarginate placenta: transition from membranous to villous chorion occurs at a distance from placental edge. **C.** Circumvallate placenta, similar to **B** except for fold in chorionic membrane. (*Reprinted with permission from* Semin Ultrasound. *Grune & Stratton; 1980; 1:293*).

forms a ring that may be flat (circummarginate) or folded (circumvallate) (Fig. 9–6). This ring may be partially or totally circumferential. The fold of membranes can be seen on sonography (Fig. 9–7); we have not detected them beyond the second trimester. The circummarginate placenta has no clinical significance, whereas a complete circumvallate placenta may be associated with a higher incidence of premature labor, threatened abortion, perinatal mortality, and marginal hemorrhage.[1,14,15] Intra-amniotic hemorrhage secondary to circumvallate placenta has been reported.[15A]

Other variations of placental shape that are of clinical significance include the annular or ring-shaped placenta

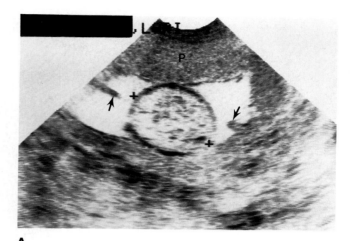

A

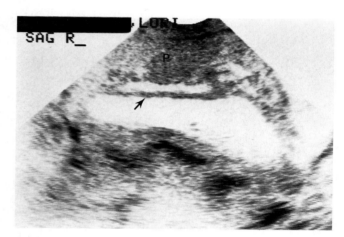

B

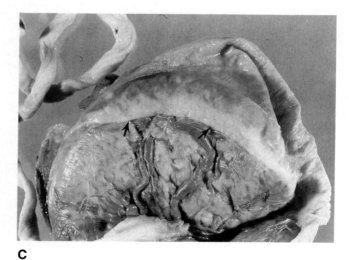

C

Fig. 9–7. A. Transverse and **B.** sagittal scans at 17 weeks show thick membranous fold (*arrows*) involving one portion of placenta (P). **C.** At delivery a partial circumvallate placenta was found. (*Arrows* indicate fold.)

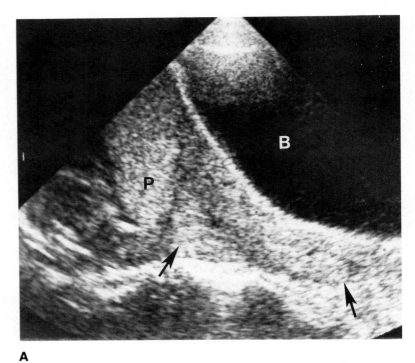

A

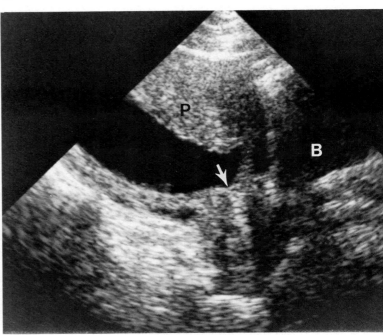

Fig. 9–8. A. Sagittal sector scan at 18.5 weeks shows elongated cervix (*arrows*) with anterior placenta (P) covering the area of cervix. **B.** Post-void scan shows placenta (P) to be well away from internal os (*arrow*) of cervix. B = maternal bladder.

B

and the placenta membranacea, in which chorionic villi cover most or all of the surface of the amniotic sac. These are both associated with antepartum and postpartum hemorrhage. They have not been documented sonographically.

Placenta accreta is a condition associated with a deficiency of the decidua basalis, in which the placenta is adherent to the myometrium.[1] The condition is divided into three categories: placenta accreta vera, in which the villi attach to but do not invade the myometrium; placenta increta, wherein the muscle is invaded; and placenta percreta, in which the villi fully penetrate the myometrium. Placenta accreta can result in antepartum and postpartum bleeding, and failure of the placenta to separate during the third stage of labor.

While we have not seen it, placenta accreta has been diagnosed sonographically.[16,17] The ultrasound diagnosis was based on the absence of the usual retroplacental hypoechoic zone of myometrium.

Temporary

The appearance of the placenta and myometrium may vary with different degrees of bladder filling.[6,18] This effect occurs most commonly in the second trimester. The full bladder compresses the anterior portion of the lower uterine segment against the posterior wall, artificially elongating the cervix. It may be necessary to repeat the examination following voiding to exclude the presence of a placenta previa (Fig. 9–8).

Transient myometrial thickening results from normal uterine contractions (Braxton-Hicks) which are imperceptible to the mother. They most commonly occur in the second trimester, but can be seen earlier (Fig. 9–9). Scanning over a short period of time (20 to 30 minutes) may demonstrate the appearance or disappearance of a thickened area of placenta, myometrium, or both. It is often possible to follow a contraction as it moves along the uterus (Fig. 9–10), causing localized thickening of placenta and/or myometrium that changes with respect to time. A contraction may mimic a placenta previa, and should be followed over time to exclude that diagnosis (Fig. 9–11). A contraction should also be distinguished from a leiomyoma, which would not change over time (Fig. 9–12).

UMBILICAL CORD

Umbilical cords insert either on the fetal surface or on the membranes. While cords may uncommonly attach at the center of the placental disc, most insert eccentrically. A placenta with a marginally inserted cord is often referred to as a "battledore placenta" (Fig. 9–13). The most important variation of umbilical cord attachment is the rare velamentous insertion. This occurs when the fetal vessels attach to the membranes at a variable distance from the fetal surface. Velamentous insertion is potentially hazardous since the fetal vessels are less protected and may be damaged during labor. In addition, fetal vessels running intramembranously across the internal os (vasa previa) may tear, leading to fetal blood loss. Such vessels traversing the internal os may be seen sonographically.[55]

PLACENTAL CALCIFICATION

Placental calcium deposition is a normal physiologic process that occurs throughout pregnancy.[1] During the first 6 months, microscopic calcification occurs. Macroscopic plaques appear in the third trimester, most commonly after 33 weeks.[19,20] The calcium is primarily deposited in the basal plate and septa, but is also found in the perivillous and subchorionic spaces. Plaques of calcium are readily detected by sonography as strong intraplacental echoes that do not produce significant acoustic shadows (Fig. 9–14). Septal calcifications result in the circular configuration seen in heavily calcified placentas. This has been incorrectly described as a cotyledonous pattern,[21] but it in fact reflects the lobes as defined by the maternal septa.

Placental calcification has been studied by histologic,[22,23] chemical,[24] radiographic[19] and sonographic[20] techniques, with the following conclusions: The incidence of placental calcification increases exponentially with increasing gestational age, beginning at about 29 weeks[19,20,22,24] (Fig. 9–15). More than 50% of placentas show some degree of calcification after 33 weeks. There is no increased calcification in postmature placentas.[1,20,22,24] Placental calcification is more common in women of lower parity.[19,20,22] It is likely related to maternal serum calcium levels.[1,25] Placental calcification is more common in late summer and early fall deliveries, at which times maternal serum calcium levels are highest.[20,23,25]

Thus far, there is no proof that placental calcification has any pathologic or clinical significance.[1,26,27]

MACROSCOPIC LESIONS OF THE PLACENTA

Table 9–1 lists the more common macroscopic lesions of the placenta (Fig. 9–16). Of these, subchorionic fibrin deposition, intervillous thrombosis, perivillous fibrin deposition, hydatidiform change, and chorioangioma have been diagnosed sonographically.

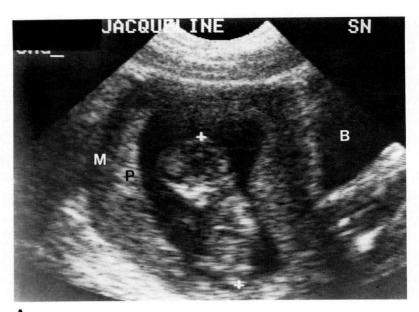

A

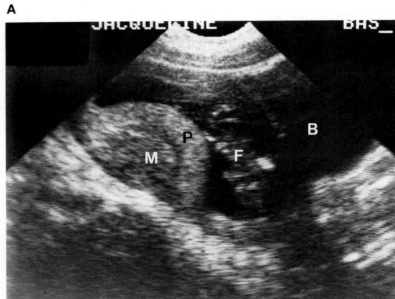

Fig. 9–9. **A.** Sagittal sector scan at 12 weeks shows posterior placenta (P). **B.** Scan in same location 20 minutes later shows contraction involving placenta (P) and myometrium (M). F = fetus; B = maternal bladder. **C.** Sagittal sector scan of another patient at 15 weeks shows contraction involving posterior placenta (P) and myometrium (M). **D.** 15 minutes later, contraction has disappeared. P = placenta.

B

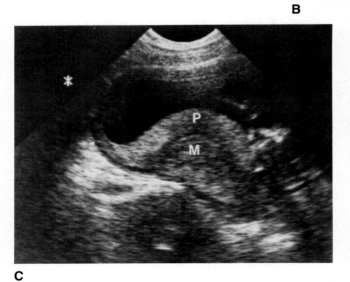

C

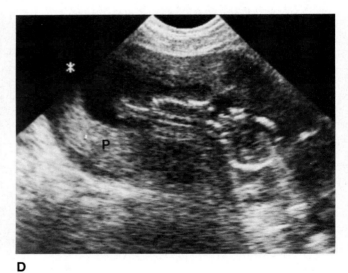

D

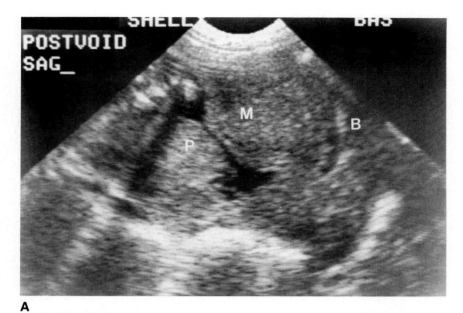

A

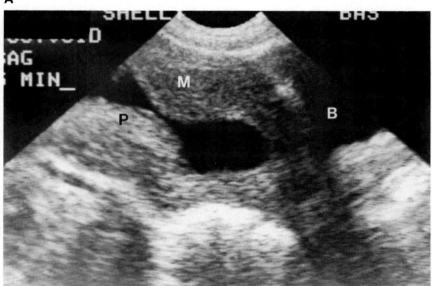

B

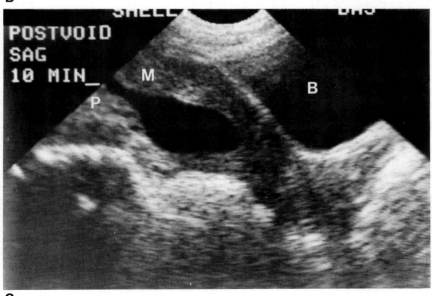

C

Fig. 9–10. A. Sagittal sector scan at 15 weeks shows contraction involving posterior placenta (P) and anterior myometrium (M) in lower segment of uterus. B = maternal bladder. **B.** 5 minutes later, contraction is less pronounced. **C.** 10 minutes later, placenta and anterior myometrium appear smooth.

141

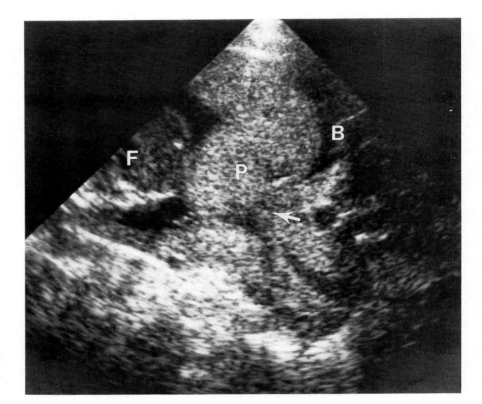

Fig. 9–11. Sagittal scan at 18.5 weeks shows anterior placenta (P) covering internal os (*arrow*). Maternal bladder is empty. This is same patient as in **Fig. 9–8,** at different time during same examination. B = maternal bladder; F = fetus.

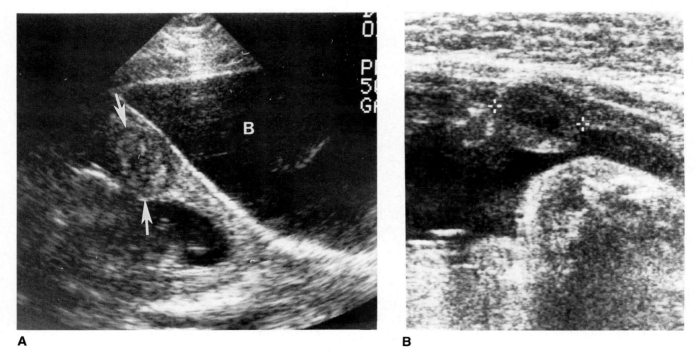

Fig. 9–12. A. Sagittal sector scan at 14.5 weeks shows round solid mass (*arrows*) in anterior wall of uterus, consistent with leiomyoma. B = maternal bladder. **B.** Linear scan at 29 weeks confirms presence of leiomyoma (*cursors*).

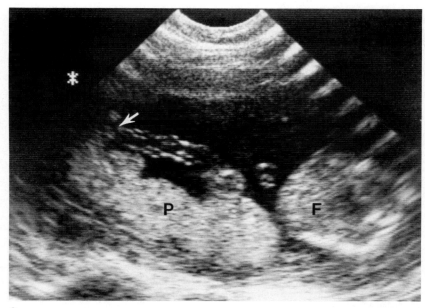

A

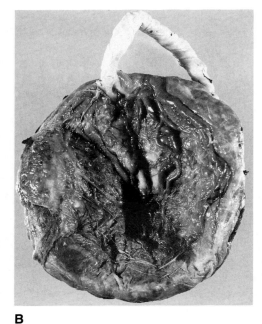

B

Fig. 9–13. A. Transverse scan at 20 weeks shows posterior placenta (P) with marginal cord insertion (*arrow*). F = fetus. **B.** Gross photograph of placenta confirms marginally-inserted umbilical cord.

Subchorionic Fibrin Deposition

Subchorionic anechoic or hypoechoic (sonolucent) areas may be demonstrated in approximately 10 to 15% of obstetric sonograms (Fig. 9–17).[1] These correspond to areas of subchorionic fibrin deposition in the term placenta,[28] and have no clinical significance.[1,29] Subchorionic fibrin refers to a laminated collection of fibrin between the chorionic plate and placental villi. It is a result of pooling and stasis of maternal blood in the intervillous space beneath the chorion, which leads to thrombosis and secondary fibrin deposition. It is often seen beneath the insertion of the umbilical cord.

A rare pathologic entity described in the literature that might produce a subchorionic sonolucent lesion is

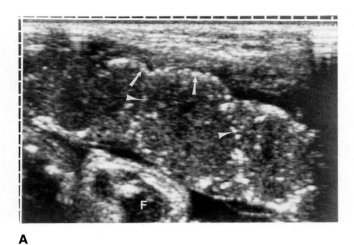

A

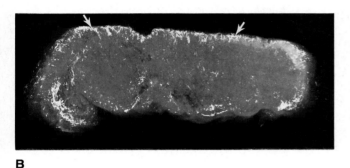

B

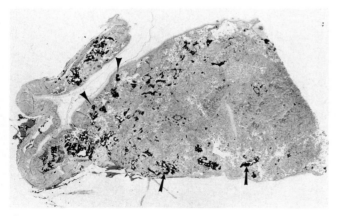

C

Fig. 9–14. A. Anterior placenta at 39 weeks contains prominent calcifications, especially in basal plate (*arrows*) and septa (*arrowheads*). F = fetus. **B.** Radiograph of tissue slice confirms presence of calcification. (*Arrows* indicate basal plate.) **C.** Photomicrograph of tissue stained for calcium shows deposits along basal plate (*arrows*), in subchorionic area (*arrowheads*), and in pervillous space (*open arrows*).

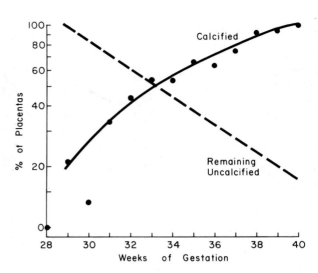

Fig. 9–15. Placental calcification versus gestational age. (*Reprinted with permission from* Radiology. *1982; 142:707.*)

massive subchorial thrombosis (Breus' mole). This entity often leads to premature delivery, and a large, fresh subchorionic hematoma is found on gross examination. The pathogenesis is thought to be extensive venous obstruction leading to massive pooling and stasis.[1] This process is considered by Fox to be unrelated to the mechanism that produces subchorionic fibrin deposition.[1]

Intervillous Thrombosis

Intervillous thromboses are intraplacental areas of hemorrhage, with a variable gross appearance depending on the age of the lesion. Fresh lesions are dark red, but with aging change to brown, yellow, and finally white. Usually, there are visible laminations that microscopically consist of layers of fibrin. Both fetal and maternal red blood cells are present, suggesting that a leakage of fetal cells from a villous tear stimulates maternal coagulation.[30] Intervillous thromboses have been found in up to 50% of term placentas from uncomplicated pregnancies.[1] In Fox's own series, 36% of full-term placentas from uncomplicated pregnancies contained intervillous thromboses.[1]

Intervillous thromboses appear sonographically as sonolucent intraplacental lesions that vary in size from a few millimeters to several centimeters[31,32] (Figs. 9–18 and 9–19). They may extend to the subchorionic space or the basal plate. These lesions have been documented by sonography as early as 19 weeks.[32] The incidence of intervillous thrombosis is increased in cases of Rh isoimmunization,[31,33,34] suggesting that the presence of intervillous thrombosis in these mothers might lead to sensitization.

Recent studies have suggested that intraplacental sonolucent lesions may be associated with elevated ma-

TABLE 9–1. MACROSCOPIC LESIONS OF THE PLACENTA

	Incidence[a] (%)	Etiology	Microscopic description	Clinical significance
Intervillous thrombosis	36[b]	Bleeding from fetal vessels	Laminated fibrin and red cells surrounded by villi	Fetal-maternal hemorrhage
(Massive) perivillous fibrin deposition	22[b]	Pooling and stasis of blood in intervillous space	Fibrosed villi entrapped in fibrin	None
Septal cyst	19[b]	Obstruction of septal venous drainage by edematous villi	Small cyst (5–10 mm) within septum containing accellular fluid	None
Infarct	25[b]	Disorder of maternal vessels; retroplacental hemorrhage	Coagulation necrosis of villi	Dependent on extent and associated maternal condition
Subchorionic fibrin deposition	20[b]	Pooling and stasis of blood in subchorionic space	Laminated subchorionic fibrin without villi; secondary cyst formation may occur	None
Massive subchorial thrombus (Breus' mole)	Undetermined (rare)	Massive pooling and stasis due to extensive venous obstruction	Fresh thrombus with no villi	Abortion or premature onset of labor
Hydatidiform change		1. Complete mole	Generalized swelling of all villi	Predisposes to choriocarcinoma
		2. Triploidy; partial mole	Mild to moderate swelling of some villi	Associated with symptoms of preeclampsia
Chorioangioma	1[b]	Vascular malformation	Multiple capillaries in a loose stroma	Usually none, dependent on size
Teratoma	Rare	?	Tissue elements of three embryonic germ layers	None
Metastatic lesions	Rare	Melanoma, CA breast, CA bronchus most frequent		

[a] Full term, uncomplicated pregnancies.
[b] Reference 1.

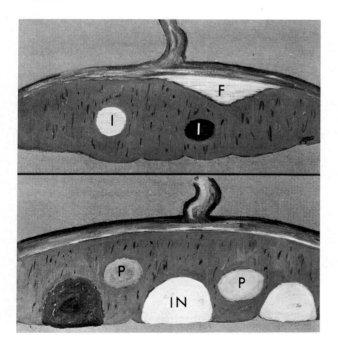

Fig. 9–16. Common macroscopic lesions of placenta. Subchorionic fibrin deposition (F) appears as laminated yellow-white plaques, sometimes associated with fresh clot and secondary cyst formation. Intervillous thrombosis (I) appears as round to oval lesions varying from red to laminated white, depending on age. Perivillous fibrin deposition (P) is seen as nonlaminated plaques varying from brown to white depending on age. True infarcts (IN) appear as dark red to white nonlaminated lesions adjacent to basal plate.

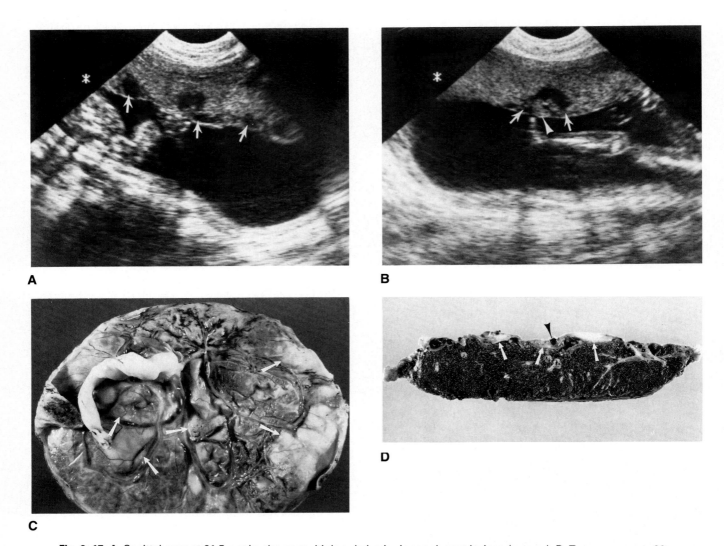

Fig. 9–17. A. Sagittal scan at 21.5 weeks shows multiple subchorionic sonolucent lesions (*arrows*). **B.** Transverse scan 90 degrees to central lesion in **A** shows subchorionic lesion (*arrows*) with vessel overlying it (*arrowhead*). **C.** Gross photograph of placenta shows multiple deposits of subchorionic fibrin corresponding to lesions seen on sonography (*arrows*). **D.** Section of placenta shows subchorionic fibrin deposition (*arrows*) corresponding to lesions in **A**. Note vessel (*arrowhead*) overlying central lesion (see **B**).

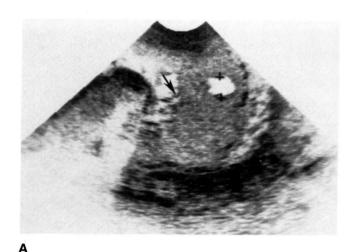

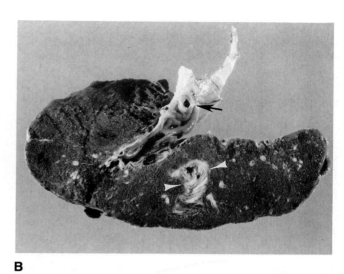

Fig. 9–18. A. Sector scan at 36.5 weeks shows intraplacental sonolucent lesion (*cursors*). *Arrow* = umbilical cord insertion. **B.** Corresponding section of placenta shows intervillous thrombus (*arrowheads*) with characteristic laminated fibrin. *Arrow* = umbilical cord. (*Reprinted with permission from* Prenatal Ultrasound: A Color Atlas with Anatomic and Pathologic Correlation. *New York, NY: Churchill Livingstone; 1987.*)

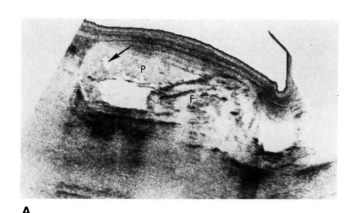

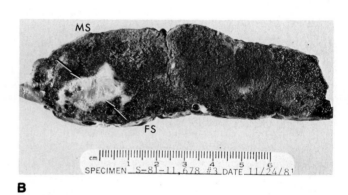

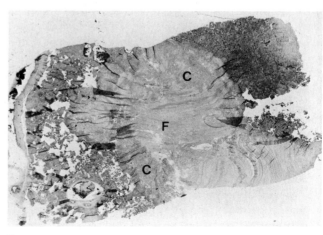

Fig. 9–19. A. Longitudinal sonogram at 29.5 weeks demonstrates sonolucent intraplacental lesion (*arrow*) in superior aspect of placenta (P). F = fetus. **B.** Gross specimen cut at right angle through lesion in **A** shows lesion (*arrows*) is composed of laminated fibrin. MS = maternal surface; FS = fetal surface. **C.** Microscopic section shows laminated bands of fibrin (F). (C) represents coagulation necrosis of surrounding villi. (*Reprinted with permission from* Radiology. *1983; 147:197.*)

ternal serum alpha-fetoprotein levels in patients with normal-appearing fetuses.[35,36] However, none of the studies provides pathologic evaluation of the lesions seen on the antenatal sonographic examination. We suspect that if the correlation is valid, it would be true only in the case of intervillous thromboses, since these are the only macroscopic placental lesions which are known to contain fetal blood.

Perivillous Fibrin Deposition

Perivillous fibrin deposition results from pooling and stasis of blood in the intervillous space. The lesions are seen as nonlaminated plaques, varying in color from brown to white depending on age. Sonographically, they appear as intraplacental sonolucent lesions (Fig. 9–20). Almost all full-term placentas contain some degree of perivillous fibrin deposition.[1] In approximately 22%, the plaques are large enough to be seen macroscopically.[1] Perivillous fibrin deposition is of no clinical significance.[26]

Maternal Lakes

"Maternal lakes" are sonolucent lesions in the placenta which correspond to blood-filled spaces at delivery. This entity is not described in the pathology literature. We believe that maternal lakes represent an early stage of intervillous thrombosis and/or perivillous fibrin deposition before the fibrin is laid down. Flow can be demonstrated in some of these lesions on real-time sonography. It is likely that in those lesions with particularly active flow, less fibrin is deposited so that the lesion is "empty" on gross inspection at delivery (Figs. 9–21 and 9–22).

Infarcts

Placental infarcts result from coagulation necrosis of villi and occur most commonly at the base of the placenta; they vary in size from a few millimeters to many centimeters. Although small infarcts are found in 25% of placentas of uncomplicated pregnancies, they occur with increased frequency in pregnancies complicated by preeclampsia and essential hypertension. Small infarcts have no clinical significance. However, extensive infarction, involving more than 10% of the placental parenchyma, is a reflection of maternal vascular disease.[26]

We have as yet been unable to document placental infarcts sonographically. We suspect that this is due to the composition of infarcts; ie, villi, even "ghost villi" that are present in infarcts, are echogenic. The sonolucent lesions that we have documented have been composed of either fibrin or blood.

Hydatidiform Change

Multiple diffuse intraplacental sonolucent lesions are abnormal and usually represent hydatidiform change.[28,37] Hydatidiform change can be separated into two groups.

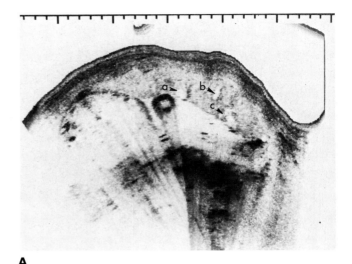

A

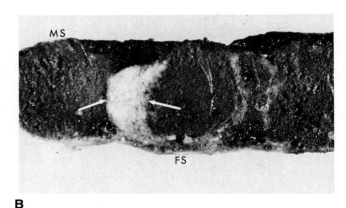

B

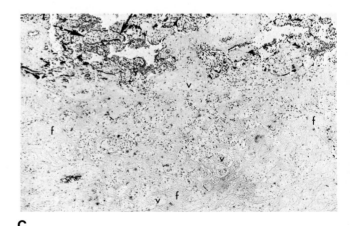

C

Fig. 9–20. A. Transverse sonogram at 31 weeks shows three intraplacental sonolucent lesions (a,b,c). B. This placenta contained multiple areas of perivillous fibrin deposition. Gross specimen at right angles to lesion "a" in A shows irregular, nonlaminated collection of perivillous fibrin (*arrows*). FS = fetal surface; MS = maternal surface. C. Fibrin (f) separates villi (v) and obliterates intervillous space. Normal villi surrounded by maternal red cells are present at the periphery (*arrows*). (H&E, X 55.)

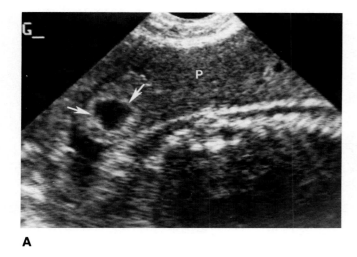

A

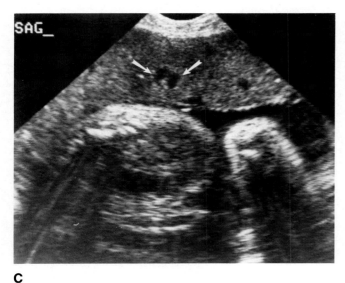

C

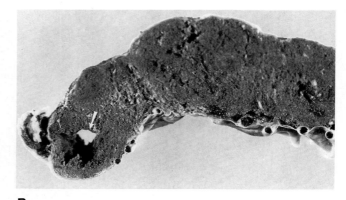

B

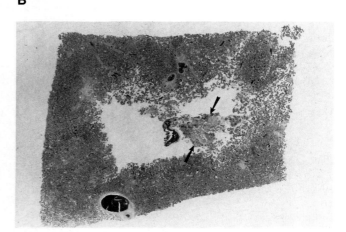

D

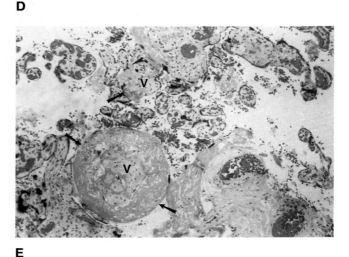

E

Fig. 9–21. A. Sector scan at 35 weeks shows intraplacental sonolucent lesion (*arrows*). P = placenta. **B.** At delivery, lesion (*arrow*) contained blood which fell out upon sectioning. **C.** Sector scan of same placenta at 35 weeks shows another intraplacental sonolucent lesion (*arrows*) with echogenic focus within. **D.** Following term delivery, corresponding microscopic section of placenta shows avillous space and area of focal villi surrounded by fibrin (*arrows*). **E.** Higher magnification demonstrates perivillous fibrin (*arrows*). V = villi.

The first is the complete or classical mole (Fig. 9–23) where there is hydatidiform swelling of all villi, a diploid karyotype, and absence of an embryo. A viable fetus may coexist with a true mole in the case of a twin pregnancy with one twin surviving (Fig. 9–24). The second is the partial mole, showing areas of molar change alternating with normal villi (Fig. 9–25). A fetus may be present and is often triploid (69 chromosomes) (Fig. 9–26). Micro-

scopically, both show trophoblastic hyperplasia, although it is usually less prominent in the partial mole which has other distinctive microscopic features.[38–41]

Clinically, partial moles may present with early onset of preeclampsia in the second trimester. Careful pathologic study, including cytogenetic analysis and monitoring of chorionic gonadotropin levels, is warranted in such cases. A few cases of partial moles that progressed to trophoblastic disease requiring chemotherapy have been reported.[41–43]

Primary Neoplasm (Chorioangioma)

There are two nontrophoblastic primary tumors of the placenta: the relatively common chorioangioma and the

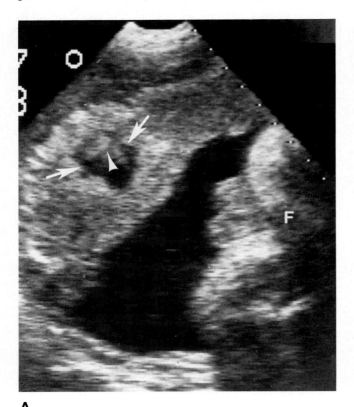

A

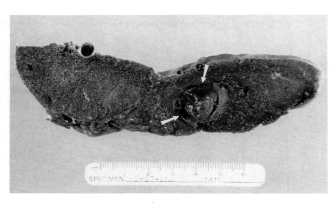

B

Fig. 9–22. A. Sagittal scan at 37 weeks shows sonolucent intraplacental lesion (*arrows*) with flow within (*arrowhead*) seen in real-time. F = fetus. (*Courtesy of Dr. John McKennan, Mohawk Valley General Hospital, Ilion, NY.*) **B.** Corresponding section of placenta following term delivery shows intraparenchymal collection of semiliquid blood and peripheral fibrin (*arrows*). Microscopic examination confirmed diagnosis of intervillous thrombosis.

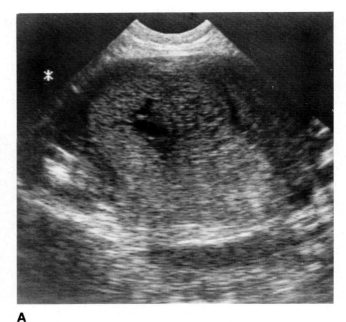

A

B

Fig. 9–23. A. Sonogram of hydatidiform mole showing vesicular echo pattern. **B.** Gross specimen shows multiple grape-like cysts. (*Courtesy of Dr. David Jones, Department of Pathology, SUNY Upstate Medical Center, Syracuse, New York. Reprinted with permission from* AJR. *1978; 131:961.*)

rare teratoma. The chorioangioma is a vascular malformation seen in approximately 1% of carefully studied placentas.[1] Small tumors occur within the placenta while large tumors may protrude from the fetal surface. The microscopic appearance is that of proliferating capillaries present in a loose fibrous stroma.

Sonographically, large chorioangiomas appear as well-circumscribed intraplacental mass lesions with a complex echo pattern[44] (Fig. 9–27). Large lesions are

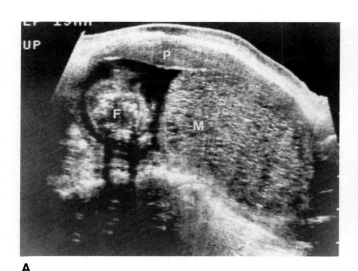
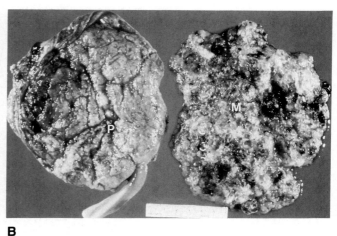

Fig. 9–24. A. Sagittal scan at 26 weeks shows anterior placenta (P) and fetus (F), with coexisting mole (M). **B.** At delivery, hydatidiform mole and placenta were separate. (*Reprinted with permission from* Prenatal Ultrasound: A Color Atlas with Anatomic and Pathologic Correlation. *New York, NY: Churchill Livingstone; 1987.*)

associated with fetal hydrops, cardiomegaly and congestive heart failure, low birth weight, premature labor, or fetal demise,[45–47] while small lesions usually have no associated problems.

THE PLACENTA IN MATERNAL AND FETAL DISORDERS

"Placental insufficiency" is a nonspecific clinical term which has no known morphologic basis. The placenta can lose up to 30% of its surface area and still maintain its function.[1,26] However, maternal vascular problems may induce a placental response to the anoxia which results from decreased uteroplacental blood flow. It is the decreased uteroplacental circulation which is believed to play a role in intrauterine growth retardation (IUGR).[26] Prior to Doppler sonography, human uteroplacental blood flow could not be studied noninvasively. As more data are obtained, Doppler evaluation of the uteroplacental circulation will likely provide useful information for the detection and management of some cases of IUGR.

The most constant placental abnormality in cases of Rh incompatibility, diabetes, anemia, and preeclampsia is variation in size. Visual assessment is usually sufficient

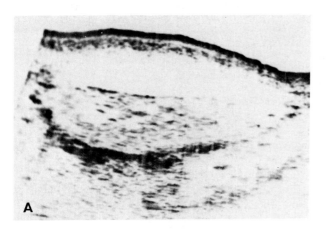
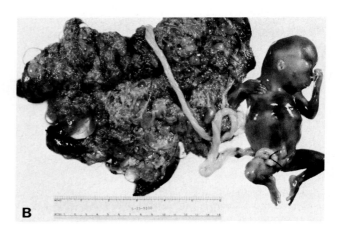

Fig. 9–25. A. Longitudinal sonogram of pre-eclamptic patient at 17 weeks shows multiple intraplacental sonolucent areas. Fetal movement was present. **B.** Patient became severely hypertensive and a hysterotomy was performed. Placenta contained areas of cystic (hydatidiform) change alternating with normal placental tissue. Chromosomes were not obtained. (*Reprinted with permission from* AJR. *1978; 131:961.*)

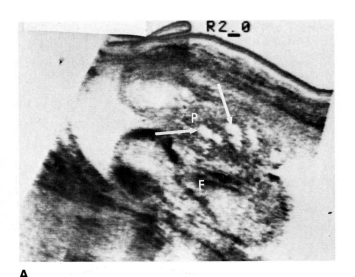

A

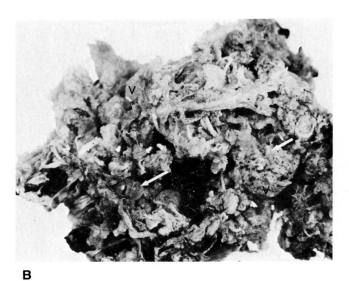

B

Fig. 9–26. A. Longitudinal sonogram at 20 weeks shows multiple sonolucent lesions (*arrows*) in placenta (P). F = fetus. A hysterotomy was performed because of severe maternal hypertension; a triploid female infant with multiple anomalies was delivered. (*Courtesy of Dr. Edward Bell, Crouse Irving Memorial Hospital, Syracuse, NY.*) **B.** Gross photograph of placenta shows areas of normal villi (V) coexisting with areas of hydatidiform change (*arrows*). (*Reprinted with permission from* Semin Roentgenol. *Grune & Stratton; 1982; 17:219.*)

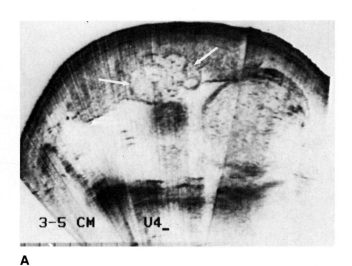

A

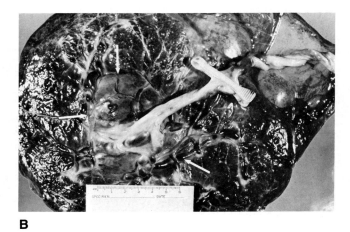

B

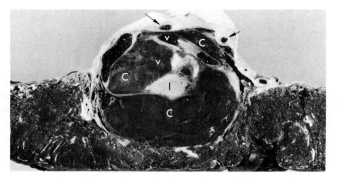

C

Fig. 9–27. A. Transverse sonogram at 24 weeks shows large solid subchorionic mass (*arrows*). **B.** At delivery, large subchorionic chorioangioma was found beneath cord insertion (*arrows*). **C.** Cross section of tumor shows vessels (v) of varying size within lesion. C = chorioangioma; I = infarct. (*Arrows* indicate vessels from cord.) (*Reprinted with permission from* AJR. *1980; 135:1273.*)

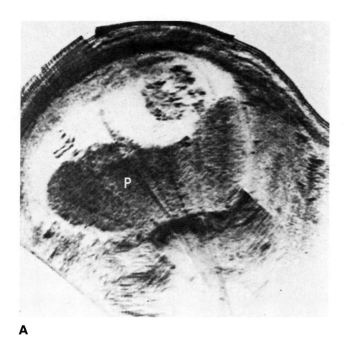

A

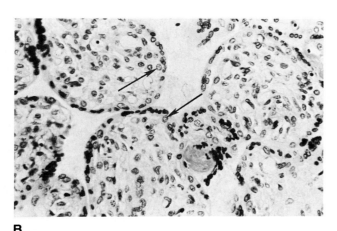

B

Fig. 9–28. A. Maternal-fetal Rh incompatibility. Transverse scan at 28 weeks shows grossly enlarged placenta. Marked fetal ascites present. (*Courtesy of Dr. Edward Bell, Crouse Irving Memorial Hospital, Syracuse, NY.*) **B.** Microscopically, villi are hypercellular with persistence of cytotrophoblasts (*arrows*). Mild edema is present. (H&E, X 100.)

to judge whether a placenta is too large or too small.

The placenta may be markedly enlarged in cases of hemolytic disease of the newborn. This appears to be secondary both to villous edema and to hyperplasia of the villous tree.[1,11] The amount of villous edema may vary in different areas of the same placenta. Sonographic examination shows a large placenta (Fig. 9–28) with an echo pattern that is similar to that of normal placentas.

Septal cysts are frequent, due to mechanical obstruction of septal venous drainage by the villous edema.[1] These have not been diagnosed sonographically.

Placentas of diabetic mothers are often unduly large due to villous edema.[1,11] Septal cysts are more frequent in these placentas as well. Placentas of mothers who are severely anemic also tend to be large but histologically normal.[1]

Placentas from preeclamptic mothers tend to be slightly smaller than the norm.[1] There is a high incidence of placental infarction in such patients, ranging from 33% of mild cases to 60% of severely affected patients. In half of the latter group, placental infarcts involving more than 5% of the placental tissue are present. This has not as yet been well documented sonographically.

There is an increased incidence of retroplacental hematomas in preeclamptic patients,[1] which undoubtedly accounts in part for the increased incidence of infarction in these patients. Placental abruption has been reported in association with cocaine abuse, which is known to have hypertensive and vasoconstrictive effects.[48]

RETROPLACENTAL HEMORRHAGE

Bleeding from placenta previa usually occurs near or at term, while retroplacental or marginal hemorrhage may occur as early as the first trimester. Retroplacental hemorrhage may manifest itself in three ways: (1) external bleeding without formation of a significant intrauterine hematoma; (2) formation of a retroplacental or marginal hematoma with or without external bleeding; and (3) formation of a submembranous clot at a distance from the placenta, with or without external bleeding (Fig.

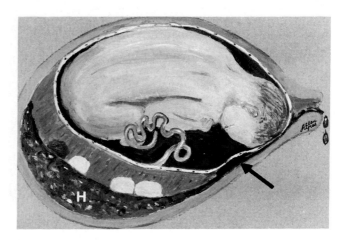

Fig. 9–29. Artist's drawing of retroplacental hematoma (H) with submembranous dissection (*arrow*) and external bleeding. Placental infarcts are present.

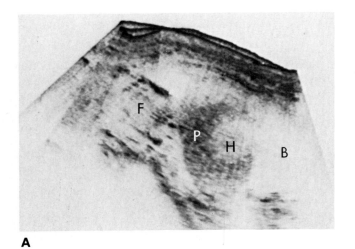

A

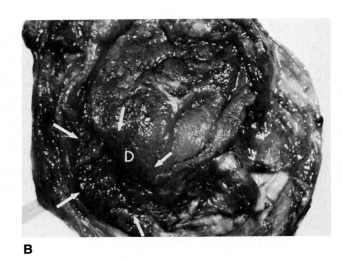

B

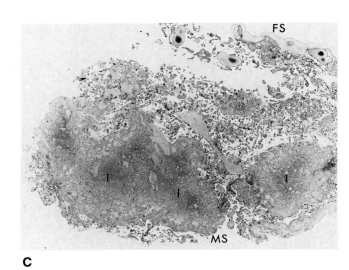

C

Fig. 9–30. A. Midline longitudinal scan at 18 weeks shows 3.5-cm retroplacental mass (H). P = placenta; B = bladder; F = fetus. **B.** Hysterotomy was performed due to severe disseminated intravascular coagulation. An area of hemorrhage was found, covering lateral portion of basal plate and extending to placental margin and over chorionic membrane (*arrows*). A depression in placenta (D) was present at hematoma site. **C.** Microscopic section through area (D) shows infarcts (I) based on maternal surface (MS) at hematoma site. FS = fetal surface. (*Reprinted with permission from* J Clin Ultrasound. *1981; 9:208.*)

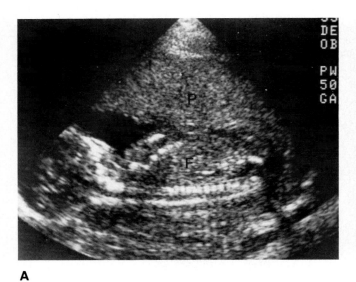

A

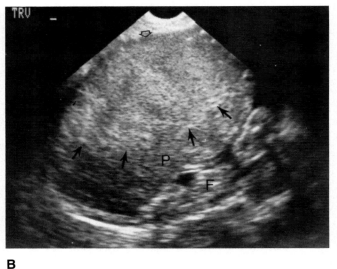

B

Fig. 9–31. A. Real-time sector scan at 17 weeks shows anterior placenta (P). F = fetus. **B.** At 35 weeks, patient presented with vaginal bleeding and hypotension. An inhomogeneous hyperechoic collection (*arrow*) is present between placenta (P) and myometrium (*open arrows*). F = fetus. At caesarian section, a 75% abruptio placenta was found. (*Courtesy of Dr. Michael Oliphant, Crouse-Irving Memorial Hospital, Syracuse, NY.*)

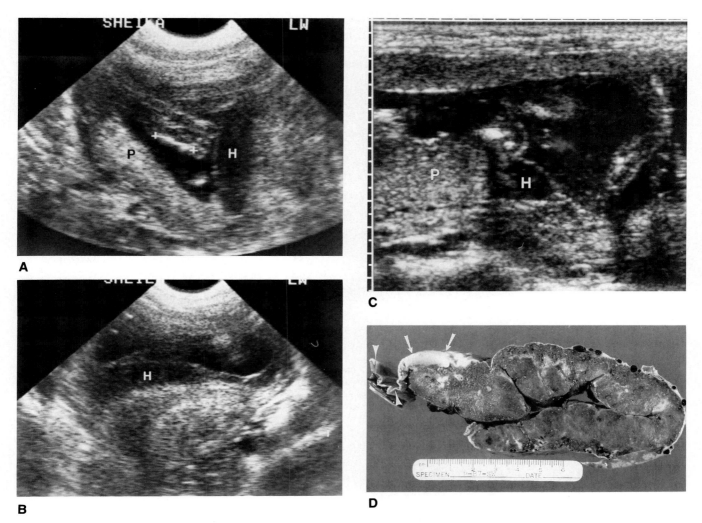

Fig. 9–32. A. Sagittal and **B.** transverse sector scans at 13 weeks in patient with vaginal bleeding show subchorionic collection (H) containing low level echoes, adjacent to posterior placenta (P). **C.** Follow-up sagittal scan at 21 weeks shows subchorionic sonolucent collection (H) adjacent to placenta (P). Collection has decreased in size. **D.** Section of placenta shows subchorionic fibrin (*arrows*) at margin of placenta adjacent to insertion of fetal membranes (*arrowheads*).

9–29). Sonographic examination in cases of antepartum bleeding will be negative if most of the bleeding is external.

A significant retroplacental or marginal hematoma will appear as a hypoechoic or complex mass on sonography[49–51] (Figs. 9–30 and 9–31). A hematoma that collects beneath the placental membranes at a distance from the placenta will appear as an anechoic, hypoechoic or mixed collection beneath the elevated membranes[49] (Figs. 9–32 and 9–33).

The size of the hematoma may be followed by serial ultrasound examinations. Even if follow-up study indicates that the lesion has disappeared, careful examination of the placenta following delivery will show a thin layer of organized hematoma or fibrin along the membranes.

The incidence of marginal hemorrhage, which may be associated with either circumvallate placenta or low-lying placenta, is approximately 1.9%.[1] Marginal hemorrhage in cases of low implantation of the placenta is thought to be due to traction of the myometrial fibers during obliteration of the lower uterine segment. This causes separation of the spongy and compact layers of decidua, leading to hemorrhage.[52]

The clinical significance of retroplacental hemorrhage is dependent upon the size and extent of the lesion.[53,54] Disseminated intravascular coagulation may occur in cases of retroplacental hemorrhage as a result of tissue injury.

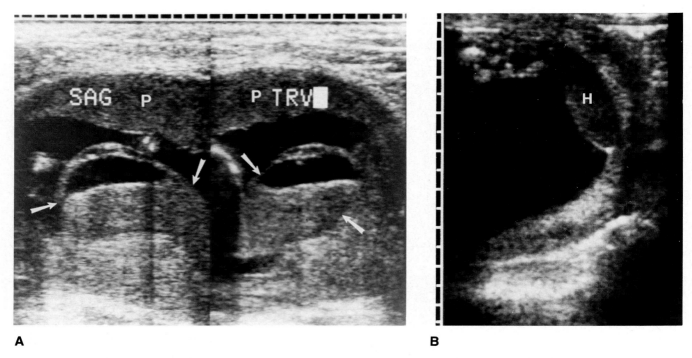

Fig. 9–33. A. Sagittal and transverse images at 17 weeks show complex subchorionic collection (*arrows*) opposite anterior placenta (P). Patient had vaginal bleeding. **B.** Follow-up transverse scan at 28 weeks shows small residual subchorionic hematoma (H). (*Courtesy of Medical Imaging Department, Crouse Irving Memorial Hospital, Syracuse, NY.*)

REFERENCES

1. Fox H. *Pathology of the Placenta*. Philadelphia: Saunders; 1978.
2. Crawford JM. Vascular anatomy of the human placenta. *Am J Obstet Gynecol*. 1962; 84:1543.
3. Ramsey EM, Corner GW, Donner MW. Serial and cineradioangiographic visualization of maternal circulation in the primate (hemochorial) placenta. *Am J Obstet Gynecol*. 1963; 86:213.
4. Wigglesworth JF. Vascular anatomy of the human placenta and its significance for placental pathology. *J Obstet Gynaecol Br Commonw*. 1969; 76:979.
5. Ramsey EM. Circulation in the maternal placenta of the Rhesus monkey and man with observations on the marginal lakes. *Am J Anat*. 1956; 98:159.
6. Spirt BA, Kagan EH, Rozanski R. Sonographic anatomy of the normal placenta. *J Clin Ultrasound*. 1979; 7:204.
7. Smith DF, Foley DW. Real-time ultrasound and pulsed doppler evaluation of the retroplacental clear area. *J Clin Ultrasound*. 1982; 10:215.
8. Winsberg F. Echographic changes with placental aging. *J Clin Ultrasound*. 1973; 1:52.
9. Fisher CC, Garrett W, Kossoff G. Placental aging monitored by gray scale echography. *Am J Obstet Gynecol*. 1976; 124:483.
10. Haney AS, Trought WS. The sonolucent placenta in high-risk obstetrics. *Obstet Gynecol*. 1980; 55:38.
11. Perrin EVDK, Sander CH. Introduction: How to examine the placenta and why. In: Perrin EVDK, ed. *Pathology of the Placenta*. New York, NY: Churchill Livingstone; 1984.
12. Earn AA. Placental anomalies. *Can Med Assoc J*. 1951; 65:118.
13. Torpin R, Hart BF. Placenta bilobata. *Am J Obstet Gynecol*. 1941; 42:38.
14. Scott JS. Placenta extrachorialis (placenta marginata and placenta circumvallate): A factor in antepartum hemorrhage. *J Obstet Gynaecol Br Commonw*. 1960; 67:904.
15. Naftolin F, Khudr G, Benirschke K, et al. The syndrome of chronic abruptio placentae, hydrorrhea, and circumvallate placentae. *Am J Obstet Gynecol*. 1973; 116:347.
15A. Cutillo DP, Swayne LC, Schwartz JR. Intra-amniotic hemorrhage secondary to placenta circumvallate. *J Ultrasound Med*. 1989; 8:399.
16. Pasto ME, Kurtz AB, Rifkin MD, et al. Ultrasonographic findings in placenta increta. *J Ultrasound Med*. 1983; 2:155.
17. deMendonca LK. Sonographic diagnosis of placenta accreta: Presentation of six cases. *J Ultrasound Med*. 1988; 7:211.
18. Zemlyn S. The effect of the urinary bladder in obstetrical sonography. *Radiology*. 1978; 128:169.
19. Tindall VR, Scott JS. Placental calcification. A study of 3,025 singleton and multiple pregnancies. *J Obstet Gynaecol Br Commonw*. 1965; 72:356.
20. Spirt BA, Cohen WN, Weinstein HM. The incidence of

placental calcification in normal pregnancies. *Radiology*. 1982; 142:707.

21. Grannum PAT, Berkowitz RL, Hobbins JC. The ultrasonic changes in the maturing placenta and their relation to fetal pulmonic maturity. *Am J Obstet Gynecol*. 1979; 133:915.

22. Wentworth P. Macroscopic placental calcification and its clinical significance. *J Obstet Gynaecol Br Commonw*. 1965; 72:215.

23. Fujikura D. Placental calcification and seasonal difference. *Am J Obstet Gynecol*. 1963; 87:46.

24. Jeacock MK. Calcium content of the human placenta. *Am J Obstet Gynecol*. 1963; 87:34.

25. Mull JW, Bill AH. Variations in serum calcium and phosphorus during pregnancy. *Am J Obstet Gynecol*. 1934; 27:510.

26. Fox H. Pathology of the placenta. *Clinics in Obstet and Gynecol*. 1986; 13:501.

27. Spirt BA, Gordon LP. The placenta as an indicator of fetal maturity—fact and fancy. *Semin Ultrasound*. 1984; 5:290.

28. Spirt BA, Kagan EH, Rozanski RM. Sonolucent areas in the placenta: sonographic and pathologic correlation. *AJR*. 1978; 131:961.

29. Benirschke K, Driscoll SG. *The Pathology of the Human Placenta*. New York, NY: Springer; 1967.

30. Kaplan C, Blanc WA, Elias J. Identification of erythrocytes in intervillous thrombi: A study using immunoperoxidase identification of hemoglobins. *Hum Pathol*. 1982; 13:554.

31. Hoogland HJ, de Haan J, Vooys GP. Ultrasonographic diagnosis of intervillous thrombosis related to Rh isoimmunization. *Gynecol Obstet Inves*. 1979; 10:237.

32. Spirt BA, Gordon LP, Kagan EH. Intervillous thrombosis: Sonographic and pathologic correlation. *Radiology*. 1983; 147:197.

33. Javert CT, Reiss C. The origin and significance of macroscopic intervillous coagulation hematomas (red infarcts) of the human placenta. *Surg Gynecol Obstet*. 1952; 94:257.

34. Devi B, Jennison RF, Langley FA. Significance of placental pathology in transplacental hemorrhage. *J Clin Path*. 1968; 21:322.

35. Perkes EA, Baim RS, Goodman KJ, Macri JN. Second-trimester placental changes associated with elevated maternal serum fetoprotein. *Am J Obstet Gynecol*. 1982; 144:935.

36. Fleischer AC, Kurtz AB, Wapner RJ, et al. Elevated alpha-fetoprotein and a normal fetal sonogram: association with placental abnormalities. *AJR*. 1988; 150:881.

37. Naumoff P, Szulman AE, Weinstein B, et al. Ultrasonography of partial hydatidiform mole. *Radiology*. 1981; 140:467.

38. Szulman AE, Surti U. The syndromes of hydatidiform mole. I: Cytogenetic and morphologic correlations. *Am J Obstet Gynecol*. 1978; 131:665.

39. Szulman AR, Surti U. The syndromes of hydatidiform mole. II: Morphologic evolution of the complete and partial mole. *Am J Obstet Gynecol*. 1978; 132:20.

40. Szulman AE, Philippe E, Boue JG, et al. Human triploidy: Association with partial hydatidiform moles and nonmolar conceptuses. *Hum Pathol*. 1981; 12:1016.

41. Szulman A. Trophoblastic disease: Complete and partial hydatidiform mole. In: Perrin EVDK, ed. *Pathology of the Placenta*. New York, NY: Churchill Livingstone; 1984.

42. Berkowitz RS, Goldstein DP, Marean AR, et al. Proliferative sequelae after evacuation of partial hydatidiform mole. *Lancet*. 1979; 2:804. Letter.

43. Szulman AE, Wong LC, Hsu C. Residual trophoblastic disease in association with partial hydatidiform mole. *Obstet Gynecol*. 1981; 57:392.

44. Spirt BA, Gordon LP, Cohen WN, et al. Antenatal diagnosis of chorioangioma of the placenta. *AJR*. 1980; 135:1273.

45. Battaglia MC, Woolever CA. Fetal and neonatal complications associated with recurrent chorioangiomas. *Pediatrics*. 1967; 41:62.

46. Wallenburg HCS. Chorioangioma of the placenta. *Obstet Gynecol Surg*. 1971; 26:411.

47. Leonidas JC, Beatty EC, Hall RT. Chorioangioma of the placenta. *Radiology*. 1975; 123:703.

48. Townsend RR, Laing FC, Jeffrey RB. Placental abruption associated with cocaine abuse. *AJR*. 1988; 150:1339.

49. Spirt BA, Kagan EH, Rozanski RM. Abruptio placenta: sonographic and pathologic correlation. *AJR*. 1979; 133:877.

50. Spirt BA, Kagan EH, Aubry RH. Clinically silent retroplacental hematoma: Sonographic and pathologic correlation. *J Clin Ultrasound*. 1981; 9:203.

51. Nyberg DA, Cyr DR, Mack LA, et al. Sonographic spectrum of placental abruption. *AJR*. 1987; 148:161.

52. Pratola D, Wilkin P. The placenta, umbilical cord, and amniotic sac. In: Gompel S, Silverberg SG, eds. *Pathology in Gynecology and Obstetrics*, 3rd ed. Philadelphia: Lippincott; 1985.

53. Nyberg DA, Mack LA, Benedetti TJ, et al. Placental abruption and placental hemorrhage: Correlation of sonographic findings with fetal outcome. *Radiology*. 1987; 164:357.

54. Stabile I, Campbell S, Grudzinskas JG. Threatened miscarriage and intrauterine hematomas: Sonographic and biochemical studies. *J Ultrasound Med*. 1989; 8:289.

55. Reuter KL, Davidoff A, Hunter T. Vasa previa. *J Clin Ultrasound*. 1988; 16:346.

10 Sonography of the Umbilical Cord and Intrauterine Membranes

David Graham • Arthur C. Fleischer • Glynis A. Sacks

Because the umbilical cord and membranes share similar developmental origins, they will both be considered in this chapter. With the recent increased use of percutaneous umbilical cord blood sampling and Doppler studies, there has been renewed interest in the sonographic evaluation of the umbilical cord. Intrauterine membranes can be delineated with sonography in patients who have bleeding episodes as well as in some uncomplicated pregnancies. This chapter will discuss the sonographic distinction between intrauterine membranes that can be associated with poor pregnancy outcome and those that cannot. It also discusses and illustrates the sonographic depiction of the umbilical cord with emphasis on normal and abnormal morphology.

FORMATION OF THE UMBILICAL CORD

The umbilical cord is formed in the early weeks of embryogenesis from a fusion between the body stalk (which contains the umbilical arteries, umbilical veins, and allantois) and the yolk stalk (which contains the omphalomesenteric stalk and remnant of the original yolk sac attachment). During this process, the two umbilical veins fuse to form a single vessel and the omphalomesenteric vessels are obliterated. The result is an umbilical cord, covered by amnion and containing a single umbilical vein, and two umbilical arteries supported in Wharton jelly, a gelatinous substance that consists mainly of collagen in addition to elastin and muscle. Although the walls of the umbilical vessels have a large proportion of muscle, they lack collagen and elastin and so are able to change configuration with changes in osmotic pressure in the amniotic fluid.

STRUCTURE AND FUNCTION OF THE UMBILICAL CORD

The umbilical cord is quite variable in length, and normally contains two umbilical arteries and a single larger umbilical vein surrounded by a clear gelatinous Wharton jelly. A layer of amnion covers the umbilical cord except near the fetal insertion, where an epithelial covering is substituted. The arteries wind around the umbilical vein in a spiral fashion and, because the vessels are longer than the cord itself, there are a number of foldings and tortuosities producing protrusions or false knots on the cord surface. The umbilical vein provides oxygenated blood to the fetus and, on reaching the fetal abdominal wall, passes through the liver posteriorly and cephalad to terminate at the portal sinus (the main left portal vein). Deoxygenated blood from the fetal aorta passes to the hypogastric arteries, which wind superiorly and medially to enter the cord as the umbilical arteries.

The Wharton jelly that surrounds the vessels apparently has a protective function protecting the vessels from undue torsion and compression.[1]

Although the site of cord insertion is usually central into the placenta, eccentric cord insertion may occur in 48 to 75% of placentas.[2,3] In 5 to 6% of cases, marginal or velamentous insertion of the cord may occur.[4]

SONOGRAPHIC ANATOMY OF THE NORMAL CORD

The umbilical stalk and the yolk sac may occasionally be seen in the late first trimester, adjacent to the anterior abdominal wall of the fetus (Fig. 10–1). In the second and third trimesters, the cord is much more readily visualized, especially where there is excess amniotic fluid. In longitudinal section, a portion of the cord will be seen as a series of parallel lines (Fig. 10–2), while in transverse section, the arteries and umbilical vein may be seen as three separately circular luciencies (Figs. 10–3 and 10–4).

Pulsations, occurring at the same rate as fetal heart rate may be seen in real time. More commonly, several portions of cord are visualized, giving a "stack of coins" appearance.

Because there are different directions of flow in the umbilical cord, color Doppler image will demonstrate one color in the vein and another in the arteries. (Fig. 10–5, found on the color plate).

Where there is oligohydramnios, the cord may be

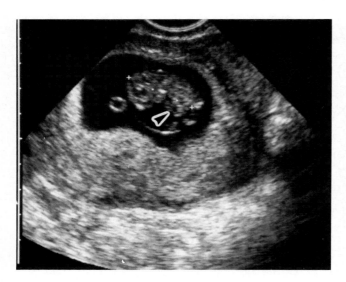

Fig. 10–1. Developing umbilical cord at 8 weeks. There is a suggestion of bowel herniating into the base of the cord (*arrowhead*). Yolk sac is extra-amniotic.

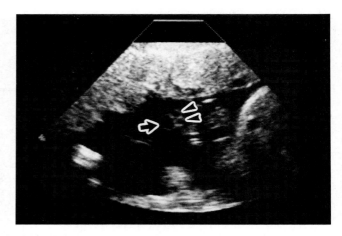

Fig. 10–3. Sonographic image of normal umbilical cord depicted in true short axis showing two arteries (*arrowheads*) adjacent to the single umbilical vein (*large arrow*).

difficult or impossible to visualize sonographically, even in late pregnancy.

By scanning near the center of the placenta, the insertion site of the cord may be demonstrated as a V- or U-shaped sonolucent area adjacent to the chorionic plate. At the insertion of the cord into the anterior abdominal wall of the fetus, the origins of the umbilical vein and hypogastric arteries may be seen (Fig. 10–6).

CORD ABNORMALITIES

Abnormalities of Cord Length

Although the average cord length is 55 cm, a normal range of cord length of 30 to 120 cm may be seen.[5] Extremes of cord length may occur from apparently no cord (achordia)[6] to lengths up to 300 cm.[5] Excessively long cords may predispose to vascular occlusion by

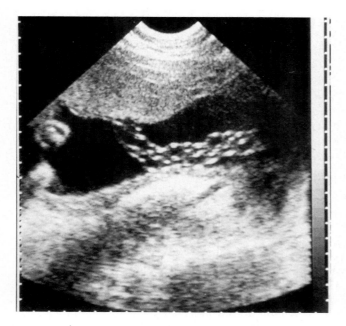

Fig. 10–2. Long axis of umbilical cord in 20-week pregnancy, demonstrating spiral course of umbilical arteries.

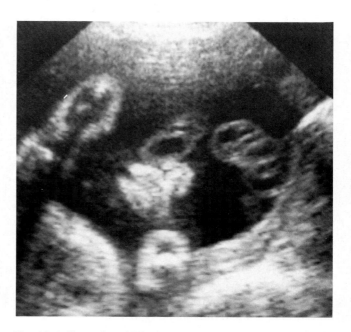

Fig. 10–4. Normal umbilical cord adjacent to fetal face demonstrating vein and two arteries in oblique section.

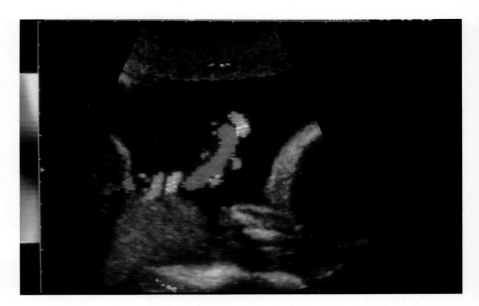

Fig. 10–5. Color Doppler image of normal umbilical cord with vein depicted as red and arteries depicted as blue.

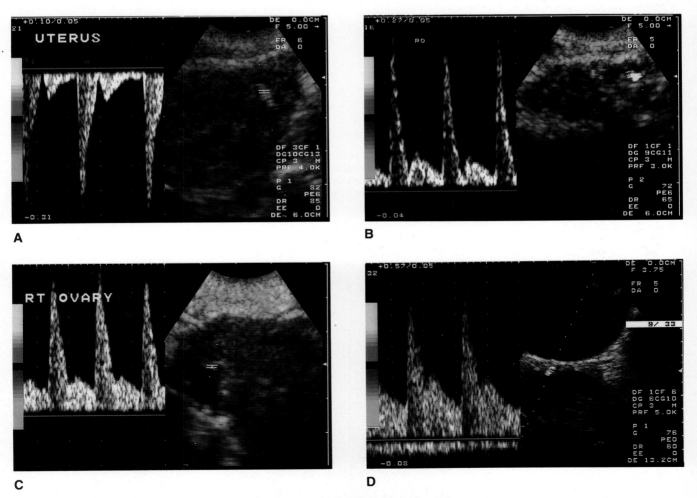

A

B

C

D

Fig. 11–1. Normal uterine and ovarian vessels with TV/CDS. **A.** Main uterine artery as it enters the myometrium (in red and blue) with accompanying arterial waveform. **B.** Main ovarian artery (shown in red) of right ovary with accompanying waveform. **C.** Same as **B** during maximal luteal function as noted by increased diastolic flow. **D.** Hemorrhagic corpus luteum. Complete torsion excluded by demonstration of arterial flow.

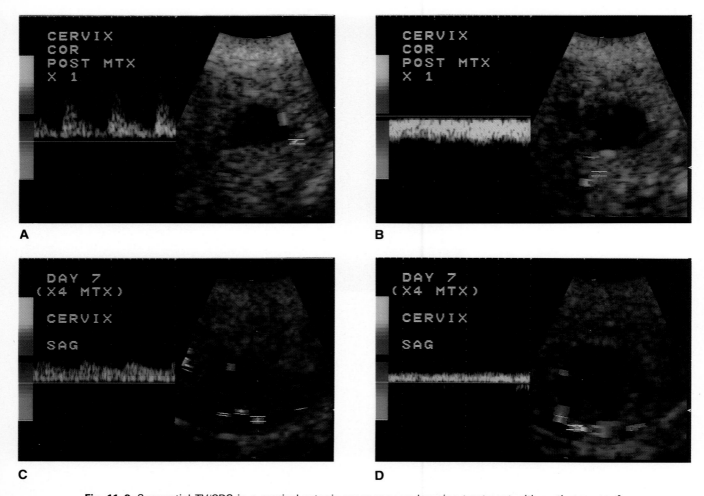

Fig. 11–2. Sequential TV/CDS in a cervical ectopic pregnancy undergoing treatment with methotrexate. **A.** Arterial flow 1 day post-initiation of methotrexate treatment. **B.** Same as **A** showing venous flow. **C.** Arterial flow after 4 doses of methotrexate treatment. **D.** Same as **C** showing venous flow. Both arterial and venous flow have decreased prior to sloughing of the remaining necrotic choriodecidua.

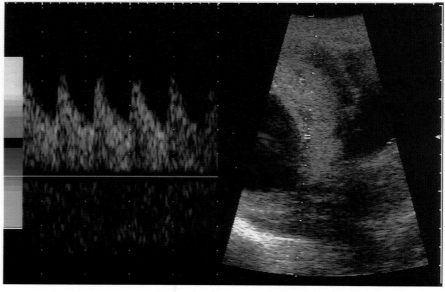

Fig. 11–3. For legend, see following page.

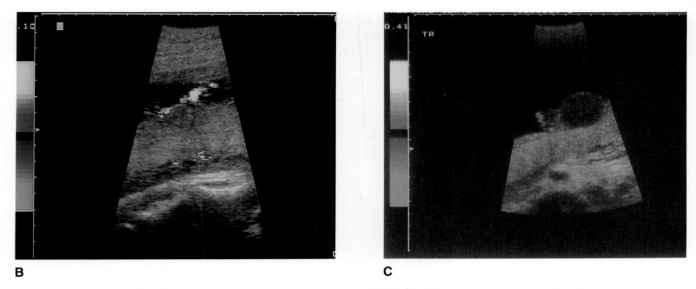

Fig. 11–3. TA/CDS of placental vessels. **A.** Arterial vessels overlying the chorionic plate. **B.** Umbilical cord origin from placenta. **C.** Chorioangioma appearing as hypovascular mass adjacent to cord origin.

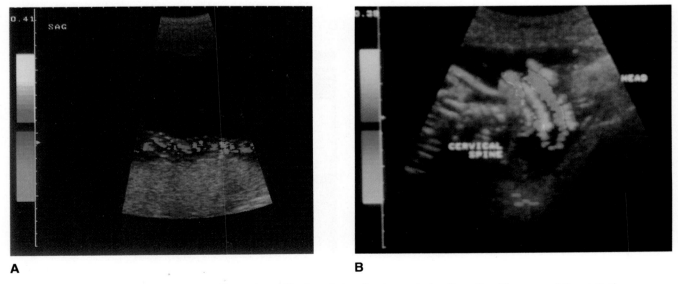

Fig. 11–4. Umbilical cord. **A.** Normal umbilical cord showing two arteries (in red) coiling around the central single vein. **B.** Nuchal cord.

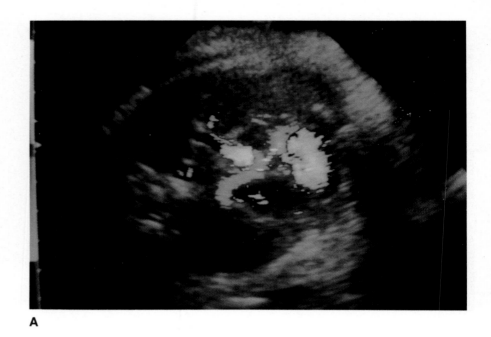

A

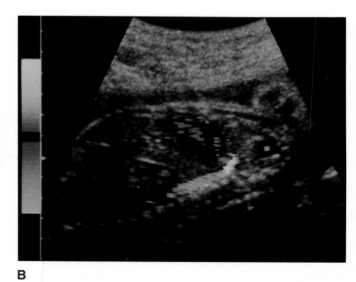

B

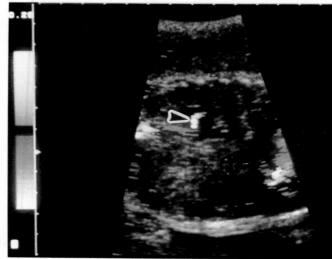

C

Fig. 11–5. Fetal heart. **A**. Normal heart, four chamber view. **B**. Aortic arch. **C**. Renal artery (*arrow*).

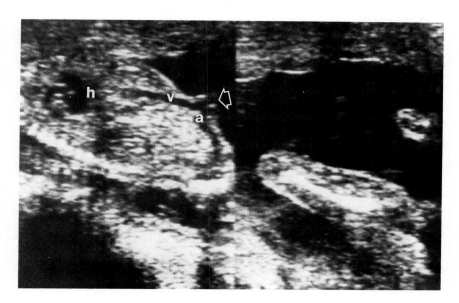

Fig. 10–6. Insertion of cord into fetus. Sagittal section of midtrimester fetus showing insertion of the cord (*arrow*) into the anterior abdominal wall. Division into the umbilical vein (v) and hypogastric artery (a) is shown. h = heart.

thrombi and by true knots, and also to cord prolapse during labor. Rarely, excessively short umbilical cords may be responsible for abruptio placentae, uterine inversion, or intrafunicular hemorrhage.[5] Although abnormalities of cord length may predispose to a number of these pathologic entities, it is impossible to determine umbilical cord length prior to delivery with current sonographic techniques.

Abnormalities of Cord Position

Normally, loops of umbilical cord lie anterior to the fetal abdominal wall and adjacent to the limbs. In a number of instances, however, they may be loopings of the cord around the fetal neck or limbs or, alternatively, loops of cord may lie between the fetal presenting part and the lower uterine segment (funic presentation). The most important umbilical cord malpositions include prolapses, knots, and neck, body, and shoulder loopings. Kamina and deTourris,[7] in a series of 1,750 deliveries, found 4 prolapses, 232 neck loopings, 45 shoulder loopings, and 13 cord knots. Walker and Pye found an incidence of nuchal cord of 17% at delivery.[8] This is not clinically diagnosable until delivery but has been recognized prenatally with ultrasound by demonstration of a loop of cord passing around the fetal neck (Fig. 10–7).[7,9–11] Although in singletons coiling of the cord around the neck is an uncommon cause of fetal death, in monoamniotic twins a significant portion of the high perinatal mortality rate is attributed to umbilical cord problems.[5]

Occasionally, loops of the cord may be seen lying between the fetal presenting part and the lower segment. It is important to recognize this because such a position predisposes to cord prolapse and possible fetal death at the time of rupture of the membranes. Funic presentation is more common with malpresentations such as breech or transverse lie.

Knotting of the cord, which usually occurs secondary to excessive fetal motion, occurs in approximately 1.1% of deliveries, and has an associated perinatal loss of 6.1%. True knot of the cord has not as yet been reported as being diagnosed prenatally.

Single Umbilical Artery (SUA)

Although the normal umbilical cord contains two umbilical arteries, a single umbilical artery may be seen in approximately 1% of all singleton births, 5% of twins, and 2.5% of abortuses (Fig. 10–8).[12] Bernischke and Brown first described a relationship between SUA and fetal malformations showing an increased incidence of genitourinary tract anomalies.[12,13] The incidence of SUA has been found to be increased in pregnancies subsequently ending in abortion, trisomy D or E, in offspring of diabetic mothers, and in black patients.[13,14]

Although there is a fourfold increase in perinatal mortality associated with SUA,[15] some of these deaths may be secondary to the major congenital malformations associated with SUA, while others remain unexplained. In following infants with SUA, Froehlich and Fujikura[16] found a high mortality (14%) but, in those who survived infancy, serious anomalies were no more common than in a control group. On the other hand, Bryan and Kohler,[17] following 98 infants, found that previously unrecognized malformations become apparent in ten.

Prenatal sonographic diagnosis of SUA in two fetuses at 34 and at 36 weeks has been reported by Jassani and Brennan.[13] The first infant subsequently died in utero and the second showed evidence of mild left hydronephrosis.

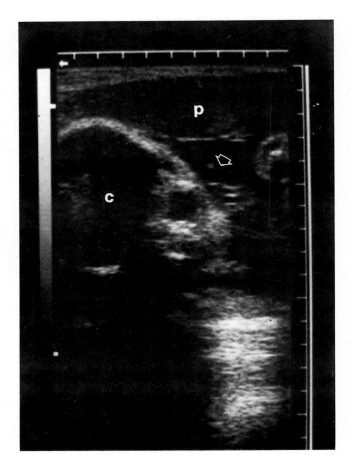

Fig. 10–7. Nuchal cord. In this third-trimester fetus with demonstrated variable decelerations on a nonstress test, there is sonographic evidence of a loop of cord (*arrow*) wrapped around the fetal neck. c = fetal cranium; p = placenta.

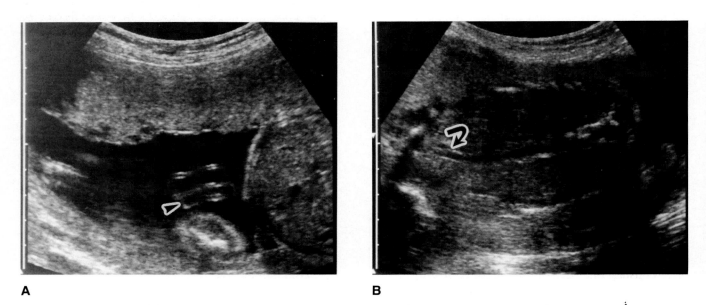

A

B

Fig. 10–8. Single umbilical artery. **A.** Long axis of cord demonstrating umbilical vein and single umbilical artery (*arrowhead*). **B.** Long axis image of iliac vessels demonstrating unilateral agenesis of the left hypogastric artery with preservation of the right (*arrow*). (*Courtesy of Philippe Jeanty, MD, PhD.*)

Umbilical Cord Masses

Masses of the umbilical cord, which are quite uncommon, have diverse etiologies. Such masses, or apparent masses, may be caused by:

1. False knots
2. True knots
3. Hematoma
4. Allantoic duct cyst
5. Neoplasms
6. Umbilical hernia
7. Omphalocele or gastroschisis

False knots, which clinically have no importance, essentially represent a varix of the umbilical vessels and are recognized grossly by a protrusion from the cord. Sonographically, they may be recognized by irregular protrusions from the cord.

True knots are thought to be caused by excessive fetal movement and may, if they become tight, lead to vascular occlusion with fetal death in utero (FDIU). They have not been described sonographically in utero and their diagnosis would most likely be serendipitous.

Umbilical cord hematoma is a rare occurrence in late pregnancy and labor[18-20] and has been reported by Dippel,[20] in a comprehensive review, to have an incidence of 1 in 5,505 deliveries. Such hematomas must commonly occur from rupture of the wall of the umbilical vein and may occur secondary to mechanical trauma between fetal and maternal tissues, traction on a short cord, or on loops of cord around the fetus or a rare congenital weakness in a vessel wall.[18] Umbilical cord hematoma is associated with a very high perinatal loss—in Dippel's series 47% of the infants were stillborn. One mechanism of FDIU may be compression of umbilical vessels by the increased pressure of blood filling the Wharton jelly in the substance of the cord.[18]

Prenatal diagnosis of umbilical cord hematoma has been reported by Ruvinsky and Wiley[19] in a patient referred at 32 weeks of gestation with FDIU. The ultrasound examination showed a 6 × 8 cm sonolucent, septated intrauterine mass adjacent to the fetal abdomen.

Hemangiomas of the umbilical cord are rare but may appear as echogenic masses related to the cord.[42] They may be associated with elevated α-fetoprotein values.

Allantoic duct cysts may occur along the course of the cord and may be either true cysts or false cysts.[5] True cysts are usually quite small and represent remnants of the umbilical vesicle or of the allantois, whereas false cysts result from liquefaction of Wharton jelly and may reach considerable size (Fig. 10–9). Such allantoic cysts, even when large, usually do not jeopardize fetal circulation. Sachs[21] has reported the prenatal diagnosis of a 5-cm cystic mass within the umbilical cord, several centimeters from the abdominal wall, at 21 weeks of ges-

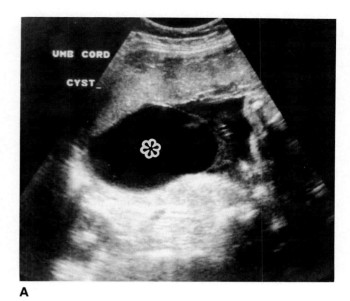

A

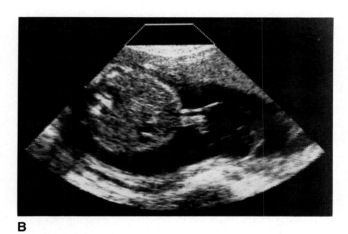

B

Fig. 10–9. Allantoic cyst. **A.** Large cystic structure (*) within umbilical cord representing allantoic cyst. **B.** Multiple-loculated cysts within umbilical cord representing allantoic cyst.

tation. Visualization of vessels in the lateral wall of the mass and an intact anterior abdominal wall allowed exclusion of other pathologies.

Neoplasms of the umbilical cord, which are quite rare, are usually angiomyxomas, myxosarcomas, dermoids, and teratomas, of which the most common is the angiomyxoma.[22] These more commonly occur in a location near the placental margin. Hemangioma of the cord has been reported as a cause of increased amniotic fluid α-fetoprotein.[23]

Umbilical hernia, which is one of the most commonly encountered abnormalities in early infancy,[24] is especially common in black and low-birth-weight infants.[25-27] Umbilical hernias are usually not significant clinically and close spontaneously in the first 3 years of life. Umbilical hernia has been reported as being more common in trisomy 21, congenital hypothyroidism, mucopolysaccharidoses, and Beckwith syndrome.[24]

Sonographically, umbilical hernia may be recognized as a protrusion from the anterior abdominal wall, with a normal insertion of the umbilical vessels.

Omphalocele and gastroschisis represent abnormalities of closure of the anterior abdominal wall. With omphalocele there is a midline umbilical defect with protrusion of abdominal structures such as bowel and liver into the base of the umbilical cord (Fig. 10–10), producing a sonographic appearance of a mass adjacent to the anterior abdominal wall, covered with a membrane and into the apex of which the umbilical cord appears to insert. There is a high incidence of other anomalies, e.g., intestinal, cardiac, and renal anomalies.

With gastroschisis, a paraumbilical abdominal wall defect results in protrusion of bowel and other intraabdominal contents into the amniotic fluid. The cord inserts normally and the gastroschisis will therefore appear as a complex mass adjacent to the base of the cord.

UMBILICAL VEIN DIAMETER AS A PREDICTOR OF FETAL DISEASE

Measurement of the diameter of the umbilical vein, both in the amniotic fluid and as it passes through the liver,

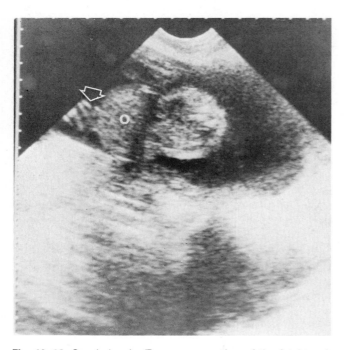

Fig. 10–10. Omphalocele. Transverse section of the fetal trunk showing a large omphacele (o). The umbilical cord (*arrow*) is implanted at the apex of the omphalocele.

has been proposed by Mayden[28] and by DeVore[29] as a predictor of the severity of Rhesus or other isoimmunization. The umbilical vein diameter in the amniotic fluid was consistently found to be the larger of the two measurements. It was suggested that the umbilical vein might dilate within the liver and in the amniotic fluid in response to severe Rh disease and that this dilatation might precede any rise in the ΔOD 450. In a subsequent communication, it appeared that the measurement was only of predictive value when increased and that normal values might be obtained in severely affected infants. Witter and Graham,[30] in a study of severely affected infants, found that, although in no instance was the umbilical vein diameter outside the normal range quoted by DeVore, in several normal patients idiopathic enlargement of umbilical vein diameter was obtained.

INTRAUTERINE MEMBRANES

Development of Amnion and Chorion

Differentiation of the trophoblastic cells from the embryo precursors occurs at approximately 5 days following conception. The trophoblast is further differentiated into two components: the cytotrophoblast and the syncytiotrophoblast. The former is mononuclear; the latter is multinuclear. The syncytiotrophoblast secretes human chorionic gonadotrophin and is responsible for proteolytic invasion into the decidua.

The chorion results from the fusion of the trophoblast and extra-embryonic mesenchyme. The chorionic villus comprises the major functioning unit of the placenta. Atrophy of the villi associated with the decidua capsularis results in the chorion laeve, which eventually becomes the chorionic membrane. The remaining villi establish the chorion frondosum, the fetal component of the placenta. The maternal component of the placenta arises from the decidua basalis. The chorion frondosum can be recognized sonographically in the first trimester as echogenic tissue surrounding the gestational sac.

The blastocyst implants into the decidualized endometrium approximately one week following fertilization. A layer of cells then separates, forming the extracelomic membrane and creating the primary yolk sac. Simultaneously, the amniotic cavity forms. The embryonic disc lies between the yolk sac and the amniotic sac, allowing real-time visualization of embryonic cardiac pulsation even prior to demonstration of the embryo. With development of the secondary yolk sac, the primary yolk sac shrinks.

While the chorion is closely related to the placenta, the amnion attaches to the embryo along its ventral aspect and envelops the umbilical cord. The amniotic cavity progressively emerges until the chorionic cavity is obliterated at 12 to 14 weeks.

The superior resolution afforded by the higher frequency, near-field focussed transvaginal approach has significantly altered the sonographic "milestones" of normal early intrauterine pregnancies. The first milestone, the chorionic mass, appears as a 2- to 3-mm hypoechoic complex within the thickened decidualized endometrium. This may be seen as early as 5 weeks and 4 days following conception. The secondary yolk sac is consistently demonstrated in a normal intrauterine pregnancy at 5 to 5½ weeks (Fig. 10–11A).

The thin amniotic membrane is delineated from 7 to 16 weeks (Fig. 10–11B, C, D). The embryo is seen to lie within the amniotic sac whereas the yolk sac is excluded from its confines.

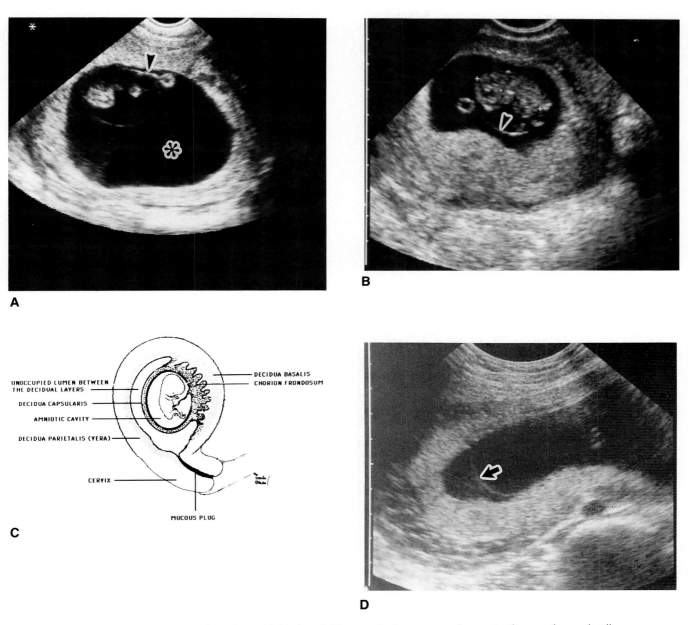

Fig. 10–11. Development of amnion and chorion. **A.** Transvaginal sonogram demonstrating amnion and yolk sac with yolk stalk (*arrowhead*). Also note that fluid in the extracelomic space (∗) is more echogenic than within the amniotic cavity. **B.** Transvaginal sonogram of 9-week intrauterine pregnancy demonstrating amnion (*arrowhead*). **C.** Diagram showing relationship of amniotic cavity to decidua and chorion prior to fusion. (*Drawn by Charles Odwin, RT, RDMS, and printed with permission.*) **D.** Unfused chorio-amnion (*arrow*) at 14 weeks.

Retrochorionic Hemorrhage

The fact that choriomyometrial separation can be associated with vaginal bleeding between 10 and 20 weeks has become more apparent with the increased use of sonography.[31,32] The sonographic features associated with retrochorionic hemorrhage include an elevated layer of chorion with an extrachorionic crescent-shaped fluid collection, which may appear purely cystic or complex if organized thrombus is present (Fig. 10–12). The prognosis of such abnormalities relates to the size of the hem-

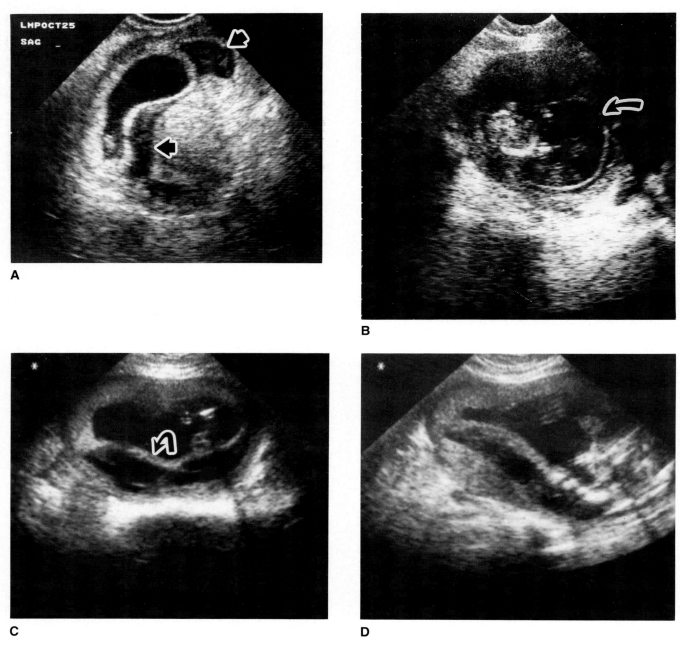

Fig. 10–12. Retrochorionic hemorrhage. **A.** TV US of elevated chorion with two areas of retrochorionic hemorrhage at 8 weeks. **B.** Extensive elevation of chorion (*curved arrow*) and separation from surrounding myometrium at 12 weeks associated with fetal demise. **C.** Transverse transabdominal sonogram of 20-week pregnancy demonstrating elevated chorion (*arrow*) with retrochorionic hemorrhage. **D.** Long-axis image of **C** demonstrating elevated chorion with retrochorionic hemorrhage. The elevated chorion interface is thicker than amnion.

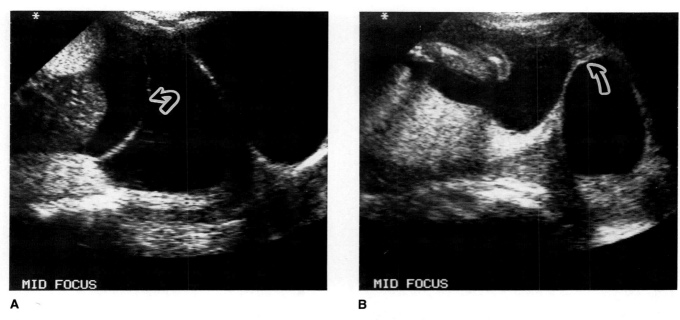

Fig. 10–13. Abnormal amnion. **A.** Thin intrauterine interface (*arrow*) corresponding to an amniotic band not involving a fetal part. **B.** Amniotic sheet probably draped over an intrauterine synechia (*curved arrow*).

orrhage, particularly as it compares to the size of the gestational sac. Those patients with small hemorrhages have an excellent chance of a favorable outcome but those patients with a hemorrhage exceeding 60 cc, or greater than 40% of the gestational sac, have a less favorable outcome, even if potential viability is demonstrated at the initial exam.[33]

It may be difficult to distinguish sonographically between a retrochorionic hemorrhage and a "vanishing" twin in the first trimester. The latter diagnosis can be made only if embryos are seen in both sacs.

The presence of an intrauterine membrane or interface can be detected in patients with a history of vaginal bleeding or as an incidental finding on an obstetrical sonogram. An intrauterine membrane arising from the unfused amnion is a normal finding up to 16 weeks gestation, at which time it should fuse with the chorion. In patients who experience bleeding in the late first and early second trimester, it is not uncommon to find areas of elevated chorion representing areas of hemorrhage. The hypoechoic space may extend to the area of the cervix, allowing for passage of blood vaginally. Areas of elevated chorion are usually thicker than areas of disrupted amnion, which tend to be more centrally located within the amniotic cavity. Typically, patients with retrochorionic hemorrhage have episodes of bleeding; but if the hemorrhage does not extend behind the placenta to involve the basal plate, these areas may regress as pregnancy progresses.

Other Conditions

Amniotic band syndrome is thought to be a sequela of rupture of the amnion, with formation of fibrous bands that may cross fetal parts and can cause significant maldevelopment (Fig. 10–13A).[34] The entrapped fetal part typically is entangled within the area of the membrane. Amniotic band syndrome has been associated with craniospinal malformations as well as gastroschisis and limb and finger amputation.[35,36] Therefore, it is important to document the integrity of only the fetal part that lies in proximity to the disrupted amnion.

A thin interface within the uterus may be encountered in patients where the amniotic membrane is draped over a uterine synechia. This uterine malformation has been termed an "amniotic sheet" and has not been associated with an increased incidence of fetal malformation (Fig. 10–13B).[37]

Uterine septae tend to be thicker than the interfaces created by amnion and chorion (Fig. 10–14). The septae may consist of either myometrium, a fibrous septation, or both, which typically have a vertical orientation within the uterus. Implantation can occur on the septum and probably accounts for the high incidence of spontaneous abortion.[38]

As mentioned in the chapter on twin pregnancies, it is important to document the presence of a membrane between fetuses of a multifetal pregnancy. The thickness of the membrane can be evidence of either monochorionic or dichorionic twin pregnancy. Membranes are

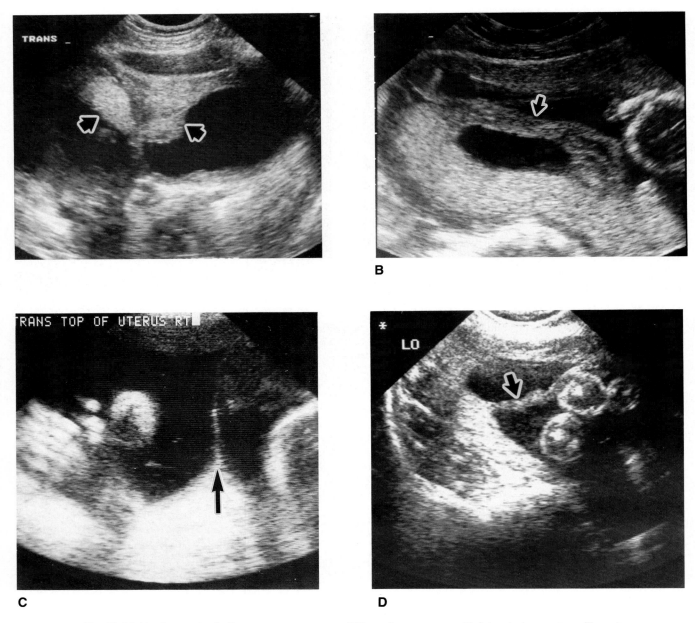

Fig. 10–14. Uterine septa. **A.** Transverse sonogram of 12-week pregnancy with intrauterine septum. Placenta (*arrows*) has implanted on both sides of septum. **B.** Long axis of edge of septum (*arrow*) coursing in a more vertical plane than that in **A. C.** Uterine septum with fetal extremities in lower part. **D.** Transverse sonogram demonstrating thin intrauterine septum (*arrow*) in a near-term pregnancy. The placenta and fetal head on the left side of septum, the fetal extremities on the right. (*Courtesy of Carl Zimmerman, MD.*)

typically dichorionic if they are well defined and have a definite measurable width (usually greater than 1 mm) (Fig. 10–15).[39–41] Conversely, monochorionic membranes tend to be thin or hairlike and visualized in short segments. Prenatal sonographic determination of the makeup of the membrane has importance in that dichorionic diamniotic gestations have the best prognosis.

Monochorionic monoamniotic have the poorest. However, sonographic demonstration of either a single placental cite, or inability to show membrane, may occur in any of the types of twinning. Intertwining of umbilical cords, conjoined twins, or more than three vessels in the umbilical cord occur only with monochorionic monoamniotic twinning.

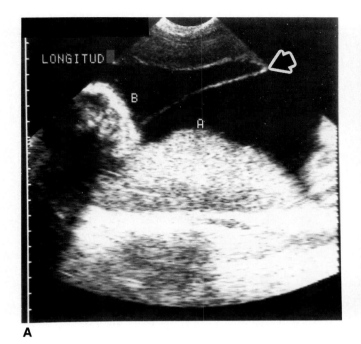

A

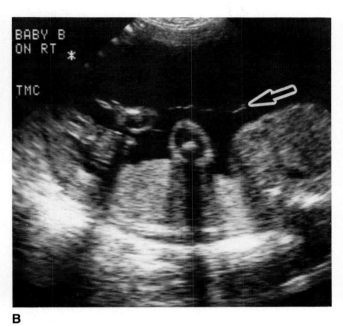

B

Fig. 10–15. Membranes in twin intrauterine pregnancy. **A.** Diamniotic, dichorionic thick membrane (*arrow*). **B.** Thin, diamniotic monochorionic membrane (*arrow*).

SUMMARY

This chapter has illustrated the sonographic depiction of the umbilical cord and intrauterine membranes. Although disorders of these structures occur relatively rarely, sonographic depiction of the type and extent of the disorder can aid management in these complicated pregnancies.

REFERENCES

1. Browne FJ. Abnormalities of the umbilical cord which may cause fetal death. *J Obstet Gynaec Br Emp*. 1925;32:17.
2. Kohorn EI, Walker RMS, et al. Placental localization. *Am J Obstet Gynecol*. 1969;103:868.
3. Purola E. The length and insertion of the umbilical cord. *Ann Chir Gynecol*. 1968;57:621.
4. Fox H. *Pathology of the Placenta*. Philadelphia: Saunders; 1978;426–457.
5. Pritchard JA, MacDonald PC. *Williams Obstetrics*, 16 ed. New York: Appleton-Century-Crofts; 1980.
6. Browne FJ. On the abnormalities of the umbilical cord which may cause antenatal death. *J Obstet Gynaecol Br Emp*. 1925;32:17.
7. Kamina P, DeTourris H. The diagnosis of umbilical cord complications with the help of ultrasonic tomography. *Electromedica*. 1977;2:50.
8. Walker CW, Pye BG. The length of the human umbilical cord: A statistical report. *Brit Med J*. 1960;1:546.
9. Spellacy WN, Gravem H, et al. The umbilical cord complications of true knots, nuchal coils and cords around the body. *Am J Obstet Gynecol*. 1966;94:1136.
10. Vintzileos AM, Nochimson DJ, et al. Ultrasonic diagnosis of funic presentation. *J Clin Ultrasound*. 1983;11:510.
11. Jouppila P, Kirkinen P. Ultrasonic diagnosis of nuchal encirclement by the umbilical cord: A case and methodological report. *J Clin Ultrasound*. 1982;10:59.
12. Benischke K, Driscoll SG. *The Pathology of the Human Placenta*. New York: Springer; 1967.
13. Jassani MN, Brennan JN, et al. Prenatal diagnosis of single umbilical artery by ultrasound. *J Clin Ultrasound*. 1980;8:447.
14. Peckham CH, Yerushalmy J. Aplasia of one umbilical artery: Incidence by race and certain obstetric factors. *Obstet Gynecol*. 1965;26:359.
15. Froehlich LA, Fujikura T. Significance of a single umbilical artery. *Am J Obstet Gynecol*. 1966;94:274.
16. Froehlich L, Fujikura T. Follow-up of infants with single umbilical artery. *Pediatrics*. 1973;52:6.
17. Bryan EM, Kohler HG. The missing umbilical artery. II. Pediatric follow-up. *Arch Dis Child*. 1975;50:714.
18. Roberts-Thomson ME. The hazards of umbilical cord haematoma. *Med J Aust*. 1973;1:648.
19. Ruvinsky ED, Wiley TL, et al. In utero diagnosis of umbilical cord hematoma by ultrasonography. *Ann J Obstet Gynecol*. 1981;140:833.

20. Dippel AL. Hematomas of the umbilical cord. *Surg Gynecol Obstet.* 1940;70:51.

21. Sachs L, Fourcroy JL, et al. Prenatal detection of umbilical cord Allantoic cyst. *Radiol.* 1982;45:445.

22. Novak ER, Woodruff JD. *Novak's Gynecologic and Obstetric Pathology.* Philadelphia: Saunders; 1967.

23. Barnson AJ. Donnai P, et al. Hemangioma of the cord: Further cause of raised maternal serum and liquor alphafetoprotein. *B Med J.* 1980;281:1251.

24. Bell MJ. Umbilical and other abdominal wall hernias. In: Holder TM, Ashcroft KW, eds. *Pediatric Surgery.* Philadelphia: Saunders; 1980.

25. Crump EP. Umbilical hernia: I. Occurrence of the infantile type in negro infants and children. *J Pediatr.* 1952;40:214.

26. Evans A. The comparative incidence of umbilical hernias in colored and white infants. *J Natl Med Assoc.* 1941;33:158.

27. Jackson DJ, Moglen LH. Umbilical hernia: a retrospective study. *Calif Med.* 1970;113:8.

28. Mayden K. The umbilical vein diameter in Rhesus isoimmunization. *Med Ultrasound.* 1980;4:119.

29. DeVore GR, Mayden K, et al. Dilatation of the fetal umbilical vein in rhesus hemolytic anemia: A predictor of severe disease. *Am J Obstet Gynecol.* 1981;141:464.

30. Witter FR, Graham D. The utility of ultrasonically measured umbilical vein diameters in isoimmunized pregnancies. *Am J Obstet Gynecol.* 1983;146:225.

31. Kaufman AJ, Fleischer AC, Thieme GA, Shah DM, James AE. Separated chorioamnion and elevated chorion: Sonographic features and clinical significance. *J Ultrasound Med.* 1985;4:119–125.

32. Burrows PE, Lyons EA, Phillips HJ, Oates I. Intrauterine membranes: Sonographic findings and clinical significance. *J Clin Ultrasound.* 1982;10:1–8.

33. Sauerbrei EE, Phan DH. Placental abruption and subchorionic hemorrhage in the first half of pregnancy: US appearance and clinical outcome. *Radiology.* 1986;160:109–112.

34. Torpin R. *Fetal Malformations Caused by Amnion Rupture During Gestation.* Springfield, Ill: Charles C Thomas; 1968:6.

35. Worthen NJ, Lawrence D, Bustillo M. Amniotic band syndrome: Antepartum ultrasonic diagnosis of discordant anencephaly. *J Clin Ultrasound.* 1980;8:453–455.

36. Hill LM, Kislak S, Jones N. Prenatal ultrasound diagnosis of a forearm constriction band. *J Ultrasound Med.* 1988;7:293–295.

37. Randel SB, Filly RA, Callen PW, Anderson RL, Golbus MS. Amniotic sheets. *Radiology.* 1988;166:633–636.

38. Fedele L, Dorta M, Brioschi D, Giudici MN, Candiani GB. Pregnancies in septate uteri: Outcome in relation to site of uterine implantation as determined by sonography. *AJR.* 1989;152:781–784.

39. Mahony BS, Filly RA, Callen PW. Amnionicity and chorionicity in twin pregnancies: Prediction using ultrasound. *Radiology.* 1985;155:205–209.

40. Hertzberg BS, Kurtz AB, Choi HY, et al. Significance of membrane thickness in the sonographic evaluation of twin gestations. *AJR.* 1987;148:151–153.

41. Townsend RR, Simpson GF, Filly RA. Membrane thickness in ultrasound prediction of chorionicity of twin gestations. *J Ultrasound Med.* 1988;7:327–332.

42. Pollack M, Boind L. Hemangioma of the umbilical cord: Sonographic appearance. *J Ultrasound Med.* 1989;8:163–166.

11 Color Doppler Sonography: Current and Potential Clinical Applications in Obstetrics and Gynecology

Arthur C. Fleischer • Bhaskara K. Rao •
Donna M. Kepple

In general, color Doppler sonography (CDS) facilitates duplex Doppler examinations of vascular structures. Color Doppler sonography, also called color flow mapping, is particularly helpful in evaluating vessels within organs or those that are not readily delineated with conventional scanning. The information obtained by color Doppler sonography is rarely diagnostic by itself, but it greatly facilitates a more complete assessment of the vascularity of a particular organ or region than is possible with conventional duplex scanning.

The principles and techniques used in color Doppler sonography have been covered in various review articles.[1-3] In general, CDS uses detection of mean Doppler frequency shifts and assigns them a color according to the mean direction and magnitude. This flow information is then superimposed on the two-dimensional real-time images to form the complete color Doppler sonogram.

The following discussion of clinical applications of color Doppler sonography is presented according to current and potential applications in obstetrics and gynecology with transabdominal and transvaginal probes.

GYNECOLOGIC APPLICATIONS

Color Doppler sonography can aid in the diagnosis of ovarian torsion, a condition that requires surgical correction immediately on diagnosis. Ovarian torsion typically occurs secondary to an intraovarian mass or exaggerated follicular development that may precipitate torsion.

Adnexal vessels may be assessed for the possibility of abnormal distension, thrombosis, or both (Fig. 11–1). Distended parauterine veins can be distinguished from

---

Figures for this chapter may be found on the color plates.

a hydrosalpinx by color Doppler sonography and directed duplex Doppler analysis. Detection of dilated parauterine vessels may have a role in monitoring treatment of the so-called "pelvic congestion syndrome."[4] Color Doppler sonography can detect pelvic arteriovenous malformations (AVM) that may arise years after instrumentation for dilatation and curettage.[5]

When there is a hemodynamically significant stenosis, the tissue distal to the stenosis may vibrate to produce an abnormal noise or bruit. The CDS equivalent of a bruit has been termed perivascular color artifact.[6] Vascular tumors such as choriocarcinoma may be detected by CDS. Color Doppler sonography may also be used as a means to serially assess the effectiveness of treatment of these tumors because the vascular areas tend to regress with successful chemotherapy.[7,8] Similarly, the vascularity of the choriodecidua can be assessed for signs of necrosis and imminent sloughing (Fig. 11–2).

Color Doppler sonography can detect abnormal ovarian flow in some vascular ovarian tumors when used on a transvaginal probe. A recent study has shown that CDS can detect neovascularity within ovarian tumors, thereby distinguishing benign from malignant lesions.[9] Our initial experience has shown that this distinction may be limited because some benign tumors (such as immature teratomas) may demonstrate neovascularity as well.[10] With better resolution of slow flow afforded by improved software, the distinction between neoplastic and inflammatory processes may become less absolute.

Similarly, CDS can assist identification of myometrial vessels that can be further evaluated by their abnormal waveforms associated with uterine hypoperfusion. This may have a role in patients whose infertility may be related to uterine hypoperfusion.[11-13] Perhaps CDS of the myometrial vessels can help distinguish endometrial tumors that are invasive from those that are significant by delineating the border between the intermediate and deep layers of myometrium.

171

OBSTETRIC APPLICATIONS

In obstetrics, color Doppler sonography can be used to evaluate the fetus, placenta, umbilical cord, and uterine structures[14,15] (Figs. 11–3; 11–4, and 11–5). Vessels around and within the placenta are detectable by color Doppler sonography (Fig. 11–3). This has particular use in evaluation of possible retroplacental hemorrhage by evaluating the subplacental vascular complex. Abnormal placental masses can be assessed by CDS for detection of vascular lesions such as chorioangiomas. CDS is also useful for detection of communicating placental vessels in patients with possible twin–twin transfusion syndrome.

Color Doppler sonography affords delineation of the size, angle of interrogation, and orientation of the umbilical vein and arteries within the umbilical cord (Fig. 11–4). These structures may be evaluated for detection of the growth-retarded or hypoxic fetus. It is possible that more accurate determinations of the volume of flow within the umbilical vein can be made with CDS. Color Doppler sonography can also delineate the umbilical cord, especially in cases where a nuchal cord, entanglement, prolapse, or an abnormal number of vessels is suspected.[16] The location of the cord is also of paramount importance prior to attempts at external version because the presence of a nuchal cord is a contraindication to the procedure.

Color Doppler sonography has a major role in evaluation of fetal cardiac malformations (Fig. 11–5). Areas of shunting, regurgitation, and overall cardiac flow dynamics can be determined with this technique. Hypoechoic lesions within the fetus, which may be vascular (such as varix or arteriovenous malformation), can also be diagnosed with CDS. Similarly, the orientation and size of the fetal aorta can be evaluated with CDS. Assessment of flow velocities in the aorta may reflect pH levels with low velocity flow occurring in a hypoxic fetus. This technique can also enhance detection of changes in the distribution of blood flow (somatic versus cerebral) in the growth-retarded fetus.

SUMMARY

Color Doppler sonography greatly increases one's ability to evaluate vascular structures within or around organs, even in vessels that may not be apparent by conventional imaging. As greater experience with the technique and further refinement of instrumentation occur, it is clear that CDS will come into routine use for sonographic evaluation of the entire body.

REFERENCES

1. Grant EG, Tessler FN, Perrella RR. Clinical Doppler imaging. *AJR*. 1989;152:707–717.
2. Lewis BD, James EM, Charboneau JW, Reading CC, Welch TJ. Current applications of color Doppler imaging in the abdomen and extremities. *RadioGraphics* 1989;9:599–617.
3. Merritt CRB. Doppler blood flow imaging integrating flow with tissue data. *Diagnostic Imaging*. November 1986;146–155.
4. Beard RW, Reginald PW, Wadsworth J. Clinical features of women with chronic lower abdominal pain and pelvic congestion. *Br J Obstet Gynecol*. 1988;95:153–161.
5. Musa AA, Hata T, Hata K, Kitao M. Pelvic arteriovenous malformation diagnosed by color flow Doppler imaging. *AJR* 1989;152:1311–1312.
6. Middleton WD, Erickson S, Melson GL. Perivascular color artifact: Pathologic significance and appearance on color Doppler US images. *Radiology* 1989;171:647–652.
7. Hata T, Hata K, Senoh D, et al. Doppler ultrasound assessment of tumor vascularity in gynecologic disorders. *J Ultrasound Med*. 1989;8:309.
8. Shimamoto K, Sakuma S, Ishigaki T, Makino N. Intratumoral blood flow: Evaluation with color Doppler echography. *Radiology* 1987;165:683–685.
9. Bourne T, Campbell S, Steer C, Whitehead MI, Collins WP. Transvaginal colour flow imaging: A possible new screening technique for ovarian cancer. *Br Med J*. 1989;299:1367–1370.
10. Fleischer AC, Kepple DM, Rao BK. Transvaginal color Doppler sonography: Preliminary experience. *Dyn Cardiovasc Imaging*. 1990. (In press.)
11. Goswamy RK, Steptoe PC. Doppler ultrasound studies of the uterine artery in spontaneous ovarian cycles. *Hum Reproduction*. 1988;3:721–726.
12. Goswamy RK, Williams G, Steptoe PC. Decreased uterine perfusion—A cause of infertility. *Hum Reproduction*. 1988;3:955–959.
13. Greiss FC, Anderson SG. Effect of ovarian hormones on the uterine vascular bed. *Am J Obstet Gynecol* 1970;107:829–836.
14. Farquhar CM, Rae T, Thomas DC, Wadsworth J, Beard RW. Doppler ultrasound in the nonpregnant pelvis. *J Ultrasound Med*. 1989;8:451–457.
15. Schaaps JP, Soyeur D. Pulsed Doppler on a vaginal probe: Necessity, convenience, or luxury? *J Ultrasound Med* 1989;8:315–320.
16. Nyberg DA, Shepard T, Mack LA, Hirsch J, Luthy D, Fitzsimmons J. Significance of a single umbilical artery in fetuses with central nervous system malformations. *J Ultrasound Med* 1988;7:265–273.

12 Obstetric Doppler Applications

Brian J. Trudinger

The use of Doppler ultrasound to study blood flow in obstetrics is of major importance because fetal inaccessibility precludes many other methods of study of the circulation. Doppler devices to detect motion of the fetal heart have been used for the past 25 years. Recent developments that have seen the growth of Doppler flow studies are the capacity to display the Doppler frequency shift spectrum (and, therefore, flow velocity waveforms) in real time, and the ability to locate and sample the Doppler spectrum from a specific vessel imaged with the conventional B-mode ultrasound scan.

DOPPLER ULTRASOUND: INSTRUMENTATION

The Doppler effect is the change in frequency (transmitted versus received) of an acoustic or ultrasound wave that results when the total path length changes between transmitting and receiving sources (Fig. 12–1).

In clinical use, the transmitting and receiving sources are stationary and the change in path length results from movement of the target either toward or away from these transducers. In studies of blood flow, the moving column of blood within the interrogated vessels is the target. The red blood cells act as scatterers, reflecting the ultrasound beam. Fetal heart detectors record movement of the heart valves and chamber walls.

In obstetric applications, both continuous-wave and pulsed Doppler ultrasound systems are used. Continuous-wave devices use separate transmitting and receiving transducers, usually mounted side by side so that reflected signals from moving targets at any point along the ultrasound beam are recorded. Such systems are relatively cheap and simple to use. Vessels may be located without prior imaging by adjusting the transducer direction until the characteristic signal of the vessel to be studied is displayed (eg, umbilical artery in the cord). This system lacks spatial resolution in that signals from all moving targets along the beam path are recorded. Pulsed Doppler devices allow position and velocity information to be recorded. A sample volume or range gate can be located on a B-mode image so that only signals from that area are displayed (eg, recording from a fetal carotid artery). Pulsed Doppler systems have a limitation on the maximum Doppler frequency shift that can be detected before aliasing occurs.

The simplest Doppler display is the audio signal. If typical values arising from clinical use are substituted in the Doppler equation, it is apparent that the Doppler frequency shifts recorded lie within the audible range. Real-time frequency spectrum analyzers are available to display the Doppler frequencies against a time base. This creates the flow velocity waveform. The Doppler information may also be stored for analysis of measures such as mean frequency.

DOPPLER ULTRASOUND: CLINICAL INFORMATION

The information about blood flow available through Doppler studies consists of the flow velocity waveform and volume blood flow.

The blood flow velocity waveform (FVW) contains information about the velocity of every blood cell within the blood vessel under interrogation by the ultrasound beam. Commonly, almost all of this information is ignored and the waveform envelope or the peak velocity is studied. This waveform has been most widely interpreted to distinguish patterns associated with high and low resistance in the vascular tree downstream from the point of recording. Indices have been developed to express this pattern change and have been used as a measure of downstream resistance. Three are in common use: the systolic:diastolic ratio, the pulsatility index, and the resistance index (Fig. 12–2).

These indices are ratios, independent of the angle between the ultrasound beam and blood vessel. This is important when the angle is not known and so absolute velocity cannot be measured. That is the case with continuous-wave ultrasound, or when the vessel is small or tortuous and, therefore, not adequately imaged (eg, umbilical artery or uterine artery). The indices were derived initially by their statistically demonstrated association with adverse clinical findings. They are commonly regarded as "resistance indices" in the belief that they reflect downstream resistance. There is now good evidence to support this theory. In the umbilical artery waveform, a high resistance pattern may be recreated by emboli-

DOPPLER MEASUREMENT OF FLOW VELOCITY

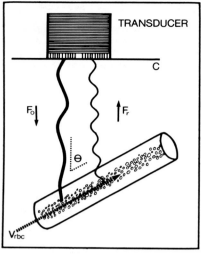

C = velocity of sound in medium

V_{rbc} = velocity of blood flow

Θ = angle between ultrasound beam and direction of flow

F_o = transmitted ultrasound frequency

F_r = reflected ultrasound frequency

F_D = Doppler shift in frequency

$\quad = F_o - F_r$

$\quad = F_o \, 2\dfrac{V_{rbc}}{c} \cos \Theta$

$F_D \propto V_{rbc}$

Fig. 12–1. Diagram of the use of Doppler principle and Doppler velocimeter to study blood flow.

zation of the vascular bed.[1] Theoretical proof is provided by mathematical analysis of a computer-based model of the umbilical vascular tree.[2] However, the resistance indices must not be considered independent of changes in other physiologic variables such as heart rate, cardiac contractility, blood pressure, and vessel wall compliance.

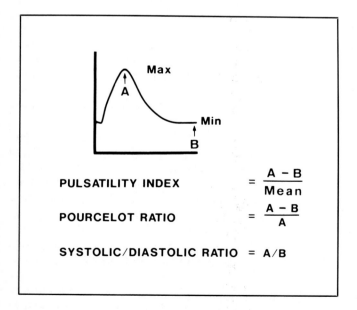

PULSATILITY INDEX $= \dfrac{A - B}{Mean}$

POURCELOT RATIO $= \dfrac{A - B}{A}$

SYSTOLIC/DIASTOLIC RATIO $= A/B$

Fig. 12–2. Three indices of downstream resistance in common use for analysis of arterial FVWs.

The three indices are highly correlated with coefficients in excess of 0.9 having been reported.[3] Such is the degree of correlation that it is unlikely one index provides different or additional information than another. The specific index used becomes a matter of personal choice. There are intrinsic errors in all which have been quantitated and lie between 10 and 20%.[4] In using the pulsatility index, it is most unlikely that the true mean velocity will be calculated accurately. The error in systolic:diastolic ratio increases as the diastolic flow velocity becomes small, but commonly values above 6 are grouped together as extremely high. The values for normal pregnancy of the systolic:diastolic ratio, and pulsatility index at any gestational age, are not normally distributed.[5] Despite all of these shortcomings, the indices serve a valuable function in providing some quantification of the changing waveform pattern that occurs with increasing downstream resistance. They should be seen as descriptors of a waveform pattern, not precise physiologic measures.

Frequently, the maximum flow velocity waveform is analyzed, and all the velocity information available in the waveform apart from peak velocity is ignored. However, it has been shown that the same resistance indices could be used to examine the mean or first-moment velocity waveform, yielding similar but more error-prone information.[6] The extra work involved in computing these waveforms does not seem justified.

Volume blood flow is measured as the product of

mean blood flow velocity and vessel area.[7] The cross-section area of the vessel is measured from a B-mode image. Good correlations have been reported between Doppler and electromagnetic flow probe measurements. In perinatal practice, only two vessels, the fetal umbilical vein and aorta, are large enough to accurately measure dimensions from the ultrasound image.

A major problem in measuring flow is the variation of blood velocity across the vessel cross-section. Because the overall flow rate is the sum of the contributions made by the blood at every point on the cross-section, it is necessary to average the velocity profile. Various approaches to this have been described.[8] They can be categorized according to whether the velocity profile is measured (using multigated pulsed Doppler) and then averaged, or averaged using a large sample volume to encompass the whole vessel.

There are several sources of error inherent in the methodology of pulsed-wave Doppler ultrasound when used for this quantitative assessment of volume blood flow:[9]

1. Measurement of the angle between the ultrasound beam and blood vessel.
2. Measurement of the vessel diameter. This is very error-susceptible. For a 6- to 8-mm vessel (eg, umbilical vein), an error of 0.4 mm in diameter produces a 10% error in calculated flow. This same measurement error for a 4-mm vessel produces a 25% error. Pulsations in arteries produce changes in diameter that have been assessed in the fetal aorta to vary as much as 19%.[10]
3. Position of the sample volume. To ensure that the vessel is uniformly insonnated, the sample volume must be larger than the vessel and positioned to completely span it. However, if the sample volume is too large, extraneous signals may be included.
4. High-pass filtering of low-amplitude signals. This is used to remove low-frequency vessel wall vibration signals, but will also remove low-flow velocities and, therefore, distort the calculation of the mean velocity. Correction factors have been introduced for this potential error.

Volume blood flow has been expressed as mL/min or normalized by estimating the fetal weight, mL/min/fetus kg. Estimates of fetal weight have been based on ultrasound mensuration formulas; these are also error-prone.

Doppler ultrasound can also be used to estimate cardiac flow. Techniques developed in adult and pediatric cardiology to estimate cardiac and ventricular output can be applied to the fetus. The sample volume of a pulsed Doppler unit can be placed in the outflow tract of one of the ventricles. Because of the high acceleration that normally occurs here during systole, the velocity profile can be assumed to be flat. It is also generally assumed that the Doppler beam is oriented parallel to the direction of flow, so that the angle Θ can be ignored ($\cos \Theta = 1$). The Doppler shift is measured, converted to a velocity using the Doppler equation, and averaged over a cardiac cycle. This average velocity is multiplied by the cross-section area of the outflow tract (which can be estimated from B- or M-mode scans) to give flow. Ventricular output has also been estimated in the fetus using ultrasonic measurements of the cardiac dimensions.

To obtain accurate and clinically useful volume flow measurement, considerable attention must be paid to methodology. With such care, measurements of the umbilical vein flow may be sufficiently accurate to permit clinical evaluation.

PHYSIOLOGY OF FETAL AND PLACENTAL CIRCULATIONS

The fetal circulation differs from the adult in a number of ways. The heart rate is higher and the cardiac output (per unit weight) is greater. Low oxygen tensions make high flow rates necessary. A high level of pumping performance by the heart is required. Blood volume is high. Despite the low systemic vascular impedance, mean systemic pressure is maintained.[11] The low-resistance umbilical placental circulation dominates, receiving some 40% of combined ventricular output. The fetal heart shows a right-ventricular dominance with the right:left ventricular output ratio being 1.3:1. The output of the left ventricle is directed mainly to the head, while the output of the right is to the trunk and placenta. Both ventricles work against systemic pressure. The output from the left ventricle is greater in the human fetus compared to many experimental animals studied; this has been attributed to the higher cerebral flow. The capacity of the fetal heart to increase output in response to an increase in filling pressure has been debated. Evidence from Doppler studies in human fetuses suggest that it does have this capacity.[12] The distribution of the fetal cardiac output is regulated by the peripheral resistance of the various vascular beds.[13]

The umbilical circulation constitutes some 40% of the combined ventricular output. It increases throughout pregnancy, although flow per unit of fetal mass decreases (fetal lamb: 0.6 gestation umbilical flow 231 mL/min/kg, term 170 mL/min/kg).[14,15] The proportion of fetal cardiac output directed to the placenta decreases in late gestation. This has been attributed to a greater decrease in resistance in other fetal vascular beds compared to the umbilical placenta. The decrease in umbilical placental resistance with gestation may be attributed to the growth of the placenta with opening of new vascular channels. Umbilical flow is increased by increases in fetal heart rate and blood pressure.[16] It does not appear that the fetus has well-developed means of regulation of umbilical circulation. The umbilical vessels are not innervated and are relatively refractory to catecholamines. Acute changes in fetal arterial blood gas tensions produce a surprisingly small effect on umbilical flow.[17] Transient compression of the umbilical cord causes fetal bradycardia and hypertension. Longer studies of continuing cord compression demonstrate that the fetus copes with a reduction in umbilical flow by increasing oxygen extraction and, indeed, can do so to maintain normal oxygen consumption until the reduction in flow exceeds 50%.[18] This information suggests that the fetus does not need to finely regulate umbilical flow, but rather can rely on variations in oxygen extraction.

Pregnancy sees marked changes in maternal cardiovascular physiology. There is a decrease in systemic vascular resistance and a fall in blood pressure with widening of the pulse pressure. Blood volume is increased. Cardiac output rises with an increase in both pulse rate and stroke volume. These changes are established in the first trimester before the low-resistance arteriovenous shunt that is the uteroplacental bed can have a significant impact. They are attributed to the steroid hormones of pregnancy.

The uterine circulation has two components, flow to the myometrium and to the placental bed. It is likely that these are under separate control. The marked increase in uterine flow that occurs in normal pregnancy is predominantly the result of increase in flow to the uteroplacental bed. This occurs in a setting of decrease in the pressure gradient across the vascular bed, and points to an even greater decrease in vascular resistance. The latter is attributed to the expansion of the uteroplacental vascular bed with an increasing number of vascular channels being incorporated into the placental bed as the placenta grows. In human pregnancy, uterine blood flow at term is estimated at 700 mL/min (10% cardiac output), of which 80% is directed to the placental bed. This flow is related to the weight of the uterus and its contents and remains constant throughout pregnancy.[19] It also has been related to oxygen consumption.[20]

During pregnancy, the spiral arteries are transformed to uteroplacental arteries in the decidua. Initially, the walls have a smudged fibrinoid outline. Later, invasion by cytotrophoblast into the lumen and wall occurs.[21–26] Further into the pregnancy, trophoblast extends down the spiral arteries to reach the myometrial segment. The uteroplacental arteries progressively expand in the decidua with loss of musculo-elastic tissue from their walls. The fully developed blood supply to the placenta is illustrated in Fig. 12–3.

Placentation brings into contact the maternal utero-

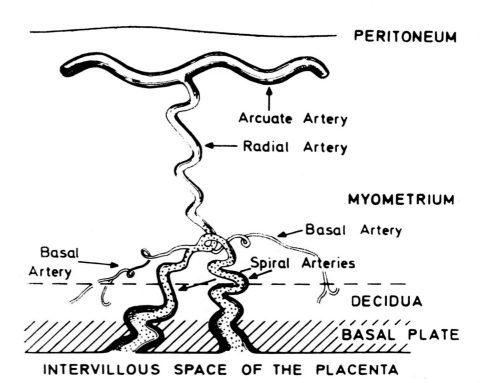

Fig. 12–3. Arterial vessels in the wall of the gravid uterus. (*Used by permission from Robertson et al.*[25])

PERITONEUM

Arcuate Artery

Radial Artery

MYOMETRIUM

Basal Artery

Basal Artery

Spiral Arteries

DECIDUA

BASAL PLATE

INTERVILLOUS SPACE OF THE PLACENTA

placental and fetal umbilical placental circulations. Uniform matching of perfusion optimizes exchange of oxygen, nutrients, and waste removal between these two circulations.[27] Both circulations seem to exert control. If uteroplacental flow is reduced by microsphere embolization, a reduction occurs in umbilical flow.[28,29] In this circumstance, the fetus redistributes cardiac output to favor vital organs.[30] The fetal umbilical circulation can influence uteroplacental perfusion. This is clearly seen after fetal death. Lowland sheep taken to high altitude maintain fetal oxygenation, due in part to increased uterine blood flow.[31] The mediation of this perfusion balance between the two placental circulations is not clear, but vasoactive prostaglandins and angiotensin have been implicated.[32]

DOPPLER STUDIES OF SPECIFIC CIRCULATIONS

Umbilical Placental Circulation

Method of Study. Flow velocity waveforms from the umbilical artery may be recorded using either a continuous-wave or pulsed Doppler system. Even with a pulsed Doppler system and B-mode imaging, it is usual to record the arterial signal by visualizing the umbilical vein and locating the sample volume adjacent to it. The spiral course of the artery means that the angle between the ultrasound beam and blood flow direction cannot be determined. With both systems, the recorded waveform is optimized by altering the line of sighting through slightly moving the transducer until the cleanest signals are obtained. Using continuous-wave systems, the waveform is identified by its characteristic shape and display of the umbilical vein flow signal in the opposite direction.

Flow waveforms should be recorded during periods of fetal inactivity. Both breathing and body movements alter the umbilical artery waveform. Fetal breathing can readily be recognized by its effect on the umbilical vein flow pattern. By insisting on fetal inactivity, possible variations due to altered state are eliminated. To establish that the fetus is not breathing, it is necessary to view a sequence of 15 to 20 cardiac cycles (8 to 10 seconds) and ensure that the waveforms are constant. Recognize that measurements from an oscilloscope screen that displays only two or three cycles are highly error-prone.

The shape of the umbilical artery waveform is not altered by the site of recording along the cord except at its two extremes. Very close to the fetal abdominal wall, the waveform may resemble the aortic waveform, which characteristically has a lower diastolic flow velocity and a more peaked systolic component. This is probably an "entrance region" flow pattern; further along the cord

the characteristic pattern is established and maintained. Recording at the point where the umbilical cord is attached to the placenta may pick up an umbilical signal after the artery has divided into branches on the placental surface. Any variation because of these factors can be checked and eliminated by recording from at least two different points along the cord.

Because of the coiling of the umbilical cord and its vessels, it is possible for the ultrasound beam to "sight" flow in the same direction in both artery and vein. In such circumstances, the flow pattern in the two vessels will be superimposed. The result may be that the umbilical vein signal covers the diastolic component of the arterial waveform and, thus, is inadvertently measured as the end diastolic velocity. This error can be eliminated and the signal checked by recording an arterial waveform with the venous signal in the opposite direction.

There are two umbilical arteries in the cord and their waveforms are often similar. It is frequently possible to locate the ultrasound beam so that flow in the two arteries is "seen" in opposite directions. In that way the waveforms can be compared. The similarity of the waveforms supports the idea that in the placenta the two umbilical arteries anastomose then branch to be distributed to overlapping areas. The result is that downstream resistance is similar. This is not invariable and occasionally two quite different waveforms are seen in association with placental infarction.[33]

It is important that the maximum-height flow waveform signal is recorded to ensure the diastolic flow is not covered by a high-pass filter. This is especially true when the diastolic component of the waveform is low. Most spectrum analyzers contain a wall-motion or thump filter that eliminates very low-frequency signals. This includes signals due to slowly moving blood cells as well as wall motion. If the beam-blood vessel angle is close to 90°, the waveform amplitude is low and diastolic flow may not be seen because it is filtered out. An ideal system should have the capacity to switch off this filter.

Waveforms should not be recorded during uterine contractions, which might affect the flow pattern. The mother should be positioned to avoid supine hypotension.

Volume blood flow can be measured in the umbilical vein as it traverses the fetal liver. The plane of scan is adjusted to obtain a longitudinal image of the umbilical vein within the fetal trunk, taking care that the point of measurement is the umbilical vein proper and not the left portal vein or ductus venous. Caliper markers are placed on the inner edge of the vessel walls to determine diameter of the lumen and spatial orientation of the vessel. It is necessary to ensure there is a clear ultrasound line of sight and a suitable angle of approach to the vessel. The range gate is adjusted so that the sample volume spans the entire vessel at its point of measurement. Flow

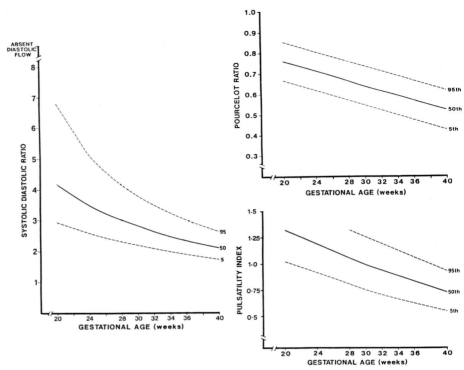

Fig. 12–4. Normal values for the umbilical artery indices of resistance. (*Based on values reported by Thompson et al.*[4])

may be calculated as the product of average velocity and area of vessel lumen.

Normal Pregnancy. The indices of "downstream" umbilical placental resistance decrease with advancing gestation, a finding that parallels direct measures of pressure flow and resistance in fetal lambs. Normal values for human pregnancy have been reported by the author[5] and others[34] and are largely in agreement (Fig. 12–4). There is a clear change in waveform shape through pregnancy. (See Figs. 12–4 and 12–5.)

There is debate about whether or not these indices should be corrected for fetal heart rate (FHR). The association with FHR is weak.[3] The correction suggested by some[35] is small when compared to inherent errors of the umbilical artery index.[4] It is noteworthy that indices derived from the aortic waveform reveal much greater dependence on heart rate and behavioral state.[36] When the fetal heart rate is outside the normal range, the reported normal ranges are not applicable.

The volume flow in the umbilical vein increases with gestation. Flow per unit fetal weight is relatively constant ($\simeq$ 110 mL/min/fetus kg), a figure much less than that measured in fetal lambs (175 mL/min/kg)[14] and other experimental animals (Fig. 12–6). In all experimental animal species studied, it has been demonstrated that flow per unit fetal weight in the second half of pregnancy is constant.[37]

Complicated Pregnancy. The two common pregnancy complications associated with abnormality of umbilical artery FVW are fetal growth retardation and pregnancy hypertension. There is much information available about the FVW, and it will be discussed in detail. Measurement of umbilical vein volume flow in complicated pregnancy is reviewed at the end of this section.

Realization of the clinical importance of umbilical artery FVWs began with the recognition of different waveform patterns in normal and complicated pregnancies. Whereas in normal pregnancy the waveform pattern is characterized by high diastolic flow velocities, the compromised fetus exhibits a waveform characterized by reduced diastolic flow velocities. This observation was first reported by the writer's laboratory in 1982[38-40] and has been confirmed by groups around the world.[41-43]

Pathophysiology of Abnormal Umbilical Doppler Studies. Pathologic and experimental studies indicate that the change in waveform pattern is associated with a change in downstream (umbilical placental circulation) vascular resistance.

The presumed explanation for the change in waveform pattern in Figure 12–7 was a change in downstream resistance. Because the umbilical placental vascular bed is downstream when the recording is from the umbilical artery, a change in the placenta is implied.

A study to correlate the umbilical artery FVW pat-

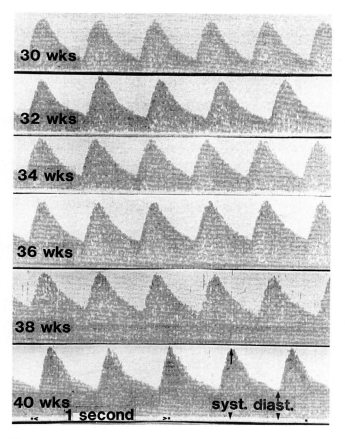

Fig. 12–5. The umbilical artery FVW recorded from one patient during the last trimester of pregnancy.

tern with the "resistance" vessels in the umbilical placental vascular tree has been carried out.[44] The major drop in arterial pressure across the umbilical placental vascular bed occurs in the small arteries and arterioles of the tertiary villi; these are the resistance vessels. Three groups of patients were compared: a normal group of uncomplicated pregnancies; a control group of potentially at-risk pregnancies with a normal umbilical artery FVW; and a third group with an abnormal umbilical artery FVW, matched by risk factor and gestation with the second group. A total of 106 patients were included. Placental arterial resistance was quantitated by counting the number of small muscular arteries (<90 μm diameter). The mode small arterial vessel count was significantly less in the group with the abnormal umbilical artery FVW (1 to 2 arteries/high power field) compared to the normal and control groups (7 to 8 arteries/field), which did not differ from one another. This work has recently been confirmed by others.[45] (See Fig. 12–8.) The antenatal Doppler umbilical artery study thus allows recognition of a specific placental lesion of vascular sclerosis with obliteration of the small muscular arteries of the tertiary stem villi. This lesion could be expected to cause an increase in flow resistance in the umbilical placenta. In the past, profound fetal growth retardation has been related to pathologic changes in the maternal uterine spiral arteries, which are referred to as placental insufficiency. The umbilical artery Doppler studies identify a lesion in the fetal placenta which could more appropriately be described as "placental insufficiency." Statements such as ". . . a pathologic basis for placental insufficiency cannot be defined"[46] result from the classification of patients by maternal disease or fetal effect, rather than dynamic blood flow patterns indicative of this pathology. Doppler umbilical studies define a placental vascular pathology.

Animal experimental studies have been carried out in fetal lambs.[1] The FVW can be recorded from the umbilical arterial circulation in the same manner as in human

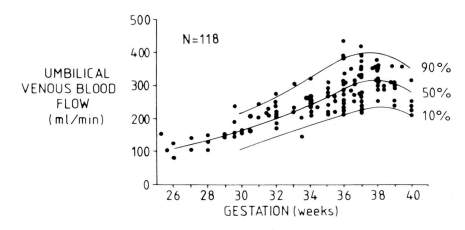

Fig. 12–6. Umbilical vein volume flow in the second half of pregnancy, measured using Doppler techniques. (*Used by permission from Gill.*[7])

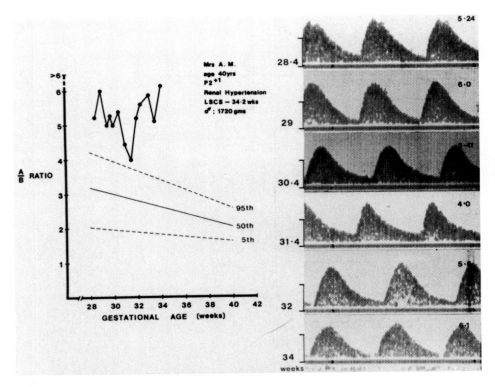

Fig. 12–7. Sequential umbilical artery FVWs recorded from a patient with renal hypertension delivering a small fetus.

pregnancy and the same change with gestation is seen.[47] Embolization of the umbilical placental circulation in fetal lambs was carried out to increase placental flow resistance and observe the effects on umbilical artery FVWs. This caused an increase in the systolic:diastolic flow velocity ratio. Blood flow to the umbilical placenta was reduced and expressed either in absolute terms or when normalized by dividing by splanchnic organ flow. This reduction, however, was not apparent until after there had been a change in the FVW. Calculated vascular resistance was increased in the umbilical circulation. This study provides experimental evidence establishing the rela-

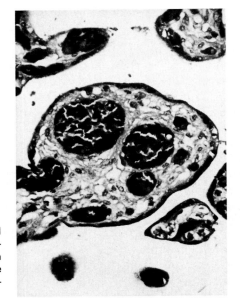
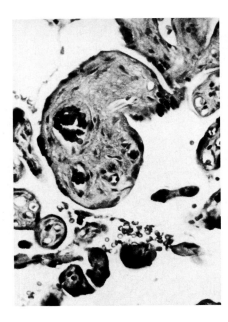

Fig. 12–8. Histomicrograph of a placental tertiary stem villus from a case with normal umbilical artery FVWs (*left*) and high resistance pattern (*right*). The difference in numbers of small arterial vascular channels in the tertiary villi is apparent.

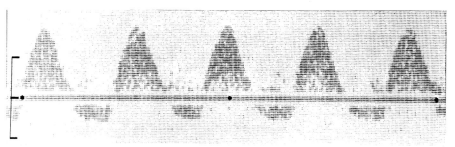

LSCS – 33·3wks
♂ ; 930 gms

Fig. 12–9. An extremely abnormal umbilical artery FVW in which there is reversal (negative) diastolic flow velocities. This patient delivered an infant of 980 g at 33 weeks.

tionship in complicated pregnancy between the high systolic diastolic ratio and a high vascular resistance.

Fetal Growth Retardation. Fetal growth retardation as evidenced by the subsequent birth of an infant small for gestational age has been consistently associated with abnormal umbilical artery FVW. In a study from the author's laboratory, 172 mothers were examined, all within 10 days of delivery.[48] There were 53 fetuses subsequently born small for gestational age (SGA) (<10th percentile); 34 had an abnormal systolic diastolic ratio (>95th percentile). These 34 pregnancies were delivered earlier (34.6 weeks) than the 19 normal-ratio SGA fetuses (37.6 weeks) (P>0.01). They required more frequent neonatal intensive care admissions (23/24 compared to 3/29, P>0.01), and included all the subsequent neonatal deaths (6 compared to 0). At the time of this study, the umbilical waveform result was not available for clinical decision making; therefore, these findings were a true correlation rather than a self-fulfilling prophecy.

Serial studies in association with fetal growth failure show a rising systolic:diastolic ratio. In some cases, diastolic flow velocities are absent or even reversed (negative) (Fig. 12–9). With a greater fraction of the vascular bed obliterated, placental resistance increases and the indices of resistance increase. The disappearance of diastolic flow is a point in this progressive change and should not be seen as a watershed of sudden change in clinical circumstances.

Pregnancy Hypertension. Independent of fetal growth retardation, severe pregnancy hypertension is associated with a high systolic:diastolic ratio.[48] In a group of 23 patients with a diastolic pressure greater than 110 mm Hg, and proteinuria in excess of 1 g/day, 17 had a high systolic:diastolic ratio. Such observations demonstrate the association between the fetal placental vascular lesion and maternal disease. In most cases, the abnormal umbilical artery waveform precedes the maternal disease. This observation has been confirmed by others.[49] In a program of routine Doppler study of all twin pregnancies at 28 weeks, it was found that if the umbilical waveform of one or both twins was abnormal, there was a 22% or four times greater likelihood that the mother would develop hypertension.

Diabetes Mellitus. Umbilical artery FVWs have also been used in the management of pregnant women with diabetes. Our experience suggests that normal results are recorded from the macrosomic fetus that is continuing to grow, but cessation of growth is associated with the development of a high resistance pattern in the umbilical artery waveform, whether the fetus is macrosomic (ie, the growth stimulus had been excessive earlier in pregnancy) or small (diabetic vascular disease developed in the maternal uterine vessels). (See Fig. 12–10.) In another report, two stillbirths from a series of 43 diabetic pregnancies were associated with high resistance waveform patterns.[50]

Multiple Pregnancy. There is an increase in perinatal mortality (three to fourfold) and morbidity for the fetal members of a twin pair. The fetal problems include prematurity, intrauterine growth failure, fetal anomaly, twin transfusion syndrome, cord entanglement, intrapartum accidents, malpresentation, and traumatic delivery. In part, the fetal problems result from difficulties in testing fetal welfare. Ultrasound mensuration is associated with technical problems: one fetus may overlie, there may be compression, or the head may be well down in the pelvis. Fetal heart rate monitoring is associated with uncertainty in identification of the twin under study. Doppler studies of twins must be carried out with simultaneous viewing of the fetal heart on a B-mode real-time image to confirm correct fetal allocation of the segment of cord being studied. Such Doppler studies have a higher sensitivity in identifying fetal growth retardation (75%) than ultrasound measurement.[51–53] It is also possible to suspect a twin transfusion situation. Here, discordancy between ultrasound measures of fetal size and cord diameter identifies

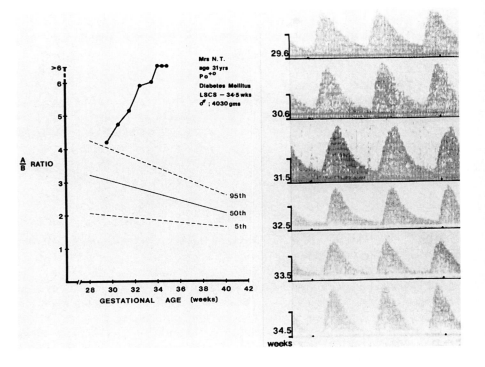

Fig. 12–10. Sequential studies of patient with maternal diabetes mellitus. The fetus was macrosomic. Delivery was indicated by decreasing maternal estrogen assays and abnormal FHR.

such a situation, especially if liquid volume in one sac is excessive while there are similar umbilical waveforms for the two fetuses.

The example shown in Figure 12–11 illustrates serial studies in association with discordant fetal growth. When one fetus is recognized as small prior to 32 weeks, management is difficult because early delivery is not in the best interests of the twin member with a normal Doppler study and normal growth.

The great value of Doppler studies in twin pregnancy management lies in the early recognition of fetal risk. An evaluation of Doppler studies assisting in the management of twin pairs was carried out. Consecutive groups of 100 twin pairs before and after the Doppler study results were made clinically available were compared.[54] The Doppler studies were done at 28 weeks and showed that fetal deaths could be significantly reduced. The perinatal mortality was reduced from 58/1,000 to 18/1,000 ($P < 0.05$). The Doppler study of abnormal fetuses identified patients who would be subjected to intensive fetal surveillance. The consequence was improved outcome.

Major Fetal Anomaly. Fetal growth retardation has been broadly divided into two groups: those fetuses that are small because of low growth potential (eg, genetic abnormality or early infection), and those that are small because of deprivation of oxygen or nutrient supply (loss of growth support). The records and outcome of 26 fetuses with major congenital malformation were examined be-

cause this group represents an example of an innate fetal disturbance.[55] In 13 of the 26 patients, the umbilical artery FVW systolic:diastolic ratio was high. It is postulated that in such patients the process of obliteration of the small arteries in the placenta is triggered by the abnormal fetus. In this series, placental weights were also examined. Those fetuses with a small placenta (low weight or low placental:fetal weight ratio) were drawn from the group with normal umbilical artery FVW pattern. It was suggested that in this group the fetus is of low growth potential and adequately supported by its small placenta. In contrast, a high placental:fetal weight ratio was present in the abnormal umbilical study group, and it was postulated that this represented placental overgrowth in an attempt to compensate for vascular obliteration. Such studies reflect the dynamics of fetal growth and fetal placental relations assessable by Doppler flow studies.

Isoimmunization and Fetal Anemia. Although Rhesus isoimmunization has decreased in frequency, there remains a small residue of isoimmunization cases due to Rh and other blood-group antigens. The systolic:diastolic ratio has been reported low in association with fetal anemia. A high umbilical vein volume flow has been seen in association with fetal hydrops.[56,57] Fetal transfusion in utero has been observed to increase the low systolic:diastolic ratio index of resistance in the umbilical placental circulation toward a more normal ratio. The high umbilical vein volume flow has been reduced in these anemic fetuses. An inverse correlation has been

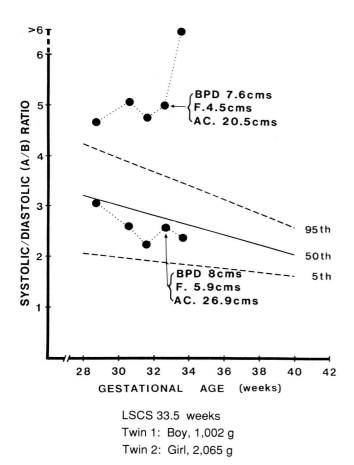

Fig. 12–11. Sequential studies in a twin pregnancy in which there was discordancy in fetal growth.

reported between the hematocrit of fetal blood and resistance index, but this is weak and not of clinical value.[58] A low systolic:diastolic ratio has also been reported in fetal anemia associated with hemoglobinopathies.

Lupus Obstetric Syndrome. A high incidence of fetal wastage both in early and late pregnancy and in maternal hypertension is associated with the presence in maternal blood of the "lupus anticoagulant." Such mothers may have systemic lupus erythematosus or other autoimmune phenomena, but in many, the obstetric manifestations are the only clinical feature. Fetal deterioration is predicted by the development of an abnormal umbilical artery waveform and these studies have aided the management of such pregnancies.[59] Frequent studies (at least weekly in the third trimester) are necessary as fetal demise may occur over a short time.

Clinical Management Incorporating Umbilical Artery FVWs. Tests of fetal welfare are required to recognize

fetal compromise and to quantitate fetal condition so that action is taken before the fetus suffers irreversible damage or dies in utero.

Doppler studies have been extensively evaluated as a means to recognize fetal compromise. Much of the data concerning this and specific clinical problems have been presented above.

Doppler umbilical FVW study has been compared to other methods of fetal surveillance. In a comparison with antenatal FHR monitoring, it was found that fetal compromise was more efficiently recognized by the study of umbilical artery waveforms.[60] The sensitivity was higher and the positive and negative predictive values were similar. Sensitivity was not achieved at the cost of an increase in false-positive findings. In this study, it was encouraging that those fetuses at risk of further morbidity were identified (18 out of 19 of the SGA infants who required admission to neonatal intensive care). Such information demonstrates the value of umbilical artery FVW as a test of recognition of fetal problems. It appears, however, that the Doppler studies do not predict the abnormal FHR monitoring study or fetal morbidity in postdate pregnancy.[61,62]

A randomized controlled clinical trial has been carried out to evaluate the influence of antenatal Doppler umbilical artery FVWs on subsequent obstetric management and fetal outcome.[63] Three hundred patients at high fetal risk were randomly assigned to an antenatal Doppler umbilical study group and a control group. The overall timing of delivery was similar in the control and Doppler study groups. However, in the Doppler study group, obstetricians allowed the pregnancies of those not selected for elective delivery to continue longer. There was no difference in the rates for elective delivery (induction of labor or cesarean section) in the two groups. However, among those allowed to labor (induced or spontaneous), emergency cesarean section was more frequent in the control group (23%) than in the report group (13%). This difference was most marked among those allowed to commence labor spontaneously (35% compared to 13%). Fetal distress was more common in the control group, accounting for the difference in cesarean section rate. This suggests that obstetric decision making was more appropriate with the aid of a Doppler umbilical artery study.

The clinical value of umbilical artery FVWs in early recognition of umbilical placental vascular lesion that leads to fetal compromise has been extended recently by the therapeutic possibility of reversing this lesion with low-dose aspirin.[64] A randomized placebo-controlled double-blind trial was carried out to evaluate the fetal benefits of low-dose aspirin (150 mg/day) in cases of umbilical placental insufficiency recognized during the last trimester. The rationale for this was the demonstrated placental vascular lesion,[44] reported alterations in placental thromboxane production,[65] and the demonstrated ability of thromboxane to increase resistance and umbilical circulation.[66] Forty-six women were included in the trial. These patients were referred for study because of concern for fetal welfare and were found to have an elevated umbilical artery waveform systolic:diastolic ratio. Mothers with severe hypertension were excluded because fetal condition would not necessarily be the dominant determinant of obstetric decision making. A distinction was made between high systolic:diastolic ratio (>95th but <99.95th percentile) and extremely high ratio (>99.95th percentile). There were 34 patients in the high ratio group and 12 in the extreme group. Aspirin therapy was associated with an increase in birthweight (mean difference 526 g, P<0.02), head circumference (1.7 cm, P<0.025), and placental weight (136 g, P<0.02) in those patients with high initial umbilical artery systolic:diastolic ratio. For the 12 women with an extremely high initial ratio, aspirin therapy did not result in a significantly different pregnancy outcome. If such treatment is to be adopted clinically, it is clear that early recognition of abnormality is most important.

Volume Blood Flow in Clinical Management. Studies of umbilical vein volume flow have been carried out in complicated pregnancies.[67] Fetal growth retardation as evidenced by birthweight below the tenth percentile was associated with reduced umbilical vein flow. Interestingly, flow was reduced when expressed both in absolute terms (mL/min) and relative to fetal weight (mL/min/kg). However, of the patients in whom a low umbilical vein flow was measured, only 40% had a birthweight below the tenth percentile. This was increased to 62% when at least two successive values were low. The relationship between umbilical artery FVW and umbilical vein volume flow measurements has been examined.[68] The FVW was more sensitive and recognized more SGA fetuses. It had a higher predictive value and similar specificity. The ratio of umbilical flow to aortic flow was also measured in this series. In normal fetuses, this was 39%. In those fetuses with an abnormal umbilical artery FVW, systolic:diastolic ratio was 25%. This result suggests that the fetus is able to maintain umbilical placental circulation, at least initially, by an increase in cardiac output. The same observation has been made in experimental growth retardation in fetal lambs.[30] Thus, there is experimental and clinical evidence to suggest that the umbilical artery FVW will detect the compromised fetus earlier than volume flow measures.

The use of volume flow in the umbilical vein to monitor fetuses affected by maternal blood group isoimmunization[56] has been mentioned above.

Aortic Blood Flow in the Fetus
Both the FVWs and volume flow have been recorded in fetal aortic circulation. The FVW may be identified using a continuous-wave Doppler system, but this is unsatisfactory because there is no information about the site of recording. A pulsed Doppler system integrated with a

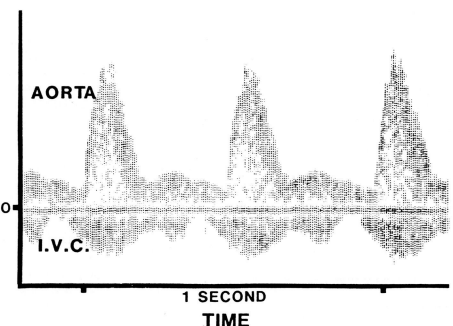

Fig. 12–12. Flow velocity waveform recorded from abdominal aorta and inferior vena cava of a normal 34-week fetus.

real-time B-mode image is preferable.[69] The same indices of downstream resistance described in the assessment of umbilical artery FVWs can be used. Volume blood flow is measured in the same way as flow in the umbilical vein. The dimensions of the aorta are measured from a "frozen" screen image. This is not entirely satisfactory because of the changing diameter with pulsatile flow. It has been estimated that this adds an error of 6% to the flow measurement.[10]

The aortic FVW shape changes with increasing distance from the heart.[70–72] The thoracic peak velocity is higher and the least diastolic velocity lower than abdominal. Therefore, mean velocity is similar and does not appear to change with gestation. The pulsatility index of the maximum velocity waveform is lower in the thoracic aorta (1.68 ± 0.28) than in the abdominal aorta (1.96 ± 0.36), but does not change with gestation (Fig. 12–12).[70,71] This index is also significantly affected by changes in fetal heart rate.[36] Within the normal FHR range there is a negative correlation with thoracic descending aorta pulsatility index (r = 0.43).[70] This pulsatility index is also affected by behavioral state. These observations are not surprising because 60% of aortic blood is distributed to nonplacental vascular beds in which vasomotor tone is regulated according to fetal behavior and metabolic states. In clinical studies, the use of a high cutoff (mean, + 2 standard deviations) to distinguish normal and abnormal eliminates the effect of FHR over the normal

range.[69] Fetal breathing movements affect the aortic flow waveform and studies should be carried out during fetal apnea to gain reproducible results.

Volume blood flow in the fetal descending thoracic aorta increases with gestation to 36 to 37 weeks when a plateau is attained, whereas flow per unit of fetal weight decreases during the third trimester.[70,71]

Studies of aortic flow velocity waveform have been evaluated as predictors of fetal growth retardation and fetal distress (diagnosed on the basis of cardiotocographic changes). A high pulsatility index in the absence of diastolic flow was the most efficient indicator in a comprehensive comparative study of many waveform parameters and volume blood flow. The results were used to support a grading score in which the degree of abnormality was quantified into "blood flow classes" (Fig. 12–13).

The high predictive capacity reported for aortic FVW for fetal growth retardation and perinatal asphyxia has been noted by others.[73,74] There is no evidence to suggest that the use of aortic FVWs provides additional information than the umbilical artery FVW. Rather, it is likely that the same cases are selected. The plausible explanation for change in aortic FVW seen in these pregnancy complications is the increase in downstream flow resistance in the placenta. Assessment of volume flow in the fetal aorta has not proved helpful.[72,75,76]

Measurements of aortic flow and the FVW have proved helpful in the assessment of fetal cardiac arrhythmias.[77–79] The most common arrhythmia, the extrasystole, is associated with a higher incidence of cardiac malformation, as are other arrhythmias. Measurements of aortic volume flow in these cases allows determination of the adequacy of ventricular output in circumstances when a high heart rate (supraventricular tachycardia) may mean insufficient time for filling, or a slow rate (eg, heart block), insufficient output. Such studies have also provided good evidence that the Frank-Starling mechanism operates in fetal life and contradicts the former belief that the fetus could only increase cardiac output by an increase in rate. The limit of fetal heart rate above which failure is imminent seems to be about 240 beats per minute.[78] At that point, cardiac output and aortic flow begin to decrease.

Fetal Cerebral Circulation

The combined use of duplex B-mode imaging and pulsed Doppler ultrasound has enabled recording of FVWs from the fetal internal carotid and cerebral arteries, and these studies have been applied to the study of human pregnancy.[80] The common carotid artery can be imaged from a longitudinal scan of the head and neck area, but may be difficult to visualize due to the often curved position of this area, particularly when the fetal spine is anterior.

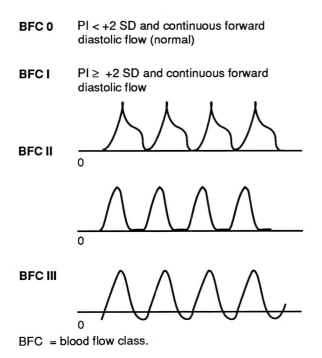

BFC 0   PI < +2 SD and continuous forward diastolic flow (normal)

BFC I   PI ≥ +2 SD and continuous forward diastolic flow

BFC II

BFC III

BFC = blood flow class.

Fig. 12–13. System for classification of fetal aortic waveforms suggested by Marsal et al.[72]

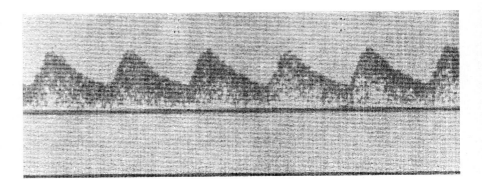

Fig. 12–14. Normal fetal internal carotid artery FVW recorded at 36 weeks' gestation.

The common carotid artery may be less representative of cerebral circulation because it also gives rise to the external carotid artery. The internal carotid artery is best located at the level of bifurcation into the middle and anterior cerebral artery.[81] This particular point can be readily identified on a transverse cross-section of the fetal cerebrum. The standard plane for measuring the biparietal diameter, which includes the thalamus and the cavum of the septum pellucidium, is visualized. The middle cerebral artery can be seen pulsating at the level of the insula. If the transducer is moved in a parallel fashion toward the base of the skull, a plane is reached that demonstrates a heart-shaped cross-section of the brain stem with the anterior lobes representing the cerebral peduncles. Anterior to this heart-shaped structure, on either side of the midline, an oblique cross-section on the internal carotid artery as it divides into its middle and anterior cerebral branches can be seen. Transducers with carrier frequencies of 3.5 and 5 MHz have been used for this. The sample volume size of the pulsed Doppler system should not exceed 3 to 4 mm. This allows clear flow-velocity signals from the internal carotid artery and reduces the likelihood of interference from other nearby vessels (such as the basilar artery).

The FVW of the fetal internal carotid artery displays a typical low-resistance pattern. With advancing gestation through the third trimester, there is a tendency for this waveform to indicate a slight fall in resistance (Fig. 12–14).

A normal range for the pulsatility index of the fetal internal carotid artery FVW has been reported. These measurements are affected by fetal breathing movements and behavioral state.[82] For clinical studies, the fetus should be inactive and apneic (Fig. 12–15).

Intrauterine fetal growth retardation is associated with a fetal internal carotid FVW pulsatility index that is lower than normal. Of 35 infants with a birthweight below the fifth percentile, 19 were observed with an internal carotid pulsatility index below the normal range (mean − 2 standard deviations).[80] These results were compared to umbilical FVWs in the same fetuses. A smaller number exhibited abnormal cerebral artery results compared to the number with a high umbilical artery pulsatility index. The presence of a normal fetal carotid FVW and a high-resistance umbilical FVW suggested the maintenance of normal cerebral flow. Later, with deteriorating fetal condition, cerebral vasodilation occurs and the cerebral FVW shows a lower pulsatility index. Whether this effect is adaptive to maintain cerebral oxygen supply or a consequence of fetal hypoxia and hy-

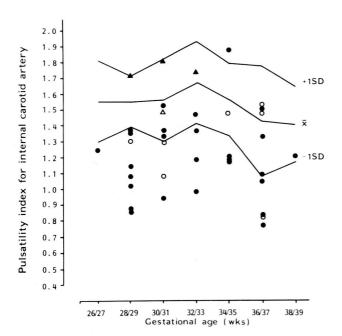

Fig. 12–15. Pulsatility index for the fetal internal carotid artery FVWs of normal pregnancy. Values for a group of fetuses subsequently born small for gestational age are plotted. Open symbol = birthweight less than 5th percentile; closed symbol = birthweight 5th to 10th percentile; circle = structurally normal; triangle = chromosomal anomaly. (*Used by permission from Waldimiroff et al.*[83])

percarbia is not known at present. It has been suggested that the ratio of umbilical to carotid-FVW pulsatility index be used to magnify the above observations. From studies in normal pregnancy, an upper limit (mean, +2 standard deviations) of 0.8 has been defined in the third trimester and used in the study of fetal growth retardation.

Maternal Uterine Circulation

The uteroplacental blood supply has been investigated invasively in the past but now can be studied using Doppler ultrasound. Signals from uteroplacental arteries can be obtained using either a duplex imaging system[83] with pulsed-wave Doppler or a continuous-wave Doppler.[84] In the latter, signals from the uteroplacental vessels are recognized by the direction of flow and the shape of the flow velocity waveform.

Method of Study. The method described by Campbell and associates[83] used a 2 MHz pulsed Doppler combined with a 3.5 MHz linear-array ultrasound imaging system. The gate and Doppler beam are displayed on the screen, allowing the operator to select areas of interest. The common iliac artery is first visualized as it bifurcates into the external and internal iliac arteries. With the Doppler transducer directed caudally, signals from these two arteries can be obtained. The FVW of the external iliac artery shows a pattern of high resistance with reverse flow in late systole and early diastole. In contrast, the FVW of the internal iliac artery shows continuous forward flow during diastole although it has a deep notch in relation to the closure of the aortic valve. With the transducer directed more medially, vessels in the lateral uterine wall can be identified. These can be visualized from 24 weeks on, and vary from 2 to 4 mm in diameter. Doppler signals from these vessels are in the opposite direction to those from the iliac arteries, indicating that the blood flow is toward the transducer.[85] It is uncertain whether these uteroplacental vessels are major branches of the uterine artery or arcuate vessels. Doppler signals are obtained from both sides of the uterus and in normal pregnancy show a typical pattern of low pulsatility with high end-diastolic frequencies.

The author and colleagues[84] use a 4 MHz continuous-wave (CW) directional Doppler to record FVWs from branches within the placental bed. A real-time ultrasound scan is first carried out to identify the site of placental implantation. The retroplacental area is then searched with the CW transducer until the characteristic sound of the uterine artery is heard. When the placenta is posterior, a more peripheral part of the bed is recorded midway along the lateral uterine margin. Most recently, a vaginal transducer has been used to record from the uterus artery in the lateral fornix.

Normal Pregnancy. In the nonpregnant uterus, end-diastolic frequencies are higher in the secretory than in the proliferative phase of the menstrual cycle. In pregnancy, there is a decrease in impedance to flow with higher end-diastolic frequencies. This can be detected in the first trimester. The decrease continues until 24 weeks' gestation; from then on, the FVW of the uteroplacental arteries has a pattern of low pulsatility with high end-diastolic velocity.[34,83,86] Throughout the last 20 weeks of pregnancy, there is a small increase in the diastolic flow velocity relative to peak systolic flow velocity. There is a difference between the placental and nonplacental sides of the uterus with a lower systolic:diastolic ratio on the side of the placental bed. Differences between records from the main uterine trunk and uteroplacental branches have been reported.[86] (Fig. 12–16.)

Complicated Pregnancy. Both severe growth retardation and maternal hypertension may be associated with uteroplacental waveforms that demonstrate a high systolic:diastolic ratio.[84] In a study of 31 patients with pregnancies complicated by hypertension or intrauterine growth retardation (IUGR), two groups were identified: those with FVWs similar to the normal population, and those who had evidence of a high impedance to flow. In this second group, there was a higher incidence of proteinuric hypertension, the time of delivery was significantly shorter, and birthweight ratio of the infants was lower (with actual birthweight/mean birthweight for gestational age corrected for sex and parity).[83] Similarly, Fleischer and coworkers[87] examined a group of 71 women with hypertensive disorders of pregnancy. An impaired placental perfusion was defined by systolic:diastolic ratio of greater than 2.6 and persistence of the notch after 26 weeks of gestation. In 28 patients with abnormal waveforms, there was a significantly higher maternal uric acid level, shorter gestation period, higher cesarean-section rate for fetal distress, and lower-birthweight infants than in the 43 patients with normal FVWs. Furthermore, in the pathologic group, there was a significantly higher incidence of SGA babies and a significant increase in stillbirths. A recent report of a similar range of uterine waveforms in normal and hypertensive pregnancies contradicts these findings.[88]

These studies have also been evaluated for screening use in early pregnancy. As trophoblast invasion has usually been completed by the 20th week, it may be possible to predict those pregnancies at risk of preeclampsia and IUGR by finding abnormal high resistance FVWs in the second trimester. In a study of 126 consecutive pregnancies screened between 16 and 18 weeks' gestation, an abnormal waveform predicted such complications with a sensitivity of 68% and specificity of 69%.[89] These preliminary results are encouraging but require confirmation

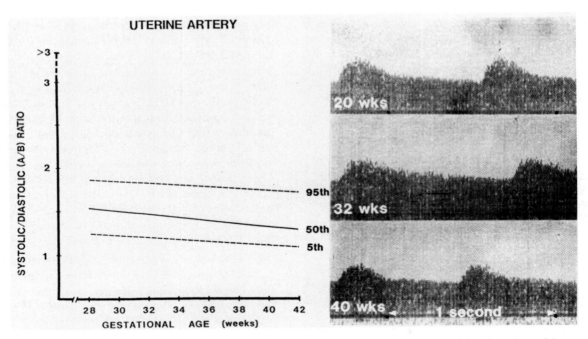

Fig. 12–16. Sequential studies of flow velocity waveform recorded from uteroplacental bed branches of the uterine artery. A normal range during the second half of pregnancy is plotted.

in larger series because there were many normal pregnancy outcomes in the large group with "abnormal" uterine waveforms.

Relationship of Umbilical and Uterine FVW Studies. The relationship between the umbilical artery and uterine artery FVW has been examined.[48] In a series of 53 SGA fetuses, it was found that three broad divisions could be created on the basis of such a study. The subgroup with normal umbilical and uterine waveforms exhibited little fetal morbidity. These fetuses did not require neonatal intensive care and were delivered later than fetuses with abnormal FVWs. In the other two subgroups characterized by abnormal uterine artery pattern, neonatal morbidity was present.

In patients with a normal uterine artery pattern, it is suggested that the primary defect is on the fetal side of the placenta. Although the uterine waveform is normal (indicating normal resistance in that branch of the uterine artery), total uterine flow may be low if the size of the uteroplacental bed (and number of branches of the uterine artery feeding it) is not large. Those fetuses with both abnormal umbilical and uterine FVWs may represent a group in which vascular disease exists in the maternal uteroplacental vascular bed, leading to constraint of the placenta and fetus.

Among 23 patients classified as severely hypertensive (with diastolic blood pressure > 110 mm Hg and proteinuria > 1 g/day), umbilical and uterine studies were performed.[48] In this group of 23 patients, the umbilical artery study result was abnormal in 17 cases. The uterine study result was abnormal in 11 cases. Ten of these 11 cases also had abnormal umbilical study results, again indicating the association between abnormal uterine and umbilical artery waveforms. Fetal morbidity occurred in the group with abnormal umbilical waveform study; even in the absence of fetal morbidity, severe maternal hypertension was more likely to be associated with abnormal umbilical study results.

SUMMARY

Doppler studies provide dynamic information about fetal and maternal circulations in pregnancy.

Flow velocity waveforms may be recorded simply from major fetal and maternal vessels and provide insight into the interaction between the heart pump upstream and the resistance vessels downstream. Most attention has focused on the interpretation of these waveforms in terms of downstream resistance. A number of indices derived from the FVW have been described for this purpose. Studies of volume blood flow require more complex equipment, and only the flow in very large vessels can be studied with a reasonable degree of accuracy. Such studies are unlikely to be clinically applicable without simpler and more accurate instrumentation. There is evidence that volume flow may be preserved despite a change in the FVW indices of resistance.

Most clinical evaluation has been carried out on the umbilical artery FVW. A high-resistance waveform pattern is seen early in the development of fetal growth failure. Such studies may be used clinically to recognize potential fetal compromise, permitting more intensive pregnancy management. Abnormal umbilical artery FVWs are also seen in severe pregnancy hypertension. The value of this early recognition has been recently enhanced by the demonstration that low-dose aspirin will improve fetal weight if administered early when abnormal FVW is recognized.

Aortic waveform studies appear to provide similar information to umbilical studies. Volume flow studies have been used to assess the adequacy of cardiac output in cases of fetal cardiac arrhythmia.

Studies of fetal cerebral circulation provide information about an important fetal vascular bed. This complements the information about placental resistance and may prove most valuable as a measure of the degree to which the fetus is compromised.

Maternal uterine studies have an uncertain clinical role. There does appear to be a problem in reproducibility as a number of different vessels are studied. At present, it is uncertain what is being defined by such studies.

REFERENCES

1. Trudinger BJ, Stevens D, Connelly A, et al. Umbilical artery flow velocity waveforms and placental resistance: The effects of embolization of the umbilical circulation. *Am J Obstet Gynecol.* 1987;157:1443–1449.
2. Thompson RS, Stevens RJ. A mathematical model for interpretation of Doppler velocity waveform indices. *Med Biol Eng Comput.* 1988. In press.
3. Thompson RS, Trudinger BJ, Cook CM. A comparison of Doppler ultrasound waveform indices in the umbilical artery, I: Indices derived from the maximum velocity waveform. *Ultrasound Med Biol.* 1986;12:835–844.
4. Thompson RS, Trudinger BJ, Cook CM. Doppler ultrasound waveform indices: AB ratio pulsatility index and Pourcelot ratio. *Br J Obstet Gynaecol.* 1988. In press.
5. Thompson RS, Trudinger BJ, Cook CM, Giles WB. Umbilical artery velocity waveforms: Normal reference values for AB ratio and Pourcelot ratio. *Br J Obstet Gynaecol.* 1988. In press.
6. Thompson RS, Trudinger BJ, Cook CM. A comparison of Doppler ultrasound waveform indices in the umbilical artery, II: Indices derived from the maximum velocity waveform. *Ultrasound Med Biol.* 1986;12:845–854.
7. Gill RW. Pulsed Doppler with B-mode imaging for quantitative blood flow measurement. *Ultrasound Med Biol.* 1979;5:223–235.
8. Gill RW. Doppler ultrasound—physical aspects. Seminars in Perinatology. 1987;11:292–299.
9. Eik-Nes SH, Marshal K, Kristoffersen K. Methodology and basic problems related to blood flow studies in the human fetus. *Ultrasound Med Biol.* 1984;10:329–337.
10. Lingman G, Gennser G, Marsal K. Ultrasonic measurements of the blood velocity and pulsatile diameter changes in the fetal descending aorta. In: Rolfe P, ed. *Fetal Physiological Measurements.* London: Butterworths; 1986:206–210.
11. Walker AM. Physiological control of the fetal cardiovascular system. In: Beard RW, Nathanielsz PW, eds. *Fetal Physiology and Medicine: The Basis of Perinatology.* London: Butterworths; 1984:287–316.
12. Tonge HM, Stewart PA, Wladimiroff JW. Fetal blood flow measurements during fetal cardiac dysrhythmia. *Early Hum Dev.* 1984;10:23–24.
13. Rudolph AM, Heymann MA. Circulatory changes during growth in the fetal lamb. *Circ Res.* 1970;26:289–290.
14. Dawes GS. The umbilical circulation. In: *Fetal and Neonatal Physiology,* Chicago: *Year Book Medical;* 1968:66–78.
15. Rudolph AM, Heymann MA. Control of the foetal circulation. In: Comline RS, Cross KW, Dawes GS, et al, eds. *Foetal and Neonatal Physiology.* London: Cambridge University Press; 1973:89.
16. Rudolph AM. Factors affecting umbilical blood flow in the lamb in utero. In: Nathanielsz PW, ed. *Animal Models in Fetal Medicine.* New York: Elsevier; 1980;1:1–58.
17. Walker AM, Oakes GK, Ehrenkranz R, et al. Effects of hypercapnia on uterine and umbilical circulations in conscious pregnant sheep. *J Appl Physiol.* 1976;41:727–733.
18. Itskovitz J, LaGamma EF, Rudolph AM. The effect of reducing umbilical blood flow on fetal oxygenation. *Am J Obstet Gynecol.* 1983;145:81–818.
19. Greiss FC. Uterine blood flow in pregnancy: An overview. In: Moawad AH, Lindheimer MD, eds. Uterine and Placental Blood Flow. New York: Masson; 1982:19–28.
20. Clapp JF. The relationship between blood flow and oxygen uptake in the uterine and umbilical circulations. *Am J Obstet Gynecol.* 1978;132:410–413.
21. Dixon HG, Robertson WB. A study of the vessels of the placental bed in normotensive and hypertensive women. *J Obstet Gynaecol Br Emp.* 1958;65:803–810.
22. Brosens I, Robertson WB, Dixon HG. The physiological response of the vessels of the placental bed to normal pregnancy. *J Path Bact.* 1967;93:569–579.
23. Boyd JD, Hamilton WJ. In: *The Human Placenta.* Cambridge, Mass: Heffer; 1970:253–266.
24. Sheppard BL, Bonnar J. The ultrastructure of the arterial supply of the human placenta in early and late pregnancy. *J Obstet Gynaecol Br Comm.* 1974;81:497–511.
25. Robertson WB, Brosen I, Dixon G. Uteroplacental vascular pathology. *Europ J Obstet Gynecol Reprod Biol.* 1975;5:47–65.

26. Robertson WB. Uteroplacental vasculature. *J Clin Path.* 1976;29(suppl 10):9–17.

27. Longo LDL. Some physiological implications of altered uteroplacental blood flow. In: Moawad AH, Lindheimer MD, eds. *Uterine and Placental Blood Flow.* New York: Masson; 1982:93–102.

28. Clapp JF, Szeto HH, Larrow R, et al. Umbilical blood flow response to embolization of the uterine circulation. *Am J Obstet Gynecol.* 1980;138:60–67.

29. Clapp JF, McLaughlin MK, Larrow R, et al. The uterine haemodynamic response to repetitive unilateral vascular embolization in the pregnant ewe. *Am J Obstet Gynecol.* 1982;144:309–318.

30. Block BSB, Llanos AJ, Creasy RK. Response of the growth retarded fetus to acute hypoxemia. *Am J Obstet Gynecol.* 1984;148:879–885.

31. Makowski EL, Battaglia FC, Meschia G, et al. Effects of maternal exposure to high altitude upon fetal oxygenation. *Am J Obstet Gynecol.* 1968;100:852–861.

32. Rankin JHG, McLaughlin MK. The regulation of placental blood flows. *J Dev Physiol.* 1979;1:3–30.

33. Trudinger BJ, Cook CM. Different umbilical artery flow velocity waveforms in one patient. *Obstet Gynecol.* 1988. In press.

34. Pearce JM, Campbell S, Cohen-Overbeek T, et al. Reference ranges and sources of variations for indices of pulsed Doppler flow velocity waveforms from the uteroplacental and fetal circulation. *Br J Obstet Gynaecol.* 1988;95:248–256.

35. Mires G, Dempster GS, Patel NB, Crawford JW. The effect of fetal heart rate on umbilical artery flow velocity waveforms. *Br J Obstet Gynaecol.* 1987;94:665–669.

36. Van Eyck J, Wladimiroff JW, Noordam MJ, Tonge HM, Prechtl HRF. The blood flow velocity waveform in the fetal descending aorta: Its relationship to fetal behavioral state in normal pregnancy at 37–38 weeks. *Early Human Devel.* 1985;12:137–143.

37. Faber JJ, Thornberg KL. *Placental Physiology.* New York: Raven Press; 1983:19.

38. Trudinger BJ, Cook CM. Fetal umbilical artery velocity waveforms. *Ultrasound Med Biol.* 1982;8(suppl 1):197.

39. Giles WB, Trudinger BJ. Umbilical artery velocity time waveforms in pregnancy. *J Ultrasound Med.* 1982;(suppl):98.

40. Trudinger BJ, Giles WB, Cook CM, et al. Fetal umbilical artery flow velocity waveforms and placental resistance: Clinical significance. *Br J Obstet Gynaecol.* 1985;92:23–30.

41. Schulman H, Fleischer A, Sterm W, et al. Umbilical velocity wave ratios in human pregnancy. *Am J Obstet Gynecol.* 1984;148:986–990.

42. Erskine RLA, Ritchie JWK. Umbilical artery blood flow characteristics in normal and growth retarded fetuses. *Br J Obstet Gynaecol.* 1985;92:605–610.

43. Reuwer PJHM, Bruinse HW, Stoutenbeek P, et al. Doppler assessment of the feto-placental circulation in normal and growth retarded fetuses. *Eur J Obstet Gynaecol Reprod Biol.* 1984;18:199–205.

44. Giles WB, Trudinger BJ, Baird P. Fetal umbilical artery flow velocity waveforms and placental resistance: Patho-

45. McCowan LM, Mullen BM, Ritchie K. Umbilical artery flow velocity waveforms and the placental vascular bed. *Am J Obstet Gynecol.* 1987;157:900–902.

46. Fox H. Pathology of the placenta. In: Bennington JL, ed. *Major Problems in Pathology.* Philadelphia: WB Saunders; 1978;8.

47. Giles WB, Trudinger BJ, Stevens D, et al. Umbilical artery flow velocity waveform analysis in normal ovine pregnancy and after carunculectomy. *J Dev Physiol.* 1988. Unpublished data.

48. Trudinger BJ, Giles WB, Cook CM. Flow velocity waveforms in the maternal uteroplacental and fetal umbilical placental circulation. *Am J Obstet Gynecol.* 1985;152:155–163.

49. Ducey J, Schulman H, Farmakides G, et al. A classification of hypertension in pregnancy based on Doppler velocimetry. *Am J Obstet Gynecol.* 1987;157:6880–685.

50. Bracero L, Schulman H, Fleischer A, et al. Umbilical artery velocimetry in diabetes and pregnancy. *Obstet Gynecol.* 1986;68:654–658.

51. Giles WB, Trudinger BJ, Cook CM. Fetal umbilical artery flow velocity time waveforms in twin pregnancies. *Br J Obstet Gynaecol.* 1985;92:490–497.

52. Farmakides G, Schulman H, Saldana LR, et al. Surveillance of twin pregnancy with umbilical arterial velocimetry. *Am J Obstet Gynecol.* 1985;153:789–792.

53. Saldana LR, Eads MC, Schaefer TR. Umbilical blood waveforms in fetal surveillance of twins. *Am J Obstet Gynecol.* 1987;157:712–715.

54. Giles WB, Trudinger BJ, Cook CM, Connelly A. Umbilical artery flow velocity waveforms and twin pregnancy outcome. *Obstet Gynecol.* 1988;47:86.

55. Trudinger BJ, Cook CM. Umbilical and uterine artery flow velocity waveforms in pregnancy associated with major fetal abnormality. *Br J Obstet Gynaecol.* 1985;92:666–670.

56. Kirkinen P, Jouppila P, Eik-Nes S. Umbilical vein blood flow in Rhesus-isoimmunisation. *Br J Obstet Gynaecol.* 1983;90:640–644.

57. Warren PS, Gill RW, Fisher CC. Doppler flow studies in Rhesus isoimmunization. *Sem Perinat.* 1987;11:375–378.

58. Rightmire DA, Nicolaides KH, Rodeck CH, et al. Fetal blood velocities in Rh-isoimmunization: Relationship to gestational age and to fetal hematocrit. *Obstet Gynecol.* 1986;68:233–236.

59. Trudinger BJ, Stewart G, Cook CM, et al. Monitoring lupus anticoagulant positive pregnancies with umbilical artery flow velocity waveforms. *Obstet Gynecol.* 1988. In press.

60. Trudinger BJ, Cook CM, Jones L. A comparison of fetal heart rate monitoring and umbilical artery waveforms in the recognition of fetal compromise. *Br J Obstet Gynaecol.* 1986;93:171–175.

61. Guidetti DA, Diven MY, Cavalieri RL, et al. Fetal umbilical artery flow velocimetry in postdate pregnancies. *Am J Obstet Gynecol.* 1987;157:1521–1523.

62. Farmakides G, Schulman H, Winter D, et al. Prenatal surveillance using non-stress testing and Doppler velocimetry. *Obstet Gynecol.* 1988;71:184–187.

63. Trudinger BJ, Cook CM, Giles WB, et al. Umbilical artery

flow velocity waveforms—A randomized control trial. *Lancet*. 1987;1:188–190.

64. Trudinger BJ, Cook CM, Thompson RS, et al. Low dose aspirin therapy improves fetal weight in umbilical placental insufficiency. *Am J Obstet Gynecol*. 1988. In press.

65. Walsh SW: Preeclampsia: An imbalance in placental prostacyclin and thromboxane production. *Am J Obstet Gynecol*. 1985;152:335–340.

66. Trudinger BJ, Connelly AJ, Giles WB, et al. The effects of prostacyclin and thromboxane analogue (U46619) on the fetal circulation and umbilical flow velocity waveforms. *J Devel Physiol*. 1988. In press.

67. Gill RW, Warren PS, Kissoff G, et al. Umbilical venous flow in normal and complicated pregnancy. *Ultrasound Med Biol* 1984;10:349–363.

68. Giles WB, Lingman G, Marsal K, Trudinger BJ. Fetal volume blood flow and umbilical artery flow velocity waveform analysis: A comparison. *Br J Obstet Gynaecol*. 1986;93:461–465.

69. Marsal K, Laurin J, Lindblad A, Lingman G. Blood flow in the fetal descending aorta. *Sem Perinat*. 1987;11:322–334.

70. Lingman G, Marsal K. Fetal central blood circulation in the third trimester of normal pregnancy, II: Aortic blood velocity waveform. *Early Hum Dev*. 1986;13:151–159.

71. Lingman G, Marsal K. Fetal central blood circulation in the third trimester of normal pregnancy, I: Aortic and umbilical blood flow. *Early Hum Dev*. 1986;13:137–150.

72. Laurin J, Marsal K, Persson PH, et al. Ultrasound measurement of fetal blood flow in predicting fetal outcome. Br J Obstet Gynaecol. In press.

73. Jouppila P, Kirkinen P. Increased vascular resistance in the descending aorta of the human fetus in hypoxia. *Br J Obstet Gynaecol*. 1984;91:853–856.

74. Hackett GA, Campbell S, Gamsu H, et al. Doppler studies in the growth retarded fetus and prediction of neonatal necrotising enterocolitis, haemorrhage, and neonatal morbidity. *Br Med J*. 1987;294:13–16.

75. Griffin D, Cohen-Overbeek T, Campbell S. Fetal and uteroplacental blood flow. *Clin Obstet Gynecol*. 1983;10:565–602.

76. Tonge HM, Wladimiroff JW, Noordam MJ, et al. Blood velocity waveforms in the descending fetal aorta: Comparison between normal and growth retarded pregnancies. *Obstet Gynecol*. 1986;67:851–855.

77. Lingman G, Lundstrom NR, Marsal K, et al. Fetal cardiac arrhythmia: Clinical outcome of 113 cases. *Acta Obstet Gynecol Scand*. 1986;65:263–267.

78. Tonge HM, Wladimiroff JW, Noordam MJ, et al. Fetal cardiac arrhythmia and its effect on volume blood flow in the descending aorta of the human fetus. *J Clin Ultrasound*. 1986;14:607–612.

79. Tonge HM, Stewart PA, Wladimiroff JW. Fetal blood flow measurements during fetal cardiac arrhythmia. *Early Hum Dev*. 1984;10:23–34.

80. Wladimiroff JW, Wijngaard JAGW vd, Degani S, et al. Cerebral and umbilical arterial blood flow velocity waveforms in normal and growth retarded pregnancies. *Obstet Gynecol*. 1987;69:705,709.

81. Wladimiroff JW, Tonge HM, Stewart PA. Doppler ultrasound assessment of cerebral blood flow in the human fetus. *Br J Obstet Gynaecol*. 1986;93:471–475.

82. Van Eyck J, Wladimiroff JW, Wijngaard JAGW vd, et al. The blood flow velocity waveform in the fetal internal carotid and umbilical artery. Its relationship to fetal behavioural states in normal pregnancy at 37–38 weeks of gestation. *Br J Obstet Gynaecol*. 1987;94:736–741.

83. Campbell S, Diaz-Recasens J, Griffin DR, et al. New Doppler technique for assessing uteroplacental blood flow. *Lancet*. 1983;1:675–677.

84. Trudinger BJ, Giles WB, Cook CM. Uteroplacental blood flow velocity-time waveforms in normal and complicated pregnancy. *Br J Obstet Gynaecol*. 1985;92:39–45.

85. Cohen-Overbeek TE, Pearce JM, Campbell S. The antenatal assessment of utero-placental and feto-placental bloodflow using Doppler ultrasound. *Ultrasound Med Biol*. 1985;11:329–339.

86. Schulman H, Fleischer A, Farmakides G, et al. Development of uterine artery compliance in pregnancy as detected by Doppler ultrasound. *Am J Obstet Gynecol*. 1986;155:1031–1036.

87. Fleischer A, Schulman H, Farmakides G, et al. Uterine artery Doppler velocimetry in pregnant women with hypertension. *Am J Obstet Gynecol*. 1986;154:806–813.

88. Hanretty KP, Whittle M, Rubin PC. Doppler uteroplacental waveforms in pregnancy induced hypertension: A reappraisal. *Lancet*. 1988;1:850–852.

89. Campbell S, Pearce JMF, Hackett G, et al. Qualitative assessment of uteroplacental bloodflow: Early screening test for high-risk pregnancies. *Obstet Gynecol*. 1986; 68:649–653.

13 Prenatal Detection of Anatomic Congenital Anomalies

*Roberto Romero • Enrique Oyarzun •
Marina Sirtori • John C. Hobbins*

The detection of anatomic congenital anomalies has become a new goal of prenatal care.[1] The information required for diagnosis and management of the obstetric patient with a fetal congenital anomaly demands knowledge in a variety of disciplines, including diagnostic imaging, obstetrics, genetics, pediatric surgery, anatomy, embryology, and teratology. Many health care professionals involved in diagnostic imaging techniques have had limited exposure to the other fields. The purpose of this chapter is to serve as an introduction to the section on congenital anomalies in this book. It will provide an overview of the definition and magnitude of the problem and pathogenic mechanisms of gross congenital anomalies. The principles behind ultrasound prenatal diagnosis and accuracy for selected anomalies will be discussed, as well as the obstetric options that such diagnosis presents.

DEFINITIONS

A congenital anomaly consists of a departure from the normal anatomic architecture of an organ or system. Anomalies may result from an intrinsically abnormal primordium or anlage of an organ, or from a normal primordium that is affected during development by extrinsic forces.[2-4] Growing interest in prenatal development, coupled with the need for a uniform nomenclature to refer to errors in morphogenesis, led an international working group to propose a set of terms useful in the classification of anatomic congenital anomalies.[2] Individual alterations of form or structure can be classified as malformations, deformations, and disruptions.

A malformation is a morphologic defect of an organ, part of an organ, or a larger area of the body resulting from an intrinsically abnormal developmental process. The term "intrinsically abnormal developmental process" refers to an abnormality in the primordium (anlage) of the organ. This abnormality may not be identifiable in early stages of development. The typical example is a limb bud that appears normal in early embryonic life but later develops an extra digit. Malformations can be considered as the result of a development arrest of the pri-

mordium (incomplete morphogenesis), redundant morphogenesis, or aberrant morphogenesis (Fig. 13–1). Examples of these types of malformations are listed in Table 13–1. Although malformations often occur during the embryonic period (until the 9th postmenstrual week,[5] some may also arise during later stages of development. A general principle is that the earlier the malformation is initiated, the more complex is the resulting anomaly (anomalies).

A deformation refers to an abnormal form, shape, or position of a part of the body caused by nondisruptive mechanical forces. The primordium of the organ is normal, but development is affected by mechanical forces that are extrinsic or intrinsic to the fetus. For example, a club foot deformity may be the result of intrauterine constraint due to oligohydramnios (extrinsic force) or lack of movement due to the neural defect associated with spina bifida (intrinsic force) (Fig. 13–2). Table 13–2 illustrates common forces leading to deformations. Four main factors influence the pathogenesis of deformations: pressure, fetal plasticity, fetal mobility, and the rate of fetal growth.[6-9] Deformations tend to occur late in gestation, as during this time there is rapid fetal growth in a potentially constraining intrauterine environment.[6-8,10,11] Removal of the mechanical force responsible for the deformation results in normalization or improvement of the anomaly. Spontaneous resolution after birth occurs in approximately 90% of deformations.[12] Table 13–3 compares malformations and deformations. In general, the term malformation describes defects that are likely to have arisen during organogenesis, whereas the term deformation is reserved for defects arising after the embryonic period.

A disruption is a morphologic defect of an organ, part of an organ, a larger region of the body resulting from a breakdown, or interference with an originally normal development process. A typical example of this type of anomaly is digital amputation associated with amniotic band syndrome (Fig. 13–3).[13-15] Disruptions are sporadic events.

Another concept frequently used by dysmorphologists is that of dysplasia, a term referring to abnormal

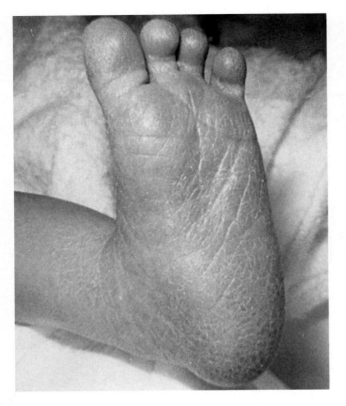

Fig. 13–1. Syndactyly (four digits on this foot), an example of malformation because of incomplete morphogenesis.

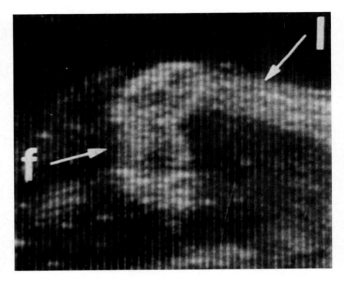

Fig. 13–2. Clubfoot, an example of deformation. l = leg; f = foot. (*Reproduced with permission from Jeanty P, Romero R. Obstetrical Ultrasound. New York: McGraw-Hill, 1984.*)

organization of cells into tissue(s) and its morphologic result(s). The term dysplasia in pathology refers to a neoplastic process. Its use in dysmorphology is broader and refers to any type of tissue disorganization. Osteogenesis imperfecta is a dysplasia in which the primary disorder affects collagen and, therefore, structures containing significant quantities of the particular type of defective collagen are affected.

It should be stressed that it is not always possible to assign an anomaly to a specific class. In fact, malformations, deformations, and disruptions may overlap (see definition of sequences later in this section).

A fetus may be affected by multiple anomalies. This association may occur simply by chance or may be part of a pathogenetically related event. A set of terms has been coined to describe the relationship between coexistent anomalies. These terms are polytopic field defect, sequence, syndrome, and association.

A polytopic field defect is a group of anomalies derived from the disturbance of a single developmental field. A developmental field is a region or part of an embryo that responds as a unit to embryonic interactions

TABLE 13–1. ABNORMAL MORPHOGENESIS RESULTING IN MALFORMATIONS

Types of Abnormal Morphogenesis	Examples of Malformation	Relative Frequency as a Class
Incomplete morphogenesis		Common
Lack of development	Absent nostril, renal agenesis	
Hypoplasia	Microcephaly, micrognathia	
Incomplete closure	Cleft palate, iris coloboma	
Incomplete separation	Syndactyly	
Incomplete septation	Ventricular septal defect	
Incomplete migration	Exstrophy of the cloaca	
Incomplete rotation	Malrotated gut	
Incomplete resolution of early form	Choanal atresia, Meckel diverticulum	
Persistence of early location	Low-set ears, undescended testes	
Redundant morphogenesis	Supernumerary ear tag, polydactyly	Uncommon
Aberrant morphogenesis	Mediastinal thyroid gland, paratesticular spleen	Rare

Reproduced with permission from: Cohen MM. The Child with Multiple Birth Defects. New York: Raven Press; 1982:2.

TABLE 13–2. CAUSES OF DEFORMATIONS

Extrinsic

Maternal

Small maternal size

Small maternal pelvis

Uterine malformation (eg, bicornuate uterus)

Uterine leyomioma

Fetal

Early pelvic engagement of the fetal head

Unusual fetal position

Oligohydramnios

Large fetus, rapid growth

Multiple fetuses

Intrinsic

Malformational

Central nervous system malformations (eg, spina bifida)

Urinary tract malformations (eg, bilateral renal agenesis or severe polycystic kidneys that may cause oligohydramnios and its sequence)

Functional

Congenital hypotonia secondary to neuromuscular disorders (eg, arthrogryposis)

Modified from: Cohen MM. The Child With Multiple Birth Defects. New York: Raven Press; 1982:10, and Smith DW. Recognizable patterns of human deformation: Identification and management of mechanical effects on morphogenesis. Major Problems in Clinical Pediatrics. Philadelphia: W.B. Saunders; 1981;21:101.

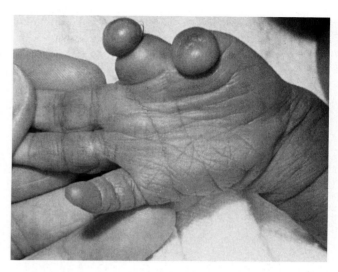

Fig. 13–3. Amputation of fingers in a fetus with amniotic band syndrome (disruption).

and results in complex or multiple anatomic structures. Opitz has discussed in detail the meaning and implications of the concept of developmental field defects.[4,16–19] The embryo is omnipotential ("the primary field") up to a certain time during which further organization and differentiation occur in a number of different developmental autonomous areas (secondary fields). Disturbances in a developmental field may result in multiple, and usually contiguous, anomalies (monotopic field defects) or multiple, distantly located anomalies (polytopic field defects). An example of a monotopic field defect is holoprosen-

cephaly where there is coexistence abnormalities of the face and of the central nervous system (Figs. 13–4 and 13–5). On the other hand, abnormalities in the acro-renal field are frequently cited as illustrative examples of polytopic field defects. There are at least 24 different genetic conditions in which both kidneys and limbs are involved. This has been explained by invoking a relationship between the mesonephros and limb buds during embry-

TABLE 13–3. COMPARISON OF MALFORMATIONS AND DEFORMATIONS

	Malformation	Deformation
Time of occurrence	Embryonic period	Fetal period
Level of disturbance	Organ	Region
Indicence before 20th week	5% (esti.)	0.1%
Incidence after 28th week	3.7%	2.0%
Perinatal mortality	+ (41%)	− (6%)
Spontaneous correction	−	+
Correction by posture	−	+

Modified from: Cohen MM. The Child With Multiple Birth Defects. New York: Raven Press; 1982:15, and Dunn PM. Congenital postural deformities: Perinatal associations. Proc Roy Soc Med. 1972;65:735.

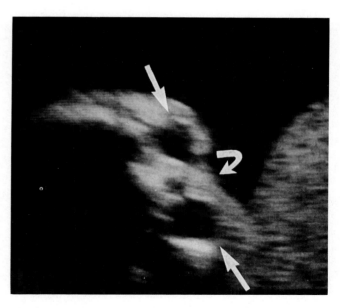

Fig. 13–4. Axial scan at the level of the orbits in a holoprosencephalic fetus, revealing hypotelorism (*between straight arrows*) and absence of the nasal bridge (*curved arrow*). (*Reproduced with permission from Pilu G, et al. Am J Perinatol. 1987:4;41.*)

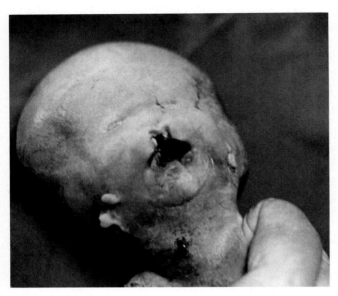

Fig. 13–5. Postnatal appearance of the infant, revealing the classic stigmata of holoprosencephaly with median cleft palate. (*Reproduced with permission from Pilu G, et al. Am J Perinatol. 1987;4;41.*)

of hypoplasia of the median central structures (cyclopia, ethmocephaly, cebocephaly, and median cleft lip).

Severe oligohydramnios may lead to intrauterine constraint and a typical deformation sequence that includes abnormal positioning of limbs (club foot), breech presentation, Potter facies, growth deficiency, amnion nodosum, and pulmonary hypoplasia.[20–24]

Early amniotic rupture with the formation of amniotic bands may lead to a disruption sequence including amputations of fingers, bizarre facial clefts, and asymmetric encephaloceles (Fig. 13–6).[15,25–32]

A syndrome is a pattern of multiple anomalies thought to be pathogenetically related and not known to represent a single sequence or a polytopic field defect. The term syndrome is frequently employed to refer to a single cause such as Down's syndrome. The difference between a malformation sequence and a malformation syndrome is best understood with an example. Isolated holoprosencephaly is a malformation sequence. However, if holoprosencephaly occurs with other anomalies in an infant with trisomy[13] or Meckel syndrome, the condition is a malformation syndrome.

An association refers to a nonrandom occurrence in

ogenesis. This is supported by the proximity between these two structures in early life and by experiments showing an inductive effect of mesonephros on proliferation and differentiation of limb bud cartilage. A complete map of the developmental fields of the human embryo is not available but could be constructed by classifying all human malformations and searching for causal heterogeneity among them. Opitz has proposed that each time a certain malformation is seen in at least two causally different conditions, a developmental field has been identified. This is so because identical structures mean identical development independent of differences in causal mechanisms. Mammalian primordia have only a limited number of responses to various dysmorphogenetic insults. The existence of developmental fields limits the possibility of independent responses from different structures of the organisms.

A sequence is a pattern of multiple anomalies derived from a single known or presumed prior anomaly or mechanical factor. Thus, there are malformation, deformation, and disruption sequences. The spectrum of anomalies of holoprosencephaly is an example of a malformation sequence. The precordal mesoderm is responsible for cleavage of the prosencephalon and normal development of the median facial structures. A primary defect of the precordal mesoderm leads to defects in both the brain and the face. In the brain, there is incomplete division of the cerebral hemispheres and underlying structures. Anomalies of the face include varying degrees

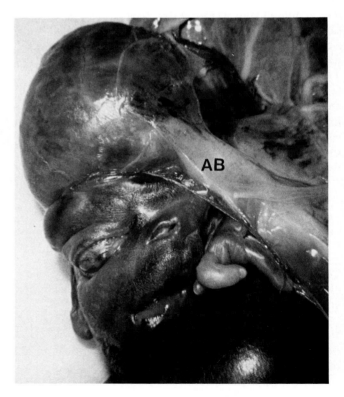

Fig. 13–6. Amniotic band syndrome. An amniotic band is seen inserting on the fetal head. There is great division of the fetal face. The hand is forced against the fetal face and deformed. AB = amniotic band.

TABLE 13–8. MORTALITY AND MORBIDITY RATES IN INFANTS WITH CONGENITAL ANOMALIES AGAINST NO-ANOMALIES GROUPS

	Postnatal Mortality to 7 yr	Neurologic Abnormality 1 to 7 yr	Psychiatric Deficits at age 7	Major Surgery to 7 yr
Total population	0.030	0.054	0.183	—
No anomaly	0.026	0.035	0.049	0.162
Minor only	0.015[a]	0.046[b]	0.059[c]	0.196[a]
Single major	0.058[a]	0.064[a]	0.069[a]	0.367[a]
Multiple major	0.116[a]	0.109[a]	0.152[a]	0.492[a]
Sequences	0.442[a]	0.211[a]	0.159[a]	0.583[a]
Syndromes	0.288[a]	0.733[a]	0.720[a]	0.378[a]
All anomalies	0.052[a]	0.069[a]	0.078[a]	0.292[a]
Major anomalies, sequences, syndromes	0.087[a]	0.092[a]	0.097[a]	0.386[a]

[a] $P \le 0.001$
[b] $P \le 0.01$
[c] $P \le 0.05$

Reproduced with permission from: Chung CS, Myrianthopoulos NC. Congenital anomalies: Mortality and morbidity, burden and classification. Am J Med Genet. *1987;27:510.*

nucleus family. The incidence of divorce and sibling social maladjustment is greater in families of children with spina bifida than in families of infants without congenital anomalies.[55,56]

ULTRASOUND DIAGNOSIS OF CONGENITAL ANOMALIES

The first reports of prenatal recognition of congenital anomalies with ultrasound were published in 1961 by Donald,[57] and in 1964 by Sunden.[58] The latter author documented identification of three cases of "acrania." Subsequently, the first prenatal diagnosis of a congenital anomaly with ultrasound that altered obstetric management was reported by Campbell and associates in 1972.[59]

The cardinal principle behind the diagnosis of congenital anomalies with ultrasound is recognition of a departure from normal fetal anatomy. Congenital anomalies are generally recognized with ultrasound by one of the following means: (1) absence of a normal anatomic structure; (2) a disruption of the contour, shape, location, sonographic texture, or size of a normal anatomic structure; (3) presence of an abnormal structure; (4) abnormal fetal biometry; or (5) abnormal fetal motion.

Inability to identify a normal structure such as the fetal stomach or calvarium suggests esophageal atresia and anencephaly or acrania, respectively. A localized defect in the calvarium indicates the presence of a cephalocele. A displaced stomach into the chest is diagnostic of a diaphragmatic hernia. This condition is suspected because of a displacement of the heart within the chest even before visualization of the stomach or intestine in an abnormal location. Duodenal atresia is diagnosed by

identifying a "double-bubble" sign (abnormal morphology of the stomach). Fetal tumors are typically identified when an additional structure is visualized that alters fetal anatomy. Abnormal biometry is used for the recognition of disorders characterized by fetal disproportion such as skeletal dysplasias and microcephaly. Absence of motion also identifies infants at risk for arthrogryposis multiplex congenita or other neuromuscular congenital disorders.

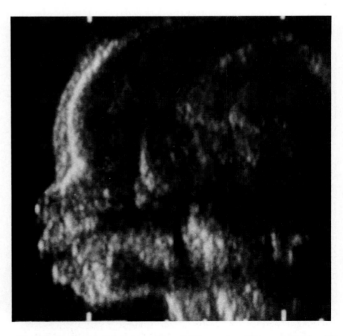

Fig. 13–7. Normal fetal profile at 25 weeks. (*Reproduced with permission from Pilu G, et al. Am J Obstet Gynecol. 1986:155; 45.*)

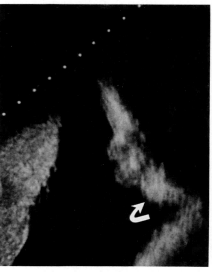
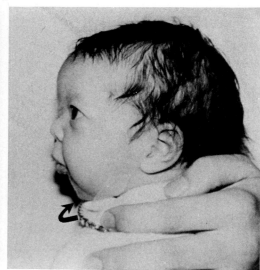

Fig. 13–8. Midsagittal scan of the face of a 35-week fetus with Robin anomaly. Micrognathia is evident. A side view of the infant is provided for comparison. (*Reproduced with permission from Pilu G, et al. Am J Obstet Gynecol. 1986:154;630.*)

A   B

The sonographic recognition of congenital anomalies depends on knowledge of normal fetal anatomy, ultrasound resolution, and the natural history of the disorder (Figs. 13–7 and 13–8). Minor anomalies recognized by a body surface examination of the newborn may not be identified sonographically because their size is beyond the spatial resolution of current equipment. Morphologic details of the external ear are not visible until the third trimester, and even then they are not consistently dem-

onstrated.[60,61] Thus, reliable diagnosis of external ear minor anomalies would be extremely difficult. Another limitation to diagnosis is imposed by the embryologic timetable. It is now possible to detect the physiologic herniation of the fetal intestine into the umbilical cord during the first trimester of pregnancy. The bowel returns to the abdominal cavity at 10 to 12 weeks. Therefore, a first trimester diagnosis of an omphalocele before the tenth week is not possible except for extremely large defects[62,63] (Figs. 13–9 and 13–10). The natural history of a disease is also important. The diagnosis of infantile polycystic kidney disease (IPKD) is possible by recognizing signs of in utero renal failure, such as oligohydramnios and a nonvisualized bladder, coupled with en-

Fig. 13–9. Longitudinal scan showing the insertion of the umbilical cord in the abdomen of a first-trimester fetus.

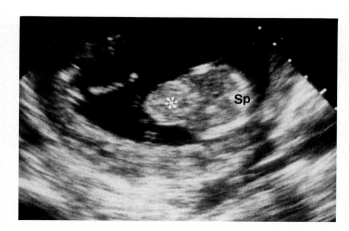

Fig. 13–10. Prenatal diagnosis of an omphalocele at 15 weeks of gestation. Transverse scan of the abdomen at the level of the umbilicus, demonstrating the lesion (*). Sp = spine.

TABLE 13–9. ANOMALIES IDENTIFIED BY ULTRASOUND

CNS

Hydrocephalus
Monolateral ventriculomegaly
Aqueductal stenosis
Communicating hydrocephalus
Dandy-Walker malformation
Choroid plexus papilloma
Spina bifida
Anencephaly
Encephalocele
Porencephaly
Hydranencephaly

Meningo (myelo) cele

Hypertelorism
Hypotelorism
Microphthalmia-anophthalmia
Cyclopia
Retinal detachment
Arhinia
Proboscis

Cystic hygroma
Goiter

Atrial septal defects
Ventricular septal defects
Atrioventricular septal defects
Univentricular heart
Ebstein's anomaly
Hypoplastic left heart syndrome
Hypoplastic right ventricle
Tetralogy of Fallot
Complete transposition of the great arteries
Corrected transposition of the great arteries
Double outlet right ventricle
Truncus arteriosus
Coarctation and tubular hypoplasia of the aortic arch
Pulmonic stenosis

Chylothorax
Congenital cystic adenomatoid malformation of the lung
Lung sequestration

Diaphragmatic hernia
Omphalocele
Gastroschisis

Esophageal atresia with/without tracheoesophageal fistula
Duodenal atresia
Bowel obstruction
Jeunal atresia
Hepatomegaly
Splenomegaly

Bilateral renal agenesis
Infantile polycystic kidney disease
Multicystic kidney disease
Ureteropelvic junction obstruction
Megaureter
Posterior urethral valves
Pelvic kidney

Microcephaly
Macrocephaly
Holoprosencephaly
Iniencephaly
Lissencephaly
Intracranial arachnoid cysts
Intracranial tumors
Acrania
Choroid plexus cyst
Aneurysm of the vien of Galen
Absent cerebellum

Spinal

Sacrococcygeal teratoma

Face

Macroglossia
Facial clefting
Median cleft lip
Epignathus
Robin anomaly
Otocephaly

Neck

Teratoma of the neck
Fetal nuchal skin thickening

Heart

Aortic stenosis
Left atrial isomerism with asplenia
Mitral atresia
Cardiomyopathies
Total anomalous pulmonary venous return
Tumors of the heart
Ectopia cordis
Cardiosplenic syndromes
Endocardial fibroelastosis
Premature atrial and ventricular contractions
Supraventricular tachyarrhythmias
Atrioventricular block
Pericardial effusion
Intrapericardial teratoma

Lung

Bronchogenic cysts
Pleural effusions

Abdominal Wall

Body stalk anomaly
Bladder exostrophy and cloacal exostrophy

Gastrointestinal Tract

Asplenia
Meconium peritonitis
Hirschsprung's disease
Hepatic hemangioma
Choledochal cyst
Mesenteric, omental and retroperitoneal cysts

Urinary Tract

Prune-belly syndrome
Megacystic-microcolon-intestinal hypoperistalsis syndrome
Meckel syndrome
Isolated renal cysts
Congenital mesoblastic nephroma
Congenital adrenal neuroblastoma
Congenital adrenal hyperplasia

(continued)

TABLE 13–9. *(continued)*

Ambiguous genitalia	**Genital Tract**
Edema of the labia majora	Hydrometrocolpos
Hydrocele	Ovarian cysts
	Skeleton
Cloverleaf skull	Scoliosis, kyphosis
Frontal bossing	Sacral agenesis
Hypoplasia of the clavicles	Curved or bowed long bone
Long, narrow thorax	Aplasia or hypoplasia of long bone
Short thorax	Hypoplastic scapulae
Hypoplastic thorax	Sirenomelia
Short ribs	Bone fractures
Vertebral disorganization	Bone demineralization
Hemivertebrae	Phocomelia
	Hand and Foot
Post-axial polydactyly	Rocker-bottom foot
Pre-axial polydactyly	Acheiria
Syndactyly	Apodia
Ectrodactyly	Acheiropodia
Brachydactyly	Joint contractures
Hitchhiker thumb	Contracture deformities of the upper and lower extremities
	Skeletal Dysplasias
Achondrogenesis	Kniest dysplasia
Achondroplasia	Larsen's syndrome
Apert's syndrome	Mesomelic dysplasia
Asphyxiating thoracic dysplasia (Jeune's syndrome)	Metatropic dysplasia
Arthrogryposis multiplex congenita	Osteogenesis imperfecta
Campomelic dysplasia	Otopalatodigital syndrome, type II
Carpenter syndrome	Pena-Shokeir syndrome
Chondrodysplasia punctata	Roberts' syndrome
McKusik's syndrome (cartilage-hair hypoplasia)	Short rib-polydactyly syndromes
Ellis-van Crevald syndrome	Spondylo-epiphyseal dysplasia (atelosteogenesis)
Diastrophic dysplasia	Spondylo-thoracic dysplasia (Jarcho-Levin syndrome)
Dyssegmental dysplasia	Thanatophoric dysplasia
Fibrochondrogenesis	Thrombocytopenia with absent radius syndrome (TAR
Hypophosphatasia	syndrome)
	Umbilical Cord
Single umbilical artery	Hemangiomas of the umbilical cord
Omphalomesenteric cyst	Hematoma of the umbilical cord
Allantoid cyst	True knots of the umbilical cord
Thrombosis of the umbilical vessels	
	Twin
Conjoined twins	Twin-to-twin transfusion
Acardius (acephalus acardia)	
	Other
Amniotic band syndrome	Vascular hamartomatosis
Nonimmune hydrops fetalis	

larged hyperechogenic kidneys. However, sonographic observations have demonstrated that kidney measurements and function may be normal in early fetal life when IPKD is present. Therefore, the diagnosis of IPKD is not always possible before the 24th week of gestation.[64,65]

A detailed discussion of the diagnosis of specific conditions is beyond the scope of this chapter, and the reader is referred to specialized textbooks[42] or relevant chapters in this book for further information. Table 13–9 lists the most important congenital disorders diagnosed with ultrasound. It includes conditions that have been identified antenatally, but the accuracy of sonography (sensitivity, specificity, positive and negative predictive values) is only known for a small number of conditions.

The development and clinical application of a diagnostic imaging technique in clinical practice follows several stages. First, the normal anatomy of an organ or region is described. Subsequently, gross deviations from the normal anatomy are recognized and often documented in the literature in the form of case reports. As experience grows, more cases are identified and case series are published. Once the diagnostic capability of the imaging technique is established, studies of a population at risk for a given condition allow determination of the accuracy of the diagnostic modality in recognizing a specific disorder. Prenatal diagnosis of anatomic congenital anomalies with obstetric ultrasound is still in its early stages. Although fetal anatomy has been described in great detail and the list of anomalies recognized with ultrasound is growing rapidly, the accuracy of ultrasound is only known for a handful of conditions, such as spina bifida and infantile polycystic kidney disease. Moreover, this information has been gathered in populations at risk for these disorders: patients with elevated maternal serum alpha-fetoprotein and a positive family history.[66-69] The only available data of the accuracy of a prenatal screening program for congenital anomalies is that of King's College Hospital in London, where ultrasound is routinely performed at 16 to 18 weeks on all patients. Fifty-four fetal malformations were detected in 16,670 patients scanned. The sensitivity of sonography in the detection of congenital anomalies was 84%, and the specificity was 99.9%.[70] However, more information is required regarding screening programs in other institutions. Such documentation is important if detection of congenital anomalies with ultrasound is to become one of the objectives of routine prenatal care. A false-positive diagnosis may lead to termination of a pregnancy with a normal fetus, while a false-negative diagnosis may leave the family with the emotional, medical, social, and economic burdens imposed by a child born with a congenital anomaly. Although inaccuracy is intrinsic to the diagnostic process in medicine and cannot be completely eradicated, it is imperative to inform patients of what to expect from our diagnostic tools. The problem is compounded by the improvement and variability in equipment resolution and operator skills, as has been shown in spina bifida. Roberts and colleagues[71] demonstrated that with the introduction of better equipment and increased operator experience, the sensitivity of ultrasound in detection of this anomaly improved from 36% to 80%, and the rate of false-positive decreased from 90% to 20%.

MANAGEMENT PRINCIPLES IN THE DETECTION OF PRENATAL DIAGNOSIS

The following issues need to be considered in a program of prenatal diagnosis of anatomic congenital anomalies.

Offering prenatal diagnosis. When a patient seeks prenatal diagnosis for a specific congenital anomaly, it is imperative to learn if this type of prenatal diagnosis has

ever been reported. Gestational age and specific sonographic findings used for the diagnosis must be carefully reviewed. Caution is advised when reading the literature. In many instances, the title of case reports claims that a specific prenatal diagnosis has been made when, actually, only recognition of an abnormal finding without a precise antenatal diagnosis has occurred. Knowledge of the spectrum of the disease, including associated anomalies and natural history of the disorder, is also required. Unless there is a great deal of experience (eg, spina bifida), patients must be informed that the diagnostic accuracy of ultrasound for that specific disorder is not known and that false-positive and false-negative diagnoses may occur. The implications of these potential diagnostic errors must also be discussed. For medicolegal considerations, it may be wise to document such discussions in the medical record.

Work-up of an abnormal finding. One of every five newborns affected with a birth defect has more than one major anatomic abnormality, and this association is often of critical prognostic importance.[46,50] Therefore, the identification of any anomaly in a fetus must prompt a careful search for other associated abnormalities. Echocardiography and fetal karyotype determinations must be considered. The association between congenital heart disease and extracardiac anomalies is demonstrated by a recent series showing that 23% of fetuses referred for echocardiography because of an extracardiac anomaly had congenital heart disease. The relationship between different types of congenital heart disease and various extracardiac anomalies has been reviewed elsewhere.[72,73] Chromosome abnormalities had been previously documented in the pediatric literature in infants with congenital anomalies. Recent studies support the view that approximately one-third of fetuses with structural anomalies have a chromosome disorder.[74-77] The information derived from amniocentesis may allow more informed counseling and influence obstetric management. Amniocentesis has been the standard method for obtaining material for karyotype determination, but percutaneous fetal blood sampling is the method of choice in cases where a rapid answer is desired or additional studies from fetal blood are indicated.[78,79]

Pregnancy termination. In a country where pregnancy termination is available for social as well as medical reasons, this option is offered to mothers carrying an anomalous fetus. The gestational age limit at which termination of pregnancy can be offered varies among countries and even among States of the United States. We subscribe to the opinion that elective termination of pregnancy in the third trimester can be offered to some mothers carrying a child with a uniformly lethal condition for which prenatal diagnosis is certain (ie, anencephaly). A list of these conditions is presented in Table 13–10. Recently, these infants have become a potential source of organs for transplantation, an option that raises serious ethical and practical medical questions.[80,81]

Site, mode, and timing of delivery. Delivery of fetuses with congenital anomalies should ideally occur in a center with a newborn special care unit. Pediatricians may face unexpected complications posed by nondiagnosed associated anomalies. An interdisciplinary team composed of specialists in maternal–fetal medicine, diagnostic imaging, neonatalogy, and human genetics should be available for consultation. Depending on the specific nature of the anomaly, other specialists such as a pediatric surgeon, pediatric cardiologist, cardiovascular surgeon, and neurosurgeon may also be required. Paramedic personnel, such as a social worker, are also important in providing emotional support to the family.

Some anomalies may alter the method of delivery. Conjoined twins, giant omphaloceles, giant sacrococcygeal tumors, and severe hydrocephaly are examples of these conditions. The optimal method of delivery for other anomalies such as omphaloceles, gastroschisis, and myelomeningocele has not been determined.[82–86] Finally, some disorders, which are not uniformly lethal but are frequently associated with neonatal death or serious neurologic handicap, require careful discussion with the parents to define management in the event fetal distress occurs during labor. For these conditions, we favor a nonaggressive management approach indicating our analysis of the risk-benefit ratio is slanted toward maternal well-being; and, therefore, we would advise against a cesarean section. However, the final decision rests with the parents.

Delivery of an infant with a congenital anomaly should ideally occur at term. Surgical corrective procedures would be delayed in the face of respiratory distress syndrome or other problems of prematurity. Early delivery may be considered for some rare conditions that worsen in utero.

Surgical fetal therapy. Initial excitement over the possibilities offered by fetal therapy for the treatment of hydrocephaly and obstructive uropathy has been tempered. The Fetal Medicine and Surgery Society has rec-

ommended that in utero treatment of hydrocephaly with ventriculo-amniotic shunts be considered a highly experimental procedure in view of the poor results reported to the International Registry.[87,88] For obstructive uropathy, careful case-selection is advocated before placement of vesico-amniotic shunts. Available experience has indicated this procedure can be performed with relative safety for both mother and fetus, although the benefits of such an intervention have not been established with a randomized clinical trial.[89–92]

SHOULD EVERY PREGNANT PATIENT HAVE AN ULTRASOUND EXAMINATION?

There has been an ongoing debate concerning the routine use of ultrasound in obstetrics. While some, including a consensus conference sponsored by the National Institutes of Health,[93] have favored selective use of ultrasound for a number of indications, other have proposed its routine use during pregnancy. Our bias lies with with the second option, and we presented our reasoning elsewhere.[94] Attempts to answer this question with randomized clinical trials have failed to demonstrate the efficacy of routine ultrasound in reducing perinatal mortality.[95–99] However, these trials included only 1,600 patients. Lilford and Chard[100] calculated that a trial designed to detect a reduction in perinatal mortality from 10/10,000 to 8/10,000 will require 46,820 mothers. Thus, the trials do not have the sample size necessary to answer this question.

A different approach to this issue is to define the goals of prenatal care. If detection of congenital anomalies is one of these goals, it seems that routine ultrasound examination is the best available tool to accomplish this objective. Prenatal diagnosis of congenital anomalies affords several advantages. Diagnosis before viability may allow pregnancy termination. Other infants may benefit by the diagnosis of anomalies whose prognosis is affected by early recognition and treatment. For example, prenatal identification of duodenal atresia allows immediate correction in the neonatal period and may prevent the complications caused by aspiration of gastric contents, perforation, and electrolyte imbalance before surgical correction.[101] The sudden deterioration of infants with ductus-dependent congenital heart disease can be avoided by preventing ductal closure until surgical correction can be performed. In another group of uncorrectable disorders, such as some skeletal dysplasias, prenatal diagnosis allows the parents to be prepared to face the birth of a physically handicapped child.

If part of the justification for routine obstetric scanning is the detection of congenital anomalies, the current concept of what constitutes a routine scan must change.

TABLE 13–10. LETHAL MALFORMATIONS

CNS
Anencephaly
Acrania
Alobar holoprosencephaly
Iniencephaly
Face
Otocephaly
Abdomen
Body stalk anomaly

The standard level 1 examination will no longer suffice.[102] Currently, it is possible to comply with these guidelines without documenting the presence of all four extremities! Ultrasound needs to be exploited as a tool capable of providing information about the fetal phenotype. We anticipate that, in the future, routine sonography will include a basic echocardiographic examination because cardiac structural defects are one of the most common types of congenital anomalies.[103,104] Recently, Benaceraff and associates[105] demonstrated that of 49 infants born with congenital anomalies, 28 were correctly identified with echocardiography. Furthermore, 29 of these patients did not have any risk factors for the presence of cardiac anomalies. It is clear that inclusion of echocardiography as part of a normal routine ultrasound will demand a significant improvement in the current level of expertise and training.

Acknowledgments

This study was supported by a grant from the Walter Scott Foundation for Medical Research.

REFERENCES

1. Romero R, Oyarzun E, Sirtori M, Hobbins J. *The detection of congenital anomalies: A new goal of prenatal care.* Unpublished data.

2. Spranger J, Benirschke K, Hall J, et al. Errors of morphogenesis: Concepts and terms. *J Pediatr.* 1982;100:160–165.

3. Smith DW. Recognizable patterns of human deformation: Identification and management of mechanical effects on morphogenesis. In: Schaffer AJ, Markowitz M, eds. *Major Clinical Problems in Clinical Pediatrics.* Philadelphia: Saunders; 1981;21:97–144.

4. Opitz JM, Herrman J, Petterson JC, Bersu ET, Colacino SC. Terminological, diagnostic, nosological, and anatomical-developmental aspects of developmental defects in man, I: Terminological and epistemological considerations of human malformations. *Am J Med Genetics.* 1979;3:71–107.

5. Moore KL. *The Developing Human: Clinically Oriented Embryology.* Philadelphia: Saunders; 1982:1–26.

6. Dunn PM. Congenital postural deformities: Perinatal associations. *Proc Roy Soc Med.* 1972;65:735–738.

7. Dunn PM. Congenital postural deformities: Further perinatal associations. *Proc Roy Soc Med.* 1974;67:32–36.

8. Dunn PM. Congenital sternomastoid torticollis: An intrauterine postural deformity. *Arch Dis Child.* 1974;49:824–825.

9. Hall JG. In utero movement and use of limbs are necessary for normal growth: A study of individuals with arthrogryposis. In: *Endocrine Genetics and Genetics of Growth.* New York: Alan R. Liss; 1985;155–162.

10. Cohen MM. *The Child With Multiple Birth Defects.* New York: Raven Press; 1982:1–26.

11. Romero R, Chervenak FA, Devore G, Tortora M, Hobbins JC. Fetal head deformation and congenital torticollis associated with a uterine tumor. *Am J Obstet Gynecol.* 1981;141:839–840.

12. Dunn PM. Congenital postural deformities. *Br Med Bull.* 1976;32:71–76.

13. Baker CJ, Rudolph AJ. Congenital ring constrictions and intrauterine amputations. *Am J Dis Child.* 1971;121:393–400.

14. Torpin R. *Fetal Malformations Caused by Amnion Rupture During Gestation.* Springfield, Ill: Charles C. Thomas; 1968.

15. Higginbottom MC, Jones KL, Hall BD, Smith DW. The amniotic band disruption complex: Timing of amniotic rupture and variable spectra of consequent defects. *J Pediatr.* 1979;95:544–549.

16. Opitz JM. The developmental analysis of human congenital anomalies. In: Papadatos CJ, Bartsocas CS, eds. *Skeletal Dysplasias.* New York: Alan R. Liss; 1982:15–43.

17. Opitz JM. What the general pediatrician should know about developmental anomalies. *Pediatr Rev.* 1982;3:267–271.

18. Opitz JM. The developmental field concept in clinical genetics. *J Pediatr.* 1982;101:805–809.

19. Opitz JM, Lewin SO. The developmental field concept in pediatric pathology—Especially with respect to fistular alhypoplasia and the DiGeorge anomaly. *Birth Defects.* 1987;23:277–292. Original Article Series.

20. Smith DW. Recognizable patterns of human deformation: Identification and management of mechanical effects on morphogenesis. In: Schaffer AJ, Markowitz M, eds. *Major Clinical Problems in Clinical Pediatrics.* Philadelphia: Saunders; 1981;21:85–87.

21. Smith DW, Jones KL. Recognizable patterns of human malformation: Genetic, embryologic and clinical aspects. In: Markowitz M. *Major Problems in Clinical Pediatrics.* Philadelphia: Saunders; 1982;12:484–485.

22. Sivit CJ, Hill MC, Larsen JW, Kent SG, Lande IM. The sonographic evaluation of fetal anomalies in oligohydramnios between 16 and 30 weeks gestation. *AJR* 1986;146:1277–1281.

23. Perlman M, Levin M. Fetal pulmonary hypoplasia, anuria, and oligohydramnios: Clinicopathologic observations and review of the literature. *Am J Obstet Gynecol.* 1974;118:1119.

24. Thomas IT, Smith DW. Oligohydramnios, cause of the nonrenal features of Potter's syndrome, including pulmonary hypoplasia. *J Pediatr.* 1974;84:811.

25. Smith DW. Recognizable patterns of human deformation: Identification and management of mechanical effects on morphogenesis. In: Schaffer AJ, Markowitz M, eds. *Major Clinical Problems in Clinical Pediatrics.* Philadelphia: Saunders; 1981;21:90–93.

26. Smith DW, Jones KL. Recognizable patterns of human malformation: Genetic, embryologic and clinical aspects. In: Markowitz M, ed. *Major Problems in Clinical Pediatrics.* Philadelphia: Saunders; 1982;12:488–495.

27. Fiske CE, Filly RA, Golbus MS. Prenatal ultrasound diagnosis of amniotic band syndrome. *J Ultrasound Med.* 1982;1:45.

28. Hughes RM, Benzie RJ, Thomson CL. Amniotic band syndrome causing fetal deformity. *Prenat Diagn.* 1984;4:447.

29. Mahony BS, Filly RA, Callen PW, et al. The amniotic band syndrome: Antenatal sonographic diagnosis and potential pitfalls. *Am J Obstet Gynecol.* 1985;152:63.

30. Seeds JW, Cefalo RC, Herbert WN. Amniotic band syndrome. *Am J Obstet Gynecol.* 1982;144:243.

31. Torpin R. Amniochorionic mesoblastic fibrous strings and amniotic bands: Associated constricting fetal malformation or fetal death. *Am J Obstet Gynecol.* 1965;91:65.

32. Worthern NJ, Lawrence D, Bustillo M. Amniotic band syndrome: Antepartum ultrasonic diagnosis of discordant anencephaly. *J Clin Ultrasound.* 1980;8:453.

33. Jones KI, Jones MC. A clinical approach to the dysmorphic child. In: Emery AEH, Rimoin DL, eds. *Principles and Practice of Medical Genetics.* Edinburgh: Churchill Livingstone; 1983:152–61.

34. Opitz JM, Herrman J, Petterson JC, Bersu ET, Colacino SC. Terminological, diagnostic, nosological, and anatomical developmental aspects of developmental defects in man, II: Patient evaluation, delineation, and nosology of developmental defects—an overview. *Am J Med Genetics.* 1979;3:107–164.

35. Epstein CJ. *The Consequence of Chromosome Imbalance: Principles, Mechanisms, and Models.* Cambridge, England: Cambridge University Press; 1986:1–486.

36. Marden PM, Smith DW, McDonald MJ. Congenital anomalies in the newborn infant, including minor variations: A study of 4,412 babies by surface examination for anomalies and buccal smear for sex chromatin. *J Pediatr.* 1964;64:358–371.

37. Emery AEH, Rimoin D, eds. *Principles and Practice of Medical Genetics.* Edinburgh: Churchill Livingstone; 1983:1–702.

38. Kaback MM. *Genetic Issues in Pediatric and Obstetric Practice.* Chicago: Year Book Medical Publishers; 1981:1–604.

39. Smith DW, Jones KL. Recognizable patterns of human malformation: Genetic, embryologic and clinical aspects. In: Markowitz M, ed. *Major Problems in Clinical Pediatrics.* Philadelphia: Saunders; 1982;7:1–653.

40. Harrison MR, Golbus MS, Filly RA. *The Unborn Patient: Prenatal Diagnosis and Treatment.* Orlando: Grune & Stratton; 1984:1–455.

41. Cohen MM. *The Child With Multiple Birth Defects.* New York: Raven Press; 1982:1–189.

42. Romero R, Pilu G, Jeanty P, Ghidini A, Hobbins JC. *Prenatal Diagnosis of Congenital Anomalies.* Norwalk, Conn: Appleton & Lange; 1988:1–466.

43. Milunsky A, ed. *Genetic Disorders and the Fetus: Diagnosis, Prevention and Treatment.* 2nd ed. New York: Plenum; 1986:1–895.

44. Papadatos CJ, Bartsocas CS, eds. Endocrine genetics and genetics of growth. In: Back N, Brewer GJ, Eijsvoogel VP, eds. *Progress in Clinical and Biological Research.* New York: Alan R. Liss; 1985;200:1–375.

45. Hook EB, Marden PM, Reiss NP, Smith DW. Some aspects of the epidemiology of human minor birth defects and morphological variants in a completely ascertained newborn population (Madison study). *Teratology.* 1976;13:47–56.

46. Myrianthopoulos NC, Chung CS. Congenital malformations in singletons: Epidemiologic survey. In: Bergsma D, ed. *Birth Defects.* New York: Stratton Inter-cont Med Book Corp; 1974:x11:1–22. Original Article Series.

47. Christianson RE, van den Berg BJ, Milkovich L, Oechsli FW. Incidence of congenital anomalies among white and black live births with long-term follow-up. *Am J Public Health.* 1981;71:1333–1340.

48. Greenberg F, James LM, Oakley GP. Estimates of birth relevance rates of spina bifida in the United States from computer-generated maps. *Am J Obstet Gynecol.* 1983;145:570–573.

49. Terry PB, Bissenden JG, Condie RG, Mathew PM. Ethnic differences in congenital malformations. *Arch Dis Child.* 1985;60:866–879.

50. Chung CS, Myrianthopoulos NC. Congenital anomalies: Mortality and morbidity, burden and classification. *Am J Med Gen.* 1987;27:505–523.

51. Manning FA, Lempe R, Morrison I, Harmon CR. Determination of fetal health: Methods for antepartum and intrapartum fetal assessment. *Curr Probl Obstet Gynecol.* 1983;7.

52. Leck I. Fetal malformations. In: Barron SL, Thomson AM, eds. *Obstetrical Epidemiology.* London: Academic Press; 1983;263–318.

53. Oakely GP. Incidence and epidemiology of birth defects. In: Kaback MM, ed. *Genetic Issues in Pediatric and Obstetric Practice.* Chicago: Year Book Medical Publishers; 1981:25–43.

54. Emery AEH, Rimoin D. Nature and incidence of genetic disease. In: Emery AEH, Rimoin D, eds. *Principles and Practice of Medical Genetics.* Edinburgh: Churchill Livingstone; 1983:1–3.

55. Lorber J. The effect of spina bifida on family life. In: Beard RW, ed. *Diagnosis and Management of Neural Tube Defects.* London: Royal College of Obstetricians and Gynaecologists; 1978:133.

56. Main DM, Mennuti MT. Neural tube defects: Issues in prenatal diagnosis and counselling. *Obstet Gynecol.* 1986;67:1–16.

57. Donald I, Brown TG. Localization using physical devices, radioisotopes and radiographic methods, I: Demonstration of tissue interfaces within the body by ultrasonic echo sounding. *Br J Radiol.* 1961;34:539–546.

58. Sunden B. In the diagnostic value of ultrasound in obstetrics and gynecology. *Acta Obstet Gynecol Scand.* 1964;43:121–123.

59. Campbell S, Holt EM, Johnstone FD, May P. Anencephaly: Early ultrasonic diagnosis and active management. *Lancet.* 1972;2:1226–1227.

60. Jeanty P, Romero R, Staucach A, Hobbins JC. Facial anatomy of the fetus. *J Ultrasound Med.* 1986;5:607–616.

61. Birnholz JC. Ultrasound imaging of fetal anatomy. In: Putnam CE, Ravin CE, eds. *Textbook of Diagnostic Imaging.* Philadelphia: Saunders; 1988:1941–1957.

62. Schmidt W, Yarkoni S, Crelin ES, Hobbins JC. Sono-

graphic visualization of physiologic anterior abdominal wall hernia in the first trimester. *Obstet Gynecol.* 1987;69:911–915.

63. Curtis JA, Watson L. Sonographic diagnosis of omphalocele in the first trimester of fetal gestation. *J Ultrasound Med.* 1988;7:97–100.

64. Romero R, Cullen M, Jeanty P, et al. The diagnosis of congenital renal anomalies with ultrasound, II: Infantile polycystic kidney disease. *Am J Obstet Gynecol.* 1984;150:259.

65. Simpson JL, Sabbagha RE, Elias S, et al. Failure to detect polycystic kidneys in utero by second trimester ultrasonography. *Hum Genet.* 1982;60:295.

66. Campbell J, Gilbert WM, Nicolaides KH, Campbell S. Ultrasound screening for spina bifida: Cranial and cerebellar signs in a high-risk population. *Obstet Gynecol.* 1987;70:247–250.

67. Grannum P, Pilu G. In utero neurosonography: Neuroembryologic and encephaloclastic lesions. *Sem Perinatol.* 1987;11:98–111.

68. Sabbagha RE, Sheikh Z, Tamura RK, et al. Predictive value, sensitivity, and specificity of ultrasonic targeted imaging for fetal anomalies in gravid women at high risk for birth defects. *Am J Obstet Gynecol.* 1985;152:822–827.

69. Manchester DK, Pretorius DM, Avery C, et al. Accuracy of ultrasound diagnoses in pregnancies complicated by suspected fetal anomalies. *Prenat Diagn.* 1988;8:109–117.

70. Nicolaides KH, Campbell S. Diagnosis of fetal abnormalities by ultrasound. In: Milunsky A, ed. *Genetic Disorders and the Fetus.* 2nd Ed. New York: Plenum; 1986:521.

71. Roberts CJ, Hibbard BM, Roberts EE, et al. Diagnostic effectiveness of ultrasound in detection of neural tube defect. *Lancet.* 1983;2:1068.

72. Copel JA, Pilu G, Kleinman CS. Congenital heart disease and extracardiac anomalies: Associations and indications for fetal echocardiography. *Am J Obstet Gynecol.* 1986;154:1121–1132.

73. Copel JA, Pilu G, Green J, Hobbins JC, Kleinman CS. Fetal echocardiographic screening for congenital heart disease: The importance of the four-chamber view. *Am J Obstet Gynecol.* 1987;157:648–655.

74. Platt LD, DeVore GR, Lopez E, Herbert W, Falk R, Alfi O. Role of amniocentesis in ultrasound-detected fetal malformations. *Obstet Gynecol.* 1986;68:153–155.

75. Williamson RA, Weiner CP, Patil S, Benda J, Varner MW, Abu-Yousef MM. Abnormal pregnancy sonogram: Selective indication for fetal karyotype. *Obstet Gynecol.* 1987;69:15–20.

76. Palmer CG, Miles JH, Howard-Peebles PN, Magenis RE, Patil S, Friedman JM. Fetal karyotype following ascertainment of fetal anomalies by ultrasound. *Prenatal Diagnosis.* 1987;7:551–555.

77. Epstein CJ. *The Consequences of Chromosome Imbalance: Principles, Mechanisms, and Models.* Cambridge, England: Cambridge University Press; 1986:3–8.

78. Romero R, Hobbins JC, Mahoney MJ. Fetal blood sampling and fetoscopy. In: Milunsky A, ed. *Genetic Disorders and the Fetus.* New York: Plenum; 1986:571–598.

79. Nicolaides KH, Rodeck CH, Gosden CM. Rapid karyotyping in non-lethal fetal malformations. *Lancet.* 1986;1:283–287.

80. Holgreve W, Beller FK, Buchholz B, et al. Kidney transplantation from anencephalic donors. *N Engl J Med.* 1987;316:1069.

81. McCullagh P. *The Foetus as Transplant Donor: Scientific, Social and Ethical Perspectives.* Chichester, England: Wiley; 1987.

82. Hill LM. Sonographic detection of fetal gastrointestinal anomalies. *Ultrasound Quarterly.* 1988;6:35–67.

83. Chervenak FA, Duncan C, Ment L, et al. Perinatal management of meningomyelocele. *Obstet Gynecol.* 1985;63:376.

84. Ralis ZA. Traumatizing effect of breech delivery on infants with spina bifida. *J Pediatr.* 1975;87:613.

85. Stark G, Drummond M. Spina bifida as an obstetric problem. *Dev Med Chil Neurol.* 1970;22(suppl):157.

86. Bensen JT, Dillard RG, Burton BK. Open spina bifida: Does cesarean section delivery improve prognosis? *Obstet Gynecol.* 1988;71:532.

87. Manning FA, Harrison MR, Rodeck C, et al. Catheter shunts for fetal hydronephrosis and hydrocephalus. *N Eng J Med.* 1986;315:336–340.

88. Manning FA. International fetal surgery registry: 1985 update. *Clin Obstet Gynecol.* 1986;29:551–578.

89. Harrison MR, Golbus MS, Filly RA. Medical considerations. In: *The Unborn Patient: Prenatal Diagnosis and Treatment.* Orlando: Grune & Stratton; 1984:145–158.

90. Appelman Z, Golbus MS. The management of fetal urinary tract obstruction. *Clin Obstet Gynecol.* 1986;29:483–489.

91. Elias S, Annas GJ. Fetal and gene therapy. *Curr Probl Obstet Gynecol Fertil.* 1987;10:99–130.

92. Purkiss S, Brereton RJ, Wright VM. Surgical emergencies after prenatal treatment for intra-abdominal abnormality. *Lancet.* 1988;1:289–291.

93. *Diagnostic ultrasound imaging in pregnancy.* Washington, D.C.: National Institutes of Health; 1984:667.

94. Jeanty P, Romero R, Hobbins JC. Routine use. In: McGahan JP, ed. *Controversies in Ultrasound.* New York: Churchill Livingstone; 1987:113–122.

95. Eik-Nes SH, Okland O, Aure JC. Ultrasound screening in pregnancy: A randomized controlled trial. *Lancet.* 1984;1:1347.

96. Bakketeig LS, Eik-Nes SH, Jacobsen G, et al. Randomized controlled trial of ultrasonographic screening in pregnancy. *Lancet.* 1984;2:207.

97. Bakketeig LS, Eik-Nes SH, Jacobsen G, et al. Randomized controlled trial of ultrasonographic screening in pregnancy. *Lancet.* 1984;2:207.

98. Wladimiroff JW, Laar J. Ultrasound measurement of fetal body size: A randomized controlled trial. *Acta Obstet Gynecol Scand.* 1980;59:177.

99. Bennett MJ, Little G, Dewhurst J, et al. Predictive value of ultrasound measurement in early pregnancy: A randomized controlled trial. *Br J Obstet Gynaecol.* 1982;89:338.

100. Lilford RJ, Chard T. The routine use of ultrasound. *Br J Obstet Gynaecol.* 1985;92:434.

101. Romero R, Ghidini A, Costigan K, Touloukian R, Hobbins JC. Prenatal diagnosis of duodenal atresia: Does it make any difference? *Obstet Gynecol.* In press.

102. Sabbagha RE, Tamura RK, Dal Compo S. Antenatal ultrasonic diagnosis of genetic defects: Present status. *Clin Obstet Gynecol.* 1981;24:1103–1119.

103. Layde PM, Dooly K, Erickson JK, Edmonds LD. Is there an epidemic of ventricular septal defects in the U.S.A.? *Lancet.* 1980;1:407–408.

104. Hoffman JIE, Christianson R. Congenital heart disease in a cohort of 19,502 births with long-term follow-up. *Am J Cardiol.* 1978;42:641–647.

105. Benacerraf BR, Pober BR, Sanders SP. Accuracy of fetal echocardiography. *Radiology.* 1987;165:847–849.

14 Prenatal Diagnosis of Cerebro-Spinal Anomalies

Gianluigi Pilu • Roberto Romero • Nicola Rizzo • Sandro Gabrielli • Antonella Perolo • Luciano Bovicelli

The overall incidence of congenital anomalies of the central nervous system (CNS) is about 1 in 100 births.[1,2] Much higher frequencies have been described in spontaneous abortions,[3-5] suggesting that these defects have a very high intrauterine fatality rate.

The CNS was probably the first fetal apparatus to be investigated in utero by diagnostic ultrasound. Anencephaly was the first congenital anomaly to be recognized by this technique before viability.[6] Anomalies of the CNS are currently among the fetal malformations most frequently encountered by obstetric sonographers. Modern high-resolution ultrasound equipment yields a unique potential in evaluating normal and abnormal anatomy of the fetal neural axis in very early stages of development.[7-12] Yet, identification of selected anomalies such as hydrocephalus and spina bifida remains a challenge in many cases, demanding that the sonographers have a thorough knowledge of normal and abnormal neuroanatomy.

In this chapter the sonographic investigation of the fetal brain and the prenatal diagnosis of CNS anomalies will be reviewed.

NORMAL INTRACRANIAL ANATOMY OF THE FETUS

Sonographers should be aware that the fetal cerebrum undergoes profound developmental modifications throughout the entire gestation. This section will mainly focus on the second trimester because ultrasound evaluation of fetal anatomy is usually performed at this time. The interested reader is referred to specific works on this subject.[13-15]

In the early second trimester, the lateral ventricles and the brightly echogenic choroid plexuses are the most prominent intracranial structures on sonography.[16] In the following weeks, the size of the lateral ventricles, compared to the mass of the hemispheres, decreases steadily. Although many scanning planes along different orientations are possible and may be required from time to time to better define subtle details of intracranial anatomy, a satisfying survey of brain morphology can be carried out by using three essential axial views that are easily and rapidly obtained in most pregnancies (Fig. 14-1). From rostrad to caudad, these views demonstrate the lateral ventricles and choroid plexuses, the diencephalon and surrounding structures, and the posterior fossa.

The clinical role of sonographic biometry of the fetal cranium is well established. Measurement of the biparietal diameter (BPD)[17-19] and head circumference (HC)[19,20] is currently used both for assessing gestational age and fetal growth and for identifying cranial abnormalities. Measurement of the transverse diameter of the cerebellum (CTD) has recently been suggested for similar purposes.[21-23] Table 14-1 presents a nomogram of these biometric parameters throughout gestation.

HYDROCEPHALUS

The incidence of congenital hydrocephalus ranges from 0.3 to 1.5 in 1,000 births in different epidemiologic surveys.[2]

The optimal approach to antenatal diagnosis of this condition with sonography is still an unresolved issue. First attempts to identify hydrocephalus in utero with sonography were made by demonstrating a gross enlargement of the head.[24] Head measurements are obviously unreliable for an early diagnosis, as hydrocephalic fetuses usually do not develop macrocrania until late in gestation.[25] At present, the sonographic identification of fetal hydrocephalus depends on the direct demonstration of the enlargement of the ventricular system. Confusion may arise at times because the relative size of ventricles and cortex undergoes important modifications throughout gestation. Both qualitative and quantitative criteria have been suggested for recognizing ventriculomegaly.

Qualitative evaluation mainly depends on the observation that in normal fetuses the large choroid plexus almost entirely fills the lumen of the lateral ventricle at the level of the atrium, being closely apposed to both the medial and lateral walls. In early hydrocephalus, the choroid plexus is shrunken and anteriorly displaced, thus being clearly detached from the medial wall of the ventricle (Fig. 14-2).[26] This simple rule is very effective in

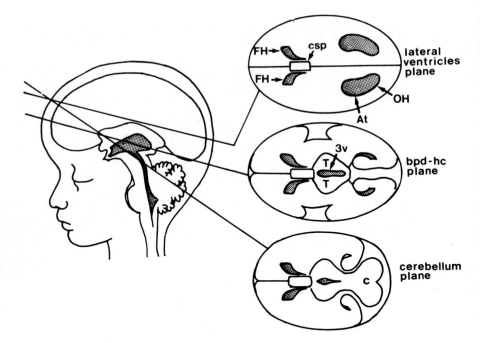

Fig. 14–1. Schematic representation of three scanning planes that allow visualization of the relevant intracranial fetal anatomy. From rostrad to caudad, the first plane demonstrates the lateral ventricles; the second plane is used to measure BPD and HC; the third plane reveals the cerebellum within the posterior fossa. FH = frontal horns; csp = cavitas septi pellucidum; T = thalami; 3v = third ventricle; C = cerebellum.

TABLE 14–1. NOMOGRAM OF BIOMETRIC PARAMETERS THROUGHOUT GESTATION ACCORDING TO PERCENTILE DISTRIBUTION

Gestational Age (weeks)	BPD (mm)			HC (mm)			CTD (mm)		
	10%	50%	90%	10%	50%	90%	10%	50%	90%
15	30	33	35	120	126	128	10	14	16
16	34	35	38	123	125	141	14	16	17
17	36	38	43	134	138	160	16	17	18
18	38	42	44	142	154	169	17	18	19
19	42	45	48	145	159	178	18	19	22
20	45	47	53	146	173	190	18	20	22
21	48	50	57	185	191	211	19	22	24
22	50	53	55	193	193	203	21	23	24
23	53	56	60	203	206	222	22	24	26
24	56	60	64	219	224	230	22	25	28
25	61	63	68	219	234	251	23	28	29
26	63	65	67	235	241	246	26	29	32
27	64	68	70	237	243	246	26	30	32
28	68	70	72	246	253	264	27	30	34
29	71	74	79	254	274	301	29	34	38
30	72	75	79	253	277	298	31	35	40
31	75	76	83	274	291	303	32	38	42
32	75	80	84	275	288	308	33	38	42
33	80	81	87	292	297	322	32	40	44
34	81	84	91	326	326	327	33	40	44
35	78	87	93	300	301	303	31	40	47
36	84	88	91	309	313	318	36	43	55
37	87	89	92	303	313	324	37	45	55
38	87	90	94	—	—	—	40	48	55
39	92	92	92	—	—	—	52	52	55

Modified with permission from Goldstein I, Reece EA, Pilu G, et al. Cerebellar measurements using sonography in the evaluation of fetal growth and development. Am J Obstet Gynecol. 1987;156:1065.

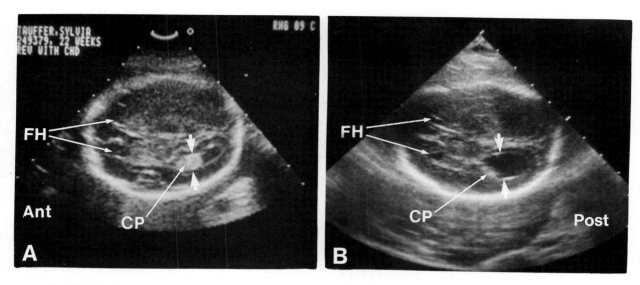

Fig. 14–2. Axial scans at similar levels in a normal fetus and in a fetus with hydrocephalus. **A.** Normalcy is indicated by brightly echogenic choroid plexus (CP) that entirely fills the lumen of the atrium, being closely apposed to both medial and lateral walls of the ventricle (*arrowheads*). **B.** Hydrocephalus is attested by anterior displacement of the shrunken choroid plexus that appears clearly detached from the medial wall of the ventricle. FH = frontal horns of lateral ventricles; Ant = anterior; Post = posterior.

screening for fetal hydrocephalus. However, we have found that in a finite number of normal fetuses, there is some disproportion between the choroid plexus and atrial lumen.

Under these circumstances, a quantitative evaluation of ventricular dimensions is required. Nomograms of the normal size of the frontal horns,[27,28] bodies[7,29] temporal horns,[27] and atria[28] of the lateral ventricles are now available. Measurement of the lateral ventricular ratio at the level of the bodies has probably been most commonly used, but the value of this determination has recently been questioned. There is evidence indicating that the linear echoes originally thought to arise from the lateral wall of the midbody actually represent white matter tracks (Fig. 14–3).[30] We favor the measurement of the atria of lateral ventricles. Due to the presence of the brightly echogenic choroid plexus, this portion of the ventricular system is easy to demonstrate. Our experience is in agreement with other reports indicating that the internal diameter of the atrium does not vary in the second half of gestation.[31] We have found that from 16 weeks to term a measurement of 1 cm or less is indicative of normalcy (Fig. 14–4). However, as an evolutive course is a distinctive feature of fetal hydrocephalus, caution is necessary. Dubious cases may require serial examination.

Hydrocephalus can result from pathologic entities that differ both in etiology and clinical course. In a pediatric series, aqueductal stenosis was found in 43% of cases, communicating hydrocephalus in 38%, and Dandy-Walker malformation (DWM) in 13%.[32] However, pediatric data may not apply to cases recognized prior to birth. In all the second-trimester fetuses with hydrocephalus electively terminated in our institution, autopsy failed to identify aqueductal obstruction. It may well be that aqueductal stenosis does not exist as a separate entity, but that it is the final result of communicating hydrocephalus. Clinical evidence would seem to support such a view.[33]

We believe that a different classification of hydrocephalus is clinically more relevant for cases diagnosed in utero. In our experience, fetal ventriculomegaly will usually enter one of three main entities: triventricular hydrocephalus; DWM; and hydrocephalus associated with other cerebral anomalies, most frequently neural tube defects, disorders of ventral induction, and porencephaly.

Triventricular hydrocephalus is featured by the simultaneous enlargement of the lateral and third ventricles in the presence of a normal posterior fossa (Fig. 14–5). In our institution, fetuses with triventricular hydrocephalus diagnosed in utero were found at birth to have either aqueductal stenosis or communicating hydrocephalus.

Dandy-Walker malformation is characterized by the presence of a retrocerebellar cyst communicating with the fourth ventricle through a defect of the cerebellar vermis (Fig. 14–6).[34] In many cases, the lateral ventricles are not enlarged in utero and hydrocephalus appears for unknown reasons months or years after birth.[34,35]

Neural tube defects, disorders of ventral induction,

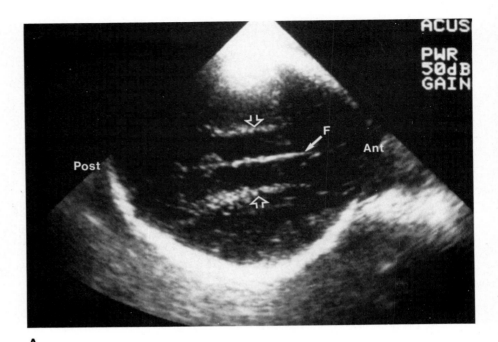

A

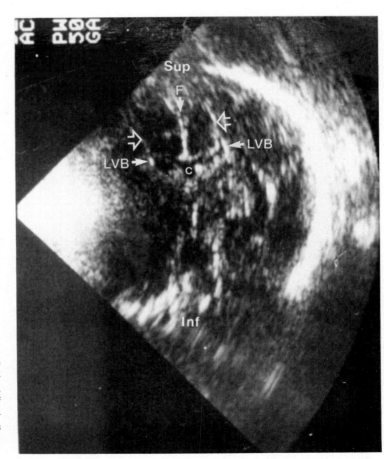

Fig. 14–3. A. Axial scan of fetal head at the level of the falx cerebrii (F). The two lines that run parallel to the midline (*open arrows*) do not pertain to the ventricular system, but arise within the cerebral cortex. **B.** Coronal scan of the head in the same fetus confirms the two lines (*arrowheads*) arise rostrad to the bodies of lateral ventricles (LVB). C = cavitas septi pellucidum; Ant = anterior; Post = posterior; Sup = superior; Inf = inferior.

B

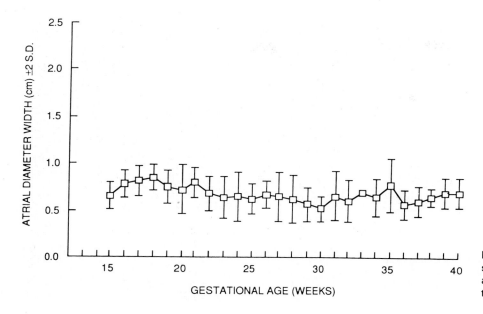

Fig. 14–4. Normal values (mean and two standard deviations) of the internal diameter of the atrium throughout gestation.

and destructive brain lesions will be separately considered.

The prognosis of fetal hydrocephalus is still uncertain. The extrapolation of data from available pediatric series has limited value. The available series of cases diagnosed in utero are biased by the inclusion of a large number of fetuses with spina bifida, ventral induction disorders, or multiple congenital anomalies.[36] Our experience with 20 consecutive cases of isolated hydrocephalus diagnosed in utero (triventricular or DWM), with a follow-up ranging from 5 years to 3 months, includes 3 cases (15%) of neonatal death, 8 infants (40%) that are developing normally, and 9 (45%) that have mild to severe handicaps.

Intrauterine treatment of fetal hydrocephalus by ventriculo-amniotic shunting has been suggested,[37] and experimental studies on animal models are promising.[38] The preliminary experience on human fetuses is less encouraging. The Registry of the International Society of Fetal Medicine and Surgery indicates that out of a total of 44 fetuses who underwent shunting between 1982 and 1985, the procedure-related death rate was 10%. Fifty-

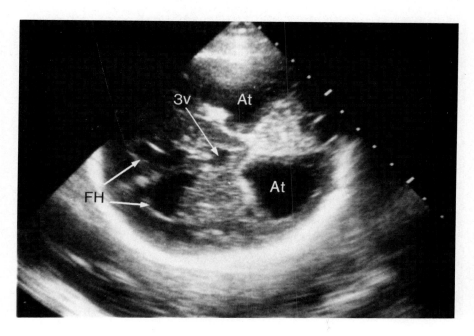

Fig. 14–5. Simultaneous distension of lateral and third ventricles (3v) in the presence of a normal posterior fossa. This is triventricular hydrocephalus. (FH = frontal horns; At = atria of lateral ventricles.)

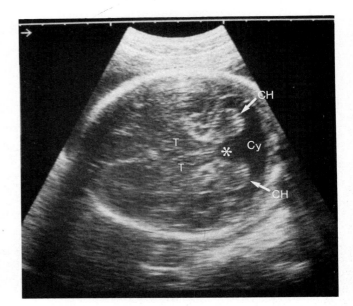

Fig. 14–6. The fourth ventricle (*) amply communicates with a cystic cisterna magna (Cy) through a wide defect of the cerebellar vermis. Cerebellar hemispheres (CH) are widely separated. This is Dandy-Walker malformation. T = thalami.

three percent of survivors have severe handicaps, 12% mild handicaps, and only 35% were developing normally at follow-up.

NEURAL TUBE DEFECTS

The average incidence of neural tube defects (NTD) is 1 to 2 in 1,000 births, with a peak of 7 in 1,000 in South Wales.[39,40] The multifactorial etiology of these anomalies is well established. The recurrence risk after the birth of one affected child is 3 to 5%.

Anencephaly is featured by the absence of the cranial vault, cerebral hemispheres, and diencephalic structures. Sonographic prenatal diagnosis is easy (Fig. 14–7). Because the fetal head can be consistently identified with modern ultrasound equipment starting at 10

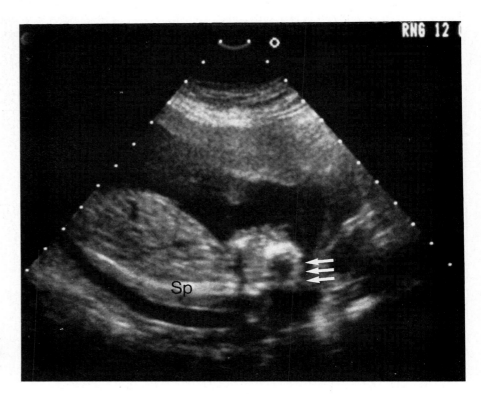

Fig. 14–7. Longitudinal view of midtrimester fetus with anencephaly, demonstrating absence of the cranial vault (*arrows*). Sp = spine.

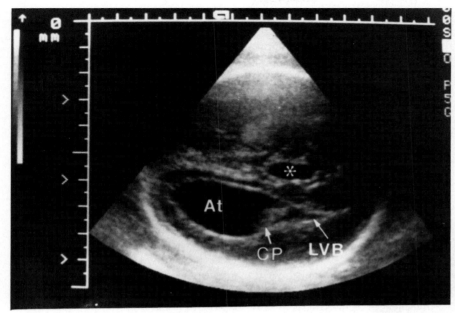

Fig. 14–15. Axial view of the head demonstrating a striking enlargement of the atria (At) and wide separation of the bodies (LVB) of lateral ventricles. Cystic structure on midline (*) is the upwardly displaced third ventricle. This is agenesis of the corpus callosum. CP = choroid plexus.

cephaly can be identified by demonstrating fusion and squaring of the roof of the frontal horns (Fig. 14–14).[62]

Alobar holoprosencephaly is fatal within the first days or weeks of life. Semilobar holoprosencephaly may be compatible with longer survival, but infants are virtually amented.[53] The outcome of infants with lobar holoprosencephaly is uncertain.[63]

The incidence of *agenesis of the corpus callosum* (ACC) is highly controversial. Figures ranging from almost 1 in 100 to 1 in 19,000 have been reported.[64] The etiology is unclear. Agenesis of the corpus callosum may be found in association with chromosomal aberrations, particularly trisomy 18. A Mendelian inheritance with autosomal dominant and autosomal recessive, as well as sex-linked transmission has been documented on several occasions.[65] Also, ACC is a part of several genetic syndromes, including Aicardi, Andermann, acrocallosal, and F.G. syndrome.[65] Anatomic anomalies including central nervous system malformations (abnormal convolutional patterns, DWM, microcephaly, aplasia, or hypoplasia of pyramidal tracts), and a wide variety of non-nervous deformities is frequently found, suggesting that ACC may be a part of a widespread developmental disturbance.[66]

Agenesis of the corpus callosum is invariably associated with a typical alteration of the intracranial architecture that includes a marked lateral separation of the bodies of lateral ventricles and enlargement of the atria and occipital horns. Such rearrangement of the ventricular morphology is commonly referred to as colpocephaly. The third ventricle is frequently enlarged and displaced upward in the position normally occupied by the corpus callosum.[64,67]

Prenatal diagnosis of ACC is possible.[68,69] The most consistent sonographic finding is colpocephaly, which is invariably found in all cases of ACC. Upward displacement of the third ventricle is highly specific of ACC, but it is only present in 50% of cases (Fig. 14–15).[69] In those cases in which coronal scans of good quality can be obtained, direct demonstration of the absence of the corpus callosum is also possible (Fig. 14–16).[69]

Many patients with ACC suffer from mental retardation, neurologic abnormalities, and are psychologically abnormal. However, the condition can be entirely asymptomatic.[64] No specific risk figures are available at present. Association with other anomalies increases the likelihood of a poor outcome. Our own experience includes six cases of isolated ACC diagnosed prior to birth with a postnatal follow-up ranging from 3 months to 5 years. All infants are remarkably normal at the time of this writing.

DESTRUCTIVE CEREBRAL LESIONS

Congenital *porencephaly* is defined as the presence of cystic cavities within the cerebral matter. The cavities

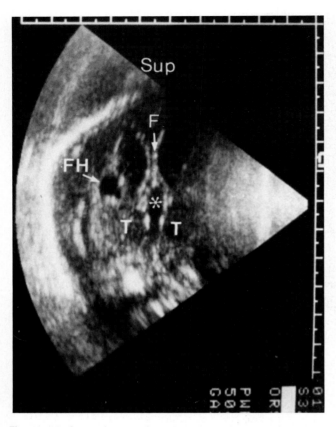

Fig. 14–16. Coronal scan of the head in the same case as Fig. 14–15. Absence of corpus callosum is clearly demonstrated by visualization of the falx cerebrii (F) that comes in close contact with the upwardly displaced third ventricle (*). Note the wide distance between midline and frontal horn (FH), distal to the transducer. T = thalami; Sup = superior.

may communicate with the ventricular system, subarachnoid space, or both. Loss of cerebral tissue may derive from primary maldevelopment of the brain (schizencephaly). More frequently, it is the consequence of a destructive process usually on an anoxic basis (encephaloclastic porencephaly).[70,71] Schizencephaly is characterized by bilateral and symmetric clefts within the cerebral substance and is frequently associated with microcephaly. Encephaloclastic porencephaly is usually a unilateral lesion that may be associated with impairment of cerebrospinal fluid, circulation, and hydrocephalus. *Hydranencephaly* can be regarded as an extreme form of encephaloclastic porencephaly. Most of the cerebral hemispheres are replaced by a cystic cavity that the brain stem and rhombencephalic structures are usually spared. Hydranencephaly has been reported in association with congenital infections, including toxoplasmosis and cytomegalovirus, and intrauterine occlusion or atresia of the internal carotid arteries.[72]

Cystic cavities within the fetal brain are easily demonstrated with ultrasound (Fig. 14–17) but, at present, it is inclear if a differential diagnosis between porencephaly and intracranial cysts of a different nature (such as arachnoid cysts and congenital cystic tumors) is possible. The fluid-filled cranial cavity typical of hydranencephaly is easily detected by antenatal ultrasound, but a specific identification of this anomaly may be difficult. The differential diagnosis includes severe hydrocephalus and holoprosencephaly. One of the most valuable sonographic findings in hydranencephaly is the demonstration of the intact brain stem which, in the absence of the

Fig. 14–17. Porencephaly. There is gross distortion of intracranial anatomy and a conspicuous shift of midline echo (*arrows*). A fluid-filled collection replaces the cerebral hemisphere close to the transducer and amply communicates with contralateral lateral ventricle (LV).

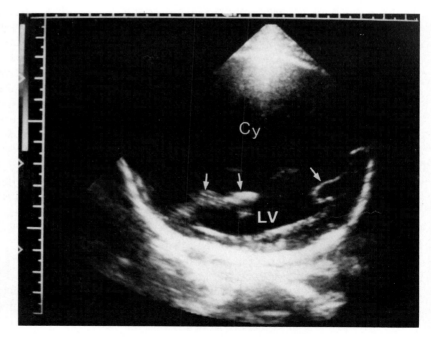

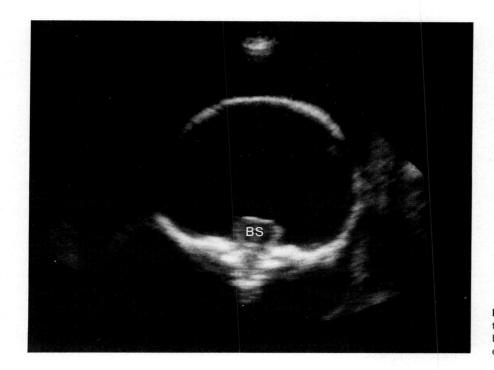

Fig. 14–18. Coronal scan of the head of a third-trimester fetus. Brain stem (BS) bulges within fluid that fills the intracranial cavity. This is hydranencephaly.

surrounding cortex, bulges inside the fluid-filled intracranial cavity (Fig. 14–18). Such findings somewhat resemble the bulb-like appearance of the hypoplastic thalami that can be seen in alobar and semilobar holoprosencephaly; however, in the latter condition, it is usually possible to demonstrate the pancacked frontal cortex.

The outcome for infants with congenital brain disruptions is dictated by the size and location of the lesion. Extensive porencephaly and hydranencephaly have a dismal prognosis.

DISORDERS OF NERVE CELL PROLIFERATION

The association between decreased head size and reduction of both brain mass and total cell number in microcephalic infants is well established.[73] However, there is disagreement with regard to the clinical threshold of abnormalcy. Some authors have suggested employing head circumference below −2 standard deviations from the mean as the diagnostic criterion.[74] Others prefer to consider head circumference below −3 standard deviations as abnormal.[75] The incidence of microcephaly obviously varies in different surveys, depending on the definition used to identify the lesion.

Microcephaly should not be considered as a separate clinical entity, but rather as a symptom of many etiologic disturbances. The clinical subdivision suggested by Book and associates[75] distinguishes between those cases resulting from environmental insults (anoxia, infections, radiations, and so forth) and genetic microcephaly, which includes all cases in which microcephaly is transmitted as a Mendelian trait, either alone or as one of a number of syndromes.

Microcephaly is featured by a typical disproportion between the skull and the face. The forehead is sloping. The brain is small (microencephaly) because the cerebral hemispheres are affected to a greater extent than the diencephalic and rhombencephalic structures. Abnormal convolutional patterns, including macrogyria, microgyria, and agyria, are frequently found. The ventricles may be dilated. Microcephaly is frequently seen in cases of porencephaly, lissencephaly, and holoprosencephaly.

Many difficulties arise in attempting to identify fetal microcephaly. The utility of head measurements alone may be hampered by incorrect dating or intrauterine growth retardation. Furthermore, the natural history of fetal microcephaly is largely unknown. A progressive intrauterine development of the lesion interfering with early recognition has been described.[76] A comparison of biometric parameters, such as the ratio of HC to abdominal circumference and the ratio of femur length to BPD, has been suggested. Chervenak and associates[77] have provided useful nomograms. Nevertheless, both false-positive and false-negative diagnoses have been reported.[77] It is clear that the predictive value of ultrasound at present

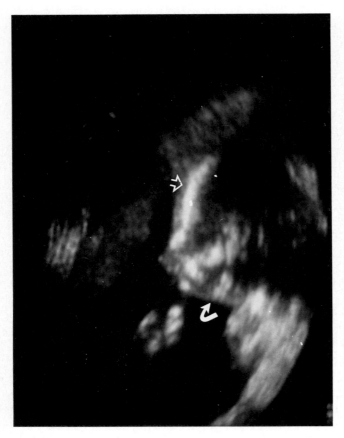

Fig. 14–19. In this midtrimester fetus with microcephaly and multiple anomalies, a sagittal view of the face reveals a sloping forehead and striking micrognathia. (*Reproduced with permission from Romero R, Pilu G, Jeanty P, Ghidini A, Hobbins JC. Prenatal Diagnosis of Congenital Anomalies. Norwalk, Conn: Appleton & Lange; 1987.*)

has some limitations and that further investigation is required. A qualitative evaluation of the intracranial anatomy is a very useful adjunct to biometry because many cases of microcephaly are associated with morphologic derangement, particularly with ventriculomegaly, schizencephaly, and disorders of ventral induction.[78] A nomogram of the normal measurements of the frontal lobes has been developed[79] and may prove useful in dubious cases. Demonstration of a sloping forehead increases the index of suspicion (Fig. 14–19).

The final outcome of microcephaly is controversial. In one series of 134 infants with a head circumference below −2 standard deviations from the mean, only one had a normal intelligence.[74] More recent studies are in disagreement with these observations. In a group of 28 infants with head circumference below −2 standard deviations from the mean, only 50% were found to have mental retardation.[80] In another study, infants with a head circumference between −2 and −3 standard deviations from the mean were mentally retarded in 18% of cases, and infants with a head circumference below −3 standard deviations from the mean were mentally retarded in 72% of cases.[81] It is hard to derive precise prognostic figures from these data. However, it is clear that a small head does not necessarily imply intellectual impairment.

The clinical significance of *megalencephaly* is unclear. An abnormally large brain is usually found in individuals of normal and even superior intelligence, but it may be associated with mental retardation and neurologic impairment.[82] Megalencephaly is also a part of congenital anomalies and syndromes such as Beckwith-Wiedemann syndrome, achondroplasia, neurofibromatosis, and tuberous sclerosis.[82] Obstetric and pediatric

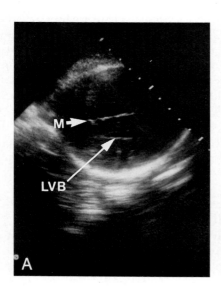
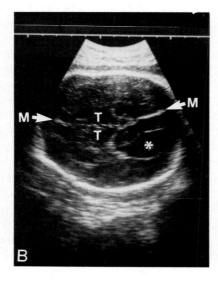
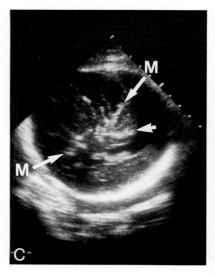

Fig. 14–20. Unilateral megalencephaly. A composition of figures demonstrating shift of the midline echo (M), unilateral distension of the occipital horn (*) and wide, irregular sulcus (*arrowhead*) within the surface of the predominant hemisphere. LVB = bodies of lateral ventricle; T = thalami.

sonographers are frequently challenged by the problem of megalencephaly, a condition that should be suspected in the presence of abnormally large head measurements without evidence of hydrocephalus or intracranial masses. In such cases, examination of the parents may be of help, as asymptomatic megalencephaly is frequently familial.

Unilateral megalencephaly is a rare anomaly of unknown etiology characterized by overgrowth of one lobe or an entire hemisphere,[83] reported occasionally in association with hemigigantism of the body.[84] Anatomic dissection reveals aberrant convolutional patterns, ectopic nodules of gray matter, and a diffuse increase in neuronal size. Sonographic findings include: enlargement of one cerebral hemisphere in the absence of mass effect, a shift of the midline structures, and mild ipsilateral ventriculomegaly (Fig. 14–20).[85] Albeit a rare condition, unilateral megalencephaly should be considered in the differential diagnosis of conditions associated with a shift of the midline, which also include porencephaly and congenital brain tumors. Mental retardation and uncontrollable seizures have been described in affected infants.[86]

ABNORMALITIES OF THE CHOROID PLEXUS

Choroid plexus papillomas (CPPs) are neuroectodermal neoplasms that are frequently congenital in their occurrence. With the exception of malignant cases, CPPs are histologically identical to the normal choroid plexus. They are most frequently found within the lateral ventricles at the level of the atria, but they have been described within the third and fourth ventricles as well. Choroid plexus papillomas are frequently associated with hydrocephalus that may arise from one of two mechanisms: intraventricular obstruction, or overproduction of cerebrospinal fluid.[87] Prenatal diagnosis of CPP associated with communicating hydrocephalus has been reported.[88]

Choroid plexus papillomas carry a severe prognosis: the mortality rate is about 30% and survivors developed a normal intelligence in approximately 60% of cases.[89,90]

Prenatal sonographic identification of *choroid plexus cysts* has been reported with increasing frequency over the last years (Fig. 14–21).[91,92] While other authors have reported a very low incidence of fetal choroid plexus cysts,[92] we have documented this finding in 4% of routine second trimester sonograms. We have never seen choroid plexus cysts beyond 28 weeks of gestation.

Although the pediatric literature indicates that small choroid plexus cysts have no clinical significance,[93] it would seem that their detection in utero may increase the risk of chromosomal aberrations, specifically of trisomy 18. However, only limited series are available at present.[94,95] Our experience includes 42 cases of fetal choroid plexus cysts that underwent karyotyping. Tri-

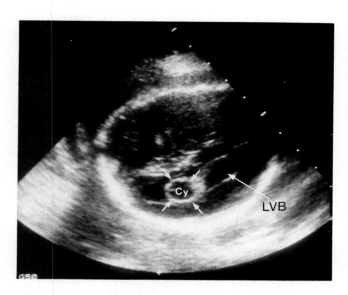

Fig. 14–21. Choroid plexus cyst (Cy) in a midtrimester fetus. (*Reproduced with permission from Romero R, Pilu G, Jeanty P, Ghidini A, Hobbins JC. Prenatal Diagnosis of Congenital Anomalies. Norwalk, Conn: Appleton & Lange; 1987.*)

somy 18 was found in three (7%). We were not able to document any difference in the sonographic appearance of the cysts in normal and trisomic fetuses. Disappearance of the cysts is not reassuring because this occurred in two of the three fetuses with abnormal chromosomes in our series. In the presence of a normal karyotype, choroid plexus cysts should be considered benign and the parents should be reassured. However, serial sonographic examinations are suggested because a disproportionate increase in size of the cyst, with symptoms of intracranial pressure, has occasionally been described.[96]

REFERENCES

1. McIntosh R, Merritt KK, Richards MR, et al. The incidence of congenital anomalies: A study of 5,964 pregnancies. *Pediatrics*. 1954;14:505.
2. Myrianthopoulos NC. Epidemiology of central nervous system malformations. In: Vinken PJ, Bruyn GW, eds. *Handbook of Clinical Neurology.* Amsterdam: Elsevier, 1977:139–171.
3. Singh RP, Carr DH. Anatomic findings in human abortions of known chromosome constitution. *Obstet Gynecol.* 1967;29:806.
4. Nishimura H. Incidence of malformations in abortions. In: Fraser FC, McKusick VA, eds. *Congenital Malformations.* New York: Excerpta Medica; 1970:275–283.
5. Creasy MC, Alberman ED. Congenital malformations of the central nervous system in spontaneous abortions. *J Med Genet.* 1976;13:9.

6. Campbell S, Johnstone FD, Holt EMT, et al. Anencephaly: Early ultrasound diagnosis and active management. *Lancet.* 1972;2:1226.

7. Johnson ML, Dunne MG, Mack LA, et al. Evaluation of fetal intracranial anatomy by static and real-time ultrasound. *J Clin Ultrasound.* 1980;8:311.

8. Fiske CE, Filly RA. Ultrasound evaluation of the normal and abnormal fetal neural axis. *Radiol Clin North Am.* 1982;20:285.

9. Chervenak FA, Berkowitz RL, Romero R, et al. The diagnosis of fetal hydrocephalus. *Am J Obstet Gynecol.* 1983;147:703.

10. Chervenak FA, Berkowitz RL, Tortora M, et al. The diagnosis of ventriculomegaly prior to fetal viability. *Obstet Gynecol.* 1984;64:652.

11. Grannum P, Pilu G. In utero neurosonography—the normal fetus and variations in cranial size. *Semin Perinatol.* 1987;11:85.

12. Grannum P, Pilu G. In utero neurosonography—neuroembryologic and encephaloclastic lesions. *Semin Perinatol.* 1987;11:98.

13. Pilu G, De Palma L, Romero R, et al. The fetal subarachnoid cisterns. An ultrasound study with report of a case of congenital communicating hydrocephalus. *J Ultrasound Med.* 1986;5:365.

14. Romero R, Pilu G, Jeanty P, et al. *Prenatal Diagnosis of Congenital Anomalies.* Norwalk, Conn: Appleton & Lange; 1987.

15. Isaacson G, Mintz MC, Crelin ES. *Atlas of Fetal Sectional Anatomy.* New York: Springer-Verlag; 1986.

16. Crade M, Patel J, McQuown D. Sonographic imaging of the glycogen stage of the fetal choroid plexus. *Am J Neuroradiol.* 1981;2:345.

17. Kurtz AB, Wagner RJW, Kurtz RJ. Analysis of biparietal diameter as an accurate indicator of gestational age. *J Clin Ultrasound.* 1980;8:319.

18. Hadlock FP, Deter RL, Harrist RB. Fetal biparietal diameter: A critical re-evaluation of the relation to menstrual age by means of real-time ultrasound. *J Ultrasound Med.* 1982;2:97.

19. Jeanty P, Cousaert E, Hobbins JC, et al. A longitudinal study of fetal head biometry. *Am J Perinatol.* 1984;1:118.

20. Campbell S, Thoms A. Ultrasound measurement of the fetal head to abdomen circumference ratio in the assessment of growth retardation. *Br J Obstet Gynaecol.* 1982;89:165.

21. MacLeary RD, Kuhus LR, Bozz MJ. Ultrasonography of the fetal cerebellum. *Radiology.* 1984;151:439.

22. Goldstein I, Reece EA, Pilu G, et al. Cerebellar measurements using sonography in the evaluation of fetal growth and development. *Am J Obstet Gynecol.* 1987;156:1065.

23. Reece EA, Goldstein I, Pilu G, et al. Fetal cerebellar growth unaffected by intrauterine growth retardation: A new parameter for prenatal diagnosis. *Am J Obstet Gynecol.* 1987;157:632.

24. Freeman RK, McQuown DS, Secrist LJ, et al. The diagnosis of fetal hydrocephalus before viability. *Obstet Gynecol.* 1977;49:109.

25. Callen PW, Chooljian D. The effect of ventricular dilatation upon biometry of the head. *J Ultrasound Med.* 1986;5:17.

26. Chinn DH, Callen PW, Filly RA. The lateral cerebral ventricle in early second trimester. *Radiology.* 1983;148:529.

27. Denkhaus H, Winsberg F. Ultrasonic measurement of the fetal ventricular system. *Radiology.* 1979;131:781.

28. Pearce JM, Little D, Campbell S. The diagnosis of abnormalities of the fetal central nervous system. In: Sanders RC, James AE, eds. *The Principles and Practice of Ultrasound in Obstetrics and Gynecolocy*, 3rd ed. Norwalk, Conn: Appleton-Century-Crofts; 1985:243–256.

29. Jeanty P, Dramaix-Wilmet M, Delbeke D, et al. Ultrasonic evaluation of fetal ventricular growth. *Neuroradiology* 1981;21:127.

30. Bowerman RA, DiPietro MA. Erroneous sonographic identification of fetal lateral ventricles. Relationship to the echogenic periventricular "blush." *Am J Neuroradiol.* 1987;8:661.

31. Siedler DE, Filly RA. Relative growth of the higher fetal brain structures. *J Ultrasound Med.* 1987;6:573.

32. Varadi V, Csecsei K, Szeifert GT, et al. Prenatal diagnosis of X-linked hydrocephalus without aqueductal stenosis. *J Med Genet.* 1987;24:207.

33. Burton BK. Recurrence risks in congenital hydrocephalus. *Clin Genet.* 1979;16:47.

34. Pilu G, Romero R, De Palma L, et al. Antenatal diagnosis and obstetrical management of Dandy-Walker syndrome. *J Reprod Med.* 1986;31:1017.

35. Hirsch JF, Pierre Kahn A, Reiner D, et al. The Dandy-Walker malformation: A review of 40 cases. *J Neurosurg.* 1984;61:515.

36. Chervenak FA, Berkowitz RL, Tortora M, et al. The management of fetal hydrocephalus. *Am J Obstet Gynecol.* 1985;151:933.

37. Clewell WH, Johnson ML, Meier PR, et al. A surgical approach to the treatment of fetal hydrocephalus. *N Engl J Med.* 1982;306:1320.

38. Michejda M, Hodgen GD. In utero diagnosis and treatment of nonhuman primate fetal skeletal anomalies. I: Hydrocephalus. *JAMA.* 1981;246:1093.

39. Laurence KM, Carter CO, David PA. Major central nervous system malformations in South Wales. I: Incidence, local variations, and geographical factors. *Brit J Prev Soc Med.* 1968;22:146.

40. Laurence KM, Carter CO, David PA. Major central nervous system malformations in South Wales. II: Pregnancy factors, seasonal variation, and social class effects. *Brit J Prev Soc Med.* 1968;22:212.

41. Hashimoto BE, Mahony BS, Filly RA, et al. Sonography, a complementary examination to alpha-fetoprotein testing for neural tube defects. *J Ultrasound Med.* 1985;4:307.

42. Nicolaides KH, Campbell S, Gabbe SG, et al. Ultrasound screening for spina bifida: Cranial and cerebellar signs. *Lancet.* 1986;2:72.

43. Pilu G, Romero R, Reece EA, et al. Subnormal cerebellum in fetuses with spina bifida. *Am J Obstet Gynecol.* In press.

44. Naidich TP, Pudlowski RM, Naidich JB. Computed tomographic signs of the Chiari II malformation. III: Ventricles and cisterns. *Radiology.* 1980;134:657.

45. Babcock DS, Han BK. Cranial sonographic findings in meningomyelocele. *AJR.* 1981;135:563.

16 Sonographic Evaluation of Abnormalities of the Fetal Gastrointestinal Tract

Barbara S. Hertzberg • James D. Bowie

The spectrum of fetal gastrointestinal anomalies diagnosed by ultrasound has widened rapidly in recent years, and abnormalities are being detected at earlier and earlier stages of gestation. One of the most difficult tasks for the sonographer is distinguishing normal from abnormal findings. Due to the wide range of appearances of normal bowel, this is particularly true of the gastrointestinal tract. This chapter will examine the types of gastrointestinal anomalies that can be recognized in utero, emphasizing potential areas of overlap between normal and abnormal patterns.

GENERAL PRINCIPLES

Our examination of the fetus begins with a general survey of the uterus in which we systematically examine the uterine wall and placenta, assess amniotic fluid volume, and subsequently image the fetus in detail. This survey may provide clues to the presence of a gastrointestinal anomaly, such as polyhydramnios, fetal ascites, too many fluid-filled structures in the abdomen, or absence of a fluid-filled fetal stomach.

Polyhydramnios is frequently unexplained. An easy-to-remember (although slightly inaccurate) summary is that mild to moderate polyhydramnios is idiopathic in 60% of cases, has maternal causes (diabetes, Rh incompatibility, and so forth) in 20%, and fetal causes in 20%.[1] However, in the presence of severe polyhydramnios, the incidence of fetal anomalies rises to approximately 75%.[2] Gastrointestinal abnormalities account for 20 to 30% of polyhydramnios cases with a fetal cause. Polyhydramnios is more common with high obstructions than with low obstructions to the gastrointestinal tract.

Fetal ascites may be seen in association with immune and nonimmune hydrops, in utero infection, high-grade renal obstruction with perforation, tumors, and bowel perforation. Fetal ascites must be distinguished from "pseudoascites," which is a normal echo-free area just inside the outer margin of the fetal abdominal wall (Fig. 16–1). Pseudoascites is thought to represent the fetal abdominal wall musculature and can sometimes be traced to muscular insertions on rib endings. True ascites tends to surround organs, collect in peritoneal recesses, and may "outline" parts of the umbilical vein, falciform ligament, or greater omentum (Figs. 16–2 and 16–3).[3–5]

Fluid-filled structures normally detected in the fetal abdomen include the stomach, gallbladder, urinary bladder, and portal vein. An attempt should be made to photograph and explain every echo-free area within the fetal abdomen. When an extra cystic structure or structures are seen, an important rule of thumb is to first determine if the abnormality is renal in origin because the vast majority of such areas will represent renal lesions. Even if the lesion is not renal, it is important to attempt to show the organ of origin, as this aids in narrowing the differential diagnosis. A wide variety of organs and pathologic processes other than the bowel may account for such areas, including ovary (cyst or teratoma), uterus (hydrometrocolpos), obstructed urinary bladder, spine (anterior meningocele or sacrococcygeal teratoma), biliary tree (choledochal cyst), omentum/mesentery (omental or mesenteric cyst), and liver (hepatic cyst). Among the clues that an abnormal area may represent dilated bowel, are presence of peristalsis, connection to the stomach, or a characteristic tubular shape. Thick-walled lesions, with or without debris, tend to be inflammatory or neoplastic, whereas areas with thinner walls are more likely to represent other processes such as cysts and obstructed urinary bladders.

Inability to identify a fluid-filled stomach suggests esophageal atresia because the stomach is usually readily imaged by 15 weeks' gestation. This is discussed in greater detail in the section on esophageal atresia and tracheoesophageal fistula.

NORMAL ANATOMY AND NORMAL VARIANTS

The fetal stomach can routinely be imaged as a fluid-filled structure in the left upper quadrant by 14 to 15 menstrual weeks. Rarely, the normal stomach is not seen in the 15- to 20-week period, but if the fetus is normal, the stomach

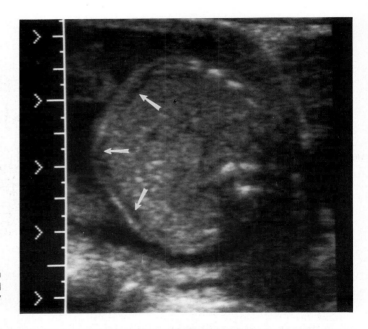

Fig. 16-1. Axial view of a normal fetal abdomen showing thin hypoechoic rim just inside the outer margin of abdominal wall (*arrows*). This echopenic area is referred to as "pseudoascites" and is thought to represent abdominal wall musculature.

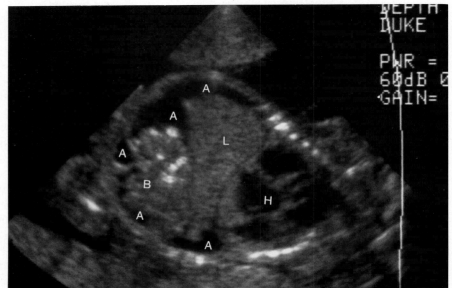

Fig. 16-2. Coronal scan of a fetus with ascites and multiple congenital anomalies, demonstrating true ascites (A) surrounding organs and collecting in peritoneal recesses. L = liver; H = heart; B = bowel.

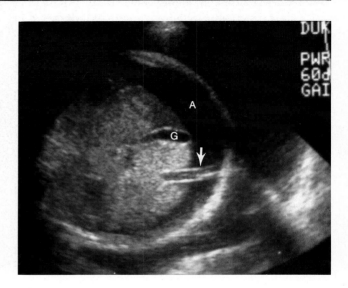

Fig. 16-3. Transverse section of fetal abdomen reveals ascites (A) surrounding umbilical vein (*arrow*). G = gallbladder.

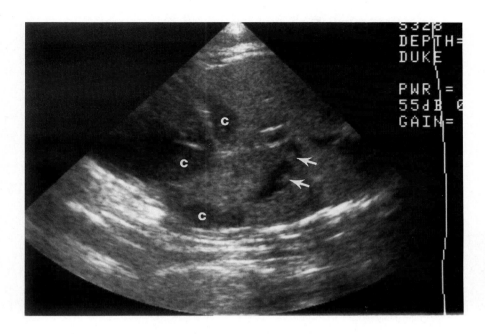

Fig. 16–4. Coronal image of a normal fetus reveals two echogenic collections (*arrows*) in the stomach. These "gastric pseudomasses" are usually a transient phenomenon without pathologic significance, although rarely they are seen in association with bowel obstruction. C = colon.

will be demonstrable on subsequent studies. Echogenic masses are sometimes observed in the fetal stomach as a transient phenomenon unassociated with pathology (Fig. 16–4).[6] Termed "gastric pseudomasses," they may be due to aggregates of swallowed cells and cell fragments, but their exact origin is not known. Occasionally, such masses are due to swallowed blood secondary to placental abruption, so careful ultrasound evaluation for placental abruption is indicated when gastric pseudomasses are seen.

Small bowel is much less commonly identified by sonography than is the stomach. Loops of small bowel are usually not seen prior to 28 weeks, and even after 34 weeks of gestation are seen in only 30% of fetuses.[7] Individual small bowel loops should not exceed approximately 7 mm in diameter or 15 mm in length. They are located centrally in the abdomen, and often exhibit peristalsis. Because these loops are usually visualized only transiently, the presence of fixed segments may suggest pathology if they remain unchanged over several examinations.

The colon appears as a hypoechoic tubular structure around the perimeter of the abdomen (Fig. 16–5). It has been detected as early as 22 menstrual weeks, and by 28

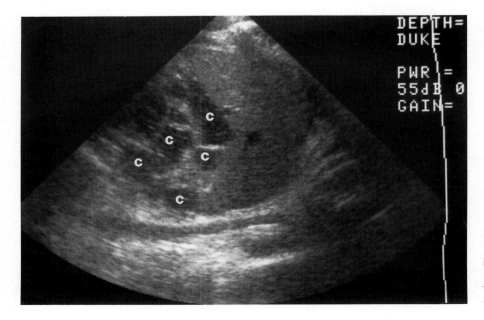

Fig. 16–5. Coronal scan of a normal fetus near term, demonstrating meconium-filled colon (C). Note how prominent the colon can be late in the third trimester.

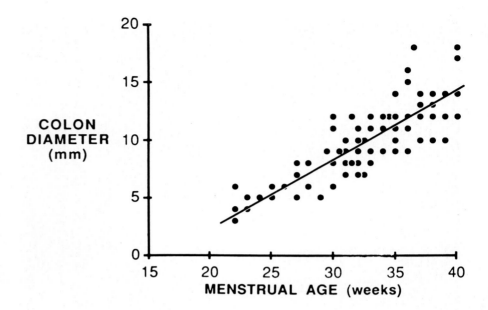

Fig. 16–6. Plot of maximal colon diameter as a function of gestational age in normal fetuses. The mean diameter of the colon increases approximately linearly as gestation progresses, but there is considerable variation in maximal colonic diameter at any given gestational age. (*Reprinted with permission of Nyberg DA, Mack LA, Patten RM, et al.* J Ultrasound Med. 1987;6:3–6.)

weeks portions of the colon may be identified in almost all fetuses.[7] The mean diameter of the normal colon increases approximately linearly with menstrual age, but the variation in size at any given age is wide and overlaps with the size range seen in an abnormally distended colon

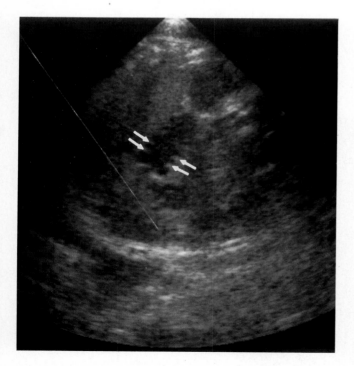

Fig. 16–7. Oblique sonogram of a normal term fetus demonstrating colonic haustra (*arrows*).

(Fig. 16–6). Thus, the sonographic diagnosis of colonic obstruction is often difficult at best. The normal fetal colon may measure up to 18 mm or more in internal diameter, does not usually exhibit peristalsis, and contains increasing amounts of hypoechoic meconium as pregnancy progresses.[7] Near term, colonic haustra are sometimes identified (Fig. 16–7).[8]

A focal well-defined area of increased echogenicity is commonly seen in the lower fetal abdomen early in the second trimester, between 16 and 22 menstrual weeks (Fig. 16–8).[9–11] This is usually a normal variant that resolves on follow-up scans and may represent small bowel mesentery, collapsed bowel, or an accumulation of meconium. If such an area is in a typical location in the pelvis and lower abdomen, and is unassociated with abnormal findings such as fetal ascites, peritoneal calcifications, bowel dilatation, or polyhydramnios, we generally interpret it as a normal variant not requiring further workup. However, caution is advised when any of these findings is in question because areas of increased echogenicity in the fetal abdomen have been described in association with such disorders as meconium peritonitis and meconium ileus (although associated abnormalities are usually detected by sonography in such cases).

The fetal bowel migrates into the umbilical cord as a normal embryologic event early in the first trimester and returns to the abdominal cavity by 10 to 12 weeks of gestation. With carefully performed high-resolution scans, the herniated bowel is commonly visualized as a mass at the base of the umbilical cord and could conceivably be confused with an omphalocele or gastroschisis (Fig. 16–9).[12,13] As a result, these diagnoses should not

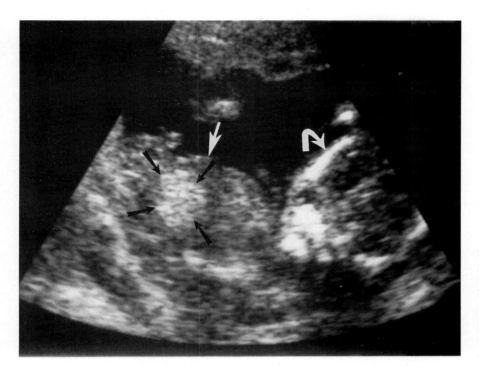

Fig. 16–8. Coronal scan of a normal 16-week fetus demonstrating a focal area of increased echogenicity (*black arrows*) in the lower abdomen. Etiology of this normal variant is not known, but it may represent collapsed bowel, mesentery, or meconium. (*Curved white arrow* = fetal head; *straight white arrow* = fetal abdomen.

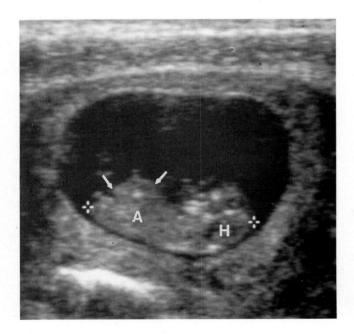

Fig. 16–9. Sagittal scan of a normal 10-week embryo reveals a mass-like protrusion from the fetal abdomen due to bowel that has migrated into the base of the umbilical cord (*arrows*). This migration occurs as a normal embryologic event during the first trimester and should not be mistaken for an omphalocele or gastroschisis. H = head; A = abdomen.

be made until after 14 menstrual weeks, and follow-up sonography should be performed in suspicious cases seen prior to that time.

ESOPHAGEAL ATRESIA AND TRACHEOESOPHAGEAL FISTULA

Esophageal atresia is associated with tracheoesophageal fistula in approximately 90% of cases. The most common form of fistula is from the trachea to the distal esophagus. Associated abnormalities occur in approximately 58% of patients and include cardiac (particularly PDA, and atrial and ventricular septal defects), chromosomal (trisomy 21), gastrointestinal (other atresias), genitourinary (most commonly unilateral renal agenesis), and central nervous system lesions.[14] The VACTERL complex of vertebral, anal, cardiovascular, tracheoesophageal, renal, radial, and limb malformations is the best known grouping of anomalies associated with tracheoesophageal lesions.

The antenatal sonographic diagnosis of esophageal atresia is based on the presence of polyhydramnios with inability to detect the fetal stomach (Fig. 16–10).[15–20] The fetal stomach can usually be readily imaged by 14 to 15 weeks' gestation and generally remains distended throughout the study. Failure to see fluid in the stomach in normal fetuses is rare beyond this stage, except in the presence of severe oligohydramnios. In that case, the

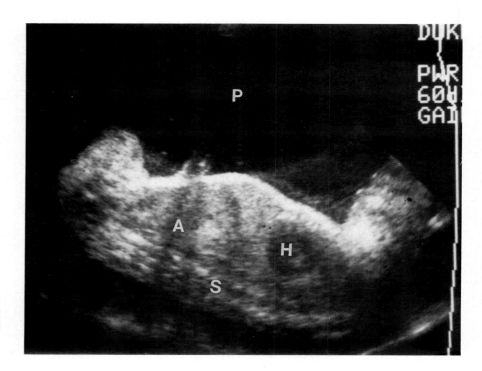

Fig. 16–10. Parasagittal scan to left of midline. Note marked polyhydramnios (P) and absence of fluid-filled stomach in this fetus with esophageal atresia. A = abdomen; H = heart; S = spine.

lack of gastric fluid is due to the paucity of fluid available for the fetus to swallow. Polyhydramnios occurs in 62 to 91% of gestations associated with esophageal atresia but esophageal atresia accounts for only a small proportion of cases of polyhydramnios.[19] Despite the presence of a fistula, the fetal stomach is not seen in up to one third of fetuses with tracheoesophageal fistulas. Therefore, it is thought that amniotic fluid flows into the stomach through some, but not all, fistulas.[18,19] A fluid-filled stomach can rarely be identified in fetuses with esophageal atresia without a distal fistula. It is thought that in these cases, gastric secretions are sufficient to permit moderate stomach distension.[19]

Although the cardinal sonographic features of esophageal atresia are polyhydramnios combined with inability to visualize the fetal stomach, other signs are also occasionally identified. They include direct visualization of a dilated proximal pouch (Fig. 16–11), which may be seen to alternately fill and empty, and observation of fetal vomiting or regurgitation, which is thought to indicate the presence of a high gastrointestinal obstruction.[20–22]

DUODENAL ATRESIA

Duodenal atresia is the most common type of congenital small-bowel obstruction. Most cases are thought to represent an alteration in embryologic development in which there is failure to recanalize the duodenal lumen during the 11th week of gestation. The diagnosis is suggested in utero by sonographic demonstration of polyhydramnios and a fluid-filled "double bubble" in the fetal abdomen (Fig. 16–12.A).[16,22–30] The sonographic double bubble corresponds to the double bubble sign seen on radiographs of infants with duodenal atresia. It consists of

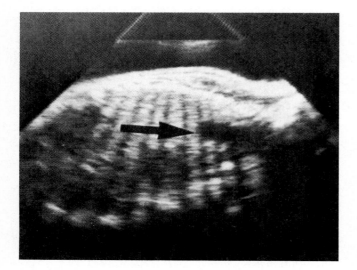

Fig. 16–11. Longitudinal scan of a fetus with esophageal atresia, demonstrating fluid in esophagus proximal to the level of the atresia (*arrow*). (*Reprinted with permission from Eyheremendy E, Pfister M. J Clin Ultrasound. 1983;11:395–397.*)

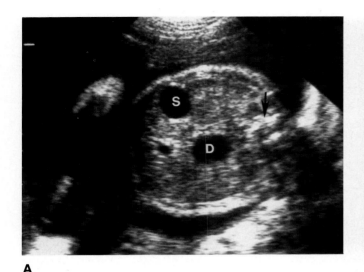
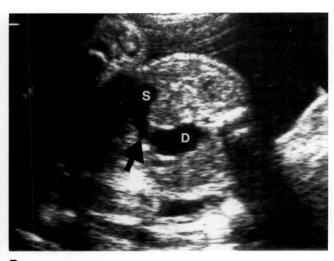

A   **B**

Fig. 16–12. A. The "double bubble" sign. Axial sonogram through the abdomen of a fetus with duodenal atresia reveals polyhydramnios and two distended fluid-filled structures, representing the obstructed duodenum (D) and stomach (S). *Black arrow* = spine. (*Reprinted with permission from Nelson LH. In: Putman CE, Ravin CE, eds.* Textbook of Diagnostic Imaging. *Philadelphia: W.B. Saunders; 1988;3:1984–1990.*) **B.** Axial sonogram through the abdomen of the same fetus, taken at a slightly more caudal level, reveals interconnection (*arrow*) between dilated duodenum (D) and stomach (S).

visualization of a distended stomach in the left upper quadrant, connecting with an enlarged duodenum located on the right (Fig. 16–12.B). However, the double bubble sign is not specific for duodenal atresia. In newborns, it can be seen in association with other forms of duodenal obstruction such as duodenal web, annular pancreas, duodenal stenosis, Ladd's bands, volvulus, and obstruction from intestinal duplications. The antenatal ultrasound diagnosis of duodenal atresia has been suggested as early as 19 menstrual weeks but may not be recognizable until much later in pregnancy.[14]

There are several potential pitfalls in diagnosing a double bubble sign. Although cystic renal abnormalities might be confused with a dilated stomach and duodenum, when the kidney is in its usual location most renal abnormalities will be located closer to the spine than the fetal stomach. A choledochal cyst situated adjacent to the stomach could potentially simulate the appearance of dilated duodenum, but in such cases it should not be possible to demonstrate a communication between the two cystic masses.[31] Finally, in coronal scan planes it may be possible to bisect an otherwise normal fetal stomach, giving the appearance of a double bubble. This error can be overcome by scanning the abdomen in a transverse plane.[32]

Duodenal atresia is associated with a high incidence of other associated anomalies, including congenital heart disease, esophageal atresia, imperforate anus, small bowel atresias, biliary atresias, and renal and vertebral anomalies. In addition, approximately 25 to 30% of patients with duodenal atresia have trisomy 21.

SMALL BOWEL OBSTRUCTION

The most common form of jejunal and ileal obstruction is atresia, which usually occurs secondary to an in utero vascular accident. The sonographic diagnosis of small bowel obstruction relies on the demonstration of multiple interconnecting overdistended bowel loops, the number of loops seen depending on the level of obstruction (Fig. 16–13).[33–38] In the normal fetus, individual loops of small bowel should not exceed approximately 7 mm in diameter or 15 mm in length, and are usually not seen prior to 28 menstrual weeks.[7] Even then they are only occasionally visualized. The stomach is also frequently overdistended, but gastric distention is difficult to judge because the normal fetal stomach varies much in size. Strong peristaltic movements can sometimes be identified in association with small bowel obstruction, and their recognition helps confirm that an abnormal process is related to the bowel.[33,34] A false-positive diagnosis of small bowel obstruction has been reported, so caution is advised in questionable cases.[39]

Polyhydramnios is seen in conjunction with some cases of jejunal or ileal obstruction and becomes more common as the level of the obstruction becomes higher. Although obstructions due to fetal volvulus or intussus-

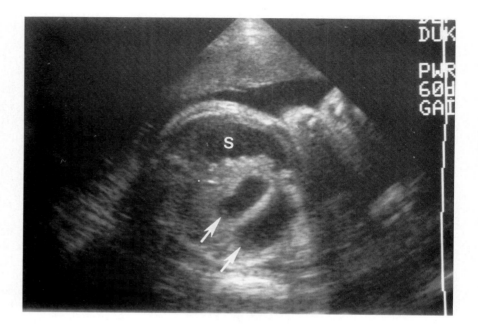

Fig. 16–13. Transverse image of a fetus with jejunal atresia. Several dilated loops of small bowel (*arrows*) are demonstrated. These were seen to interconnect and peristalse during real-time evaluation. S = stomach.

ception have been detected antenatally, the sonographic findings associated with these entities appear to be non-specific.[34,36,40,41] If intestinal perforation occurs in association with small bowel obstruction of any cause, fetal ascites and sonographic changes related to meconium peritonitis may be seen.

MECONIUM PERITONITIS AND MECONIUM PSEUDOCYST

Meconium peritonitis is a chemical peritonitis resulting from intrauterine bowel perforation of any cause. Common underlying disorders include small-bowel atresia, meconium ileus, volvulus, and intussusception, but some cases are idiopathic. Because fetal meconium is sterile, in utero leakage of bowel contents does not lead to bacterial contamination.[42]

Multiple reports of the in utero detection of meconium peritonitis describe a wide spectrum of sonographic findings.[42–54] The ultrasound changes detected depend on whether the bowel perforation seals as well as on the underlying disorder. Following leakage of bowel contents, an intense peritoneal inflammatory reaction ensues, leading to formation of dense fibrotic tissue that often calcifies. This form of meconium peritonitis is the fibroadehesive type, and is identified in utero by characteristic intraperitoneal calcifications also seen on postnatal abdominal radiographs. In antenatal sonography, these calcifications appear as highly echogenic linear or

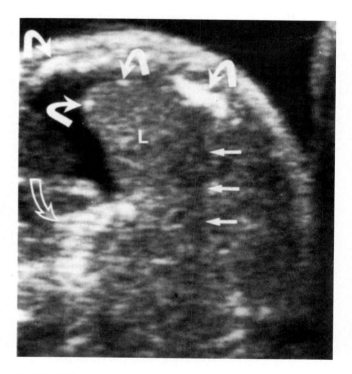

Fig. 16–14. Transverse sonogram through the abdomen of a fetus with meconium peritonitis reveals multiple calcific foci lining the visceral and parietal peritoneum (*curved arrows*) and a large calcific deposit near the root of the mesentery (*open arrow*). *Straight arrows* delineate acoustic shadowing from a calcific focus on liver surface. L = liver. (*Reprinted with permission from Foster MA, Nyberg DA, Mahony BS, et al. Radiology. 1987;165:661–665.*)

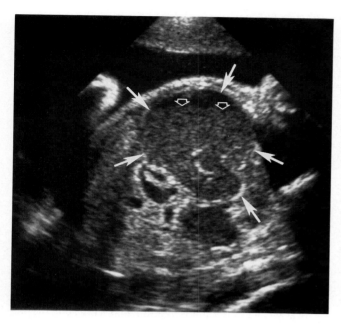

Fig. 16–15. Oblique image through the abdomen of a fetus with meconium peritonitis demonstrating a large meconium pseudocyst (*solid arrows*) with a fluid debris level (*open arrows*).

clumped foci in the abdomen or pelvis, some of which may exhibit posterior acoustic shadowing (Fig. 16–14).[43,44]

If a bowel perforation remains patent, the cystic form of meconium peritonitis results from continued spillage of intestinal contents into a cavity consisting of matted bowel loops and fibrous tissue around the perforation site. With antenatal sonography a meconium pseudocyst appears as an irregular thick-walled cystic abdominal mass that often contains internal debris, septations, and wall calcifications (Fig. 16–15).[45–50] Although the differential diagnosis of a cystic mass in the fetal abdomen or pelvis is broad and includes such entities as obstructed bladder, ovarian cyst, pararenal pseudocyst, teratoma, omental cyst, hydrometrocolpus, gastrointestinal duplication, and so forth, the presence of associated peritoneal calcifications strongly supports the diagnosis of meconium pseudocyst. Other sonographic findings that may be seen in conjunction with meconium peritonitis include dilated bowel loops, fetal ascites, echogenic ascites with mass effect on adjacent organs, and polyhydramnios.[43]

MECONIUM ILEUS AND MECONIUM PLUG SYNDROME

Meconium ileus is obstruction of the distal small bowel by meconium. It occurs almost exclusively in conjunction with cystic fibrosis, due to the abnormally thick and viscous meconium of infants with this disorder. When meconium ileus is accompanied by bowel perforation, meconium peritonitis results and the antenatal sonographic findings are as discussed above.

The in utero sonographic appearance of uncomplicated meconium ileus has been described.[55–58] Findings include abnormal areas of increased echogenicity in the fetal abdomen and dilatation of small bowel in association with polyhydramnios. Areas of increased abdominal echogenicity are thought to emanate from abnormal intraluminal meconium and range in appearance from a single echogenic mass in the lower abdomen to multiple scattered hyperechoic regions.[55,56] However, because the specificity of these hyperechoic areas is suspect, caution is advised in interpreting such regions. For instance, a single echogenic mass-like area in the lower abdomen occurs transiently as a normal finding during the second trimester (Fig. 16–8).[9,11] Similarly, small bowel dilatation is a nonspecific finding that has been described in association with many entities other than meconium ileus, including atresia, stenosis, congenital bands, midgut volvulus, duplication, internal hernias, and Hirschsprung's disease.[57]

In the meconium plug syndrome, a collection of meconium in the distal colon causes transient colonic obstruction with failure to pass meconium in the first days of life. Although dilated colon has been identified antenatally in some patients with meconium plug syndrome,[57,59] this should be considered a nonspecific finding that can also occur in normal fetuses and those with anorectal malformations and Hirschsprung's disease.

ANORECTAL MALFORMATIONS

Anorectal malformation (ARM) refers to a spectrum of abnormalities of hindgut termination including imperforate anus, anal agenesis, anorectal agenesis, and rectal atresia. These lesions are associated with a high incidence of other anomalies, most commonly as components of the VACTERL syndrome (vertebral, anal, cardiovascular, tracheoesophageal, renal, radial, and limb malformations) or the caudal regression syndrome. They also occur with other complex abnormalities of cloacal development.[60–62] The malformations are divided into two groups depending on the location of atresia. High lesions terminate above the levator sling, are commonly associated with a fistula to the genitourinary system, and require abdominal surgery. Low malformations terminate below the levator sling in an orifice on the perineum or inside the posterior vaginal fourchette, and are usually treated with perineal surgery.

Antenatal ultrasound reveals dilated fetal colon in

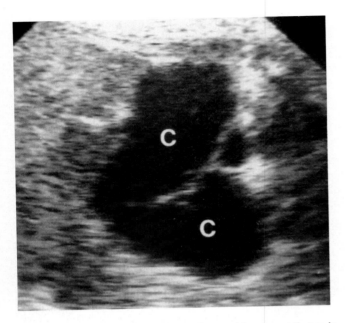

Fig. 16–16. Coronal sonogram of a fetus with anorectal atresia and multiple congenital anomalies reveals a V-shaped segment of dilated colon (C) in the pelvis. (*Reprinted with permission from Harris RD, Nyberg DA, Mack LA, et al. AJR. 1987;149:395–409.*)

some, but not all, cases of anorectal malformations.[60–64] However, the reader is cautioned that the normal colon is quite prominent late in pregnancy, so it is possible to overcall colonic obstruction when the loops of bowel are only moderately distended. The incidence of sonographic visualization of dilated bowel in association with anorectal malformations increases as pregnancy progresses.[60] The presence of a dilated V- or U-shaped segment of bowel in the fetal pelvis or lower abdomen is thought to be particularly suggestive of anorectal malformation (Fig. 16–16).[60] Intraluminal intestinal calcifications occur in some newborns with imperforate anus and have also been identified in utero.[65,66]

HIRSCHSPRUNG'S DISEASE

Hirschsprung's disease is due to congenital absence of the ganglion cells of the myenteric plexus, extending proximally from the anus to involve a variable segment of bowel. Because the aganglionic segment is unable to transmit peristaltic contractions normally, a functional obstruction occurs that results in dilation of bowel proximal to the affected segment. The disease usually is not apparent prior to birth, although two cases of antenatal detection have been described, with polyhydramnios and multiple loops of dilated fetal bowel seen in both.[67,68] It

should be stressed that this appearance is uncommon and nonspecific.

VENTRAL ABDOMINAL WALL DEFECTS

The two main types of abdominal wall defects detected by antenatal sonography are omphalocele and gastroschisis.[69–82] Both are associated with external herniation of abdominal contents, but in omphalocele the defect is in the midline at the site of the umbilicus, whereas gastroschisis is a paraumbilical defect usually located to the right of midline.

Distinction between these two conditions can usually be made in utero. This is of prognostic value because gastroschisis is essentially an isolated entity rarely associated with anomalies other than intestinal malrotation and secondary gastrointestinal lesions. Fetuses with omphalocele are at high risk for other abnormalities that include cardiac anomalies (ventricular and atrial septal defects, tetralogy of Fallot) in up to 47%, genitourinary abnormalities in up to 40%, neural tube defects in up to 39%, gastrointestinal anomalies, and trisomies in 35 to 58%.[69] Omphaloceles are found in conjunction with several syndromes, including the Beckwith-Wiedemann syndrome (omphalocele, macroglossia, organomegaly, and neonatal hypoglycemia) and pentalogy of Cantrell (midline supraumbilical abdominal defect, sternal defect,

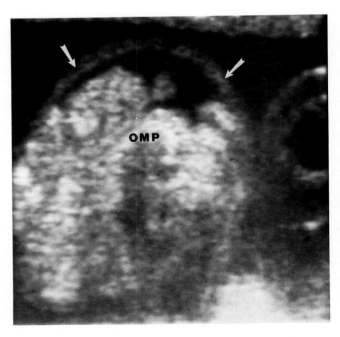

Fig. 16–17. Oblique scan through herniated mass of an omphalocele (OMP) demonstrating a membrane surrounding herniated contents (*arrows*).

deficiency of diaphragmatic pericardium, deficiency of anterior diaphragm, and intracardiac anomaly).[83-86] Prenatal diagnosis of an omphalocele should prompt a careful search for additional abnormalities as well as consideration of amniocentesis.

In omphalocele the umbilical cord inserts into the membrane surrounding the herniated mass, whereas in gastroschisis the cord inserts normally into the fetal abdomen. A membrane consisting of amnion and peritoneum surrounds the herniated contents of an omphalocele (Fig. 16–17); but gastroschisis represents a full-thickness abdominal wall defect without a covering membrane, so the herniated bowel loops float freely in the amniotic fluid. Unprotected by a membrane, and at risk for ischemic events, the eviscerated bowel is prone to secondary complications, including thickening and fibrosis (Fig. 16–18). The membrane surrounding an omphalocele occasionally ruptures, in which case it may be difficult to distinguish between a ruptured omphalocele and gastroschisis.[87] However, the ruptured membrane can sometimes be identified by tracing the umbilical cord to its insertion on the membrane. In most fetuses with gastroschisis, only the small bowel is eviscerated, whereas omphaloceles more commonly involve liver and other organs in addition to intestinal loops (Fig. 16–19). Therefore, sonographic demonstration that liver has herniated through an abdominal wall defect is considered strong evidence for an omphalocele.[70] When gastroschisis is associated with evisceration of organs other than bowel or when the defect is in an unusual location, the amniotic band syndrome should be considered and the spine and extremities carefully examined for anomalies. Finally, fetal ascites should be visualized only with an omphalocele because the absence of a covering membrane in gastroschisis allows ascites to escape into the surrounding amniotic fluid.[70]

There are several potential sources of false-positives in the antenatal sonographic diagnosis of omphalocele and gastroschisis. If the fetal abdomen is compressed between the uterine walls, secondary to oligohydramnios or a uterine contraction, it may become elongated, giving the spurious impression of an abdominal wall defect (a "pseudoomphalocele") (Fig. 16–20).[71,88] A similar appearance may result if the abdomen is scanned obliquely. However, a true omphalocele should form an acute angle with the abdominal wall; with a pseudoomphalocele, the angle between the apparent "mass" and abdominal wall is obtuse. Another potential source of false-positive is confusion between the umbilical cord or an umbilical cord mass and bowel, but Doppler evaluation may be helpful in distinguishing between these possibilities.[71] Finally, the fetal bowel migrates into the umbilical cord as a normal embryologic event during the first trimester and returns to the abdominal cavity by 10 to 12 menstrual weeks

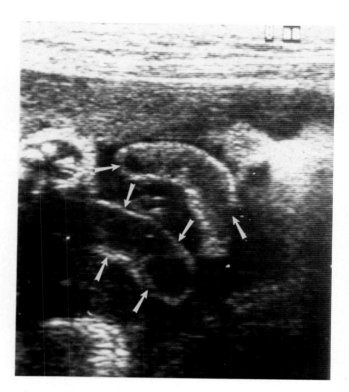

Fig. 16–18. Fetus with gastroschisis. Sonogram reveals dilated thick-walled bowel loops floating freely in amniotic cavity without a covering membrane. (*Courtesy of Mary Warner, MD.*)

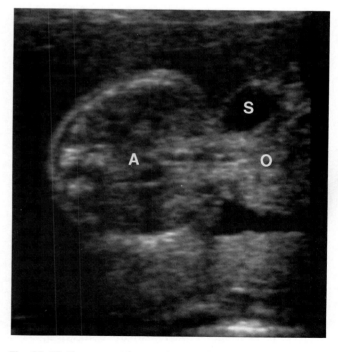

Fig. 16–19. Transverse image through the abdomen of a fetus with an omphalocele revealing exteriorization of the stomach. O = omphalocele; S = stomach; A = abdomen.

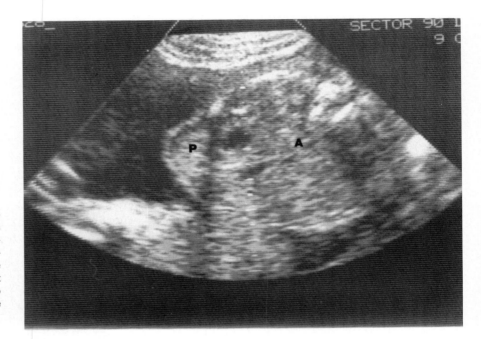

Fig. 16–20. Transverse section demonstrating a "pseudo-omphalocele." This normal variant occurs when the fetal abdomen is scanned obliquely or is compressed between the uterine walls. Note the obtuse angle between apparent "mass" and the abdomen and compare to Fig. 16–19, which reveals the acute angle characteristic of true omphaloceles. A = abdomen; P = pseudo-omphalocele.

(Fig. 16–9).[12,13] The herniated bowel can be routinely visualized by high-resolution sonography. Therefore, to avoid confusing this normal process with omphalocele or gastroschisis and to allow for possible errors in dating, it is recommended that the sonographic diagnosis of an abdominal wall defect not be made prior to 14 weeks' gestation, and suspicious cases be rescanned at this time.[12]

CONGENITAL DIAPHRAGMATIC HERNIA

Diaphragmatic hernias may be detected in utero, based on the sonographic recognition of distended loops of bowel in the thoracic cavity. They are discussed in more detail in Chapter 15.

LIVER AND SPLEEN

A nomogram of normal fetal liver lengths is available for evaluation of suspected abnormalities of liver size.[89] The liver is among the first organs affected in fetal growth abnormalities, being abnormally decreased in size with intrauterine growth retardation. Hepatomegaly occurs with severe isoimmunization disorders, fetal congestive heart failure, and macrosomia. There is also preliminary evidence suggesting that hepatosplenomegaly may correlate with the severity of isoimmunization disorders.[90,91] In the fetus, the left lobe of the liver is disproportionately large compared to the right lobe. This is thought to relate to fetal vascular anatomy, the left lobe receiving more oxygenated blood than the right due to direct drainage of the umbilical vein into the left portal vein.[92]

Various fetal liver masses have been detected in utero. There are at least three reported cases of benign vascular tumors (hemangioendotheliomas or cavernous hemangiomas), each identified between 29 and 33 weeks of gestation. Two of these masses appeared as homogeneous hypoechoic areas within the liver without evidence of fetal hydrops.[93,94] In the third case, a large hyperechoic mass occupying most of the liver was detected in conjunction with fetal demise and hydrops (Fig. 16–21).[95] Other hepatic masses identified antenatally have included a solitary unilocular hepatic cyst first seen at 27 weeks of gestation, and a mesenchymal hamartoma which was identified at 33 weeks.[96,97] Although we know of no antenatally detected cases of hepatoblastoma, this is the most common hepatic malignancy in young children and could potentially be identified in utero. In children, these tumors are generally heterogeneous in echogenicity.

Hepatic calcifications are occasionally identified antenatally and may be due to intrauterine infection or fetal tumors, but are sometimes idiopathic.[14]

The fetal spleen may be visualized on transverse scans as a homogeneous solid structure posterolateral to the stomach (Fig. 16–22). Normal values are available for splenic measurements. Splenomegaly has been detected in utero in conjunction with congenital syphilis, cytomegalovirus infection, and severely affected Rh-isoimmunized fetuses.[14,91,98]

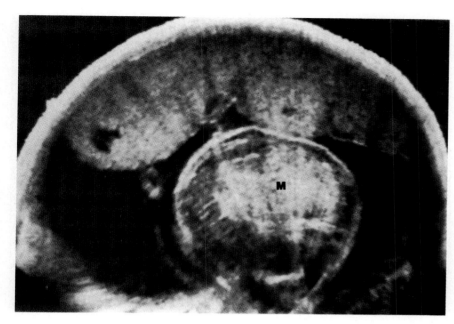

Fig. 16–21. Axial sonogram of a fetus with a hepatic hemangioma, revealing large hyperechoic mass (M) within the liver. Fetal demise and hydropic changes were also demonstrated during the examination. (*Reprinted with permission from Nakamoto SK, Dreilinger A, Dattel B, et al. J Ultrasound Med. 1983;2:239–241.*)

GALLBLADDER AND BILE DUCTS

In transverse scans, the fetal gallbladder can frequently be seen as an ovoid fluid-filled structure between the right and left lobes of the liver. The gallbladder is thought to play a relatively passive role in fetal gastrointestinal physiology and does not exhibit significant volume changes following administration of a glucose load or fatty meal to the fasting mother.[99] Although cholelithiasis is extremely rare in utero, the antenatal sonographic demonstration of gallstones has been described in a 36-week fetus and was confirmed by a scan performed postnatally.[100] Interestingly, the stones could no longer be identified one month following birth, and may have passed or dissolved.

A choledochal cyst is a localized dilatation of the biliary system, most commonly cystic dilatation of the common bile duct. Several reports describe the antenatal sonographic appearance of choledochal cysts.[101–104] In each of these cases, a fluid-filled mass was identified in the right upper quadrant. The gallbladder can sometimes be identified adjacent to a choledochal cyst, giving the impression of two fluid-filled right upper quadrant masses, but the gallbladder can usually be distinguished from other fluid-filled structures by its typical ovoid configuration and location. A common problem is confusing gallbladder with the umbilical portion of the portal vein, but when the typical configuration and location of these structures is considered, such differentiation should not be difficult (Fig. 16–23). The differential diagnosis of a

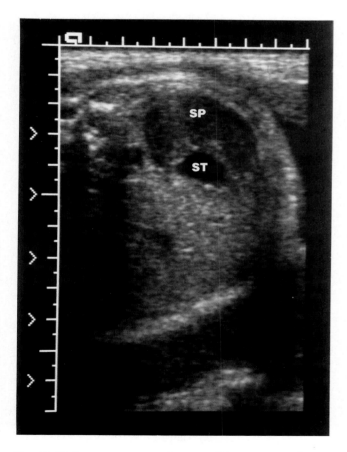

Fig. 16–22. Transverse scan of a normal fetus at term demonstrates the spleen (SP) posteriolateral to the fetal stomach (ST).

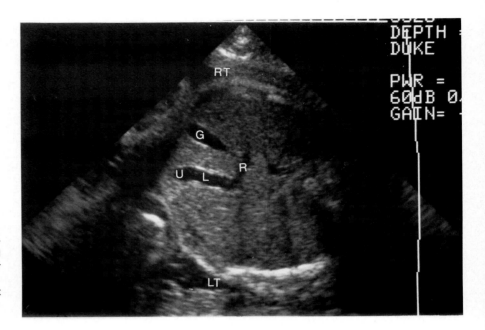

Fig. 16–23. Axial scan through the abdomen of a normal fetus revealing typical configuration and location of gallbladder and portal veins. G = gallbladder; U = umbilical portion of portal vein; RT = right side of fetus; LT = left side of fetus; L = left portal vein; R = right portal vein.

cystic mass in the right upper quadrant includes choledochal cysts, duodenal atresia, renal, omental, ovarian, pancreatic, and mesenteric and hepatic cysts. In duodenal atresia, peristalsis is sometimes observed, and there should be clear-cut communication between the right upper quadrant "cyst" and the dilated fluid-filled stomach.[14] In addition, the specific diagnosis of choledochal cyst is suggested when tubular structure(s) representing dilated bile ducts are identified communicating with the cystic mass, but this finding is more commonly seen postpartum than in utero.[102,103]

OTHER CONDITIONS INVOLVING THE GASTROINTESTINAL TRACT

Congenital duplication cysts may occur anywhere along the gastrointestinal tract, and duplications of both the stomach and ileum have been detected by ultrasound in utero.[105,106] A specific sonographic appearance has not been described in conjunction with such duplications; rather, they appear as tubular or cystic structures in the fetal abdomen and the differential diagnosis depends on their location. For example, the differential diagnosis of a gastric duplication includes choledochal cyst and duodenal atresi; whereas with an ileal duplication mesenteric, omental, and ovarian cysts are among the diagnostic considerations.

A complex mass representing a sterile appendiceal abscess has been detected by antenatal sonography, but this can be expected to be an extremely rare cause of a fetal right lower-quadrant mass because appendicitis is very unusual in the fetus and neonate.[107] More commonly, a complex mass in this location would be due to a meconium pseudocyst or a teratoma.

Additionally, mesenteric and omental cysts could potentially be detected in utero and should be considered in the differential diagnosis of a cystic intraabdominal lesion in the fetus.[14] They are usually multilocular and single, and their etiology is unknown.

REFERENCES

1. Alexander ES, Spitz HB, Clark RA. Sonography of polyhydramnios. *AJR.* 1982;138:343.
2. Barkin SZ, Pretorius DH, Beckett MK, et al. Severe polyhydramnios: Incidence of anomalies. *AJR.* 1987;148:155.
3. Rosenthal SJ, Filly RA, Callen PW, et al. Fetal pseudoascites. *Radiology.* 1979;131:195.
4. Hashimoto BE, Filly RA, Callen PW, et al. Fetal pseudoascites: Further anatomic observations. *J Ultrasound Med.* 1986;5:151.
5. Gross BH, Callen PW, Filly RA. Ultrasound appearance of fetal greater omentum. *J Ultrasound Med.* 1982;1:67.
6. Fakhry J, Shapiro LR, Schechter A, et al. Fetal gastric pseudomasses. *J Ultrasound Med.* 1987;6:177.
7. Nyberg DA, Mack LA, Patten RM, et al. Fetal bowel: Normal sonographic findings. *J Ultrasound Med.* 1987;6:3.
8. Zilianti M, Fernandez S. Correlation of ultrasonic images of fetal intestine with gestational age and fetal maturity. *Obstet Gynecol.* 1983;62:569.
9. Fakhry J, Reiser M, Shapiro LR, et al. Increased echogenicity in the lower fetal abdomen: A common normal

variant in the second trimester. *J Ultrasound Mea.* 1986;5:489.

10. Lince DM, Pretorius DH, Manco-Johnson ML, et al. The clinical significance of increased echogenicity in the fetal abdomen. *AJR.* 1985;145:683.

11. Manco LG, Nunan FA, Sohnen H, et al. Fetal small bowel simulating an abdominal mass at sonography. *J Clin Ultrasound.* 1986;14:404.

12. Cyr DR, Mack LA, Schoenecker SA, et al. Bowel migration in the normal fetus: US detection. *Radiology.* 1986;161:119.

13. Schmidt W, Yarkoni S, Crelin E, et al. Sonographic visualization of physiologic anterior abdominal wall hernia in the first trimester. *Obstet Gynecol.* 1987;69:911.

14. Romero R, Pilu G, Jeanty P, et al. The gastrointestinal tract and intraabdominal organs. In: *Prenatal Diagnosis of Congenital Anomalies.* Norwalk, Conn: Appleton & Lange; 1988:233.

15. Farrant P. The antenatal diagnosis of oesophageal atresia by ultrasound. *Br J Radiology.* 1980;53:1202.

16. Jassani MN, Gauderer MWL, Fanaroff AA, et al. A perinatal approach to the diagnosis and management of gastrointestinal malformations. *Obstet Gynecol.* 1982;59:33.

17. Zemlyn S. Prenatal detection of esophageal atresia. *J Clin Ultrasound.* 1981;9:453.

18. Rahmani MR, Zalev AH. Antenatal detection of esophageal atresia with distal tracheoesophageal fistula. *J Clin Ultrasound.* 1986;14:143.

19. Pretorius DH, Drose JA, Dennis MA, et al. Tracheoeophageal fistula in utero: Twenty-two cases. *J Ultrasound Med.* 1987;6:509.

20. Eyheremendy E, Pfister M. Antenatal real-time diagnosis of esophageal atresia. *J Clin Ultrasound.* 1983;11:395.

21. Bowie JD, Clair MR. Fetal swallowing and regurgitation: Observation of normal and abnormal activity. *Radiology.* 1982;144:877.

22. Weinberg B, Diakoumakis EE. Three complex cases of foregut atresia: Prenatal sonographic diagnosis with radiographic correlation. *J Clin Ultrasound.* 1985;13:481.

23. Nelson LH, Clark CE, Fishburne JI, et al. Value of serial sonography in the in utero detection of duodenal atresia. *Obstet Gynecol.* 1982;59:657.

24. Jouppila P, Kirkinen P. Ultrasonic and clinical aspects in the diagnosis and prognosis of congenital gastrointestinal anomalies. *Ultrasound Med Biol.* 1984;10:465.

25. Boychuk RB, Lyons EA, Goodhand TK. Duodenal atresia diagnosed by ultrasound. *Radiology.* 1978;127:500.

26. Houlton MCC, Sutton M, Aitken J. Antenatal diagnosis of duodenal atresia. *J Obstet Gynaecol Br Commwlth.* 1974;81:818.

27. Clark JFJ, Hales E, Ma P, et al. Duodenal atresia in utero in association with Down's syndrome and annular pancreas. *J Natl Med Assoc.* 1984;76:190.

28. Loveday BJ, Barr JA. The intra-uterine demonstration of duodenal atresia by ultrasound. *Br J Radiology.* 1975;48:1031.

29. Zimmerman HB. Prenatal demonstration of gastric and duodenal obstruction by ultrasound. *J Can Assoc Radiol.* 1978;29:138.

30. Barss VA, Benacerraf BR, Frigoletto FD. Antenatal sonographic diagnosis of fetal gastrointestinal malformations. *Pediatrics.* 1985;76:445.

31. Dewbury KC, Chir AM, Birch SJ, et al. Prenatal ultrasound demonstration of a choledochal cyst. *Br J Radiol.* 1980;53:906.

32. Gross BH, Filly RA. Potential for a normal fetal stomach to simulate the sonographic "double bubble" sign. *J Can Assoc Radiol.* 1982;33:39.

33. Kjoller M, Holm-Nielsen G, Meiland H, et al. Prenatal obstruction of the ileum diagnosed by ultrasound. *Prenat Diagn.* 1985;5:427.

34. Samuel N, Dicker D, Feldberg D, et al. Ultrasound diagnosis and management of fetal intestinal obstruction and volvulus in utero. *J Perinat Med.* 1984;12:333.

35. Nikapota VLB, Loman C. Gray scale sonographic demonstration of fetal small-bowel atresia. *J Clin Ultrasound.* 1979;7:307.

36. Lyrenas S, Cnattingius S, Lindberg B. Fetal jejunal atresia and intrauterine volvulus: a case report. *J Perinat Med.* 1982;10:247.

37. Osler GE, Dumaresq L, Becker H. Ultrasonic demonstration in utero of surgically correctable fetal small-bowel obstruction. *SA Med J.* 1982;62:83.

38. Fletman D, McQuown D, Kanchanapoom V, et al. "Apple peel" atresia of the small bowel: Prenatal diagnosis of the obstruction by ultrasound. *Pediatr Radiol.* 1980;9:118.

39. Skovbo P, Smith-Jensen S. Hyperdistended fluid-filled bowel loops mimicking gastrointestinal atresia. *J Clin Ultrasound.* 1981;9:463.

40. Cloutier MG, Fried AM, Selke AC. Antenatal observation of midgut volvulus by ultrasound. *J Clin Ultrasound.* 1983;11:286.

41. Baxi LV, Yeh MN, Blanc WA, et al. Antepartum diagnosis and management of in utero intestinal volvulus with perforation. *N Eng J Med.* 1983;308:1519.

42. Brugman SM, Bjelland JJ, Thomasson JE, et al. Sonographic findings with radiologic correlation in meconium peritonitis. *J Clin Ultrasound.* 1979;7:305.

43. Foster MA, Nyberg DA, Mahony BS, et al. Meconium peritonitis: Prenatal sonographic findings and their clinical significance. *Radiology.* 1987;165:661.

44. Nancarrow PA, Mattrey RF, Edwards DK, et al. Fibroadhesive meconium peritonitis: In utero sonographic diagnosis. *J Ultrasound Med.* 1985;4:213.

45. McGahan JP, Hanson F. Meconium peritonitis with accompanying pseudocyst: Prenatal sonographic diagnosis. *Radiology.* 1983;148:125.

46. Fleischer AC, Davis RJ, Campbell L. Sonographic detection of a meconium-containing mass in a fetus: A case report. *J Clin Ultrasound.* 1983;11:103.

47. Clair MR, Rosenberg ER, Ram PC. Prenatal sonographic diagnosis of meconium peritonitis. *Prenat Diagnosis.* 1983;3:65.

48. Silverbach S. Antenatal real-time identification of meconium cyst. *J Clin Ultrasound.* 1983;11:455.

49. Lauer JD, Cradock TV. Meconium pseudocyst: Prenatal sonographic and antenatal radiologic correlation. *J Ultrasound Med.* 1982;1:333.

50. Schwimer SR, Vanley GT, Reinke RT. Prenatal diagnosis of cystic meconium peritonitis. *J Clin Ultrasound.* 1984;12:37.

51. Diakoumakis EE, Weinberg B, Beck R, et al. A case of meconium peritonitis with ileal stenosis: Prenatal sonographic findings with radiologic correlation. *Mt Sinai J Med.* 1986;53:152.

52. Williams J, Nathan RO, Worthen NJ. Sonographic demonstration of the progression of meconium peritonitis. *Obstet Gynecol.* 1984;64:822.

53. Shalev J, Frankel Y, Avigad I, et al. Spontaneous intestinal perforation in utero: Ultrasonic diagnostic criteria. *Am J Obstet Gynecol.* 1982;144:855.

54. Skoll MA, Marquette GP, Hamilton EF. Prenatal ultrasonic diagnosis of multiple bowel atresias. *Am J Obstet Gynecol.* 1987;156:471.

55. Denholm TA, Crown HC, Edwards WH, et al. Prenatal sonographic appearance of meconium ileus in twins. *AJR.* 1984;143:371.

56. Muller F, Aubry MC, Gasser B, et al. Prenatal diagnosis of cystic fibrosis. II: Meconium ileus in affected fetuses. *Prenat Diagn.* 1985;5:109.

57. Nyberg DA, Hastrup W, Watts H, et al. Dilated fetal bowel. A sonographic sign of cystic fibrosis. *J Ultrasound Med.* 1987;6:257.

58. Goldstein RB, Filly RA, Callen PW. Sonographic diagnosis of meconium ileus in utero. *J Ultrasound Med.* 1987;6:663.

59. Samuel N, Dicker D, Landman J, et al. Early diagnosis and intrauterine therapy of meconium plug syndrome in the fetus: Risks and benefits. *J Ultrasound Med.* 1986;5:425.

60. Harris RD, Nyberg DA, Mack LA, et al. Anorectal atresia: Prenatal sonographic diagnosis. *AJR.* 1987;149:395.

61. Lande IM, Hamilton EF. The antenatal sonographic visualization of cloacal dysgenesis. *J Ultrasound Med.* 1986;5:275.

62. Meizner I, Bar-Ziv J. In utero prenatal ultrasonic diagnosis of a rare case of cloacal exstrophy. *J Clin Ultrasound.* 1985;13:500.

63. Bean WJ, Calonje MA, Aprill CN, et al. Anal atresia: A prenatal ultrasound diagnosis. *J Clin Ultrasound.* 1978;6:111.

64. Claiborne AK, Blocker SH, Martin CM, et al. Prenatal and postnatal sonographic delineation of gastrointestinal abnormalities in a case of the VATER syndrome. *J Ultrasound Med.* 1986;5:45.

65. Shalev E, Weiner E, Zuckerman H. Prenatal ultrasound diagnosis of intestinal calcifications with imperforate anus. *Acta Obstet Gynecol Scand.* 1983;62:95.

66. Berdon WE, Baker DH, Wigger HJ, et al. Calcified intraluminal meconium in newborn males with imperforate anus. Enterolithiasis in the newborn. *AJR.* 1975;125:449.

67. Vermesh M, Mayden KL, Confino E, et al. Prenatal sonographic diagnosis of Hirschsprung's disease. *J Ultrasound Med.* 1986;5:37.

68. Wrobleski D, Wesselhoeft C. Ultrasonic diagnosis of prenatal intestinal obstruction. *J Pediat Surg.* 1979;14:598.

69. Romero R, Pilu G, Jeanty P, et al. The abdominal wall. In: *Prenatal Diagnosis of Congenital Anomalies.* Norwalk, Conn: Appleton & Lange; 1988:209.

70. Bair JH, Russ PD, Pretorius DH, et al. Fetal omphalocele and gastroschisis: a review of 24 cases. *AJR.* 1986;147:1047.

71. Lindfors KK, McGahan JP, Walter JP. Fetal omphalocele and gastroschisis: Pitfalls in sonographic diagnosis. *AJR.* 1986;147:797.

72. Nelson PA, Bowie JD, Filston HC, et al. Sonographic diagnosis of omphalocele in utero. *AJR.* 1982;138:1178.

73. Roberts C. Intrauterine diagnosis of omphalocele. *Radiology.* 1978;127:762.

74. Fink IJ, Filly RA. Omphalocele associated with umbilical cord allantoic cyst: Sonographic evaluation in utero. *Radiology.* 1983;149:473.

75. Cameron GM, McQuown DS, Modanlou HD, et al. Intrauterine diagnosis of an omphalocele by diagnostic ultrasonography. *Am J Obstet Gynecol.* 1978;131:821.

76. Schaffer RM, Barone C, Friedman AP. The ultrasonographic spectrum of fetal omphalocele. *J Ultrasound Med.* 1983;2:219.

77. Davidson JM, Johnson TRB, Rigdon DT, et al. Gastroschisis and omphalocele: prenatal diagnosis and perinatal management. *Prenat Diagn.* 1984;4:355.

78. Holmgren G, Sigurd J. Prenatal diagnosis of two cases of gastroschisis following alpha-fetoprotein (AFP) screening. *Acta Obstet Gynecol Scand.* 1984;63:325.

79. Grossman M, Fischermann EA, German J. Sonographic findings in gastroschisis. *J Clin Ultrasound.* 1978;6:175.

80. Youngblood JP, Franklin DW, Stein RT. Omphalocele: early prenatal diagnosis by ultrasound. *J Clin Ultrasound.* 1983;11:339.

81. Yaghoobian J, Chaudary R, Pinck RL. Antenatal diagnosis of omphalocele by ultrasound. Case report with a brief review of the literature. *J Reprod Med.* 1981;26:274.

82. Giulian B, Alvear D. Prenatal ultrasonographic diagnosis of fetal gastroschisis. *Radiology.* 1978;129:473.

83. Weinstein L, Anderson C. In utero diagnosis of Beckwith-Wiedmann syndrome by ultrasound. *Radiology.* 1980;134:474.

84. Koontz WL, Shaw LA, Lavery JP. Antenatal sonographic appearance of Beckwith-Wiedemann syndrome. *J Clin Ultrasound.* 1986;14:57.

85. Baker ME, Rosenberg ER, Trofatter KF, et al. The in utero findings in twin pentalogy of Cantrell. *J Ultrasound Med.* 1984;3:525.

86. Fried AM, Woodring JH, Shier RW, et al. Omphalocele in limb/body wall deficiency syndrome: Atypical sonographic appearance. *J Clin Ultrasound.* 1982;10:400.

87. Cand LKH, Pederson SA, Kirstoffersen K. Prenatal rupture of omphalocele. *J Clin Ultrasound.* 1987;15:191.

88. Salzman L, Kuligowska E, Semine A. Pseudoomphalocele: Pitfall in fetal sonography. *AJR.* 1986;146:1283.

89. Vintzileos AM, Neckles S, Campbell WA, et al. Fetal liver ultrasound measurement during normal pregnancy. *Obstet Gynecol.* 1985;66:477.

90. Vintzileos AM, Campbell WA, Storlazzi E, et al. Fetal liver ultrasound measurements in isoimmunized pregnancies. *Obstet Gynecol.* 1986;68:162.

91. Schmidt W, Yarkoni S, Jeanty P, et al. Sonographic meas-

urements of the fetal spleen: Clinical implications. *J Ultrasound Med.* 1985;4:667.

92. Gross BH, Harter LP, Filly RA. Disproportionate left hepatic lobe size in the fetus: Ultrasonic demonstration. *J Ultrasound Med.* 1982;1:79.

93. Platt LD, DeVore GR, Benner P, et al. Antenatal diagnosis of a fetal liver mass. *J Ultrasound Med.* 1983;2:521.

94. Horgan JG, King DL, Taylor KJW. Sonographic detection of prenatal liver mass. *J Clin Gastroenterol.* 1984;6:277.

95. Nakamoto SK, Dreilinger A, Dattel B, et al. The sonographic appearance of hepatic hemangioma in utero. *J Ultrasound Med.* 1983;2:239.

96. Chung WM. Antenatal detection of hepatic cyst. *J Clin Ultrasound.* 1986;14:217.

97. Foucar E, Williamson RA, Yiu-Chiu V, et al. Mesenchymal hamartoma of the liver identified by fetal sonography. *AJR.* 1983;140:970.

98. Eliezer S, Esler F, Ehud W, et al. Fetal splenomegaly, ultrasound diagnosis of cytomegalovirus infection: A case report. *J Clin Ultrasound.* 1984;12:520.

99. Jouppila P, Heikkinen J, Kirkinen P. Contractility of maternal and fetal gallbladder: An ultrasonic study. *J Clin Ultrasound.* 1985;13:461.

100. Beretsky I, Lankin DH. Diagnosis of fetal cholelithiasis using real-time high-resolution imaging employing digital detection. *J Ultrasound Med.* 1983;2:381.

101. Frank JL, Hill MC, Chirathivat S, et al. Antenatal observation of a choledochal cyst by sonography. *AJR.* 1981;137:166.

102. Dewbury KC, Aluwihare MC, Birch SJ, et al. Prenatal ultrasound demonstration of a choledochal cyst. *Br J Radiol.* 1980;53:906.

103. Elrad H, Mayden KL, Ahart S, et al. Prenatal ultrasound diagnosis of choledochal cyst. *J Ultrasound Med.* 1985;4:553.

104. Howell CG, Templeton JM, Weiner S, et al. Antenatal diagnosis and early surgery for choledochal cyst. *J Pediat Surg.* 1983;18:387.

105. Bidwell JK, Nelson A. Prenatal ultrasonic diagnosis of congenital duplication of the stomach. *J Ultrasound Med.* 1986;5:589.

106. vanDam LJ, deGroot CJ, Hazebroek FWS, et al. Intrauterine demonstration of bowel duplication by ultrasound. *Europ J Obstet Gynecol Reprod Biol.* 1984;18:229.

107. Hill LM, Breckle R, Avant RF. Sonographic findings associated with a sterile fetal appendiceal abscess. *J Ultrasound Med.* 1982;1:257.

17 Sonography of Fetal Genitourinary Anomalies

Calliope Fine • Peter M. Doubilet

The genitourinary tract is one of the organ systems in which congenital anomalies most frequently occur, and one particularly well suited to sonographic evaluation. A knowledge of the embryology, physiology, and anatomy of the genitourinary tract provides an understanding of the origin of anomalies and the patterns in which they occur, thus allowing one to make accurate prenatal sonographic diagnoses. Because genitourinary anomalies are often not evident at birth, prenatal sonography plays an important role in early diagnosis and timely treatment.

EMBRYOLOGY

There are three ontogenic stages in the development of the human kidney.[1,2] These stages are sequential and result in the appearance and disappearance of two primitive kidneys, the pronephros and mesonephros, before the final kidney, the metanephros, appears. All three kidneys arise from intermediate mesoderm (the nephrogenic cord) located between the lateral surface of the somite and the coelom.

The *pronephros* is the first excretory organ in the human embryo. It appears in the middle of the third week (from date of conception) and consists of a series of about seven tubules that appear, and almost immediately disappear, in a cephalocaudal sequence. Each pronephric tubule fuses with the tubule immediately caudal to it to form the pronephric duct. The pronephric duct continues to grow caudally to become the mesonephric duct. The pronephros is of no significance as a functioning excretory organ.

The *mesonephros* develops immediately caudal to the pronephros. The pronephric duct, now called the mesonephric duct, continues to grow toward the cloaca. Each mesonephric nephron consists of a simple glomerulus and a short tubule that attaches directly to the mesonephric duct. In embryos of 10 to 15 mm, the mesonephroi form prominent elongated masses in the posterior abdominal cavity close to the spinal column. The mesonephron is capable of producing urine.[3] It remains active during early development of the metanephros and then degenerates in a cephalocaudal sequence.

As the mesonephroi disappear, parts of the tubules persist. In the male, the more cranial tubules become the efferent ductules of the testis through which the seminiferous tubules communicate with the epididymis. The mesonephric duct becomes the epididymis and the ductus deferens. In the female, the mesonephric tubules persist as small functional remnants in the mesosalpinx, ie, epioopheron, paraoopheron, and Walthard rests.[2] The mesonephros has regressed completely by the 11th to 12th week.

The final kidney, or *metanephros*, can only develop when two types of cells of differing potentialities, the ureteric bud and the metanephric blastema, come into contact with each other and interact in a normal manner.

A *ureteric bud* arises from the distal end of the mesonephric duct just at the point where it swings ventrally and medially to join the cloaca. It undergoes a series of dichotomous branchings, ultimately forming the collecting system of the kidney (ureter, renal pelvis, calyces, and collecting tubules). The actively growing tip of each ureteral bud branch is the ampulla.

The *metanephric blastema* originates in the most caudal portion of the nephrogenic cord. Initially, the cells of the metanephric blastema form a discrete zone around the ampulla of the ureteral bud, and they proliferate only when in direct contact with the ampullae. Ampullae are responsible for inducing the metanephric blastema to form nephrons and for establishing communication with these nephrons. Later, cells of the metanephric blastema will proliferate independently and form a more diffuse zone. In this zone, cells immediately surrounding the ampullae are stimulated to differentiate into nephrons, and those further away differentiate into connective tissue.

The first three to five generations of tubules produced by ampullary division form the renal pelvis; the next three to five generations form the minor calyces, papillae, and cribriform plates; and the next six to nine generations become the collecting tubules. Accumulation of urine (ie, the presence of functioning nephrons) seems to be essential for the conversion of the primitive renal pelvis and calyces into their definitive forms.[2]

The ampullae divide rapidly until 14 to 15 weeks, and then at a slower rate until 19 to 20 weeks. Division is rare from 20 to 32 weeks and ceases between 32 and 36 weeks. Their capacity for nephron induction is constant between 8 to 10 and 32 to 36 weeks. If birth occurs prematurely, ampullary activity continues as if the fetus were still in the uterus.[2]

The segment of mesonephric duct between the ureteral bud and the future urogenital sinus is called the common excretory duct or trigone precursor.[4] This becomes absorbed into the urogenital sinus and contributes mesenchyme to the muscularization of the trigone. The ureteral bud and mesonephric duct thus acquire separate openings, and the tissue between the orifices is the future trigone. Further development results in the ureter migrating cranially and laterally and the mesonephric duct migrating inferiorly and medially to terminate eventually in the posterior urethra. The mesonephric duct becomes the vas deferens, seminal vesicle, and ejaculatory duct in the male and vestigial structures in the female.

A familiarity with normal embryology helps in the understanding of the pathogenesis of many anomalies of the genitourinary tract. For example, several lower ureteral abnormalities (eg, primary reflux, ectopic ureter, ureteral duplication, and ureterocele) probably result from abnormalities in the location and number of ureteral buds which, in turn, influence the length of the common excretory duct or trigone precursor.[4] The embryologic bases of these and other anomalies are presented in the sections devoted to specific anomalies.

PHYSIOLOGY

Tubules of the pronephros never become functional in mammalian embryos. The mesonephros functions to a greater or lesser degree in all mammals including man. Mesonephric urine represents a glucose- and protein-free fluid similar to fetal plasma.[5] The fetal metanephric kidney elaborates true urine in that its composition differs from a simple protein-free ultrafiltrate of plasma. It is slightly acidic, free of glucose and protein, and hypotonic to plasma. It has a higher concentration of urea to creatinine than does fetal plasma.[5]

Gersh[3] concluded that renal function begins in the human fetus at about 32 mm, or between 9 and 11 weeks. In embryos younger than the 35-mm stage, a definite membrane can be seen to stretch across the anatomic junction of the ureter and urogenital sinus. The opening of this membrane coincides in time with the onset of renal function and probably results from the hydrostatic pressure generated from renal secretion. Prior to opening of the membrane, fetal urine cannot contribute to the amniotic fluid volume. Once patency of the urethra is established, fetal urination becomes a source of amniotic fluid and influences its volume and composition through-

out the rest of gestation.[5] The relative amount of amniotic fluid, therefore, can provide information on the status of fetal renal function. Oligohydramnios due to diminished fetal urination may become evident sonographically by 15 to 16 weeks.

Fetal kidneys are not responsible for fluid and electrolyte balance in the fetus. This function is primarily regulated by the placenta. Immediately after birth, the kidneys are called on to assume the homeostatic functional demands of extrauterine life. It appears to take approximately 24 hours for newborn infants to adapt their glomerular filtration rate to the extrauterine environment. In the first 12 hours of life, the glomerular filtration rate is approximately 15% of the adult level. Then, glomerular filtration rate and renal blood flow follow a similar postnatal pattern with values more than doubling in the first two weeks of life.[6] In preterm neonates, the same pattern applies but values start at lower levels. Adult levels of glomerular filtration rate are achieved at 1 to 2 years of age.[6]

THE POTTER SEQUENCE

In 1946, Potter described characteristic facial, limb, and lethal pulmonary abnormalities due to bilateral renal agenesis.[7] This became known as the Potter syndrome. It is now recognized that the Potter "syndrome" is the result of severe oligohydramnios, and that the same spectrum of anomalies may be due to any condition resulting in longstanding severe oligohydramnios (eg, bilateral urologic abnormalities associated with renal functional impairment, intrauterine growth retardation, early premature rupture of membranes).[8–10] The term now used to describe these anomalies is the Potter sequence or oligohydramnios sequence.

Facial anomalies include a prominent fold of skin that begins above each eye and extends down over the inner canthus onto the cheek, a nose turned down at the tip, a prominent depression between the lower lip and chin, low set ears, and a prematurely senile appearance. Limb abnormalities include abnormal positioning of hands and feet, hyperextension or bowing of legs, clubbed or fused feet, and hip dislocation. The lungs are small and hypoplastic, which may lead to death from pulmonary insufficiency after birth.

ABNORMALITIES OF THE KIDNEYS

Bilateral Renal Agenesis
Bilateral renal agenesis is a fatal anomaly that occurs with an incidence of approximately 0.3 per 1,000 births.[11] There is a male predominance of 2.5 to 1. Absence of

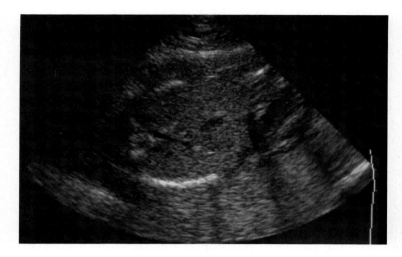

Fig. 17–1. Bilateral renal agenesis (21 weeks). Transverse view through the fetal abdomen demonstrates oligohydramnios and no evidence of fetal kidneys. A more caudal view, not shown here, failed to demonstrate a fetal bladder.

fetal urine production initiates the Potter sequence (see preceding discussion) so that death usually occurs shortly after delivery as a result of pulmonary hypoplasia.

Bilateral renal agenesis may be due to absence of the nephrogenic ridge on both sides of the coelomic cavity,[12] or to bilateral failure of the ureteric bud to reach the metanephric blastema, or for differentiation of the blastema to occur. Both kidneys and ureters may be entirely absent, or blind-ending ureters may be found together with fragments of nonfunctioning renal tissue.[12]

Most often, bilateral renal agenesis is an isolated abnormality (aside from those abnormalities resulting from oligohydramnios, as discussed in the section on Potter sequence). On occasion, it may be associated with other abnormalities or occur as part of a syndrome. These other abnormalities may involve adjacent organs, including lower bowel, anus, genital tract, or the lower spine and lower extremities as in the sirenomelic deformity. They may also involve other organ systems, including cardiovascular, musculoskeletal, central nervous system, or gastrointestinal tract. A single umbilical artery may be present.

Sonographic findings include nonvisualization of the fetal kidneys and bladder and severe oligohydramnios (Fig. 17–1).[13,14] The fetal thorax may be abnormally small for gestational age, especially in the mid-to-late third trimester. The condition is usually diagnosable by 16 to 20 weeks' gestation.

As with any other severe fetal anomaly, the diagnosis should be made only after careful sonographic evaluation. In particular, three potential pitfalls must be avoided. First, the fetal adrenals are often enlarged in the second trimester and take on a discoid configuration, and they may be mistaken for kidneys.[13,14] With careful scanning, it can be noted that adrenals tend to be hypoechoic, there is not a well-defined capsule, and a fluid-filled central

renal pelvis cannot be seen. Second, because one or both fetal kidneys may reside in an ectopic location, nonvisualization of kidneys in the renal fossae is an insufficient criterion to diagnose bilateral agenesis; instead, a careful search for an ectopic kidney must be undertaken. Third, severe oligohydramnios due to other causes (eg, ruptured membranes or intrauterine growth retardation) hinders delineation of fetal anatomy and can make identification of the kidneys more difficult. The use of furosemide administered to the mother intravenously has been suggested as an adjunctive diagnostic tool in cases of oligohydramnios and nonvisualization of the fetal bladder. It has been shown, however, that furosemide may fail to induce diuresis in growth-retarded fetuses. Therefore, failure to see the fetal bladder after furosemide administration does not necessarily indicate bilateral renal agenesis.[15] With the above-mentioned pitfalls in mind, a confident and reliable diagnosis of bilateral agenesis can be made based on a constellation of findings: nonvisualization of the kidneys after careful and extensive search, absent bladder, and severe oligohydramnios.

Unilateral Renal Agenesis

Unilateral renal agenesis occurs more commonly than bilateral renal agenesis. The incidence is approximately 1 in 1,000 in autopsy series.[16] It occurs more commonly on the left than the right side. There is a male predominance of 1.8 to 1, but the diagnosis is made more frequently in females later in life because of the associated genital malformations.

The embryology is similar to bilateral renal agenesis but occurs only on one side. It may be due to unilateral absence of the nephrogenic ridge, abnormal differentiation of the distal mesonephric and ureteric buds, or failure of the ureteric bud to stimulate development of the metanephric blastema.

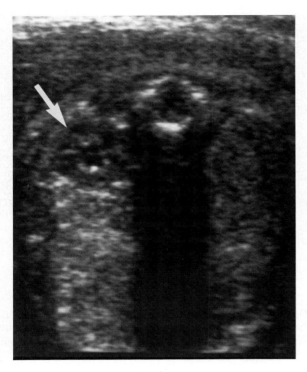

Fig. 17–2. Unilateral renal agenesis (37 weeks). Transverse view through the renal fossae demonstrates a normal left kidney (*arrow*) and no right kidney. The diagnosis of unilateral renal agenesis was made after careful examination for an ectopically located kidney.

Unilateral renal agenesis can be diagnosed sonographically by visualization of only a single fetal kidney (Fig. 17–2). Care must be undertaken to assure that there is no second kidney in an ectopic location. With unilteral agenesis, fluid should be seen in the fetal bladder and amniotic fluid volume should be normal.

Associated anomalies involving the genital tract are common. There is a high incidence of absent or malformed proximal mesonephric duct structures in the male (vas deferens, seminal vesicle, and ejaculatory duct), and müllerian duct structures in the female (uterus and fallopian tube). These genital abnormalities are more frequently observed in females (25 to 50%) than males (10 to 15%).[17,18] Conversely, 43% of females with genital anomalies have unilateral renal agenesis.[19] Other organ system abnormalities include cardiovascular system (30%), gastrointestinal (25%), and musculoskeletal (14%).[20]

Ectopic Kidney

An ectopic kidney can be found in one of the following locations: pelvic, iliac, abdominal, thoracic, and contralateral (crossed). The incidence in autopsy series is approximately 1 in 500. There is no difference between the sexes. It is slightly more common on the left side.

At the end of the 5th week, the ureteral bud and the surrounding metanephric blastema is opposite the upper sacral somites. As elongation and straightening of the embryo occurs, the developing metanephros ascends from the pelvis and medially rotates. This process of migration and rotation is complete by the end of the 8th week of gestation. Any interference of this process will result in *caudad ectopia* (ie, pelvic, iliac, or abdominal location). The kidney is usually smaller than normal and may not have the regular reniform shape. The ureter is short.

Caudad ectopic kidneys are associated with an increased incidence of contralateral agenesis and with genital anomalies (15 to 45%).[21,22] A small number of patients have anomalies of other organs, most often cardiovascular or skeletal.[23]

Prenatal sonographic detection of a pelvic kidney is relatively easy (Fig. 17–3), although occasionally the ectopic kidney may be confused with bowel. In some cases, there is mild hydronephrosis due to a malrotated and anteriorly placed pelvis and impaired drainage from the ureteropelvic junction. Anomalous vasculature may also be the cause of the hydronephrosis.

Cephalad ectopia (ie, kidney position more cranial than normal) may occur in fetuses with omphalocele. If the liver is herniated into the omphalocele sac, then the kidneys continue to ascend until they are stopped by the diaphragm (level of T-10). Ureters are excessively long.

Thoracic kidney is a very rare form of renal ectopia. It is thought to result embryologically from delayed closure of the diaphragmatic anlage, allowing for ascent of the kidneys above the level of the future diaphragm. Alternatively, the kidneys may ascend at an accelerated rate, reaching the diaphragm before normal closure.[24] The adrenal gland is usually located below the kidney. No consistent associated anomalies have been described.

Crossed ectopia refers to an ectopic kidney that is located on the opposite side of the midline from its ureteral insertion. Most crossed ectopic kidneys are fused with the opposite kidney and termed *crossed fused ectopia* (Fig. 17–4). Usually, the uncrossed kidney is normal in position and orientation, and the crossed kidney is inferior in an oblique or horizontal location with an anteriorly placed renal pelvis. Crossed fused ectopic kidneys may be S-shaped, L-shaped, or discoid in shape. Their ureters are orthotopic (ie, enter the bladder on each side in the normal location). Occasionally, the ectopic kidney is obstructed at the ureteropelvic junction and may show evidence of cystic dysplasia. Other associated anomalies are rare and include imperforate anus, skeletal, or cardiovascular abnormalities.

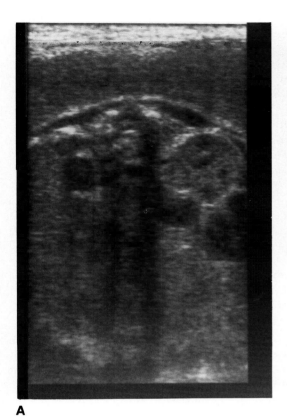

A

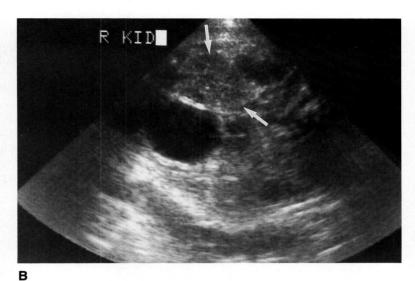

B

Fig. 17–3. Right pelvic kidney (35 weeks). **A.** Transverse view through the renal fossae demonstrates a normal left kidney and bowel in the right renal fossa. **B.** The right kidney (*arrows*) is located in the pelvis behind the bladder.

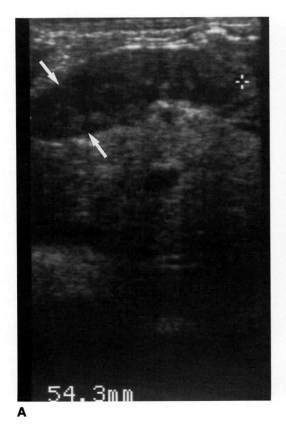

A

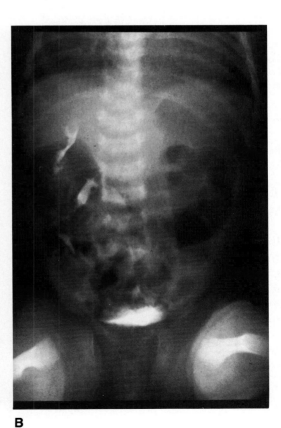

B

Fig. 17–4. Crossed fused ectopia (36 weeks). **A.** The right kidney is elongated and abnormal in shape. The bulge at the lower pole (*arrows*) represents an oblique view through the ectopic fused left kidney. **B.** Postnatal intravenous pyelogram confirms crossed fused ectopia.

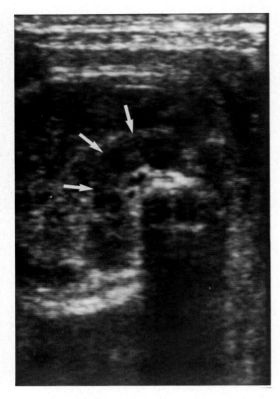

Fig. 17–5. Horseshoe kidney (34 weeks). Transverse view through the fetal abdomen demonstrates renal tissue on either side of spine and connecting across the midline (*arrows*) anterior to the inferior vena cava and aorta.

Horseshoe Kidney

Two kidneys may be joined at their lower poles by a parenchymatous or fibrous isthmus. This is known as a horseshoe kidney. The incidence is approximately 1 in 400 births, and is more common in males by a ratio of 2:1.[25]

Embryologically, the abnormality occurs after the ureteral bud meets the metanephric blastema but before ascent and rotation (4 to 6 weeks' gestation). The cause of the defect is unknown. Usually, the isthmus is located adjacent to the third or fourth lumbar vertebrae just below the junction of the inferior mesenteric artery and aorta. It is almost always anterior to the aorta and inferior vena cava, although it can occasionally pass behind these vessels. The ureters usually enter the bladder in a normal location.

Sonographically, a horseshoe kidney may be difficult to demonstrate. The lower poles are usually displaced anteriorly and connect across the midline (Fig. 17–5). Renal pelves are anterior rather than medial and may be dilated to a greater or lesser degree.

Approximately one third of cases of horseshoe kidney

have associated anomalies. These include cardiovascular, skeletal, central nervous system, and anorectal malformations. Infants with trisomy 18 or Turner's syndrome frequently have a horseshoe kidney.[26] Other genitourinary abnormalities may occur (eg, hypospadius, undescended testes, bicornuate uterus, ureteral duplication, and vesicoureteric reflux).

The prognosis depends largely on the associated malformations. If there are no associated malformations, then a horseshoe kidney may remain symptom-free. Persistent urinary tract infection or renal calculi may occur in 20% of cases.

Cystic Diseases of the Kidney

Infantile Polycystic Kidney Disease (Potter Type 1).
Infantile polycystic kidney disease is inherited as an autosomal recessive trait. The primary abnormality is in the collecting tubules, which become altered sometime during the second half of gestation resulting in saccular or cylindrical dilatation throughout. The abnormality is always bilateral. Embryologically, the ureteral bud and the metanephric blastema are normal.[2] Normal calyces and papillae are formed, indicating that early intrauterine renal function is normal. A normal number of nephrons develop although some of these may be small. The connective tissue is normal. The liver is frequently abnormal, with elongation and dilatation of the bile ducts; periportal fibrosis and portal hypertension often develop later.

The disease may present in utero. In such cases, there is oligohydramnios resulting from diminished urine production. This initiates the Potter sequence, and death may occur shortly after birth from pulmonary hypoplasia. The disease can also present postnatally at several weeks or months of life, or occasionally up to 5 years of age.[27] The earlier the presentation, the more severe the renal involvement. The later the presentation, the less severe the renal involvement and the more severe the hepatic involvement.

The sonographic findings reflect the presence of multiple microscopic cysts in the kidneys (Fig. 17–6).[28–31] The kidneys are bilaterally enlarged, maintaining their reniform shape (Fig. 17–6.A). The enlargement can be substantiated by an elevated ratio of kidney circumference to abdominal circumference.[32] The kidneys are also hyperechoic as a result of multiple cyst wall interfaces, and they demonstrate increased through-transmission due to the high fluid content of the cysts (Fig. 17–6.B). Individual cysts are frequently too small to be resolved sonographically. In severe cases, additional findings include nonvisualization of the fetal bladder, marked oligohydramnios, and a small fetal thorax.

The sonographic findings of infantile polycystic kidney disease progress with increasing gestational age.[29,30]

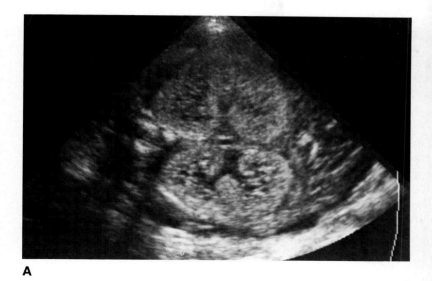

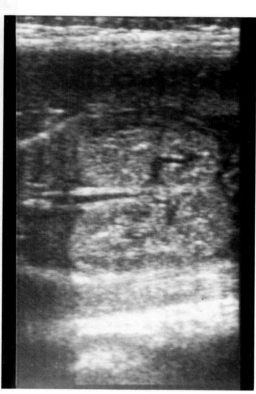

Fig. 17–6. Infantile polycystic kidney disease. **A.** Coronal view of a 21-week fetal abdomen demonstrates markedly enlarged (45 mm) echogenic kidneys that maintain a reniform shape. **B.** Another case at 22 weeks demonstrates enhanced transmission through enlarged echogenic kidneys. Severe oligohydramnios was present in both cases.

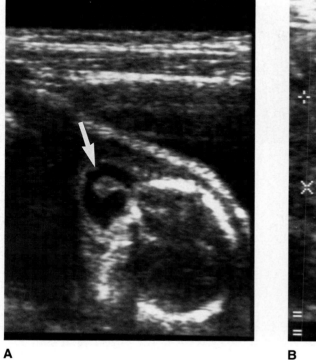

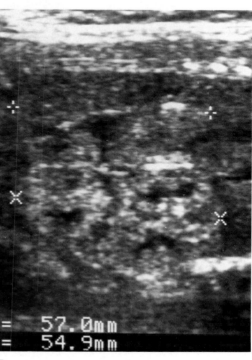

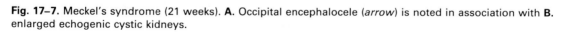

Fig. 17–7. Meckel's syndrome (21 weeks). **A.** Occipital encephalocele (*arrow*) is noted in association with **B.** enlarged echogenic cystic kidneys.

The diagnosis in some cases can be made in the second trimester, as early as 17 weeks' gestation.[28,29] In other reported cases, the kidneys appear sonographically normal in the second trimester and do not become enlarged and hyperechoic until the third trimester.[29,30,33]

Enlarged echogenic kidneys can also be seen in adult-type polycystic kidney disease (see following discussion), as well as in a number of syndromes. Polycystic kidneys are a major feature of the Meckel syndrome[34] (Fig. 17–7), an autosomal recessive disorder with other manifestations, including occipital encephalocele, polydactyly, and cleft lip and palate. Cystic disease of the kidneys is also seen in the Jeune syndrome (asphyxiating thoracic dysplasias),[35] Zellweger syndrome, short rib-polydactyly syndromes, and tuberous sclerosis.

Adult Polycystic Kidney Disease (Potter Type 3).

Adult polycystic kidney disease is an autosomal dominant dis-order. It typically presents in early adulthood, but rarely can be present in fetal life, and has been identified sonographically in utero.[36] The fetal kidneys are usually large and echogenic (similar to the appearance in infantile polycystic kidney disease) but in a minority of cases macroscopic cysts may be visualized. If symmetrically enlarged and echogenic (or cystic) kidneys are seen in utero, the key to making a diagnosis of adult-type polycystic kidney disease is a positive family history for that disorder. It must be emphasized that a prenatal scan with normal findings does not rule out adult-type polycystic kidney disease in a fetus at risk for that disorder.

Multicystic Dysplastic Kidney (Potter Type 2).

Multicystic dysplastic kidney is the most common cause of an abdominal mass in the neonate. It is typically unilateral, affecting a single kidney in its entirety, but may be bilateral or segmental. The involved renal tissue has little

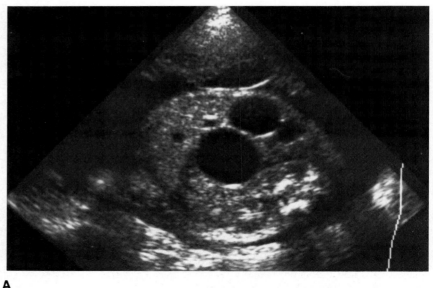

A

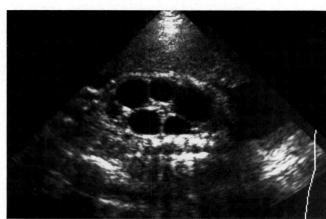

Fig. 17–8. Multicystic dysplastic kidney (28 weeks). **A.** Transverse and **B.** sagittal views of the right fetal kidney demonstrate multiple cysts of varying sizes that do not communicate with the renal pelvis.

B

or no function, and is characterized by replacement of the renal parenchyma by multiple cysts. Multicystic dysplastic kidney is thought to result from an inhibition of ampullary activity early in gestation, which then leads to decreased division of the collecting tubules, and failure of induction and maturation of nephrons.[2] The pathogenesis may be on the basis of a very early complete obstructive uropathy.[37,38]

When there is a unilateral multicystic dysplastic kidney, contralateral renal anomalies are present in 20 to 45% of cases.[38–40] These contralateral abnormalities include ureteropelvic junction obstruction, agenesis, and ureterovesicle junction obstruction. Other associated anomalies are uncommon.

The sonographic appearance consists of multiple cysts of varying sizes, with little or no normal-appearing renal parenchyma[41,42] (Fig. 17–8). In addition to the macroscopic cysts, there may be areas of hyperechoic tissue representing multiple small cysts, each of which is too small to be resolved sonographically. Careful technique may be needed to distinguish multicystic dysplastic kidney from uteropelvic junction obstruction.[43] The size of the individual cysts and of the entire multicystic dysplastic kidney may enlarge or shrink over serial scans, sometimes dramatically.[44] When unilateral, the amniotic fluid volume is most often normal, although polyhydramnios has been reported.[45] Polyhydramnios in this case is thought to be due to pressure on the gastrointestinal tract from the markedly enlarged kidney.

When a severe contralateral anomaly is present (eg, agenesis, severe ureteropelvic junction obstruction) or when there are bilateral multicystic dysplastic kidneys

(Fig. 17–9), the fetal bladder is nonvisualized and there is severe oligohydramnios. Lack of fetal urine production in these fetuses will lead to the Potter sequence.

Cystic Dysplasia Secondary to Obstruction (Potter Type 4). Obstructive uropathy very early in renal development, or interference with ampullary activity, are factors thought to be responsible for the classic form of multicystic dysplastic kidney (see preceding discussion). Renal dysplasia can also occur as a result of severe prolonged obstruction later in fetal life. The obstruction may be at any level, from the ureteropelvic junction to the urethra. The sonographic hallmarks of dysplasia in an obstructed kidney are parenchymal cysts (typically subcapsular) or increased parenchymal echogenicity[46] (Fig. 17–10). A

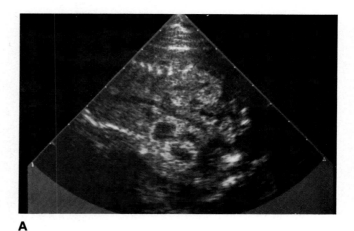

A

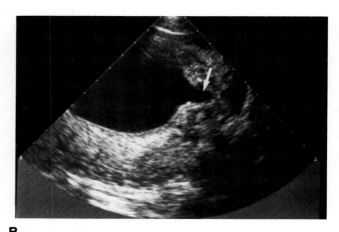

B

Fig. 17–9. Bilateral multicystic dysplastic kidneys (18 weeks). Transverse view through the fetal abdomen demonstrates a large right and small left kidney, both with multiple cysts. No normal-appearing renal tissue was seen, and oligohydramnios was present. Pathologic examination following therapeutic abortion confirmed bilateral multicystic dysplastic kidneys (right, 8.5 g; left, 1.3 g; expected, 1.5 g). Pulmonary hypoplasia was present.

Fig. 17–10. Potter type 4 cystic dysplasia in an 18-week fetus with posterior urethral valves. **A.** Kidneys are echogenic due to microscopic cysts throughout renal cortex. Bilateral hydronephrosis is less severe on the one side, presumably due to diminished renal function and less urine production. **B.** Coronal view through lower abdomen demonstrates markedly distended bladder and posterior urethra (*arrow*).

normal sonographic appearance of the renal parenchyma does not, however, rule out dysplasia in an obstructed kidney.[46] It seems that the more proximal the level of obstruction, the more likely that the cysts will be visible sonographically.[47]

Recognition of dysplastic changes in an obstructed kidney has important prognostic implications. Such a kidney will likely have little or no function even if the obstruction is relieved. For example, surgical repair of urethral valves (in utero or postnatally) will generally be futile once the kidneys have become dysplastic.

Renal Tumors

Mesoblastic Nephroma. Also called leiomyomatous hamartoma or fetal renal hamartoma, mesoblastic nephroma is the most common renal tumor in the neonate. Several cases of prenatal detection of this tumor have been reported.[48–54] Unlike Wilms' tumor, it is usually benign, unilateral, and solitary. Histologically, it can be differentiated from Wilms' tumor by the presence of mesenchymal tissue, as opposed to the epithelial tissue of Wilms' tumor. Because of its benign clinical course, it can be treated by nephrectomy alone.[55]

The sonographic appearance of mesoblastic nephroma is that of a solid mass in the renal fossa[56] (Fig. 17–11). Discrete areas of cystic degeneration may be present.[56,57] Polyhydramnios is often present.[50–52,58,59] This may be due to extrinsic pressure exerted on the gastrointestinal tract by the large renal mass. Alternatively, there may be increased renal blood flow to the mass, resulting in increased fetal urine production.[58]

The differential diagnosis includes:

1. Infantile polycystic kidney disease. This is bilateral in contrast to mesoblastic nephroma, which is usually unilateral. Furthermore, polycystic kidneys tend to maintain their reniform shape.
2. Adrenal tumor. Tissue planes can often be identified between the kidney, adrenal, and adjacent organs. The kidney may be displaced inferiorly by an adrenal tumor, but will maintain its structure and form.

The prognosis of mesoblastic nephroma is good, as it is almost always benign and easily resected. There is, therefore, no indication for premature delivery and early treatment. Local recurrences have been described,[53,60] but this is the exception rather than the rule. The more aggressive lesions tend to present after 3 months of age.[48,61]

Wilms' Tumor. Wilms' tumor differs from congenital mesoblastic nephroma by the presence of epithelial elements within the tumor and a more aggressive clinical course. It can be multifocal and, therefore, bilateral. To

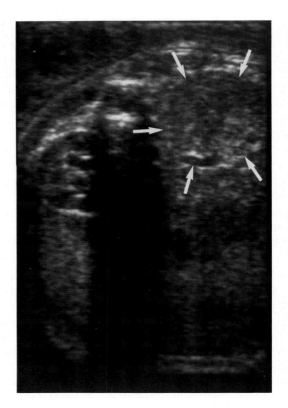

Fig. 17–11. Mesoblastic nephroma (34 weeks). Transverse view through the abdomen demonstrates a solid mass in the right renal fossa (*arrows*). This mass was separate from the adrenal and appeared to be contained within the renal capsule. Normal kidney is seen on the left.

this date, prenatal detection of this tumor has not been made. Postnatally, its sonographic appearance is identical to that of congenital mesoblastic nephroma. Statistically, however, congenital mesoblastic nephroma is more likely in the fetus and neonate. If the lesion is bilateral, then Wilms' should be considered and more aggressive obstetric management should be evaluated.

ABNORMALITIES OF THE URETERS, BLADDER, AND URETHRA (HYDRONEPHROSIS)

Hydronephrosis is the most common fetal abnormality encountered in obstetric ultrasound. Most cases are found incidentally in women scanned for routine obstetric indications, who are not at increased risk to bear a child with such malformation.

Hydronephrosis may be due to obstruction or reflux. The sites of obstruction include ureteropelvic junction, ureter, ureterovesicle junction, and urethra. Each of these conditions will be discussed separately.

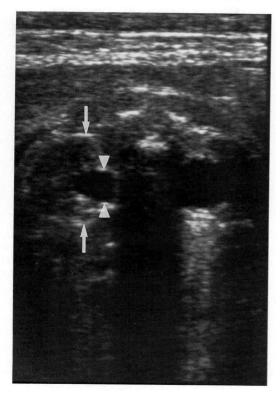

Fig. 17–12. The ratio of the anteroposterior diameter of the renal pelvis (1.2 cm) (*arrowheads*) to the anteroposterior diameter of the kidney (3 cm) (*arrows*) at the same level is less than 50%, indicating insignificant hydronephrosis. The same ratio on the opposite kidney is 1.9 to 3.0 (greater than 50%), indicating significant hydronephrosis.

Criteria for diagnosing significant hydronephrosis are important in order to identify those cases of pelviectasis that require follow-up prenatal or postnatal investigation, or both. Significant hydronephrosis should be diagnosed when at least one of the following criteria is met[62–64]:

1. An anteroposterior renal pelvic diameter of 10 mm or more. A diameter of 5 mm or less is usually normal, and one between 5 and 9 mm may be normal or due to an extrarenal pelvis.
2. A ratio of the anteroposterior diameter of the renal pelvis to the anteroposterior diameter of the kidney measured at the same level (Fig. 17–12), greater than 50%.
3. The presence of calyceal dilatation (Fig. 17–13). Calyceal dilatation in itself is an indication for postnatal investigation, regardless of the renal pelvic diameter or ratio.
4. Pelviectasis together with cystic change in the kidneys. Cystic change is the result of longstanding, severe urinary tract obstruction, and signifies severe structural damage and functional impairment (Potter type 4 cystic dysplasia) (Fig. 17–10). Because of diminished renal function and less urine production, there may be a lesser degree of distension of the collecting system.

Longstanding severe hydronephrosis will result in renal functional impairment. Experimental work has shown that the extent of renal damage at birth is proportional to the severity and duration of in utero obstruction.[65]

If a high-grade obstruction (eg, from urethral occlu-

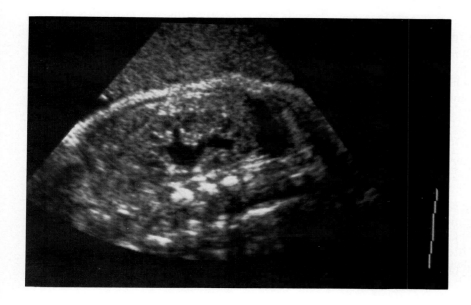

Fig. 17–13. Pelviectasis with calyceal dilatation (32 weeks). Sagittal view through the fetal kidney demonstrates mild pelviectasis, as well as calyceal dilatation. This degree of hydronephrosis, although mild, warrants postnatal evaluation. In this instance, evaluation demonstrated grade III vesicoureteric reflux.

sion) occurs early in fetal development while nephron induction is occurring, cystic dysplasia (Potter type 4) will result.[2] Back pressure of urine is exerted through the short collecting tubules to the later generation of nephrons, which are attached to and in direct alignment with the collecting tubules. (Earlier formed nephrons are attached to collecting tubules at acute angles and are not subject to the same pressure as the nephrons that have just completed their attachment and have not yet begun to differentiate.)[2] These nephrons become distended into cysts, further nephron induction is halted, and the result is a layer of cysts under the capsule. If the injury occurs more slowly, further nephron induction may occur so that a wider zone of cysts is produced.[2]

If the obstruction occurs later in fetal development, after the form of the kidney is established and nephron induction is completed, then the effect on the kidney is much the same as in the adult. The back pressure of urine will distend the renal pelvis and calyces more easily than it can distend individual tubules, and cystic dysplasia is less likely to occur. Renal function is also more likely to return to normal once the obstruction is relieved.[2]

If renal functional impairment is bilateral, oligohydramnios will result and there will be little or no urine in the fetal bladder. Amniotic fluid volume is, therefore, a good indicator of renal function in cases of bilateral hydronephrosis. In unilateral cases, amniotic fluid volume would most likely be normal. Occasionally, normal or increased amniotic fluid volume may be present in cases with bilateral poor renal function. This is usually due to a coexisting lesion that leads to polyhydramnios, eg, gastrointestinal obstruction, diaphragmatic hernia, and so forth.[66]

Occasionally, severe hydronephrosis can result in rupture of the collecting system with resultant paranephric urinoma (Fig. 17–14) or urinary ascites.[67,68] In most cases of paranephric urinoma, the ipsilateral kidney is nonfunctioning.[64,67,69] Urinomas may resolve spontaneously in utero.[69] In such cases, the prognosis for the underlying kidney is still poor.

Significant fetal hydronephrosis should be classified as mild, moderate, or severe. Hydronephrosis may progress or regress as pregnancy continues or may remain the same. Transient or intermittent hydronephrosis can occur. This may be related to the degree of bladder distension, and may be caused by vesicoureteric reflux. Maternal hydration does not appear to play a role in transient hydronephrosis.[70]

The frequency of prenatal follow-up scans depends on the severity of the hydronephrosis and whether it involves one or both sides. In cases of *unilateral* hydronephrosis, at least one follow-up scan is indicated between 30 and 35 weeks to determine progression or re-

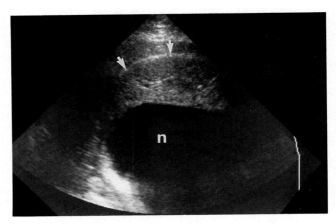

Fig. 17–14. Paranephric urinoma (30 weeks). Transverse view of the fetal abdomen (*arrows*) demonstrates a large fluid collection (u) occupying almost the entire right side of the abdominal cavity. This represents a urinoma from rupture of the collecting system in a fetus with a severe UPJ obstruction. There was a multicystic dysplastic kidney on the opposite side (not shown here) and severe oligohydramnios.

gression. If the degree of hydronephrosis is the same or worse, then postnatal evaluation is indicated. If the hydronephrosis is no longer present, both with a full and empty or partially empty fetal bladder, then no further work-up is indicated. Obstetric management should not be altered in cases of unilateral hydronephrosis, even if severe, as long as the contralateral kidney is normal. In cases of *bilateral* hydronephrosis, follow-up scans at 2 to 6 week intervals should be performed (depending on severity) in order to assess amniotic fluid volume as an index of renal function. Evidence of renal functional impairment may be an indication for preterm delivery and early surgical correction, or for fetal intervention.

The initial neonatal ultrasound examination should be performed on the 3rd to 7th day of life (Chart 17–1). If the examination is performed in the first 24 to 48 hours of life, hydronephrosis may be transiently absent.[71] This is probably due to a relative state of dehydration and decreased glomerular filtration rate in the immediate neonatal period. It has also been postulated that, after birth, dilatation may appear less prominent because the fetus is no longer exposed to progesterone-like maternal hormones which cause smooth muscle relaxation in the maternal renal collecting system and the fetal collecting system.[72–74]

Postnatal radiologic work-up should include ultrasound examination, intravenous pyelogram, voiding cystourethrogram, and, in certain cases, radionuclide scan to assess residual function. The amount of residual function is important in surgical planning. Prophylactic an-

**CHART 17–1. POSTNATAL EVALUATION OF
FETAL HYDRONEPHROSIS**

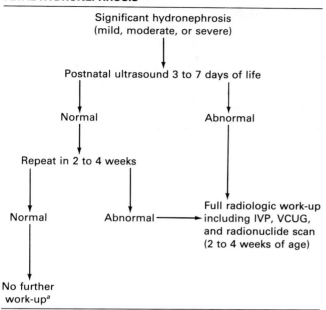

^a The pediatrician should be aware that intermittent vesicoureteric reflux may be missed in a small percentage of these cases, and that voiding cystourethrogram (VCUG) may be indicated if the infant develops a urinary tract infection.

tibiotics may be indicated during the interval between the abnormal neonatal ultrasound and the planned radiologic studies.

Ureteropelvic Junction Obstruction

Obstruction at the ureteropelvic junction (UPJ) is the most common cause of hydronephrosis in the fetal kidney. The exact etiology is unknown and several theories have been proposed based on embryologic, anatomic, histologic, and functional hypotheses. It is more common in males and, when discovered in the fetus or neonate, the male to female ratio exceeds 2:1. Left-sided lesions are more common. The lesion is bilateral in 10 to 40% of cases (Fig. 17–15), but the degrees of severity are usually different on the two sides. Anomalies of the contralateral kidney are relatively common. These include multicystic dysplastic kidney, renal agenesis, duplication, horseshoe, and ectopic kidney. Leibowitz and Blickman[75] observed minor degrees of vesicoureteric reflux in as many as 40% of affected children, possibly the result of urinary tract infection. The coexistence of UPJ and ureterovesical junction (UVJ) obstruction has been described in rare cases.[76] Anomalies of other organ systems are infrequent, and no consistent pattern of association has been found.

Sonographically, the point of obstruction at the UPJ can be identified by failure to visualize a dilated ureter. One may be able to see classic tapering at the UPJ (Fig. 17–16). Significant progression of dilatation in utero is relatively uncommon, especially in unilateral cases.[64] Even when bilateral, the condition is unlikely to be fatal,[64] but significant renal impairment can occur. The degree of dilatation does not necessarily correlate with renal functional impairment measured postnatally.[64] Occasionally, severe hydronephrosis from UPJ obstruction can result in rupture of the collecting system and the development of a paranephric urinoma (Fig. 17–14). In such cases, the underlying kidney is usually nonfunctioning.[64,67–69]

Postnatal studies are indicated in all cases in which UPJ obstruction is suspected prenatally. It is not unusual for the degree of hydronephrosis on the neonatal scan to improve due to removal of the influence of maternal hormones.

Minor degrees of UPJ obstruction may not require surgical repair, but should be followed at 3- or 6-month intervals until resolution. With more severe degrees of UPJ obstruction, the optimal time to repair the lesion is as soon as possible after birth.[77–79] Early relief of ob-

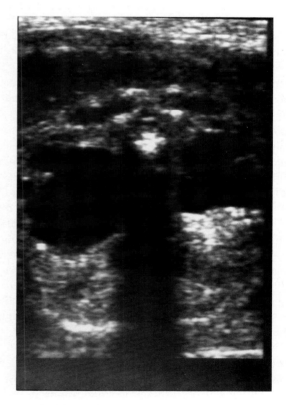

Fig. 17–15. Bilateral severe UPJ obstruction (34 weeks). Transverse view through the fetal kidneys demonstrates severe bilateral hydronephrosis. Ureters were not visible and the bladder was not distended.

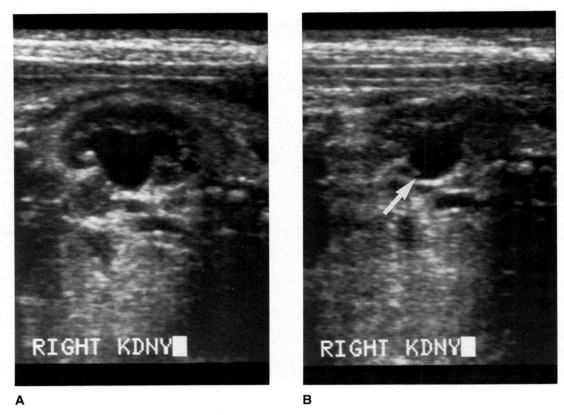

A   **B**

Fig. 17–16. Mild UPJ obstruction (35 weeks). **A.** There is mild pelviectasis and caliectasis. **B.** Classic tapering of the renal pelvis can be demonstrated (*arrow*). The ureter was not visible.

struction is associated with a significantly greater return of renal function than when surgery is performed later in life. Many cases of UPJ obstruction severe enough to require surgical decompression may go undetected on postnatal physical examination.[79] Prenatal ultrasound has proved invaluable in the detection of these cases. Bilateral, severe UPJ obstruction may require prenatal decompression or early delivery and repair, depending on the gestational age. Prenatal diagnosis also permits termination of pregnancy if a bilateral lesion is discovered early enough and is already associated with severe oligohydramnios. Unilateral UPJ obstruction, even if severe, should not alter obstetric management as long as the contralateral kidney appears normal.

Ureteral Valves or Strictures

A ureteral valve is a circumferential or semicircumferential fold of mucosa containing smooth muscle. A congenital ureteral stricture is a narrowing in the ureter located anywhere from the UPJ to the UVJ. Both are extremely rare causes of ureteric obstruction. Prenatal sonographic diagnosis can be made by noting the ureter to be dilated above the obstruction and not visible below

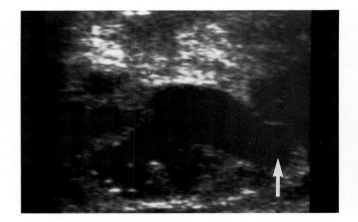

Fig. 17–17. Hydronephrosis due to a ureteral valve (33 weeks). Sagittal view through the fetal right kidney demonstrates hydronephrosis and dilatation of the upper third of the ureter (*arrow*). The distal two thirds of the ureter was not visible. This finding was persistent on several prenatal examinations. Postnatal findings were similar and at surgery a ureteral valve was found.

of abdominal muscles (prune belly), dilatation of the urinary tract, and failure of testicular descent (cryptorchidism).

The pathogenesis of prune belly has intrigued urologists and pathologists for years, and several theories have been proposed. Ives suggested that there was a primary mesodermal defect resulting in defective development of the abdominal wall and urinary tract.[96] Burton proposed a developmental arrest of mesodermal elements at 10 weeks' gestation.[97] More recently, evidence has been presented to suggest that the abdominal hypoplasia in prune belly is an etiologic nonspecific anatomic defect secondary to fetal abdominal distention of various causes. The most common cause is urethral obstruction.[98–103] Causes other than urethral obstruction include fetal ascites, abdominal masses (eg, infantile polycystic kidney disease), and visceromegaly (eg, Beckworth–Wiedeman syndrome). The complex morphogenesis of the male urethra results in an increased risk of obstructive anomalies; hence, the predominance of prune belly in boys. In some cases of prune belly with bladder outlet obstruction, no pathologic urethral lesion can be found. In these cases, Moerman and associates[104] believe that the urogenital anomalies can be attributed to a functional urethral obstruction, which in turn is the result of prostatic hypoplasia. There are many boys with posterior urethral valves and abdominal distention that do not have prune belly, so genetic factors may be involved.[105] In support of this theory is the fact that familial occurrence has been observed, and there is a high incidence of the condition in Nigeria.

The abdominal wall defect may be asymmetric or patchy in distribution. The flanks often bulge markedly and there tends to be flaring at the costal margins. Hydronephrosis and cystic dysplasia are the two renal abnormalities associated with the syndrome, and the prognosis is often determined by the degree of dysplasia. Occasionally, the kidneys are normal. The ureters are dilated and tortuous with the lower ends of the ureters more severely affected. The UVJ is abnormal and vesicoureteric reflux is present in most patients. The bladder is typically large. The urachus may be patent, especially in patients with urethral atresia. The prostatic urethra has a dilated and somewhat triangular configuration. Usually, the obstruction at this point is functional. In a few cases, there is complete atresia of the membranous urethra, and very rarely there is a true urethral valve. The prostate gland is usually hypoplastic,[104] which may be a factor in etiology.[106] The anterior urethra and penis are normal in most patients with prune belly. Bilateral cryptorchidism is characteristic of the syndrome. Failure of testicular descent may be due to a distended bladder early in gestation. This may also be the reason for abnormal intestinal rotation in many cases of prune belly.

Limb deformities may be present, resulting from fetal compression due to oligohydramnios. Ventricular septal defects, atrial septal defects, and tetralogy of Fallot occur with increased frequency in children with prune belly.[107]

ABNORMALITIES OF THE GENITAL TRACT

Hydrocele is a collection of fluid within the tunica vaginalis. This is easily diagnosed sonographically by identifying fluid within the scrotum, often outlining the testes (Fig. 17–21).[108–110] Isolated hydrocele is of no pathologic significance.

Cryptorchidism (undescended testes) can be detected sonographically by failure to visualize the testes within the scrotum.[111] The testes may not fully descend until late in pregnancy, so this finding may be present in at least 10% of fetuses in the early- to mid-third trimester.[111–113] Its incidence at term is 0.7%. While most often an isolated finding, it can be seen in a variety of syndromes, including prune belly syndrome, Noonan syndrome, and trisomies 13, 18, and 21.

Ambiguous genitalia refers to external genitalia that are not clearly of either sex. This can result from abnormal hormone levels, as in congenital adrenal hyperplasia, transplacental passage of hormones, and true hermaphroditism (presence of both ovarian and testicular tissue). Anomalies of the external genitalia that are not hormonally mediated can also occur (eg, micropenis). These latter anomalies can be isolated, they may have associated urinary tract anomalies or chromosomal abnormalities, or they may occur as one component of a multiple malformation syndrome. At least one case of prenatal ultrasound diagnosis of ambiguous genitalia has been reported.[114] Scans of the fetal perineum at 34 weeks demonstrated two rounded structures representing either labia majora

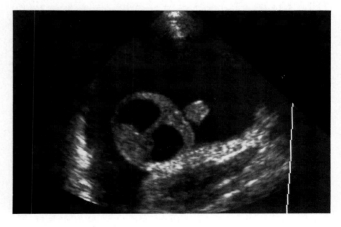

Fig. 17–21. Bilateral hydroceles in a 32-week fetus. The testes are descended and surrounded by fluid.

(without labia minora) or a bifid scrotum with undescended testes. A small structure projected from the midline of the perineum, with the appearance of either a small penis or a hypertrophied clitoris. Morphologically ambiguous genitalia were confirmed postnatally, and chromosome analysis revealed a 46XY karyotype with translocation of genetic material from chromosome 9 to chromosome 3. Congenital adrenal hyperplasia has also been diagnosed prenatally, on the basis of elevated steroid precursors in the amniotic fluid.[115]

Testicular feminization is a condition characterized by female external genitalia in conjunction with a male karyotype (46XY chromosomes). It results from a disorder in the androgen receptor, which renders the body unable to respond to testosterone. While testerosterone is produced (in fact, at above-normal levels), it has no effect and the embryo fails to virilize. Prenatal diagnosis of this disorder has been reported in a fetus undergoing genetic amniocentesis at 16 weeks gestation.[116] The sonogram demonstrated female external genitalia, and amniocentesis yielded a 46XY karyotype. These findings suggested testicular feminization, and the diagnosis was confirmed when a repeat amniocentesis reproduced the initial findings and demonstrated an elevated amniotic fluid testosterone level.

Ovarian cysts occur in approximately one third of newborn females at autopsy.[117] Most are follicular cysts; corpus luteum cysts, theca lutein cysts, paraovarian cysts, teratomas, and cystadenomas also occur.[118] Ovarian cysts are typically small and clinically insignificant, but large cysts can lead to prenatal or postnatal complications: polyhydramnios, dystocia, torsion, respiratory distress.[118–120] An association between ovarian cysts and congenital hypothyroidism has been suggested.[121] In utero sonographic findings include a simple (Fig. 17–22),[121–123]

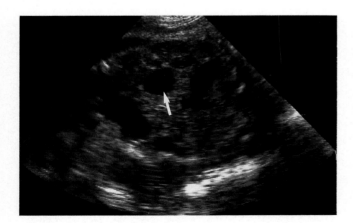

Fig. 17–22. Ovarian cyst (31 weeks). A 3-cm simple cyst is noted (*arrow*) separate from the kidney, stomach, and bladder. The differential diagnosis would include mesenteric cyst and bowel duplication cyst.

septated,[120,124] or debris-filled[125] cyst in the pelvis or lower abdomen. In one reported case, a torsed ovarian cyst presented prenatally as a complex abdominal mass with several cystic components.[119] Differential diagnosis of a fetal lower abdominal cyst includes urachal cyst, mesenteric cyst, gastrointestinal duplication cyst, and hydrometrocolpos (see discussion following). Differentiation among these is often not possible, although a multiseptated appearance should strongly suggest an ovarian cyst.

Hydrometrocolpos is a condition in which the uterus and vagina are distended with cervical and vaginal secretions due to obstruction. Causes include imperforate hymen, transverse vaginal septum, and vaginal or cervical atresia. Cases due to vaginal or cervical atresia are frequently accompanied by other abnormalities, including imperforate anus (often with rectouterine or rectovaginal fistula), unilateral renal agenesis or hypoplasia, polycystic kidneys, bicornuate uterus, polydactyly, esophageal atresia, and sacral hypoplsia.[126–128] Hydrometrocolpos is also a component of the McKusick–Kaufman syndrome, an autosomal recessive disorder of which other manifestations include polydactyly and congenital heart disease.[129] It has been described in the Ellis–van Crefeld syndrome. When large, hydronephrosis and hydroureter may result. Prenatal sonographic appearance is that of a cystic mass with low-level echoes posterior to the bladder and extending into the fetal abdomen.[130–132] In one reported case, the cystic lesion could be seen separating and protruding through the labia majora.[130] Unless this last finding is present, precise diagnosis is not possible; differential diagnosis includes other cystic lesions listed in the above discussion of ovarian cysts.

ABNORMALITIES OF THE ADRENALS

Neuroblastoma is the most common abnormality of the adrenal gland in the fetus. Prenatal ultrasound is likely to play a very important role in the early detection of such tumors because if an abdominal mass is not palpated neonatally, there may be a delay in diagnosis resulting in a poorer prognosis.

The sonographic appearance is variable. Typically, there is a mixed solid and cystic pattern because hemorrhage and necrosis are common in these tumors.[133] Cystic change may be the predominant feature[134] (Fig. 17–23). Calcification is present in a small percentage of cases.[135] Hydrops fetalis has been described associated with neuroblastoma.[136] Metastatic neuroblastoma in utero, presenting as a fetal neck mass, has been reported.[137] Adrenal masses can displace the ipsilateral kidney inferiorly. On the left side, the inferior vena cava may be displaced anteriorly.

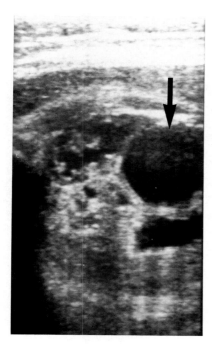

Fig. 17–23. Adrenal neuroblastoma (38 weeks). A 3.6-cm cystic suprarenal mass is seen (*arrow*), involving the fetal left adrenal gland. A cystic neuroblastoma was diagnosed at surgery performed soon after birth. No metastatic disease was found. (*Courtesy of Wane Joselow, MD, Catholic Medical Center, Manchester, NH.*)

Differential diagnoses include:

1. Adrenal hemorrhage. The sonographic appearance of an adrenal hemorrhage should undergo the typical changes of a hematoma, so a follow-up scan would differentiate it from adrenal tumor.
2. Tumor in adjacent organ. Mesoblastic nephroma or Wilms' tumor arising from the kidney tend to be more echogenic and more solid in sonographic appearance. Other tumors include liver hamartoma or hemangioma, or retroperitoneal teratoma. Sometimes, visualization of the exact origin of the tumor can be difficult. It is important, therefore, to identify tissue planes between these closely applied organs.

A large percentage of neuroblastomas release catecholamines. As these are capable of being passed through the placenta, there may be maternal symptoms and signs of nausea, vomiting, headaches, hypertension, and so forth. Such symptoms appearing for the first time in the third trimester should raise the suspicion of fetal neuroblastoma.[137]

Neuroblastoma in situ may degenerate and regress spontaneously. Spontaneous regressions of larger masses, and even metastases, have been reported.[138]

The prognosis depends on the time of diagnosis. The younger the patient, the better the prognosis. Prenatal diagnosis, therefore, should greatly enhance the prognosis.

SYSTEMATIC APPROACH TO THE DIAGNOSIS OF GENITOURINARY ANOMALIES

A systematic approach is critical to the correct identification of genitourinary tract anomalies. We present here such an approach, consisting of a series of questions that can be addressed by the sonologist or sonographer while performing and interpreting the prenatal scan. Details of the specific lesions mentioned here are omitted, as they have been included in previous sections.

1. Are the kidneys normal in size, echogenicity, and location? Norms for kidney length, width, and volume, and for ratio of kidney circumference to abdominal circumference, have been established.[32,139] Large kidneys, especially when bilateral and increased in echogenicity, suggest infantile polycystic kidney disease or related entities. When one or both kidneys are not visualized in the renal fossae, the rest of the abdomen and pelvis should be searched for an ectopic kidney.
2. If fluid spaces are seen in a kidney, do they represent parenchymal cysts or pelvocalyceal dilatation? The key to making this distinction is to thoroughly scan the kidney to establish the presence or absence of interconnections between fluid spaces (Fig. 17–24). When pelvocalyceal dilatation is present, the correct choice of scanning plane will demonstrate the interconnections between dilated calyces and the centrally located renal pelvis. Multiple cysts, as seen in a multicystic dysplastic kidney, will appear separate in all scanning planes.
3. When fluid is visualized in the renal pelvis or calyces, is it a normal finding or does it represent significant hydronephrosis? Fluid is detected in one or both fetal renal pelves in over 50% of cases and is especially common in the third trimester.[70,140] Most of these infants prove to be normal after birth. Significant hydronephrosis should be diagnosed when at least one of the following four criteria is met: (a) anteroposterior diameter of the renal pelvis 10 mm or greater in size, (b) ratio of anteroposterior diameter of the renal pelvis to the anteroposterior diameter of the kidney greater than 0.5, (c) the presence of caliectasis, and (d) the presence of pelviectasis and cystic changes in the kidneys. The degree of maternal hydration has little effect on the size of the fetal renal pelvis.[70,140]
4. If significant hydronephrosis is present, where is the point of obstruction? The fetal abdomen and pelvis

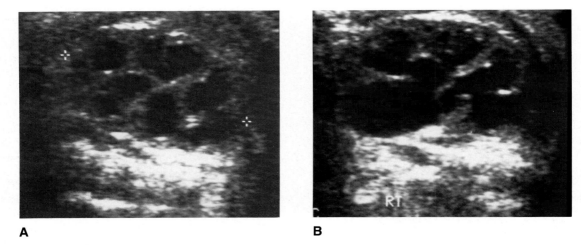

A   **B**

Fig. 17–24. Hydronephrosis versus parenchymal cysts (33 weeks). **A.** Sagittal view through the kidney demonstrates multiple separate fluid-filled spaces. **B.** Slight angulation of the transducer demonstrates that the fluid-filled spaces interconnect and are continuous with the renal pelvis, consistent with a diagnosis of hydronephrosis.

should be examined for hydroureter, distended bladder or thickened bladder wall, and dilated posterior urethra. Active peristalsis in a dilated ureter suggests obstruction rather than reflux.

5. If a lesion is detected, is it unilateral or bilateral? The answer to this question is important for both diagnostic and prognostic reasons. Some lesions are typically unilateral (eg, multicystic dysplastic kidney), whereas others affect both kidneys (eg, infantile polycystic kidney disease, urethral valve). Unilateral lesions carry an excellent prognosis in almost all cases, whereas severe bilateral abnormalities may be incompatible with life.

6. Is the amniotic fluid volume normal? In abnormalities involving both fetal kidneys or collecting systems, amniotic fluid volume is an important prognostic feature. In one series of patients with urethral obstruction, for example, 95% of cases with oligohydramnios subsequently died, whereas 74% of cases without definite oligohydramnios survived the neonatal period.[95]

7. What is the fetal sex? Determination of fetal sex can be helpful when diagnoses of posterior urethral valves and prune belly syndrome are entertained. The former occurs almost exclusively in males, and the latter occurs mainly in males.

REFERENCES

1. McCrory WW. Embryonic development and prenatal maturation of the kidney. In: Edelmann CM, ed. *Pediatric Kidney Disease.* Boston: Little, Brown; 1978:3–25.

2. Potter EL. *Normal and Abnormal Development of the Kidney.* Chicago: Year Book Medical Publishers; 1972.

3. Gersh I. The correlation of structure and function in the developing mesonephros and metanephros. *Contrib Embryol.* 1937;26:35.

4. Tanagho EA. Embryologic basis for lower ureteral anomalies: A hypothesis. *Urology.* 1976;7:451.

5. McCrory WW. *Developmental Nephrology.* Cambridge, Mass: Harvard University Press; 1972.

6. Stewart CL, Jose PA. Transitional nephrology. *Urol Clin North Am.* 1985;12:143.

7. Potter EL. Facial characteristics of infants with bilateral renal agenesis. *Am J Obstet Gynecol.* 1946;41:855.

8. Thomas IT, Smith DW. Oligohydramnios, cause of the nonrenal features of Potter's syndrome, including pulmonary hypoplasia. *J Pediatr.* 1974;84:811.

9. Fantel A, Shepard T. Potter's syndrome—non-renal features induced by oligohydramnios. *Am J Dis Child.* 1975;129:1346.

10. Perlman M, Levin M. Fetal pulmonary hypoplasia, anuria, and oligohydramnios: Clinicopathologic observations and review of the literature. *Am J Obstet Gynecol.* 1974;118:1119.

11. Potter EL. Bilateral absence of ureters and kidneys: Report of 50 cases. *Obstet Gynecol.* 1965;25:3.

12. DuBois AM. The embryonic kidney. In: Rouiller C, Muller AF, eds. *The Kidney: Morphology, Biochemistry, Physiology.* New York: Academic Press; 1969:1–59.

13. Dubbins PA, Kurtz AB, Wapner RJ, Goldberg BB. Renal agenesis: Spectrum of in utero findings. *J Clin Ultrasound.* 1981;9:189.

14. Romero R, Cullen M, Grannum P, et al. Antenatal diagnosis of renal anomalies with ultrasound, III: Bilateral renal agenesis. *Am J Obstet Gynecol.* 1985;151:38.

15. Raghavendra BN, Young BK, Greco MA, et al. Use of

furosemide in pregnancies complicated by oligohydramnios. *Radiology.* 1987;165:455.

16. Longo VJ, Thompson GJ. Congenital solitary kidney. *J Urol.* 1952;68:63.

17. Thompson DP, Lynn HB. Genital anomalies associated with solitary kidney. *Mayo Clin Proc.* 1966;41:538.

18. Smith EC, Orkin LA. A clinical and statistical study of 471 congenital anomalies of the kidney and ureter. *J Urol.* 1945;53:11.

19. Semmens JP. Congenital anomalies of the female genital tract: Functional classification based on review of 56 personal cases and 500 reported cases. *Obstet Gynecol.* 1962;19:328.

20. Emanuel B, Nachman R, Aronson N, et al. Congenital solitary kidney: A review of 74 cases. *Am J Dis Child.* 1974;127:17.

21. Malek RS, Kelalis PP, Burke EC. Ectopic kidney in children and frequency of association of other malformations. *Mayo Clin Proc.* 1971;46:461.

22. Thompson GJ, Pace JM. Ectopic kidney: A review of 97 cases. *Surg Gynecol Obstet.* 1937,64:935.

23. Downs RA, Lane JW, Burns E. Solitary pelvic kidney: Its clinical implications. *Urology.* 1973;1:51.

24. N'Guessan G, Stephens FD. Congenital superior ectopic (thoracic) kidney. *Urology.* 1984;24:219.

25. Campbell MF. Anomalies of the kidney. In: Campbell MF, Harrison JH, eds. *Urology.* Philadelphia: W.B. Saunders; 1970:1447–1452.

26. Smith DW. *Recognizable Patterns of Human Malformation.* 3rd ed. Philadelphia: W.B. Saunders; 1982.

27. Blyth H, Ockenden BG. Polycystic disease of kidneys and liver presenting in childhood. *J Med Genet.* 1971;8:257–284.

28. Habif DV Jr, Berdon WE, Yeh MN. Infantile polycystic kidney disease: In utero sonographic diagnosis. *Radiology.* 1982;142:475.

29. Romero R, Cullen M, Jeanty P, et al. The diagnosis of congenital renal anomalies with ultrasound, II: Infantile polycystic kidney disease. *Am J Obstet Gynecol.* 1984;150:259.

30. Mahoney BS, Callen PW, Filly RA, Golbus MS. Progression of infantile polycystic kidney disease in early pregnancy. *J Ultrasound Med.* 1984;3:277.

31. Boal DK, Teele RL. Sonography of infantile polycystic kidney disease. *AJR.* 1980;135:575.

32. Grannum P, Bracken M, Silverman R, et al. Assessment of fetal kidney size in normal gestation by comparison of ratio of kidney circumference to abdominal circumference. *Am J Obstet Gynecol.* 1980;136:249.

33. Luthy DA, Hirsch JH. Infantile polycystic kidney disease: Observations from attempts at prenatal diagnosis. *Am J Med Genet.* 1985;20:505.

34. Pardes JG, Engel IA, Blomquist K, Magid MS, Kazam E. Ultrasonography of intrauterine Meckel's syndrome. *J Ultrasound Med.* 1984;3:33.

35. Schinzel A, Savoldelli G, Briner J, Schubiger G. Prenatal sonographic diagnosis of Jeune syndrome. *Radiology.* 1985;154:777.

36. Pretorius DH, Lee ME, Manco-Johnson ML, Weingast

GR, Sedman AB, Gabow PA. Diagnosis of autosomal dominant polycystic kidney disease in utero and in the young infant. *J Ultrasound Med.* 1987;6:249.

37. Felson B, Cussen LJ. The hydronephrotic type of unilateral congenital multicystic disease of the kidney. *Semin Roentgenol.* 1975;10:113.

38. Griscom NT, Vawter GF, Fellers FX. Pelvoinfundibular atresia: The usual form of multicystic kidney: 44 unilateral and 2 bilateral cases. *Semin Roentgenol.* 1975;10:125.

39. Kleiner B, Filly RA, Mack L, Callen PW. Multicystic dysplastic kidney: Observations of contralateral disease in the fetal population. *Radiology.* 1986;161:27.

40. Greene LF, Feinzaig W, Dahlin DC. Multicystic dysplasia of the kidney, with special reference to the contralateral kidney. *J Urol.* 1971;105:482.

41. Hadlock FP, Deter RL, Carpenter R, Gonzalez ET, Park SK. Sonography of fetal urinary tract anomalies. *Am J Roentgenology.* 1981;137:261.

42. Stuck KJ, Koff SA, Silver TM. Ultrasonic features of multicystic dysplastic kidney: Expanded diagnostic criteria. *Radiology.* 1982;143:217.

43. Beretsky I, Lankin DH, Rusoff JH. Sonographic differentiation between the multicystic dysplastic kidney and the ureteropelvic junction obstruction in utero using high resolution real-time scanners employing digital detection. *J Clin Ultrasound.* 1984;12:429.

44. Hashimoto BE, Filly RA, Callen PW. Multicystic dysplastic kidney: Changing appearance on ultrasound. *Radiology.* 1986;159:107.

45. Henderson SC, Van Kolkin RJ, Rahatzad M. Multicystic kidney with hydramnios. *J Clin Ultrasound.* 1980;8:249.

46. Mahoney BS, Filly RA, Callen PW, Hricak H, Golbus MS, Harrison MR. Fetal renal dysplasia: Sonographic evaluation. *Radiology.* 1984;152:143.

47. Sanders RC, Nussbaum AR, Solez K. Renal dysplasia: Sonographic findings. *Radiology.* 1988;167:623.

48. Ehman RL, Nicholson SF, Machin GA. Prenatal sonographic detection of congenital mesoblastic nephroma in a monozygotic twin pregnancy. *J Ultrasound Med.* 1983;2:555.

49. Giulian BB. Prenatal ultrasonographic diagnosis of fetal renal tumors. *Radiology.* 1984;152:69.

50. Romano WL. Neonatal renal tumor with polyhydramnios. *J Ultrasound Med.* 1984;3:475.

51. Geirsson RT, Ricketts NEM, Taylor DJ, et al. Prenatal appearance of a mesoblastic nephroma associated with polyhydramnios. *J Clin Ultrasound.* 1985;13:488.

52. Howey DD, Farrell EE, Sholl J, et al. Congenital mesoblastic nephroma: Prenatal ultrasonic findings and surgical excision in a very-low-birth-weight infant. *J Clin Ultrasound.* 1985;13:506.

53. Walter JP, McGahan JP. Mesoblastic nephroma: Prenatal sonographic detection. *J Clin Ultrasound.* 1985;3:686.

54. Apuzzio JJ, Unwin W, Adhale A, et al. Prenatal diagnosis of fetal renal mesoblastic nephroma. *Am J Obstet Gynecol.* 1986;154:636.

55. Bolande RP. Congenital and infantile neoplasia of the kidney. *Lancet.* 1974;2:1497.

56. Hartman DS, Lesar MSL, Madewell JE, et al. Mesoblastic

nephroma: Radiologic-pathologic correlation of 20 cases. *AJR.* 1981;136:69.

57. Grider RD, Wolverson MK, Jagannadharao B, et al. Congenital mesoblastic nephroma with cystic component. *J Clin Ultrasound.* 1981;9:43.

58. Perlman M, Potashnik G, Wise S. Hydramnios and fetal renal anomalies. *Am J Obstet Gynecol.* 1976;125:966.

59. Blank E, Neerhout RC, Burry KA. Congenital mesoblastic nephroma and polyhydramnios. *JAMA.* 1978;240:1504.

60. Fu YS, Kay S. Congenital mesoblastic nephroma and its recurrence. *Arch Pathol.* 1973;96:66.

61. Gonzalez-Crussi F, Sotelo-Avila C, Kidd JM. Mesenchymal renal tumors in infancy: A reappraisal. *Human Pathol.* 1981;12:78.

62. Arger PH, Coleman BG, Mintz MC, et al. Routine fetal genitourinary tract screening. *Radiology.* 1985;156:485.

63. Grignon A, Jilian R, Filiatrault D, et al. Urinary tract dilatation in utero: Classification and clinical applications. *Radiology.* 1986;160:645.

64. Kleiner B, Callen PW, Filly RA. Sonographic analysis of the fetus with ureteropelvic junction obstruction. *AJR.* 1987;148:359.

65. Beck AD. The effect of intrauterine urinary obstruction upon development of the fetal kidney. *J Urol.* 1971; 105:784.

66. Harrison MR, Golbus MS, Filly RA, eds. *The Unborn Patient: Prenatal Diagnosis and Treatment.* Orlando, Fla: Grune & Stratton; 1984.

67. Callen PW, Bolding D, Filly RA, Harrison MR. Ultrasonographic evaluation of fetal paranephric pseudocysts. *J Ultrasound Med.* 1983;2:309.

68. Adzick NS, Harrison MR, Flake AW, et al. Urinary extravasation in the fetus with obstructive uropathy. *J Ped Surg.* 1985;20:608.

69. Avni EF, Thoria Y, Van Gansbeke D, et al. Development of the hypodysplastic kidney: Contribution of antenatal ultrasound diagnosis. *Radiology.* 1987;164:123.

70. Hoddick WK, Filly RA, Mahoney BS, Callen PW. Minimal fetal renal pyelectasis. *J Ultrasound Med.* 1985;4:85.

71. Laing FC, Burke VD, Wing VW, et al. Postpartum evaluation of fetal hydronephrosis: Optimal timing for follow-up sonography. *Radiology.* 1984;152:423.

72. Berman LB. The pregnant kidney. *JAMA.* 1975;230:111.

73. Waltzer WC. The urinary tract in pregnancy. *J Urol.* 1981;125:271.

74. Peake SL, Roxburgh HB, Langlois SLP. Ultrasonic assessment of hydronephrosis of pregnancy. *Radiology.* 1983;146:167.

75. Lebowitz RL, Blickman JG. The coexistence of ureteropelvic junction obstruction and reflux. *AJR.* 1983;140:231.

76. McGrath MA, Estroff J, Lebowitz RL. The coexistence of obstruction at the ureteropelvic and ureterovesical junctions. *AJR.* 1987;149:403.

77. Mayor G, Genton N, Torrado A, et al. Renal function in obstructive nephropathy: Long term effect of reconstructive surgery. *Pediatrics.* 1975;56:740.

78. McCrory WW, Shebuya M, Leumann E. Studies of renal function in children with chronic hydronephrosis. *Pediatr Clin North Am.* 1971;18:445.

79. Flake AW, Harrison MR, Sauer L, et al. Ureteropelvic junction obstruction in the fetus. *J Pediatr Surg.* 1986;21:1058.

80. Pfister RC, Papanicolaou N, Yoder IC. The dilated ureter: Refluxing, obstructing, and unobstructed megaureters. *Semin Roentgenol.* 1986;21:224.

81. Blickman JG, Lebowitz RL. The coexistence of primary megaureter and reflux. *AJR.* 1984;143:1053.

82. Malek RS, Kelalis PP, Burke EL, et al. Simple and ectopic ureterocele in infancy and childhood. *Surg Gynecol Obstet.* 1972;134:611.

83. Mandell J, Colodny AH, Lebowitz R, et al. Ureteroceles in infants and children. *J Urol.* 1980;123:921.

84. Abrams HJ, Sutton AP, Buchbinder MI. Ureteroceles in siblings. *J Urol.* 1980;124:135.

85. Ayalon A, Shapiro A, Ruben SZ, et al. Ureterocele—a familial congenital anomaly. *Urology.* 1979;13:551.

86. Stephens FD. *Congenital Malformations of the Rectum, Anus, and Genitourinary Tracts.* London: E & S Livingstone; 1963.

87. Bailey RR, James E, McLoughlin K, et al. Familial and genetic data in reflux nephropathy. *Contrib Nephrol.* 1984;39:40.

88. Blane CE, Koff SA, Bowerman RA, et al. Nonobstructive fetal hydronephrosis: Sonographic recognition and therapeutic implications. *Radiology.* 1983;147:95.

89. Sanders R, Graham D. Twelve cases of hydronephrosis in utero diagnosed by ultrasonography. *J Ultrasound Med.* 1982;1:341.

90. Baker ME, Rosenberg ER, Bowie JD, et al. Transient in utero hydronephrosis. *J Ultrasound Med.* 1983;4:51.

91. King LR. Vesicoureteral reflux: History, etiology, and conservative management. In: Kelalis PP, King LR, eds. *Clinical Pediatric Urology.* Philadelphia: W.B. Saunders; 1976;1:342–365.

92. Lenaghan D, Whitaker JG, Jensen F, et al. The natural history of reflux and long-term effects of reflux on the kidney. *J Urol.* 1976;115:738.

93. Berdon WE, Baker DH, Blanc WA, et al. Megacystis-microcolon-intestinal hypoperistalsis syndrome: A new cause of intestinal obstruction in the newborn. Report of radiologic findings in five newborn girls. *AJR.* 1976;126: 957.

94. Stephens FD. Congenital intrinsic lesions of the posterior urethra. In: *Congenital Malformations of the Urinary Tract.* New York: Praeger; 1983.

95. Mahoney BS, Callen PW, Filly RA. Fetal urethral obstruction: Ultrasound evaluation. *Radiology.* 1985;157: 221.

96. Ives EJ. The abdominal muscle deficiency triad syndrome: Experience with ten cases. *Birth Defects.* 1974;10:127.

97. Burton OC. Agenesis of abdominal musculature associated with genitourinary and gastrointestinal anomalies. *J Urol.* 1951;66:607.

98. Pagon RA, Smith DW, Shepard TH. Urethral obstruction malformation complex: A cause of abdominal muscle deficiency and the "prune belly." *J Pediatr.* 1979;94:900.

99. Nakayama DK, Harrison MR, Chinn DH, et al. The pathogenesis of prune belly. *Am J Dis Child.* 1984;138:834.

100. Wilson SK, Moore GW, Hutchins GM. Congenital cystic adenomatoid malformation of the lung associated with abdominal musculature deficiency (prune belly). *Pediatrics.* 1978;62:421.

101. Monie IW, Monie BJ. Prune belly syndrome and fetal ascites. *Teratology.* 1979;19:111.

102. Smythe AR II. Ultrasonic detection of fetal ascites and bladder dilation with resulting prune belly. *J Pediatr.* 1981;98:798.

103. Lubinsky M, Rapoport P. Transient fetal hydrops and "prune belly" in one identical female twin. *N Engl J Med.* 1983;308:256.

104. Moerman P, Fryns JP, Goddeeris P, et al. Pathogenesis of prune-belly syndrome: A functional urethral obstruction caused by prostatic hypoplasia. *Pediatrics.* 1984;73:470.

105. Adeyokunnu AA, Familusi JB. Prune belly syndrome in two siblings and a first cousin. *Am J Dis Child.* 1982;136:23.

106. Monie IW, Monie BJ. Determinants of the prune belly syndrome. *J Pediatrics.* 1979;95:1084.

107. Adebonojo FO. Dysplasia of the abdominal musculature with multiple congenital anomalies: Prune belly or triad syndrome. *J Natl Med Assoc.* 1973;65:327.

108. Vanesian R, Grossman M, Metherell A, Flynn JJ, Louscher S. Antepartum ultrasonic diagnosis of congenital hydrocele. *Radiology.* 1978;126:765.

109. Miller EI, Thomas RH. Fetal hydrocele detected in uteo by ultrasound. *Br J Radiol.* 1979;52:624.

110. Meizner I, Katz M, Zmora E, Insler V. In utero diagnosis of congenital hydrocele. *J Clin Ultrasound.* 1983;11:449.

111. Birnholz JC. Determination of fetal sex. *N Engl J Med.* 1983;309:942.

112. Scorer CG. A treatment of undescended testicle in infancy. *Arch Dis Child.* 1957;32:520.

113. Kogan SJ. Cryptorchidism. In: Kelalis PP, King LR, Belman AB, eds. *Clinical Pediatric Urology.* 2nd ed. Philadelphia: W.B. Saunders; 1985:864–887.

114. Cooper C, Mahoney BS, Bowie JD, Pope II. Prenatal ultrasound diagnosis of ambiguous genitalia. *J Ultrasound Med.* 1985;4:433.

115. Warsof SL, Larsen JW, Kent SG, et al. Prenatal diagnosis of congenital adrenal hyperplasia. *Obstet Gynecol.* 1980;55:751.

116. Stephens JD. Prenatal diagnosis of testicular feminization. *Lancet.* 1984;2:1038.

117. DeSa DJ. Follicular ovarian cysts in stillbirths and neonates. *Arch Dis Child.* 1975;50:45.

118. Carlson DH, Griscom NT. Ovarian cysts in the newborn. *AJR.* 1972;116:664.

119. Preville EJ. Presentation of an unusual complication of an ovarian cyst. *J Canad Assoc Radiol.* 1987;38:222.

120. Nguyen KT, Reid RL, Sauerbrei E. Antenatal sonographic detection of a fetal theca lutein cyst. *J Ultrasound Med.* 1986;5:665.

121. Jafri SZH, Bree RL, Silver TM, Ouimette M. Fetal ovarian cysts: Sonographic detection and association with hypothyroidism. *Radiology.* 1984;150:809.

122. Crade M, Gillooly L, Taylor KJW. In utero demonstration of an ovarian cystic mass by ultrasound. *J Clin Ultrasound.* 1980;8:251.

123. Tabsh K. Antenatal sonographic appearance of a fetal ovarian cyst. *J Ultrasound Med.* 1982;1:329.

124. Sandler MA, Smith SJ, Pope SG, Madrazo BL. Prenatal diagnosis of septated ovarian cysts. *J Clin Ultrasound.* 1985;13:55.

125. Preziosi P, Fariello G, Maiorana A, Malena S, Ferro F. Antenatal sonographic diagnosis of complicated ovarian cysts. *J Clin Ultrasound.* 1986;14:196.

126. Westerhout FC Jr, Hodgman JE, Anderson G, et al. Congenital hydrocolpos. *Am J Obstet Gynecol.* 1964;89:957.

127. Gravier L. Hydrocolpos. *J Pediatr Surg.* 1969;4:563.

128. Reed MH, Griscom NT. Hydrometrocolpos in infancy. *AJR.* 1973;118:1.

129. Robinow M, Shaw A. The McKusick–Kaufman syndrome: Recessively inherited vaginal atresia, hydrometrocolpos, uterovaginal duplications, anorectal anomalies, postaxial polydactyly, and congenital heart disease. *J Pediatr.* 1979;94:776.

130. Davis GH, Wapner RJ, Kurtz AB, Chhibber G, Fitz-Simmons J, Blocklinger AJ. Antenatal diagnosis of hydrometrocolpos by ultrasound examination. *J Ultrasound Med.* 1984;3:371.

131. Hill SJ, Hirsch JH. Sonographic detection of fetal hydrometrocolpos. *J Ultrasound Med.* 1985;4:323.

132. Russ PD, Zavitz WR, Pretorius DH, et al. Hydrometrocolpos, uterus didelphys, and septate vagina: An antenatal sonographic diagnosis. *J Ultrasound Med.* 1986;5:211.

133. Giulian BB, Chang CCN, Yoss BS. Prenatal ultrasonographic diagnosis of fetal adrenal neuroblastoma. *J Clin Ultrasound.* 1986;14:225.

134. Atkinson GO, Zaatari GS, Lorenzo RL, et al. Cystic neuroblastoma in infants: Radiographic and pathologic features. *AJR.* 1986;146:113.

135. White SJ, Stuck KJ, Blane CE, et al. Sonography of neuroblastoma. *AJR.* 1983;141:465.

136. Moss TJ, Kaplan L. Association of hydrops fetalis with congenital neuroblastoma. *Am J Obstet Gynecol.* 1978;132:905.

137. Gadwood KA, Reynes CJ. Prenatal sonography of metastatic neuroblastoma. *J Clin Ultrasound.* 1983;11:512.

138. Cassady JR. A hypothesis to explain the enigmatic natural history of neuroblastomas. *Am J Dis Child.* 1982;136:370.

139. Bertagnoli L, Lalatta F, Gallicchio R, et al. Quantitative characterization of the growth of the kidneys. *J Clin Ultrasound.* 1983;11:349.

140. Allen KS, Arger PH, Mennuti M, Coleman BG, Mintz MC, Fishman M. Effects of maternal hydration on fetal renal pyelectasis. *Radiology.* 1987;163:807.

18 Fetal Skeletal Anomalies

Roberto Romero • Apostolos P. Athanassiadis • Marina Sirtori • Mona Inati

Skeletal dysplasias are a heterogeneous group of disorders of bone growth resulting in abnormal shape and size of the skeleton. The prenatal diagnosis of these disorders is a particularly challenging task. This chapter will review the birth prevalence and classification of skeletal dysplasias and provide an approach to the diagnosis of conditions identifiable at birth.

BIRTH PREVALENCE AND CONTRIBUTION TO PERINATAL MORTALITY

The birth prevalence of skeletal dysplasias, excluding limb amputations, recognizable in the neonatal period has been estimated to be 2.4/10,000 births.[1] In a large series, 23% of affected infants were stillbirths, and 32% died during the first week of life. The overall frequency of skeletal dysplasias among perinatal deaths was 9.1/1,000. The birth prevalence of the different skeletal dysplasias and their relative frequency among perinatal deaths in this study are shown in Table 18–1. The four most common skeletal dysplasias found were thanatophoric dysplasia, achondroplasia, osteogenesis imperfecta, and achondrogenesis. Thanatophoric dysplasia and achondrogenesis accounted for 62% of all lethal skeletal dysplasias.[1] The most common non-lethal skeletal dysplasia was achonodroplasia.

In another large series reporting the prevalence and classification of lethal neonatal skeletal dysplasias in West Scotland, the prevalence was 1.1/10,000 births, and the most frequently diagnosed conditions were thanatophoric dysplasia (1/42,000), osteogenesis imperfecta (1/56,000), rhizomelic chondrodysplasia punctata (1/84,000), campomelic syndrome (1/112,000), and achondrogenesis (1/112,000).[2]

CLASSIFICATION OF SKELETAL DYSPLASIAS

The existing nomenclature for skeletal dysplasias is complicated. There is a lack of uniformity about definition criteria. For example, some disorders are referred to by eponyms (eg, Ellis–van Creveld syndrome, Larsen dysplasia), by Greek terms describing a salient feature of the disease (diastrophic [twisted], metatropic [changeable]), or by a term related to the presumed pathogenesis of the disease (eg, osteogenesis imperfecta, achondrogenesis). The fundamental problem with any classification of skeletal dysplasias is that the pathogenesis of these diseases is largely unknown. Therefore, the current system relies on purely descriptive findings of either clinical or radiologic nature.

In an attempt to develop a uniform terminology, a group of experts met in Paris in 1977 and proposed an International Nomenclature for Skeletal Dysplasias that has been recently revised (Table 18–2).[3,4] The system subdivides the diseases into five different groups: (1) osteochondrodysplasias (abnormalities of cartilage and/or bone growth and development); (2) dysostoses (malformations of individual bones singly or in combination); (3) idiopathic osteolysis (disorders associated with multifocal resorption of bone); (4) skeletal disorders associated with chromosomal aberrations; and (5) primary metabolic disorders.

A comprehensive description of these diseases is beyond the scope of this chapter and the interested reader is referred to genetic textbooks for a full discussion on the subject. This chapter will focus primarily on the osteochondrodysplasias that are recognizable at birth. Although more than 200 skeletal dysplasias have been described and more will probably be identified as distinct entities, the number that can be recognized with the use of sonography in the antepartum period is considerably smaller. Most of these disorders result in short stature, and the term dwarfism has been used to refer to this clinical condition. However, this term carries a negative connotation and for this reason the term dysplasia is used instead.

BIOMETRY OF THE FETAL SKELETON IN THE DIAGNOSIS OF BONE DYSPLASIAS

Long bone biometry has been used extensively in the prediction of gestational age. Nomograms available for this purpose use the long bone as the independent variable and the estimated fetal age as the dependent vari-

TABLE 18–1. BIRTH PREVALENCE OF SKELETAL DYSPLASIAS

	Birth Prevalence (per 10,000)	Frequency among Perinatal Deaths
Thanatophoric dysplasia	0.69	1:246
Achondroplasia	0.37	—
Achondrogenesis	0.23	1:639
Osteogenesis imperfecta type II	0.18	1:799
Osteogenesis imperfecta, other types	0.18	—
Asphyxiating thoracic dysplasia	0.14	1:3196
Chrondrodysplasia punctata	0.09	—
Campomelic dysplasia	0.05	1:3196
Chondroectodermal dysplasia	0.05	1:3196
Larsen syndrome	0.05	—
Mesomelic dysplasia (Langer's type)	0.05	—
Others	0.46	1:800
Total skeletal dysplasias	**2.44**	**1:110**

(*Reproduced with permission from Camera G, Mastroiacovo P. Birth prevalence of skeletal dysplasias in the Italian multicentric monitoring system for birth defects. In: Papadatos CJ, Bartsocas CS, eds.* Skeletal Dysplasias. *New York: Alan R Liss; 1982:441.*)

able. However, the type of nomogram required to assess the normality of bone dimensions uses the gestational age as the independent variable and the long bone as the dependent variable. For the proper use of these nomograms, the clinician must accurately know the gestational age of the fetus. Therefore, patients at risk for skeletal dysplasias should be advised to seek prenatal care at an early gestational age to assess all clinical estimators of gestational age. Tables 18–3 and 18–4 present nomograms for the assessment of limb biometry for the upper and lower extremities, respectively. For those patients presenting with uncertain gestational age, comparisons between limb dimensions and the head perimeter can be used (Figs. 18–1 and 18–2). Other authors have employed the biparietal diameter for this purpose. The head perimeter has the advantage of being shape-independent. A limitation of this approach is that it assumes that the cranium is not involved in the dysplastic process, and this may not be the case in some skeletal dysplasias.

The nomograms and figures in this chapter provide the mean, 5th, and 95th percentiles of limb biometric parameters. The reader should be aware that 5% of the general population will fall outside these boundaries. Ideally, a more stringent criterion, such as the 1st percentile of limb growth for gestational age, should be used for diagnosis. Unfortunately, none of the currently available nomograms has been based on enough patients to provide

an accurate discrimination between the 5th and the 1st percentiles. However, most skeletal dysplasias diagnosed in utero or at birth are associated with dramatic long bone shortening, and under these circumstances the precise boundary used (1st or 5th percentile) will not be critical. An exception to this is achondroplasia, in which limb biometry is mildly affected until the third trimester when abnormal growth can be detected by examining the slope of growth of femur length.[5]

TERMINOLOGY FREQUENTLY USED IN THE DESCRIPTION OF BONE DYSPLASIAS

Shortening of the extremities can involve the entire limb (micromelia), the proximal segment (rhizomelia), the intermediate segment (mesomelia), or the distal segment (acromelia). The diagnosis of rhizomelia or mesomelia requires the comparison of the dimensions of the bones of the legs and forearm with those of the thigh and arm. Figures 18–3 and 18–4 display the relationships between the humerus and ulna, and the femur and tibia, and can be used in the assessment of rhizomelia and acromesomelia. Table 18–5 presents skeletal dysplasias characterized by rhizomelia, mesomelia, acromelia, and micromelia.

Several skeletal dysplasias feature alterations of the hands and feet. Polydactyly refers to the presence of more than five digits. It is classified as postaxial if the extra digits are on the ulnar or fibular side, and preaxial if they are located on the radial or tibial side. Syndactyly refers to soft tissue or bony fusion of adjacent digits. Clinodactyly consists of deviation of a finger(s). The most common spinal abnormality seen in skeletal dysplasias is platyspondyly, which consists of flattening of the vertebrae. The antenatal detection of this sign has not been reported. Kyphosis and scoliosis can also be identified in utero (Fig. 18–5). Prenatal diagnosis of congenital hemivertebra has been recently reported (Fig. 18–6).[6]

CLINICAL PRESENTATION

The challenge of the antenatal diagnosis of skeletal dysplasias will generally present itself in one of two ways: (1) a patient who has delivered an infant with a skeletal dysplasia and desires antenatal assessment of a subsequent pregnancy, or (2) the incidental finding of a shortened, bowed, or anomalous extremity during a routine sonographic examination. The task is easier when a particular phenotype is looked for in a patient at risk. The inability to obtain reliable information about skeletal mineralization and the involvement of other systems (eg, skin)

TABLE 18–2. INTERNATIONAL CLASSIFICATION FOR DYSPLASIAS

	Mode of Transmission	Frequency		Mode of Transmission	Frequency
OSTEOCHONDRODYSPLASIAS Abnormalities of cartilage and/or bone growth and development			21. Acromesomelic dyplasia	AR	**
			22. Cleidocranial dysplasia	AD	****
A. Defects of growth of tubular bones and/or spine			23. Otopalatodigital syndrome		
Identifiable at birth			a. Type I (Langer)	XLSD	**
Usually lethal before or shortly after birth			b. Type II (André)	XLR	**
1. Achondrogenesis type I (Parenti–Fraccaro)	AR	**	24. Larsen syndrome	AR, AD	**
2. Achondrogenesis type II (Langer–Saldino)		**	25. Other multiple dislocation syndromes (Desbuquois)	AR	
3. Hypochondrogenesis		*	*Identifiable in late life*		
4. Fibrochondrogenesis	AR	*	1. Hypochondroplasia	AD	***
5. Thanatophoric dysplasia		***	2. Dyschondrosteosis	AD	***
6. Thanatophoric dysplasia with cloverleaf skull		**	3. Metaphyseal chondrodysplasia type Jansen	AD	*
7. Atelosteogenesis		*	4. Metaphyseal chondrodysplasia type Schmid	AD	**
8. Short rib syndrome (with or without polydactyly)			5. Metaphyseal chondrodysplasia type McKusick	AR	**
a. Type I (Saldino–Noonan)	AR	**	6. Metaphyseal chondrodysplasia with exocrine pancreatic insufficiency and cyclic neutropenia	AR	**
b. Type II (Majewski)	AR	*	7. Spondylometaphyseal dysplasia		
c. Type III (lethal thoracic dysplasia)	AR	*	a. Type Kozlowski	AD	**
Usually nonlethal dysplasia			b. Other forms		***
9. Chondrodysplasia punctata			8. Multiple epiphyseal dysplasia		
a. Rhizomelic form autosomal recessive	AR	**	a. Type Fairbank	AD	****
b. Dominant X-linked form; lethal in male	XLD	**	b. Other forms		***
c. Common mild form (Sheffield)			9. Multiple epiphyseal dysplasia with early diabetes (Wolcott–Rallisson)	AR	**
Exclude: symptomatic stippling (warfarin, chromosomal aberration)			10. Arthro-ophthalmopathy (Stickler)	AR	***
10. Campomelic dysplasia		**	11. Pseudoachondroplasia		
11. Kyphomelic dysplasia	AR	*	a. Dominant	AD	***
12. Achondroplasia	AD	****	b. Recessive	AR	**
13. Diastrophic dysplasia	AR	***	12. Spondyloepiphyseal dysplasia tarda (X-linked recessive)	XLR	**
14. Metatropic dysplasia (several forms)	AR, AD	**	13. Progressive pseudorheumatoid chondrodysplasia	AR	**
15. Chrondroectrodermal dysplasia (Ellis–Van Creveld)	AR	***	14. Spondyloepiphyseal dysplasia, other forms		***
16. Asphyxiating thoracic dysplasia (Jeune)	AR	**	15. Brachyolmia		
17. Spondyloepiphyseal dysplasia congenita			a. Autosomal recessive	AR	*
a. Autosomal dominant form	AD	**	b. Autosomal dominant	AD	*
b. Autosomal recessive form	AR	**	16. Dyggve–Melchior–Clausen dysplasia	AR	**
18. Kniest dysplasia	AR	**	17. Spondyloepimetaphyseal dysplasia (several forms)		***
19. Dyssegmental dysplasia	AR	*	18. Spondyloepimetaphyseal dysplasia with joint laxity	AR	**
20. Mesomelic dysplasia			19. Otospondylomegaepiphyseal dysplasia (OSMED)	AR	*
a. Type Nievegelt	AD	*	20. Myotonic chondrodysplasia (Catel–Schwartz–Jampel)	AR	**
b. Type Langer (probable homozygous dyschondrosteosis)	AR	*	21. Parastremmatic dysplasia	A	*
c. Type Robinow		*	22. Trichorhinophalangeal dysplasia	AD	**
d. Type Rheinardt	AD	*			
e. Others		***			

(cont.)

TABLE 18–2. Continued

	Mode of Transmission	Frequency
23. Acrodysplasia with retinitis pigmentosa and nephropathy (Saldino–Mainzer)	AR	**
B. Disorganized development of cartilage and fibrous components of skeleton		
1. Dysplasia epiphyseal hemimelica		**
2. Multiple cartilaginous exestoses	AD	***
3. Acrodysplasia with exostoses (Giedion–Langer)		**
4. Enchondromatosis (Ollier)		***
5. Enchondromatosis with hemangioma (Maffucci)		**
6. Metachondromatosis	AD	**
7. Spondyloenchondroplasia	AR	*
8. Osteoglophonic dysplasia		*
9. Fibrous dysplasia (Jaffe–Lichtenstein)		***
10. Fibrous dysplasia with skin pigmentation and precocious puberty (McCune–Albright)		***
11. Cherubism (familial fibrous dysplasia of the jaws)	AD	**
C. Abnormalities of density of cortical diaphyseal structure and/or metaphyseal modeling		
1. Osteogenesis imperfecta (several forms)	AD, AR	****
2. Juvenile idiopathic osteoporosis		**
3. Osteoporosis with pseudoglioma	AR	*
4. Osterpetrosis		
a. Autosomal recessive lethal	AR	**
b. Intermediate recessive	AR	**
c. Autosomal dominant	AD	***
d. Recessive with tubular acidosis	AR	**
5. Pycnodysostosis	AR	***
6. Dominant osteosclerosis type Stanescu	AD	**
7. Osteomesopycnosis	AD	**
8. Osteopoikilosis	AD	***
9. Osteopathia striata	AD	***
10. Osteopathia striata with cranial sclerosis	AD	**
11. Melorheostosis		***
12. Diaphyseal dysplasia (Camurati–Engelmann)	AD	***
13. Craniodiaphyseal dysplasia	AR	**
14. Endosteal hyperostosis		
a. Autosomal dominant (Worth)	AD	**
b. Autosomal recessive (Van Buchem)	AR	**
c. Autosomal recessive (sclerosteosis)	AR	**

	Mode of Transmission	Frequency
15. Tubular stenosis (Kenny–Caffey)	AD	*
16. Pachydermoperiostosis	AD	**
17. Osteodysplasty (Melnick–Needles)	AD	**
18. Frontometaphyseal dysplasia	XLR	**
19. Craniometaphyseal dysplasia (several forms)	AD	***
20. Metaphyseal dysplasia (Pyle)	AR or AD	**
21. Dysosteosclerosis	AR or XLR	**
22. Osteo-sctasia with hyperphosphatasia	AR	**
23. Oculo-dento-osseous dysplasia		
a. Mild type	AD	***
b. Severe type	AR	*
24. Infantile cortical hyperostosis (Caffey disease, familial type)	AD	**

DYSOSTOSES
Malformation of individual bones, singly or in combination

	Mode of Transmission	Frequency
A. Dysostoses with cranial and facial involvement		
1. Craniosynostosis (several forms)		***
2. Craniofacial dysostosis (Crouzon)		***
3. Acrocephalosyndactyly		
a. Type Apert	AD	***
b. Type Chotzen	AD	**
c. Type Pfeiffer	AD	**
d. Other types		***
4. Acrocephalopolysyndactyly (Carpenter and others)	AR	**
5. Cephalopolysyndactyly (Greig)	AD	*
6. First and second branchial arch syndromes		
a. Mandibulofacial dysotosis (Treacher Collins, Franceschetti)	AD	***
b. Acrofacial dysostosis (Nager)		**
c. Oculo-auriculo-vertebral dysostosis (Goldenhar)	AR	***
d. Hemifacial microsomia		***
e. Others (Probably parts of a large spectrum)		
7. Oculomandibulofacial syndrome (Hallermann–Streiff–François)		
B. Dysostoses with predominant axial involvement		
1. Vertebral segmentation defects (including Kippel–Feil)		**
2. Cervico-oculo-acoustic syndrome (Wildervanck)		***
3. Sprengel anomaly		***

(cont.)

TABLE 18–2. Continued

	Mode of Trans- mission	Fre- quency		Mode of Trans- mission	Fre- quency
4. Spondylocostal dysostosis			**IDIOPATHIC OSTEOLYSES**		
a. Dominant form	AD	**	1. Phalangeal (several forms)		**
b. Recessive form	AR	**	2. Tarsocarpal		
5. Oculovertebral syndrome (Weyers)		*	a. Including François form and others	AR	**
6. Osteo-onychodysostosis	AD	***	b. With nephropathy	AD	**
7. Cerebrocostomandibular syn- drome	AR	**	3. Multicentric		
			a. Hajdu–Cheney form	AD	**
C. Dysostoses with predominant in- volvement of extremities			b. Winchester form	AR	*
1. Acheiria		**	c. Torg form	AR	*
2. Apodia		**	d. Other forms		**
3. Tetraphocomelia syndrome (Robert's) (SC pseudothali- domide syndrome)	AR	**	**MISCELLANEOUS DISORDER WITH OSSEOUS INVOLVEMENT**		
4. Ectrodactyly			1. Early acceleration of skeletal maturation		
a. Isolated		***	a. Marshall–Smith syndrome		*
b. Ectrodactyly-ectodermal dysplasia, cleft palate syn- drome	AD	**	b. Weaver syndrome		*
			c. Other types		*
c. Ectrodactyly with scalp de- fects	AD	**	2. Marfan syndrome	AD	****
5. Oro-acral syndrome (aglossia syndrome, Hanhart syn- drome)		*	3. Congenital contractural arach- nodactyly	AD	**
6. Familial radioulnar synostosis		**	4. Cerebrohepatorneal syndrome (Zellweger)		**
7. Brachydactyly, types A, B, C, D, E (Bell's classification)	AD	****	5. Coffin–Lowry syndrome	SLR	**
8. Symphalangism	AD	***	6. Cockayne syndrome	AR	**
9. Polydactyly (several forms)		****	7. Fibrodysplasia ossificans con- genita	AD	***
10. Syndactyly (several forms)		****	8. Epidermal nervus syndrome (Solomon)		**
11. Polysyndactyly (several forms)		***			
12. Camptodactyly		****	9. Nevoid basal cell carcinoma syndrome		**
13. Manzke syndrome		*	10. Multiple hereditary fibromato- sis		**
14. Poland syndrome		***			
15. Rubinstein–Taybi syndrome		**	11. Neurofibromatosis	AD	****
16. Coffin–Siris syndrome		**			
17. Pancytopenia-dysmelia syn- drome (Franconi)	AR	***	**CHROMOSOMAL ABERRATIONS** Primary Metabolic Abnormalities		
18. Blackfan–Diamond anemia with thumb anomalies (Aase'e syndrome)	AR	**	**A. Calcium and/or phosphorus**		
			1. Hypophosphatemic rickets	XLD	****
19. Thrombocytopenia-radial- aplasia syndrome	AR	**	2. Vitamin D dependency or pseudodeficiency rickets		
20. Orodigitofacial syndrome			a. Type I with probable defi- ciency in 25-hydroxy vita- min D 1-alpha-hydroxlase	AR	***
a. Type Papillon–Leage; le- thal in males	XLD	**			
b. Type Mohr	AR	**	b. Type II with target-organ resistancy	AR	**
21. Cardiomelic syndromes (Holt– Oram and others)	AD	***	3. Late rickets (McCance)		**
			4. Idiopathic hypercalciuria		***
22. Femoral focal deficiency (with or without facial anomalies)		**	5. Hypophosphatasia (several forms)	AR	***
23. Multiple synostoses (includes some forms of symphalan- gism)	AD	***	6. Pseudohypoparathyroidism (normo- and hypocalcemic forms, including acrodysosto- sis)	AD	***
24. Scapulo-iliac dysostosis (Kosenow–Sinios)	AD	**			
25. Hand-foot-genital syndrome	AD	**	**B. Complex carbohydrates**		
26. Focal dermal hypoplasia (Goltz); lethal in males	XLD	**	1. Mucopolysaccharidosis type I (alpha-L-iduronidase defi- ciency)		

(cont.)

TABLE 18–2. Continued

	Mode of Transmission	Frequency		Mode of Transmission	Frequency
a. Hurler form	AR	***	11. Multiple sulfatases deficiency (Austin–Thieffry)	AR	**
b. Scheie form	AR	**	12. Isolated neuraminidase deficiency; several forms including		**
c. Other forms	AR	**	a. Mucolipidosis I	AR	
2. Mucopolysaccharidosis type II—Hunter (sulfoiduronate sulfatase deficiency)	XLR	***	b. Nephrosialidosis	AR	
3. Mucopolysaccharidosis type III—Sanfilippo		***	c. Cherry red spot myoclonia syndrome	AR	
a. Type III A (heparin sulfamidase deficiency	AR		13. Phosphotransferase deficiency; several forms including		**
b. Type III B (N-acetyl-alpha-glucosaminidase	AR		a. Mucolipidosis II (I cell disease)	AR	
c. Type III C (alpha-glucos-aminide-N-acetyl transferase deficiency)	AR		b. Mucolipidosis III (pseudo-polydystrophy)	AR	
d. Type III D (N-acetyl-glucos-amine-6 sulfate sulfatase deficiency)	AR		14. Combined neuraminidase beta-galactosidase deficiency	AR	*
4. Mucopolysaccharidosis type IV		**	15. Salla disease	AR	*
a. Type IV A—Morquio (N-acetyl-galactosamine-6 sulfate sulfatase deficiency	AR		**C. Lipids**		
b. Type IV B (beta-galactosidase deficiency)	AR		1. Niemann–Pick disease (sphingomyelinase deficiency) (several forms)	AR	***
5. Mucopolysaccharidosis type VI—Maroteaux–Lany (arylsulfatase B deficiency)	AR		2. Gaucher disease (beta-glucosidase deficiency) (several types)	AR	****
6. Mucopolysaccharidosis type VII (beta-glucuronidase deficiency)	AR	**	3. Farber disease lipogranulomatosis (ceraminidase deficiency)	AR	**
7. Aspartyl glucosaminuria (aspartylglucosaminidase deficiency)	AR	**	**D. Nucleic acids**		
8. Mannosidosis (alpha-mannosidase deficiency)	AR	**	1. Adenosine-deaminase deficiency and others	AR	**
9. Fucosidosis (alpha-fucosidase deficiency)	AR	**	**E. Amino acids**		
10. GMI-Gangliosidosis (beta-galactosidase deficiency) (several forms)	AR	**	1. Homocystinuria and others	AR	***
			F. Metals		
			1. Menkes syndrome (kinky hair syndrome and others)	AR	***

Mode of transmission: AR = autosomal recessive; XLD = X-linked dominant; AD = autosomal dominant; XLR = X-linked recessive; SLR = sex-linked recessive.
Frequency: **** = 1000+ cases; *** = 100–1000 cases; ** = 20–100 cases; * = fewer than 20 cases. Estimates of the relative frequency of these conditions are based on the compilers' experience and a review of the literature.
(*Reproduced with permission from Kozlowski K, Beighton P.* Gamut Index of Skeletal Dysplasias (An aid to Radiodiagnosis). *Berlin: Springer-Verlag; 1986.*)

with sonography is a limiting factor in the establishment of an accurate diagnosis after the identification of an incidental finding. Another limitation is the paucity of information about the in utero natural history of these disorders.

Despite these difficulties and limitations, there are good medical reasons for attempting an accurate prenatal diagnosis of skeletal dysplasias. A number of these disorders are uniformly lethal, and a confident antenatal diagnosis would present the patient with options for the termination of the pregnancy. Table 18–6 lists such disorders. Other skeletal dysplasias are associated with men-

TABLE 18–3. NORMAL VALUES FOR THE ARM (mm)

Week No.	Humerus (percentile)			Ulna (percentile)			Radius (percentile)		
	5th	50th	95th	5th	50th	95th	5th	50th	95th
12	–	9	–	–	7	–	–	7	–
13	6	11	16	5	10	15	6	10	14
14	9	14	19	8	13	18	8	13	17
15	12	17	22	11	16	21	11	15	20
16	15	20	25	13	18	23	13	18	22
17	18	22	27	16	21	26	14	20	26
18	20	25	30	19	24	29	15	22	29
19	23	28	33	21	26	31	20	24	29
20	25	30	35	24	29	34	22	27	32
21	28	33	38	26	31	36	24	29	33
22	30	35	40	28	33	38	27	31	34
23	33	38	42	31	36	41	26	32	39
24	35	40	45	33	38	43	26	34	42
25	37	42	47	35	40	45	31	36	41
26	39	44	49	37	42	47	32	37	43
27	41	46	51	39	44	49	33	39	45
28	43	48	53	41	46	51	33	40	48
29	45	50	55	43	48	53	36	42	47
30	47	51	56	44	49	54	36	43	49
31	48	53	58	46	51	56	38	44	50
32	50	55	60	48	53	58	37	45	53
33	51	56	61	49	54	59	41	46	51
34	53	58	63	51	56	61	40	47	53
35	54	59	64	52	57	62	41	48	54
36	56	61	65	53	58	63	39	48	57
37	57	62	67	55	60	65	45	49	53
38	59	63	68	56	61	66	45	49	54
39	60	65	70	57	62	67	45	50	54
40	61	66	71	58	63	68	46	50	55

tal retardation,[7] and this information is important in prenatal counseling. There is a group of disorders associated with thrombocytopenia. Vaginal delivery may expose these infants to the risk of intracranial hemorrhage.

APPROACH TO THE DIAGNOSIS OF SKELETAL DYSPLASIAS

Our approach to the diagnosis of skeletal dysplasias follows an organized plan of examination of the fetal skeleton which is performed in the following manner:

Evaluation of Long Bones. All long bones should be measured in all extremities. Comparisons with other seg-

ments should be performed to establish whether the limb shortening is predominantly rhizomelic, mesomelic, acromelic, or involves all segments (Fig. 18–7). A detailed examination of each bone is necessary to exclude the absence or hypoplasia of individual bones (fibula, tibia, scapula, radius), which are frequently absent in certain conditions.[8–11]

An attempt should be made to characterize the degree of mineralization. This can be assessed by examining the acoustic shadow behind the bone and the echogenicity of the bone itself. It should be stressed that there are limitations in the sonographic evaluation of mineralization of long bones and that other structures, such as the skull, are perhaps better suited for this assessment (Fig. 18–8). The degree of long bone curvature should be

TABLE 18–4. NORMAL VALUES FOR THE LEG (mm)

Week No.	Tibia (percentile)			Fibula (percentile)			Femur (percentile)		
	5th	50th	95th	5th	50th	95th	5th	50th	95th
12	–	7	–	–	6	–	4	8	13
13	–	10	–	–	9	–	6	11	16
14	7	12	17	6	12	19	9	14	18
15	9	15	20	9	15	21	12	17	21
16	12	17	22	13	18	23	15	20	24
17	15	20	25	13	21	28	18	23	27
18	17	22	27	15	23	31	21	25	30
19	20	25	30	19	26	33	24	28	33
20	22	27	33	21	28	36	26	31	36
21	25	30	35	24	31	37	29	34	38
22	27	32	38	27	33	39	32	36	41
23	30	35	40	28	35	42	35	39	44
24	32	37	42	29	37	45	37	42	46
25	34	40	45	34	40	45	40	44	49
26	37	42	47	36	42	47	42	47	51
27	39	44	49	37	44	50	45	49	54
28	41	46	51	38	45	53	47	52	56
29	43	48	53	41	47	54	50	54	59
30	45	50	55	43	49	56	52	56	61
31	47	52	57	42	51	59	54	59	63
32	48	54	59	42	52	63	56	61	65
33	50	55	60	46	54	62	58	63	67
34	52	57	62	46	55	65	60	65	69
35	53	58	64	51	57	62	62	67	71
36	55	60	65	54	58	63	64	68	73
37	56	61	67	54	59	65	65	70	74
38	58	63	68	56	61	65	67	71	76
39	59	64	69	56	62	67	68	73	77
40	61	66	71	59	63	67	70	74	79

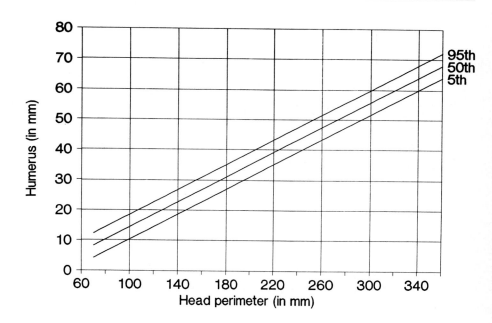

Fig. 18–1. Relationship between the head perimeter and the humerus.

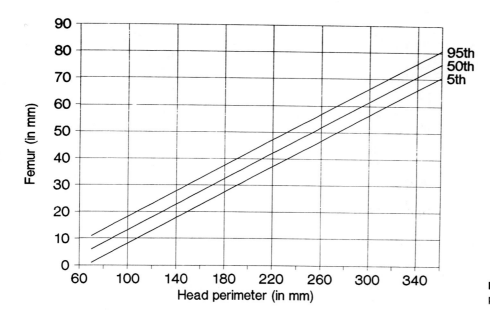

Fig. 18–2. Relationship between the head perimeter and the femur.

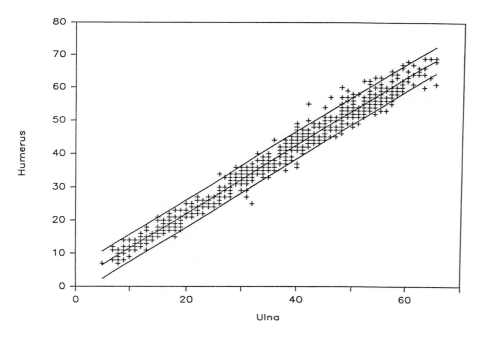

Fig. 18–3. Relationship between the ulna and the humerus.

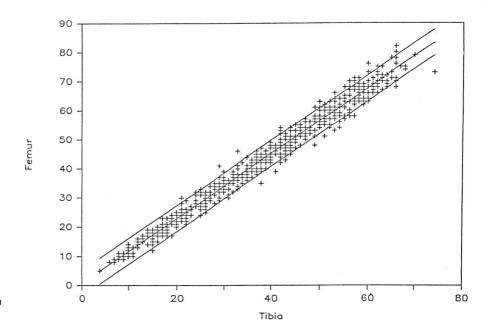

Fig. 18–4. Relationship between the tibia and the femur.

TABLE 18–5. CLASSIFICATION OF SKELETAL DYSPLASIAS BY RHIZOMELIA, MESOMELIA, ACROMELIA, AND MICROMELIA

Rhizomelia
Thanatophoric dysplasia
Atelosteogenesis
Chondrodysplasia punctata (rhizomelic type)
Diastrophic dysplasia
Congenital short femur
Achondroplasia

Mesomelia
Mesomelic dysplasia (Langer, Reinhardt, and Robinow types)
COVESDEM association

Acromelia
Ellis–van Creveld syndrome (Chondroectodermal dysplasia)

Micromelia
Achondrogenesis
Atelosteogenesis
Short rib-polydactyly syndrome (type I and type II)
Diastrophic dysplasia
Fibrochondrogenesis
Osteogenesis imperfecta (type III)
Kniest dysplasia
Dyssegmental dysplasia
Robert's syndrome

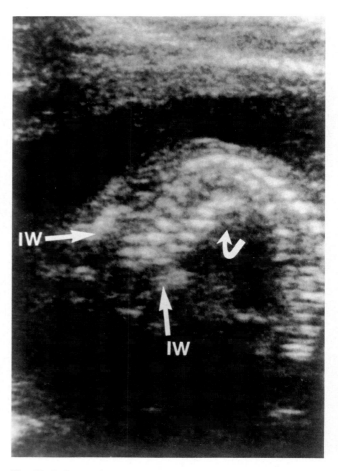

Fig. 18–5. Coronal scan demonstrating severe scoliosis (*curved arrow*). IW = iliac wings.

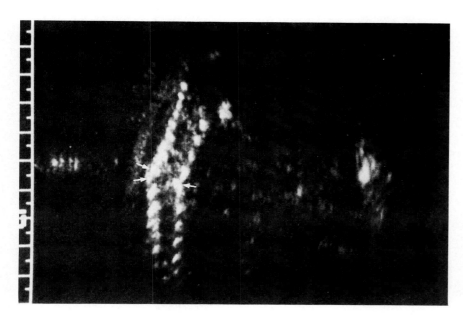

Fig. 18–6. Hemivertebra. Longitudinal view of the lower thoracic spine showing the two abnormal ossification centers of the posterior elements, opposite a single ossification center. (*Reproduced with permission from Benacerraf et al. J Ultrasound Med 1986; 5:257.*)

examined. At present, there is no objective means of assessing this sign, and experience is the only means by which the operator can discern the boundary between normality and abnormality. Campomelia (excessive bowing) is characteristic of certain disorders (eg, campomelic dysplasia). Finally, the possibility of fractures should also be considered, as they can be detected in some conditions (eg, osteogenesis imperfecta). The fractures may be extremely subtle or may lead to angulation and separation of the segments of the affected bone (Figs. 18–9 and 18–10).

Evaluation of Thoracic Dimensions. Several skeletal dysplasias are associated with a hypoplastic thorax. Such a finding is extremely important because chest restriction leads to pulmonary hypoplasia, a frequent cause of death in these conditions. The appropriateness of thoracic dimensions can be assessed by measuring the thoracic cir-

cumference at the level of the four-chamber view of the heart. The thoracic circumference can be measured or calculated using the formula: thoracic circumference = (anteroposterior diameter + transverse diameter) × 1.57. The thoracic length is measured from the boundary between the neck and the chest and the diaphragm. Tables 18–7 and 18–8 illustrate nomograms used to evaluate the thoracic dimensions in fetuses with known gestational age. When gestational age is uncertain, age-independent ratios can be used. The thoracic-to-abdominal circumference ratio (normal value: 0.77 to 1.01) and the thoracic-to-head circumference ratio (normal value: 0.56 to 1.04) permit evaluation of the transverse thoracic dimensions.[12]

Evaluation of thoracic dimensions is a critical part of the work-up because the cause of death in most lethal skeletal dysplasias is pulmonary hypoplasia secondary to an underdeveloped rib cage (Figs. 18–11 through 18–14). Table 18–9 displays skeletal dysplasias associated with alteration of thoracic dimensions.

Evaluation of Hands and Feet. Hands and feet should be examined to exclude polydactyly and syndactyly (Figs. 18–14 and 18–15) as well as extreme postural deformities such as those seen in diastrophic dysplasia (Fig. 18–16). Table 18–10 shows a nomogram of the fetal foot size throughout gestation. Table 18–11 displays disorders associated with hand and feet deformities. Disproportion between hands and feet and the other parts of the extremity may also be a sign of a skeletal dysplasia. Figure 18–17 illustrates the relationship between the femur length and foot length. The femur length:foot length ratio

TABLE 18–6. LETHAL SKELETAL DYSPLASIAS

Achondrogenesis
Thanatophoric dysplasia
Short rib polydactyly syndromes (types I, II, and III)
Fibrochondrogenesis
Atelosteogenesis
Homozygous achondroplasia
Osteogenesis imperfecta, perinatal type
Hypophosphatasia

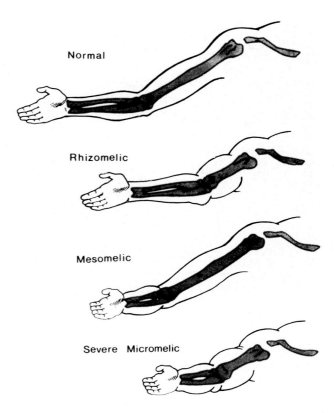

Fig. 18–7. Varieties of short limb dysplasia according to the segment involved.

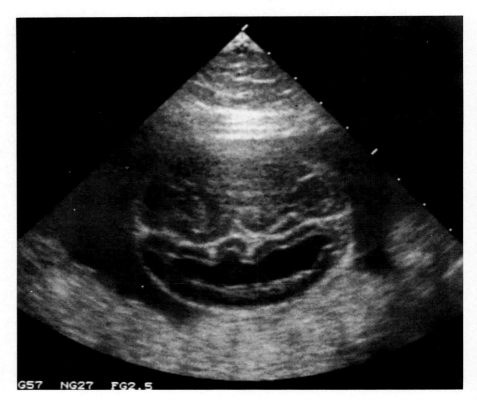

Fig. 18–8. Demineralization of the skull in a case of congenital hypophosphatasia.

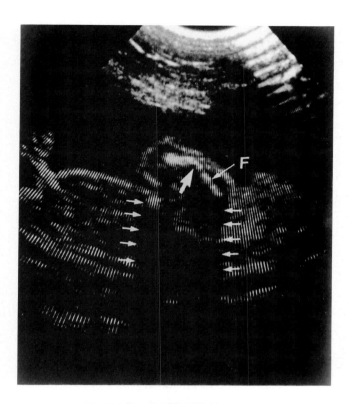

Fig. 18–9. In utero fracture in a case of osteogenesis imperfecta. The *large arrow* corresponds to the fracture site. The *small arrows* outline the decreased shadowing cast by the bone. F = femur.

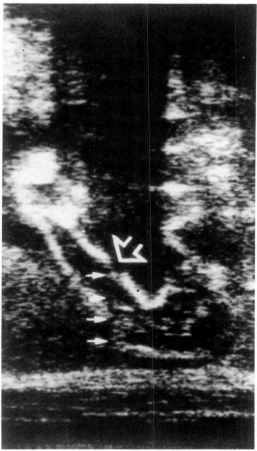

Fig. 18–10. Potential pitfall. Shadowing from an upper extremity (*arrows*) creates the false image of a femur fracture (*open arrow*).

TABLE 18–7. FETAL THORACIC CIRCUMFERENCE MEASUREMENTS (cm)

Gestational Age (wk)	Sample No.	Predictive Percentiles								
		2.5	5	10	25	50	75	90	95	97.5
16	6	5.9	6.4	7.0	8.0	9.1	10.3	11.3	11.9	12.4
17	22	6.8	7.3	7.9	8.9	10.0	11.2	12.2	12.8	13.3
18	31	7.7	8.2	8.8	9.8	11.0	12.1	13.1	13.7	14.2
19	21	8.6	9.1	9.7	10.7	11.9	13.0	14.0	14.6	15.1
20	20	9.5	10.0	10.6	11.7	12.8	13.9	15.0	15.5	16.0
21	30	10.4	11.0	11.6	12.6	13.7	14.8	15.8	16.4	16.9
22	18	11.3	11.9	12.5	13.5	14.6	15.7	16.7	17.3	17.8
23	21	12.2	12.8	13.4	14.4	15.5	16.6	17.6	18.2	18.8
24	27	13.2	13.7	14.3	15.3	16.4	17.5	18.5	19.1	19.7
25	20	14.1	14.6	15.2	16.2	17.3	18.4	19.4	20.0	20.6
26	25	15.0	15.5	16.1	17.1	18.2	19.3	20.3	21.0	21.5
27	24	15.9	16.4	17.0	18.0	19.1	20.2	21.3	21.9	22.4
28	24	16.8	17.3	17.9	18.9	20.0	21.2	22.2	22.8	23.3
29	24	17.7	18.2	18.8	19.8	21.0	22.1	23.1	23.7	24.2
30	27	18.6	19.1	19.7	20.7	21.9	23.0	24.0	24.6	25.1
31	24	19.5	20.0	20.6	21.6	22.8	23.9	24.9	25.5	26.0
32	28	20.4	20.9	21.5	22.6	23.7	24.8	25.8	26.4	26.9
33	27	21.3	21.8	22.5	23.5	24.6	25.7	26.7	27.3	27.8
34	25	22.2	22.8	23.4	24.4	25.5	26.6	27.6	28.2	28.7
35	20	23.1	23.7	24.3	25.3	26.4	27.5	28.5	29.1	29.6
36	23	24.0	24.6	25.2	26.2	27.3	28.4	29.4	30.0	30.6
37	22	24.9	25.5	26.1	27.1	28.2	29.3	30.3	30.9	31.5
38	21	25.9	26.4	27.0	28.0	29.1	30.2	31.2	31.9	32.4
39	7	26.8	27.3	27.9	28.9	30.0	31.1	32.2	32.8	33.3
40	6	27.7	28.2	28.8	29.8	20.9	32.1	33.1	33.7	34.2

(Reproduced with permission from Chitkara U, Rosenberg J, Chervenak FA, et al. Am J Obstet Gynecol. 1987;156:1069.)

is nearly constant from the 14th to 40th week. The mean is 0.99 (SD = 0.06). A ratio below 0.87 should be considered abnormal.[13] Although fetuses with skeletal dysplasias have been reported to have abnormally low ratios, more experience is required to test the diagnostic value of this method.[14] It is expected that a small proportion of normal fetuses may have an abnormal ratio. As in the cause of other limb biometric parameters, large deviations from the lower limit of normal are likely to be significant.

Evaluation of the Fetal Cranium. Several skeletal dysplasias are associated with defects of membranous ossification and, therefore, affect skull bones. Orbits should be measured to exclude hypertelorism.[15,16] Other findings that should be searched for are micrognathia,[17] short upper lip, abnormally shaped ear,[18] frontal bossing (Fig. 18–18), and cloverleaf skull deformity (Figs. 18–19 and 18–20). Table 18–12 presents abnormalities of the skull and face in the different skeletal dysplasias.

Despite all efforts to establish an accurate prenatal

diagnosis, a careful study of the newborn will be required in all instances. The evaluation should include a detailed physical examination performed by a geneticist or an individual with experience in the field of skeletal dysplasias and radiograms of the skeleton. The latter should include anterior, posterior, lateral, and Towne views of the skull and antero-posterior views of the spine and extremities, with separate films of hands and feet. Examination of the skeletal radiographs will permit precise diagnoses in the overwhelming majority of cases, because the classification of skeletal dysplasias is largely based on radiographic findings. In lethal skeletal dysplasias, histologic examination of the chondro-osseous tissue should be included, as this information may help reach a specific diagnosis. Chromosomal studies should be included because there is a specific group of constitutional bone disorders associated with cytogenetic abnormalities. Biochemical studies are helpful in rare instances (eg, hypophosphatasia). DNA restrictions and enzymatic activity assays should be considered in those cases in which the phenotype suggests a metabolic disorder such as a mucopolysaccharidosis.

TABLE 18–8. FETAL THORACIC LENGTH MEASUREMENTS (cm)

Gestational Age (wk)	Sample No.	Predictive Percentiles								
		2.5	5	10	25	50	75	90	95	97.5
16	6	0.9	1.1	1.3	1.6	2.0	2.4	2.8	3.0	3.2
17	22	1.1	1.3	1.5	1.8	2.2	2.6	3.0	3.2	3.4
18	31	1.3	1.4	1.7	2.0	2.4	2.8	3.2	3.4	3.6
19	21	1.4	1.6	1.8	2.2	2.7	3.0	3.4	3.6	3.8
20	20	1.6	1.8	2.0	2.4	2.8	3.2	3.6	3.8	4.0
21	30	1.8	2.0	2.2	2.6	3.0	3.4	3.7	4.0	4.1
22	18	2.0	2.2	2.4	2.8	3.2	3.6	3.9	4.1	4.3
23	21	2.2	2.4	2.6	3.0	3.4	3.8	4.1	4.3	4.5
24	27	2.4	2.6	2.8	3.1	3.5	3.9	4.3	4.5	4.7
25	20	2.6	2.8	3.0	3.3	3.7	4.1	4.5	4.7	4.9
26	25	2.8	2.9	3.2	3.5	3.9	4.3	4.7	4.9	5.1
27	24	2.9	3.1	3.3	3.7	4.1	4.5	4.9	5.1	5.3
28	24	3.1	3.3	3.5	3.9	4.3	4.7	5.0	5.4	5.4
29	24	3.3	3.5	3.7	4.1	4.5	4.9	5.2	5.5	5.6
30	27	3.5	3.7	3.9	4.3	4.7	5.1	5.4	5.6	5.8
31	24	3.7	3.9	4.1	4.5	4.9	5.3	5.6	5.8	6.0
32	28	3.9	4.1	4.3	4.6	5.0	5.4	5.8	6.0	6.2
33	27	4.1	4.3	4.5	4.8	5.2	5.6	6.0	6.2	6.4
34	25	4.2	4.4	4.7	5.0	5.4	5.8	6.2	6.4	6.6
35	20	4.4	4.6	4.8	5.2	5.6	6.0	6.4	6.6	6.8
36	23	4.6	4.8	5.0	5.4	5.8	6.2	6.5	6.8	7.0
37	22	4.8	5.0	5.2	5.6	6.0	6.4	6.7	7.0	7.1
38	21	5.0	5.2	5.4	5.8	6.2	6.6	6.9	7.1	7.3
39	7	5.2	5.4	5.6	6.0	6.4	6.8	7.1	7.3	7.5
40	6	5.4	5.6	5.8	6.1	6.5	6.9	7.3	7.5	7.7

(*Reproduced with permission from Chitkara U, Rosenberg J, Chervenak FA, et al. Am J Obstet Gynecol. 1987;156:1069.*)

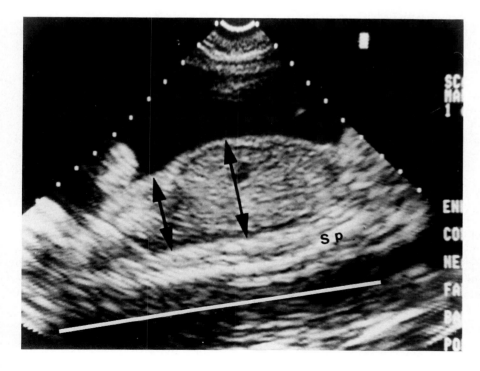

Fig. 18–11. Longitudinal section of a fetus affected with thanatophoric dysplasia. Note the significant disproportion between the chest and abdomen. Sp = spine. (*Reproduced with permission from Jeanty P, Romero R. Obstetrical Ultrasound. New York: McGraw-Hill; 1983.*)

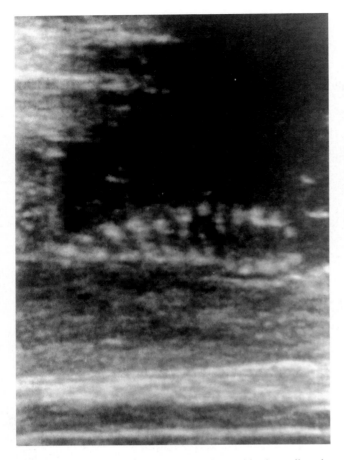

Fig. 18–12. Longitudinal section of a fetus with short rib-poly-dactyly syndrome showing the very short ribs.

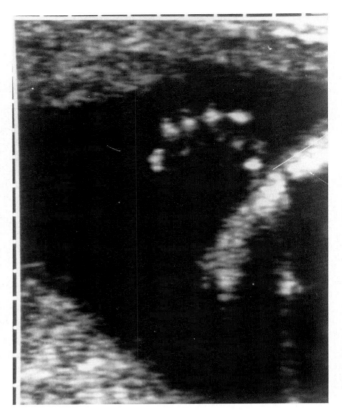

Fig. 18–14. Transverse section of a hand of a fetus with short rib-polydactyly syndrome showing post-axial polydactyly. Six digits are easily identified.

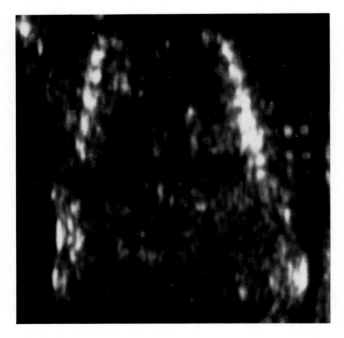

Fig. 18–13. Coronal section of a fetus with short rib-polydactyly syndrome. Note the disproportion between the thoracic and the abdominal cavities.

TABLE 18–9. SKELETAL DYSPLASIAS ASSOCIATED WITH ALTERED THORACIC DIMENSIONS

Long, narrow thorax:
  Asphyxiating thoracic dysplasia (Jeune)
  Chondroectodermal dysplasia (Ellis–van Creveld)
  Metatropic dysplasia
  Fibrochondrogenesis
  Atelosteogenesis
  Campomelic dysplasia
  Jarcho–Levin syndrome
  Achondrogenesis
  Osteogenesis imperfecta congenita
  Hypophosphatasia
  Dyssegmental dysplasia
  Cleidocranial dysplasia

Short thorax:
  Osteogenesis imperfecta (type II)
  Kniest's dysplasia (metatropic dysplasia type II)
  Pena–Shokeir syndrome

Hypoplastic thorax:
  Short rib-polydactyly syndrome (type I, type II)
  Thanatophoric dysplasia
  Cerebro-costo-mandibular syndrome
  Cleidocranial dysostosis syndrome
  Homozygous achondroplasia
  Melnick–Needles syndrome (osteodysplasty)
  Fibrochondrogenesis
  Otopalatodigital syndrome type II

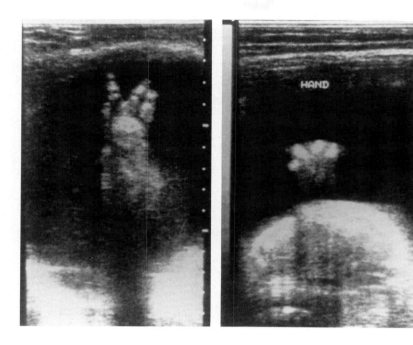

Fig. 18–15. Only four fingers are visualized. The left photograph shows a long axis view of the hand; the right photograph shows a transverse section of the hand. (*Courtesy of C Otto, MD.*)

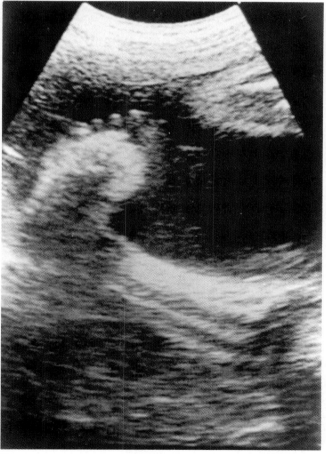

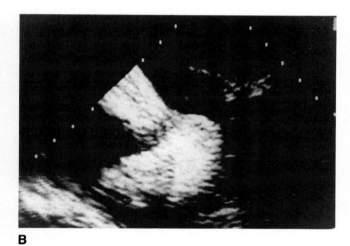

B

Fig. 18–16. **A.** Clubfoot. **B.** Rocker-bottom foot.

A

TABLE 18–10. NOMOGRAM OF FETAL FOOT SIZE THROUGHOUT GESTATION (cm)

Gestational Age (wk)	Percentile		
	10th	50th	90th
14	1.6	18	21
15	1.6	19	22
16	1.8	22	28
17	1.9	22	22
18	1.9	27	30
19	2.5	30	39
20	3.3	33	33
21	2.4	24	24
22	2.5	36	40
23	4.1	41	40
24	4.6	46	46
25	4.0	47	53
26	4.0	47	54
27	4.5	50	56
28	5.1	53	55
29	4.9	54	58
30	6.1	61	61
31	5.1	56	52
32	5.4	57	62
33	5.9	59	59
34	6.0	65	71
35	7.1	71	71

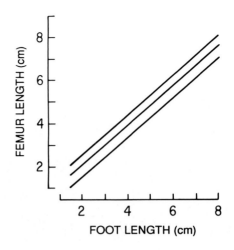

Fig. 18–17. Relationship between femur length and foot length.

TABLE 18–11. SKELETAL DYSPLASIAS ASSOCIATED WITH POLYDACTYLY AND SYNDACTYLY

Postaxial polydactyly:
  Chondroectodermal dysplasia
  Short rib-polydactyly syndrome (type I, type II)
  Asphyxiating thoracic dysplasia
  Otopalatodigital syndrome
  Mesomelic dysplasia Werner type (associated with absence of thumbs)
Preaxial polydactyly:
  Chondroectodermal dysplasia
  Short rib-polydactyly syndrome type II
  Carpenter syndrome
Syndactyly:
  Poland syndrome
  Acrocephalosyndactylies (Carpenter syndrome, Apert's syndrome)
  Otopalatodigital syndrome type II
  Mesomelic dysplasia Werner type
  TAR syndrome
  Jarcho–Levin syndrome
  Robert's syndrome
Brachydactyly:
  Mesomelic dysplasia Robinow type
  Otopalatodigital syndrome
Hitch-hiker thumbs:
  Diastrophic dysplasia
Club feet deformity:
  Diastrophic dysplasia
  Osteogenesis imperfecta
  Kniest's dysplasia
  Spondyloepiphyseal congenita

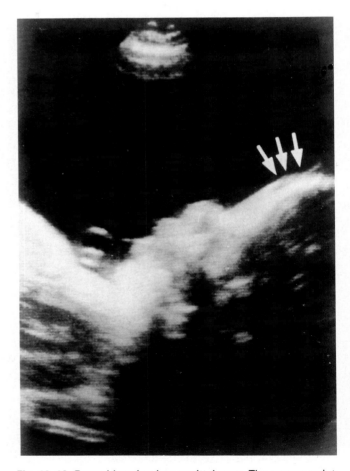

Fig. 18–18. Frontal bossing in a sagittal scan. The *arrows* point to the prominent frontal bone.

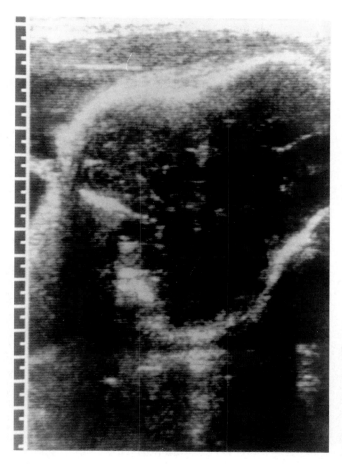

Fig. 18–19. Coronal scan of the head of a fetus with thanatophoric dysplasia with cloverleaf skull.

Although a full discussion about such disorders is beyond the scope of this text, they are well known causes of constitutional bone diseases.

OSTEOCHONDRODYSPLASIAS

A growing number of skeletal dysplasias have been recognized in utero. A complete account of each disorder is beyond the scope of this chapter, and we refer the reader to texts on the subject for further details.[19] A few of the most common disorders relevant to prenatal diagnosis are discussed below.

Thanatophoric Dysplasia, Fibrochondrogenesis, Atelosteogenesis
Thanatophoric dysplasia is the most common lethal skeletal dysplasia in fetuses and neonates. It is characterized by extreme rhizomelia, a normal trunk length with a narrow thorax, and a large head with a prominent forehead. It occurs in 0.24 to 0.69/10,000 births.[1,2] Two subtypes have been identified. Type I with typical bowed "telephone receiver" femurs without cloverleaf skull, and type 2 with cloverleaf skull and short, straight, long bones. However, mild cloverleaf skull has been described in type 1.[20] The differential diagnosis between the two depends on the radiographic findings and histology. There is no agreement regarding the pattern of inheritance of this condition. The first type seems to have an undetermined pattern of inheritance and most cases are sporadic. The second type seems to be inherited with an autosomal recessive pattern.

The prenatal sonographic findings depend on the specific variety. The association of cloverleaf skull and

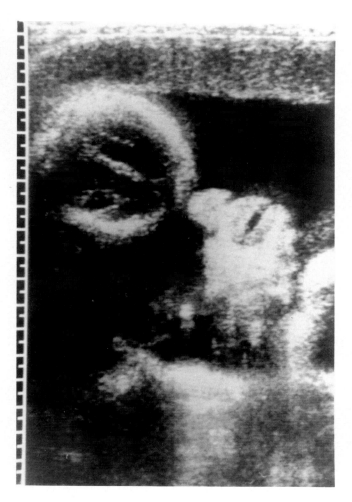

Fig. 18–20. Frontal bossing in a fetus with cloverleaf skull. Note the prominent forehead. Under normal circumstances, the forehead is not visible in a scan that allows imaging of the mouth and nose.

TABLE 18-12. SKELETAL DYSPLASIAS ASSOCIATED WITH SKULL AND FACE DEFORMITIES

Large head:
  Achondroplasia
  Achondrogenesis
  Thanatophoric dysplasia
  Osteogenesis imperfecta
  Cleidocranial dysplasia
  Hypophosphatasia
  Campomelic dysplasia
  Short rib-polydactyly syndrome type III
  Robinow mesomelic dysplasia
  Otopalatodigital syndrome

Cloverleaf skull:
  Thanatophoric dysplasia (rare variant)
  Campomelic syndrome

Other craniostenosis:
  Apert's syndrome
  Carpenter syndrome
  Hypophosphatasia

Congenital cararacts:
  Chondrodysplasia punctata

Cleft palate:
  Asphyxiating thoracic dysplasia
  Kniest's dysplasia
  Diastrophic dysplasia
  Spondyloepiphyseal dysplasia
  Campomelic syndrome
  Jarcho–Levin syndrome
  Ellis–van Creveld syndrome
  Short rib-polydactyly syndrome type II
  Metatropic dysplasia
  Dyssegmental dysplasia
  Otopalatodigital syndrome type II
  Robert's syndrome

Short upper lip:
  Chondroectodermal dysplasia

micromelia is specific for thanatophoric dysplasia. The other skeletal dysplasia associated with cloverleaf skull is campomelic syndrome. However, micromelia is not a feature of this condition. Cloverleaf skull may result from: (1) premature closure of the coronal and lambdoid sutures; (2) defective development of the cranial base with secondary synostosis; or (3) a primary developmental disorder of the brain with secondary deformation of the skull. The forehead is prominent and a saddle nose and hypertelorism may be present. Hydrocephaly and polyhydramnios are frequently present. Thanatophoric dysplasia is a uniformly lethal disorder. Prenatal diagnosis has been documented on several occasions.[21–27]

Fibrochondrogenesis and atelosteogenesis have a clinical presentation similar to that of thanatophoric dysplasia. A differential diagnosis between these disorders in utero is extremely difficult. Fibrochondrogenesis is a lethal chondrodysplasia inherited with an autosomal re-cessive pattern and characterized by rhizomelia with significant metaphyseal flaring and clefting of the vertebral bodies. Metaphyseal flaring is not a feature of thanatophoric dysplasia.[28] Atelosteogensis is also a lethal chondrodysplasia characterized by severe micromelia (with hypoplasia of the distal segments of the humerus and femur), bowing of long bones, and dislocation at the level of the elbow and knee. Clubfoot deformities may also be present.[29] Fibrochondrogenesis and atelosteogenesis are extremely rare, and only a few cases of each have been reported.

Achondrogenesis

Achondrogenesis, or anosteogenesis, is a lethal chondrodystrophy, characterized by extreme micromelia, short trunk, and macrocrania. The birth prevalence is 0.09 to 0.23/10,000 births.[1,2] The traditional classification of achondrogenesis subdivides this disorder into two types. The more severe form, achondrogenesis type I (Parenti–Fraccaro), is characterized by partial or complete lack of ossification of the calvarium and spine, very short long bones, and multiple rib fractures. Type II achondrogenesis (Langer–Saldino) is characterized by a variable degree of calcification of the calvarium and spine and by absence of fractures of the ribs (Fig. 18–20). Hypochondrogenesis had been considered a separate disorder from achondrogenesis. However, recent evidence suggests that hypochondrogenesis and achondrogenesis type II are phenotypic variants of the same disorder.[30] Recently, Whitley and Gorlin have proposed a new classification for achondrogenesis dividing the disease into four types.[31] Prenatal diagnosis should be suspected on the basis of micromelia, lack of vertebral ossification, and a large head with various degrees of ossification of calvarium.[32–37] Polyhydramnios and hydrops have been associated with achondrogenesis. However, sonographic examinations of affected fetuses do not demonstrate fluid accumulation in body cavities. The hydropic appearance of these fetuses and neonates is probably attributable to redundancy of soft-tissue mass over a limited skeletal frame. Achondrogenesis type I is inherited with an autosomal recessive pattern, while most cases of achondrogenesis type II and hypochondrogenesis have been sporadic (new autosomal dominant mutations).[37]

Achondroplasia

The most common nonlethal skeletal dysplasia is achondroplasia. It is characterized by rhizomelic dwarfism, limb bowing, lordotic spine, and enlarged head. It is inherited with an autosomal dominant pattern, and its prevalence is 1/66,000.[1] Advanced paternal age is a risk factor of achondroplasia. This disease is the result of anomalous growth of cartilage, followed by abnormal endochondral ossification, which is reponsible for the shortness of long bones. The bones of the hands and feet are short (brachydactyly). The head is large; a flattened nasal bridge, frontal bossing, and a broad mandible are frequent features. The problems in the prenatal diagnosis of this condition have been discussed in detail by Kurtz and colleagues.[38] The major difficulty in the antenatal diagnosis is that the long bone growth in this disease is not clearly appreciated in most cases until the third trimester of pregnancy. Therefore, it is not possible, in most cases, to detect this disorder in time to allow for pregnancy termination.[39,40] Heterozygous achondroplasia is compatible with a normal life. The disease is lethal in the homozygous state.

Osteogenesis Imperfecta and Hypophosphatasia

These two disorders are discussed together because they are characterized by significant skeletal demineralization.

Osteogenesis imperfecta (OI) is a heterogeneous group of collagen disorders with a prevalence of 0.18/10,000 births.[1,2] The most popular classification is that proposed by Sillence and associates.[41] In type I (autosomal dominant), patients have blue sclera and bone fragility. Type II (autosomal recessive) is also known as the perinatal variety and is uniformly lethal. There are multiple fractures in utero, and the long bones are shortened. The thorax is short but not narrow (Fig. 18–10). Type III (autosomal recessive or dominant) is characterized by blue sclera and multiple fractures present at birth. Type IV (autosomal dominant) is the mildest form. Although the sclera is blue at birth, it becomes white with time. Long bones are of normal length. Type II is subclassified into three subtypes: IIA, IIB, and IIC.[42] The prognosis for types I and IV is much better than for types II and III. Antenatal diagnosis of OI Type II has been reported several times.[43-46] Type I OI and Type III OI diagnoses have also been reported.[47-51]

Hypophosphatasia is inherited with an autosomal recessive pattern and is characterized by demineralization of bones and low alkaline phosphatase in serum and other tissues. There are four clinical forms of the disease. The neonatal form (also known as congenital or lethal) is associated with early neonatal death or intrauterine fetal demise. Prenatal diagnosis of this condition has been reported with both ultrasound[52] and by assaying alkaline phosphatase in tissue obtained by chorionic villous sampling.[53] The congenital variety is uniformly lethal.

Skeletal Dysplasias Characterized by a Hypoplastic Thorax

The dysplastic process involves the ribs and other bones of the rib cages in many skeletal dysplasias. A reduction in thoracic dimensions leads to restriction of lung growth and, consequently, pulmonary hypoplasia. Lung hypoplasia is the main cause of death in lethal skeletal dysplasias. There is a specific group of dysplasias in which thoracic hypoplasia is a cardinal feature. These include asphyxiating thoracic dysplasia, Ellis–van Creveld syndrome, and short rib polydactyly syndrome. Table 18–13 illustrates the criteria for the differential diagnoses of these conditions.

Asphyxiating Thoracic Dysplasia

This skeletal dysplasia, known as Jeune syndrome, is rare. Its prevalence is 0.14/10,000 births, and it is inherited in an autosomal recessive pattern.[1] It is characterized by a narrow and "bell-shaped" thorax, with short, horizontal ribs. Long bones are normal or mildly shortened. Polydactyly and cleft lip and/or palate can occur in association.[54-57] The disease is not uniformly lethal, and long-term survivors have been reported.[58,59]

Short Rib Polydactyly Syndromes

Short rib polydactyly syndromes are a group of disorders characterized by short limb dysplasia, constricted thorax, and postaxial polydactyly. Classically, three different types have been recognized. These conditions have been prenatally identified.[60,61] Table 18–13 illustrates the differential diagnosis and features of these conditions.

Campomelic Dysplasia

Campomelic dysplasia is characterized by bowing of the long bones of the lower extremities, hypoplastic scapulae, and several associated anomalies, such as hydrocephalus, cleft palate, micrognathia, hydronephrosis, and congenital heart defects. Campomelic syndrome has a prevalence of 0.05/10,000 births.[1] The most important feature is bowing of the femur and tibia, whereas other tubular bones are normal in length. The chest is narrow and can be "bell-shaped"; the vertebrae are hypoplastic. Differential diagnoses include OI, thanatophoric dysplasia, and hypophosphatasia. Antenatal diagnosis of this dysplasia has been reported in patients at risk.[62-65] The condition is frequently lethal, but some survivors have been reported.[66,67]

Diastrophic Dysplasia

Diastrophic dysplasia is characterized by micromelia, clubfoot, hand deformities, multiple joint flexion contractures, and scoliosis (Fig. 18–5). This disorder is inherited as an autosomal recessive trait. Due to phenotypic variability, the diagnosis may be difficult at birth and milder cases are diagnosed later.[68] The clinical features include rhizomelic type micromelia, contractures, hand deformities with abducted position of the thumbs ("hitchhiker thumb"), and severe talipes equinovarus. The head is normal, but micrognathia and cleft palate may be associated. This dysplasia is a generalized disorder of cartilage with destructive process of cartilage matrix and

TABLE 18–13. DISORDERS WITH THORACIC DYSPLASIA AND POLYDACTYLY

	Asphyxiating Thoracic Dysplasia (Jeune)	Chondro-ectodermal Dysplasia (Ellis–van Creveld)	Short Rib-Polydactyly Syndrome Type I (Saldino–Noonan)	Short Rib-Polydactyly Syndrome Type II (Majewski)	Short Rib Syndrome Type III (Davidoff)
Relative prevalence	Common	Uncommon	Common	Extremely rare	Rare
Clinical features					
Thoracic constriction	+ +	+	+ + +	+ + +	+ + +
Polydactyly	+	+ +	+ +	+ +	+ +
Limb shortening	+	+	+ + +	+	+ +
Congenital heart disease	–	+ +	+ +	+ +	–
Other abnormalities	Renal disease	Extodermal dysplasia	Genitourinary and gastrointestinal anomalies	Cleft lip and palate	Renal abnormality
Radiographic features					
Tubular bone shortening	+	+	+ + +	+ +	+ + +
Distinctive features in femora	–	–	Pointed ends	–	Marginal spurs
Short, horizontal ribs	+ +	+ +	+ + +	+ + +	+ + +
Vertical shortening of ilia and flat acetabula	+ +	+ +	+ +	–	+ +
Defective ossification of vertebral bodies	–	–	+ +	–	+
Shortening of skull base	–	–	–	–	+

+ = not common; + + = common; + + + = most common; – = absent.
(*Reproduced with permission from Cremin BJ:* Bone Dysplasias of Infancy: A Radiological Atlas. *Berlin: Springer-Verlag; 1978.*)

resulting formation of fibrous scar tissue and ossification. The latter process is responsible for the contractures. The prenatal diagnosis of diastrophic dysplasia has been found in patients at risk,[69–72] based on severe shortening and bowing of all long bones. This disorder has a wide spectrum and some cases may not be diagnosable in utero. The disease is not lethal and intellect is not affected.

LIMB DEFICIENCY OR CONGENITAL AMPUTATIONS

On occasion, the only identifiable anomaly is the absence of an extremity or a segment of an extremity. These anomalies are referred to as "limb deficiencies" or "congenital amputations" (Table 18–14). They constitute a group of disorders different from osteochondrodysplasias. The overall incidence of congenital limb reduction deformities is approximately 0.49/10,000 births (Table 18–15).[73] It has been estimated that 51% of these limb reduction defects are simple transverse reduction deficiencies of one forearm or hand without associated anomalies. The remainder consists of multiple reduction deficiencies, with an approximate 23% incidence of additional anomalies of the internal organs or craniofacial structures.[73]

Limb deficiencies can present alone or as part of a specific syndrome. An isolated limb deficiency of the upper extremity (eg, distal segment of an arm) is generally an isolated anomaly. In contrast, congenital amputation of the leg generally occurs within the context of a syndrome, as do bilateral amputations or reduction of all limbs.[74]

Isolated amputation of an extremity can be due to amniotic band syndrome, exposure to a teratogen, or a vascular accident. In most cases, the anomaly is sporadic and the risk of recurrence is negligible. However, recurrence of upper limb deficiencies has been reported.[75,76]

The syndromes associated with limb deficiencies include aglossia-adactylia syndrome and Moebius sequence. The aglossia-adactylia syndrome (also known as Hanhart syndrome or glossopalatine ankylosis) consists of transverse amputations of the limbs and malformations of the mouth (including micrognathia; vestigial tongue; or ankylosis of the tongue to the hard palate, the floor of the mouth, or the lips [glossopalatine ankylosis]). The spectrum of anomalies of the extremities is quite broad, ranging from absent digits to severe deficiencies of all four extremities. Intelligence is generally normal. The syndrome is sporadic.[77]

The Moebius sequence consists of a number of facial anomalies attributed to the paralysis of the 6th and 7th cranial nerves. Impairment of jaw mobility leads to micrognathia. Ptosis is also a common feature. The Moebius

TABLE 18–14. CONGENITAL AMPUTATIONS

Absent limb(s) only
    Single absent limb
    Multiple absent limbs
Absent limbs with rings
    Congenital ring constriction syndrome
Absent limbs and face anomaly
    Aglossia-adactylia syndromes
    Moebius syndrome
Absent limbs with other anomalies
    Ichthyosiform skin (CHILD syndrome)
    Fibula agenesis-complex brachydactyly (Dupan's syndrome)
    Splenogonadal fusion
    Skull and scalp defects (Adams–Oliver syndrome)
Phocomelia
    Thalidomide
    Thrombocytopenia with absent radii (TAR) syndrome
    Robert's pseudothalidomide-SC syndrome
    Grebe's syndrome
Proximal femoral focal deficiency
    Femoral hypoplasia-unusual facies syndrome
    Femur-fibula-ulna complex
    Femur-tibia-radius complex
Split hand/split foot (SH/SF) syndromes
    Only split hand/split foot
    SH/SF and absent long bones
    Ectrodactyly, ectodermal dysplasia, cleft lip/palate (EEC syndrome)
Others
    Split foot and triphalangeal thumb, autosomal dominant
    Split foot, or split hand and central polydactyly (see central polydactyly)
    SH/SF and congenital nystagmus (Karsch–Neugebauer syndrome)
    SH/SF and renal malformations (acrorenal syndrome)
    Split foot and mandibulofacial dysostosis (Fontaine's syndrome), autosomal dominant

(*Reproduced with permission from Goldberg MD,* The Dysmorphic Child: An Orthopedic Perspective. *New York: Raven Press; 1987.*)

sequence is generally sporadic.[78] Rare cases of a familial form have been reported.[79] The associated limb reduction anomalies are generally present in the upper extremities and range from transverse deficiencies to absent digits.

Limb Reduction Defects Associated with Other Anomalies. Congenital hemidysplasia with ichthyosiform erythroderma and limb defects (CHILD syndrome) is a defect characterized by strict demarcation of the skin lesions to one side of the midline. The presence of unilateral defects of long bones is an important feature of the syndrome. Limb deficiencies may vary from hypoplasia of phalanges or metacarpals to complete absence of an extremity. The calvarium, scapulae, or ribs may also be involved. Zellweger syndrome and warfarin embryopathy may present with similar findings. Visceral

anomalies include congenital heart disease, unilateral hydronephrosis, hydroureter, unilateral absence of the kidney, Fallopian tube, ovaries, adrenal gland, and thyroid. The CHILD syndrome predominantly affects females (ratio 19:1).[80]

Fibula aplasia-complex brachydactyly (Du Pan's syndrome) is an extremely rare condition characterized by bilateral agenesis of the fibula with abnormalities of the metacarpals and proximal phalanges. Limb reduction defects can involve the lower extremities.[81]

The splenogonadal fusion syndrome is characterized by limb reduction defects and splenogonadal fusion. A review of 14 reported cases indicates that there is some overlap between this syndrome and the agglosia-adactylia syndrome or Hanhart syndrome. Most reported cases have occurred in males. Typically, there is a mass in the scrotum, and an ectopic spleen is identified during surgery.[82]

The Adams–Oliver syndrome is an autosomal dominant disorder characterized by the association of limb reduction defects and scalp defects (aplasia cutis and deficiency of bony calvarium).[83]

In phocomelia, the extremities resemble those of a seal. Typically, the hands and feet are present, but the intervening arms and legs are absent. Hands and feet may be normal or abnormal. Three syndromes must be considered in the differential diagnosis of phocomelia: Robert's syndrome, some varieties of the thrombocytopenia with absent radius (TAR syndrome), and Grebe's syndrome. Phocomelia can also be caused by exposure to thalidomide, but this is only of historical interest.[84]

Robert's syndrome is an autosomal recessive disorder characterized by the association of tetraphocomelia and facial clefting defects or hypoplastic nasal alae. Hypertelorism may also be present. The upper extremities are generally more severely affected than the lower extremities. The spine is not involved. Polyhydramnios has been noted, and other anomalies associated with the syn-

TABLE 18–15. INCIDENCE OF DIFFERENT TYPES OF LIMB REDUCTION MALFORMATIONS IN HUNGARY, 1975–1977

Type	Total No.	Population Incidence (per 1,000 births)
Terminal transverse	79	0.14
Radial	13	0.09
Ulnar and fibular	41	0.11
Split hand and/or foot	20	0.04
Ring constriction	62	0.11
Total	**274**	**0.49**

(*Adapted from Bod M, Czeizel A, Lenz W.* Hum Genet. *1983;65:27.*)

drome include horseshoe kidney, hydrocephaly, cephalocele, and spina bifida.[85]

Grebe's syndrome is a condition described among the inbred Indian tribes from Brazil. It is an autosomal recessive disorder characterized by marked hypomelia of upper and lower limbs, increasing in severity from proximal to distal segments. In contrast to Robert's syndrome, the lower limbs are more affected than the upper extremities.[86]

TAR syndrome is discussed in detail in the section on radial clubhand deformities.

Proximal femoral focal deficiency, or congenital short femur, consists of a wide variety of congenital developmental anomalies of the femur. The disorder has been classified into five groups: type I, simple hypoplasia of the femur; type II, short femur with angulated shaft; type III, short femur with coxa vara (the most common); type IV, absent or defective proximal femur; and type V, absent or rudimentary femur.[87] One or both femurs can be affected. The right femur is more frequently involved. Anomalies of the upper limbs can also be present and do not exclude the diagnosis.[8] The proximal femoral focal deficiency syndrome may be associated with umbilical or inguinal hernias.

If both femurs are affected, it is important to examine the face carefully. The disorder may be femoral hypoplasia and unusual face syndrome.[88,89] Femoral hypoplasia-unusual facies syndrome consists of bilateral femoral hypoplasia and facial defects, including short nose with broad tip, long philtrum, micrognathia, and cleft palate. Long bone abnormalities can extend to other segments of the lower extremity (absent fibula) and also to the upper extremity. The syndrome is sporadic and has been associated with maternal diabetes mellitus. A familial form has been described.[90]

If the defect is unilateral, it may correspond to the femur-fibula unla or femur-tibia-radius complex. These two syndromes have different implications for genetic counseling; the former is nonfamilial, while the second has a strong genetic component.[91]

The term "split hand and foot syndrome" is used to refer to a group of disorders characterized by splitting of the hand and foot into two parts. Other terms include lobster-claw deformity, ectrodactyly, and aborted fingers. The conditions are classified into typical and atypical varieties.[92] The typical form consists of absence of both the finger and the metacarpal bone, resulting in a deep V-shaped central defect that clearly divides the hand into an ulnar and a radial part. It occurs in 1/90,000 live births and has a familial tendency (usually inherited with an autosomal dominant pattern).[93] The atypical variety is characterized by a much wider cleft formed by a defect of the metacarpals and the middle fingers. As a consequence, the cleft is U-shaped and wide with only thumb

and small finger remaining. It occurs in 1/150,000 live births.[93]

A complex system for the classification of these disorders, based on the distribution of remaining fingers, has been proposed.[94] However, this system is not helpful in differential diagnosis and syndrome classification.

Split hand/foot deformities can occur as isolated anomalies or as part of a more complex syndrome. The syndromic types are the ones more frequently encountered.[74]

Several syndromes are associated with split hand/foot deformities. The split hand/foot and absent long bones syndromes include two conditions in which there is split hand and aplasia of the tibia, or split foot with aplasia of the ulna. However, skeletal anomalies are not limited to these bones; the clavicle, femur, and fibula can also be affected. The pattern of inheritance of these disorders has not been clearly determined. Autosomal dominant, recessive, and X-linked recessive patterns have been proposed.[95,96] Ectrodactyly-ectodermal dysplasia-cleft lip/palate syndrome (EEC syndrome) generally involves the four extremities with more severe deformities of the hands. The spectrum of ectodermal defects is wide, including dry skin, sparse hair, and dental defects.[97] Defects of the tear duct lead to absence of lacrimal secretions, chronic kerato-conjunctivitis, and severe loss of visual acuity. The cleft lip is generally bilateral. Obstructive uropathy can also occur.[98] The pattern of inheritance is autosomal dominant. Intelligence is generally normal.[99]

There is a different group of syndromes that involves associations of the split hand/foot deformity with other anomalies. This entity includes split foot and triphalangeal thumb, split foot and hand and central polydactyly, Karsch–Neugebauer syndrome (split hand/foot with congenital nystagmus), acro-renal syndrome, and mandibulofacial dysostosis (Fontaine syndrome).[100–103]

Clubhands

Clubhand deformities are classified into two main categories: radial and ulnar. Radial clubhand includes a wide spectrum of disorders that encompass absent thumb, thumb hypoplasia, thin first metacarpal, and absent radius (Table 18–16). Ulnar clubhand is much less frequent than radial clubhand and manifestation ranges from mild deviations of the hand on the ulnar side of the forearm to complete absence of the ulna. While radial clubhand is frequently syndromatic, ulnar clubhand is usually an isolated anomaly.[74]

Whenever a clubhand is identified, it is important to conduct a thorough examination of the fetus and newborn to delineate associated anomalies that may suggest a syndrome. Fetal blood sampling procedures and fetal echocardiography are recommended. A complete blood

TABLE 18–16. RADIAL RAY DEFECTS: A DIFFERENTIAL DIAGNOSIS OF CONGENITAL DEFICIENCY OF THE RADIUS AND RADIAL RAY

I. Isolated: nonsyndromatic

II. Syndromes with blood dyscrasias
   A. Fanconi's anemia
   B. Thrombocytopenia with absent radii (TAR) syndrome
   C. Aase's syndrome: congenital anemia, nonopposable triphalangeal thumb, scaphoid and distal radius hypoplasia, radioulnar synostosis, short stature with narrow shoulders, autosomal recessive (see Diamond–Blackfan syndrome for a similar, perhaps identical, syndrome)

III. Syndromes with congenital heart disease
   A. Holt–Oram syndrome
   B. Lewis upper limb-cardiovascular syndrome: more extensive arm malformations and more complex heart anomalies than Holt–Oram, but probably not a separate syndrome, autosomal dominant

IV. Syndromes with cranio-facial abnormalities
   A. Nager acrofacial dysostosis
   B. Radial clubhand and cleft lip and/or cleft palate: sporadic
   C. Juberg–Hayward syndrome: cleft lip and palate, hypoplastic thumbs, short radius, radial head subluxation, autosomal recessive
   D. Baller–Gerold syndrome: craniosynostosis, bilateral radial clubhand, absent/hypoplastic thumb; autosomal recessive
   E. Rothmund–Thomson syndrome: prematurely aged skin changes, juvenile cataract, sparse grey hair, absent thumbs, radial clubhands, occasional knee dysplasia (see progeria syndromes)
   F. Duane-radial dysplasia syndrome: abnormal ocular movements: inability to abduct and eyeball retraction with adduction, radius and radial ray hypoplasia, vertebral anomalies, renal malformation, autosomal dominant (see Klippel–Feil variants)
   G. The IVIC syndrome (Instituto Venezolano de Investigaciones Cientificas): radial ray deficiency, hypoplastic or absent thumbs and radial clubhands, impaired hearing, abnormal movements of extraocular muscles with strabismus, autosomal dominant
   H. LARD syndrome (lacrimo-auriculo-radial-dental; Levy–Hollister): absent lacrimal structures, protuberant ears, thumb and radial ray hypoplasia, abnormal teeth, autosomal dominant.
   I. Radial defects with ear anomalies and cranial nerve 7 dysfunction
   J. Radial hypoplasia, triphalangeal thumb, hypospadias, diastema of maxillary central incisors, autosomal dominant

V. Syndromes with congenital scoliosis
   A. The VATER association
   B. Goldenhar syndrome (oculoauriculovertebral dysplasia)
   C. Klippel–Feil syndrome

VI. Radial aplasia and chromosome aberrations

VII. Syndromes with mental retardation
   A. Seckel syndrome (bird-headed dwarfism): microcephaly, beak-like protrusion of nose, mental retardation, absent/hypoplastic thumbs, bilateral dislocated hips

VIII. Thalidomide embryopathy (of historical interest, but some 60% had radial clubhand)

(Reproduced with permission from Goldberg MD. The Dysmorphic Child: An Orthopedic Perspective. New York: Raven Press; 1987.)

cell count, including platelets, is important to establish the diagnosis of Fanconi's pancytopenia, TAR syndrome, and Aase's syndrome. A fetal karyotype is indicated because several chromosomal abnormalities (eg, trisomy 18, 21, and other structural aberrations) have been reported in association with clubhand deformities. Congenital heart disease is an important feature of the Holt–Oram syndrome, and the Lewis upper limb-cardiovascular syndrome, and is also present in some cases of TAR syndrome.

The isolated radial clubhand can be present with other anomalies. This constellation may not represent a recognizable or previously described syndrome. Isolated radial clubhand is generally a sporadic disorder.[104]

The three syndromes associated with hematologic abnormalities are Fanconi's pancytopenia, TAR syndrome, and Aase's syndrome.

Fanconi's anemia (pancytopenia) is an autosomal recessive disease characterized by the association of bone marrow failure (anemia, leukopenia, and thrombocytopenia) and skeletal anomalies, including a radial clubhand with absent thumbs, radial hypoplasia, and a high frequency of chromosomal breakage (demonstrated in amniotic fluid cells or fetal lymphocytes after incubation with diepoxy-butane).[105,106] It can be associated with congenital dislocation of the hip, scoliosis, and cardiac, pulmonary, and gastrointestinal anomalies. Intrauterine growth retardation is common. Prenatal diagnosis has been reported many times.[107]

TAR syndrome is an autosomal recessive disorder characterized by thrombocytopenia (platelet count of less than 100,000/mm³) and bilateral absence of the radius. The thumb and metacarpals are always present. The ulna and humerus may be absent, and clubfoot deformities may also be present. Congenital heart disease is present in 33% of the cases (tetralogy of Fallot and septal defects). Delivery by cesarean section is recommended, as these fetuses are at risk for intracranial hemorrhage.[10,11,108]

Aase's syndrome is an autosomal recessive condition characterized by congenital hypoplastic anemia and a radial clubhand with a triphalangeal thumb and a hypoplastic distal radius. Cardiac defects (ventricular septal defects) may be present.[109,110] Other disorders associated with triphalangeal thumbs are Holt–Oram syndrome and the Nager syndrome.

The *Holt–Oram syndrome* is an autosomal dominant disorder characterized by congenital heart disease (mainly atrial septal defects, secundum type, and ventricular septal defects) and aplasia or hypoplasia of the radius. Limb defects are often asymmetric. There is no correlation between the severity of the limb defects and the cardiac anomaly. Other anomalies include hypertelorism and vertebral defects.[111] This condition has been prenatally diagnosed.[112,113] The upper limb/cardiovascular syndrome described by Lewis and colleagues[114] is probably not a separate entity from the Holt–Oram syndrome.

Craniofacial abnormalities and radial clubhand deformities form a different group of syndromes. These syndromes are sporadic and have common features that make a prenatal differential diagnosis difficult. The most common craniofacial anomaly is cleft lip and palate. Uuspaa's study of 3,225 cases with orofacial cleft showed a 2.8% association with upper extremity deformities.[115]

Radial clubhand is also associated with congenital scoliosis. The three syndromes that should be considered part of the differential diagnosis include VATER association, some cases of the Goldenhar syndrome, and the Klippel–Feil syndrome.[116,117] The VATER association includes vertebral segmentation (70%), anal atresia (80%), tracheo-esophageal fistula (70%), esophageal atresia (65%), and radial and renal defects (53%). Other anomalies include a single umbilical artery (35%) and congenital heart disease, occurring in nearly 50% of the patients. The VATER association occurs sporadically. The Goldenhar syndrome, a disorder characterized by alterations in the morphogenesis of the first and second brachial arches (microtia and hypoplasia of the malar, maxillary, and/or mandibular region), can also be associated with radial clubhand.[118]

Radial clubhand has been reported in association with several chromosomal anomalies, including trisomies 18 and 21, deletion of the long arm of 13, and ring formation of chromosome 4.[119,120]

Ulnar clubhand occurs as an isolated, nonsyndromic anomaly in most cases. It can also be associated with a variety of syndromes, for example, Poland complex (Table 18–17).[121]

Polydactyly

Polydactyly is the presence of an additional digit. The extra digit may range from a fleshy nubbin to a complete digit with controlled flexion and extension. Polydactyly can be classified as postaxial (the most common form), preaxial, and central (see Table 18–11). Postaxial polydactyly occurs on the ulnar side of the hand and fibular

---

TABLE 18–17. ULNAR RAY DEFECTS: A DIFFERENTIAL DIAGNOSIS OF CONGENITAL DEFICIENCY OF THE ULNA AND ULNAR RAY

I. Isolated: nonsyndromatic absent ulna

II. Ulna hypoplasia and skeletal deficiency elsewhere
   A. Ulna aplasia with lobster-claw deformity of hand and/or foot, autosomal dominant
   B. Femus-fibula-ulan complex

III. Syndromes with ulna deficiency
   A. Cornelia de Lange syndrome
   B. Miller syndrome (postaxial acrofacial dysostosis): absent ulna and ulnar rays and absent 4th and 5th toes: Treacher Collins mandibulofacial hypoplasia, autosomal recessive; distinguish from Nager preaxial acrofacial dysostosis
   C. Pallister ulnar-mannary syndrome: hypoplasia of ulna and ulnar rays; hypoplasia of the breast and absence of apocrine sweat glands, autosomal dominant
   D. Pillay syndrome (ophthalmo-mandibulo-melic dysplasia): absent distal third of ulna, absent olecranon, hypoplastic trochlea and proximal radius, fusion of interphalangeal joints in ulnar fingers, knee dysplasia; corneal opacities, fusion of temporomandibular joint, autosomal dominant
   E. Weyers oligodactyly syndrome: deficiency of ulna and ulnar rays, antecubital webbing, short sternum, malformed kidney and spleen, cleft lip and palate, sporadic
   F. Schnizel syndrome: absent/hypoplastic 4th, 5th metacarpals and phalanges, hypogenitalism, anal atresia, autosomal dominant
   G. Mesomelic dwarfism, Reinhardt-Pfeiffer type (ulno-fibula dysplasia): a generalized bone dysplasia but with a disproportionate hypoplasia of the ulna and fibula, autosomal dominant
   H. Mesomelic dwarfism, Langer's type: a generalized bone dysplasia, but with aplasia of the distal ulna and proximal fibula and hypoplasia of the mandible

(Reproduced with permission from Goldberg MD. The Dysmorphic Child: An Orthopedic Perspective. New York: Raven Press; 1987.)

side of the foot. Preaxial polydactyly is present on the radial side of the hand and the tibial side of the foot.

The majority are isolated conditions with an autosomal dominant mode of inheritance. Some of them are part of a syndrome, usually an autosomal recessive one. Preaxial polydactyly, especially triphalangeal thumb, is most likely to be part of a multisystem syndrome. Central polydactyly consists of an extra digit that is usually hidden between the long and the ring finger. It is often bilateral and is inherited with an autosomal mode of inheritance. It can be associated with other hand and foot malformations.[122–125]

Arthrogryposis

The term arthrogryposis multiple congenita (AMC) refers to multiple joint contractures present at birth. Normal fetal movement is important for the development of the joints; limitation of fetal joint motion leads to the development of contractures and AMC.[126] Therefore, AMC is not a specific disorder but rather a syndrome. Neurologic, muscular, connective tissue, or skeletal abnormalities or intrauterine crowding can lead to impaired fetal motion and AMC.[127] Table 18–18 illustrates disorders of the motor systems that can lead to AMC. In a series of 74 children, Banker found that the most common cause of AMC was a neurogenic disorder followed by myopathic disorders.[128] The condition is present in 0.03% of livebirths.[129]

The deformities are usually symmetric. In most cases of AMC, all four limbs are involved, followed in frequency by deformities of the lower extremities only, or bimelic involvement. The severity of the deformities increases distally in the involved limb, with the hands and feet typically being the most deformed.

There are many congenital anomalies associated with AMC. The most frequent are cleft palate, Klippe–Feil syndrome, meningomyelocele, and congenital heart disease. Ten percent of patients with AMC have associated anomalies of the central nervous system.[126]

The prenatal diagnosis of AMC with ultrasound has been reported only five times.[130–134] The cardinal findings are absent fetal movement on real-time examination and severe flexion deformities.[135]

For a complete discussion of the skeletal dysplasias, the reader is referred to Goldberg's textbook *The Dysmorphic Child*.[74]

TABLE 18–18. DISORDERS OF THE DEVELOPING MOTOR SYSTEM ON ALL LEVELS, LEADING TO IMMOBILIZATION

Disorders of the developing neuromuscular system
  Loss of anterior horn cells
  Radicular disease with collagen proliferation
  Peripheral neuropathy with neurofibromatosis
  Congenital myasthenia
  Neonatal myasthenia (maternal myasthenia gravis)
  Amyoplasia congenita
  Congenital muscular dystrophy
Central core disease
  Congenital myotonic dystrophy
  Glycogen accumulation myopathy
Disorders of developing connective tissues or connective tissue disease
  Muscular and articular connective tissue dystrophy
  Articular defects by mesenchymal dysplasia
  Increased collagen synthesis
Disorders of developing medulla or medullar disease
  Congenital spinal epidural hemorrhage
  Congenital duplication of the spinal canal
Disorders of brain development (eg, porencephaly or brain disease (eg, congenital encephalopathy)

REFERENCES

1. Camera G, Mastroiacovo P. Birth prevalence of skeletal dysplasias in the Italian multicentric monitoring system for birth defects. In: Papadatos CJ, Bartsocas CS, eds. *Skeletal Dysplasias.* New York: Alan R. Liss; 1982:441–449.
2. Connor JM, Connor RAC, Sweet EM, et al. Lethal neonatal chondrodysplasias in the west of Scotland 1970–1983 with a description of a thanatophoric, dysplasialike, autosomal recessive disorder, Glasgow variant. *Am J Med Genet.* 1985;22:243–53.
3. International Nomenclature of Constitutional Diseases of Bone. *J Pediatr.* 1978;93:614–616.
4. International Nomenclature of Constitutional Diseases of Bone. *Ann Radiol.* 1984;27:275–280.
5. Kurtz AB, Wapner RJ. Ultrasonographic diagnosis of second trimester skeletal dysplasias: A prospective analysis in a high-risk population. *J Ultrasound Med.* 1983;2:99.
6. Benaceraff BR, Greene MF, Barss VA. Prenatal sonographic diagnosis of congenital hemivertebra. *J Ultrasound Med.* 1986;5:257.
7. Coffin GS, Siris E, Wegienka LC. Mental retardation with osteocartilaginous anomalies. *Am J Dis Child.* 1966;112:205.
8. Graham M. Congenital short femur: Prenatal sonographic diagnosis. *J Ultrasound Med.* 1985;4:361.
9. Pashayan H, Fraser FC, McIntyre JM, et al. Bilateral aplasia of the tibia, polydactyly and absent thumbs in father and daughter. *J Bone Joint Surg.* 1971;53B:495.
10. Filkins K, Russo J, Bilinki I, et al. Prenatal diagnosis of thrombocytopenia absent radius syndrome using ultrasound and fetoscopy. *Prenat Diagn.* 1984;4:139.
11. Luthy DA, Hall JG, Graham CB, et al. Prenatal diagnosis of thrombocytopenia with absent radii. *Clin Genet.* 1979;15:495.
12. Chitkara U, Rosenberg J, Chervenak FA, et al. Prenatal sonographic assessment of the fetal thorax: Normal values. *Am J Obstet Gynecol.* 1987;156:1069.
13. Campbell J, Henderson A, Campbell S. The fetal femur/

foot length ratio: A new parameter to assess dysplastic limb reduction. *Obstet Gynecol.* 1989;72:181.

14. Hershey DW. The fetal femur/foot length ratio: A new parameter to assess dysplastic limb reduction. *Obstet Gynecol.* 1989;73:682.

15. Galli G. *Craniosynostosis.* Boca Raton, Fla: CRC Press; 1984.

16. Kozlowski K, Robertson F, Middleton R. Radiographic findings in Larsen's syndrome. *Aust Radiol.* 1974;18:336.

17. Pilu G, Romero R, Reece EA, et al. The prenatal diagnosis of Robin anomalad. *Am J Obstet Gynecol.* 1986;154:630.

18. Pilu G, Reece EA, Romero R, et al. Prenatal diagnosis of craniofacial malformations with ultrasonography. *Am J Obstet Gynecol.* 1986;155:45.

19. Romero R, Pilu G, Jeanty P, et al. *Prenatal Diagnosis of Congenital Anomalies.* Norwalk, Conn: Appleton & Lange; 1988:311–384.

20. Yang SS, Heidelberger KP, Brough AJ, et al. Lethal short-limbed chondrodyslasia in early infancy. In: Rosenberg HS, Boland RP, eds. *Perspectives in Pediatric Pathology.* Chicago: Year Book Medical Publishers; 1976;3:1–48.

21. Fink IJ, Filly RA, Callen PW, et al. Sonographic diagnosis of thanatophoric dwarfism in utero. *J Ultrasound Med.* 1982;1:337.

22. Beetham FGT, Reeves JS. Early ultrasound diagnosis of thanatophoric dwarfism. *J Clin Ultrasound.* 1984;12:43.

23. Burrows PE, Stannard MW, Pearrow J, et al. Early antenatal sonographic recognition of thanatophoric dysplasia with cloverleaf skull deformity. *AJR.* 1984;143:841.

24. Mahony BS, Filly RA, Callen PW, et al. Thanatophoric dwarfism with the cloverleaf skull: A specific antenatal sonographic diagnosis. *J Ultrasound Med.* 1985;4:151.

25. Elejalde BR, de Elejalde MM. Thanatophoric dysplasia: Fetal manifestations and prenatal diagnosis. *Am J Med Genet.* 1985;22:669–683.

26. Weiner CP, Williamson RA, Bonsib SM. Sonographic diagnosis of cloverleaf skull and thanatophoric dysplasia in the second trimester. *J Clin Ultrasound.* 1986;14:463–465.

27. van der Harten JJ, Brons JTJ, Dijkstra PF, et al. Some variants of lethal neonatal short-limbed platyspondylic dysplasia: A radiologic, ultrasonographic, neuropathologic and histopathologic study of 22 cases. In: Brons JTJ, van der Harten JJ, eds. *Skeletal Dysplasias, Pre- and Postnatal Identification: An Ultrasonographic, Radiologic and Pathologic Study.* Amsterdam: Free University Hospital; 1988:111–142.

28. Whitley CB, Langer LO, Ophoven J, et al. Fibrochondrogenesis: Lethal, autosomal recessive chondrodysplasia with distinctive cartilage histopathology. *Am J Med Genet.* 1984;19:265.

29. Chevernak FA, Isaacson G, Rosenberg JC, et al. Antenatal diagnosis of frontal cephalocele in a fetus with atelosteogenesis. *J Ultrasound Med.* 1986;5:111.

30. Borochowitz Z, Ornoy A, Lachman R, et al. Achondrogenesis II–hypochondrogenesis: Variability versus heterogeneity. *Am J Med Genet.* 1986;24:273–288.

31. Whitley CB, Gorlin RJ. Achondrogenesis: New nosology with evidence of genetic heterogeneity. *Radiology.* 1983;148:693.

32. Johnson VP, Yiu-Chiu VS, Wierda DR, et al. Midtrimester prenatal diagnosis of achondrogenesis. *J Ultrasound Med.* 1984;3:223.

33. Mahony BS, Filly RA, Cooperberg PL. Antenatal sonographic diagnosis of achondrogenesis. *J Ultrasound Med.* 1984;3:333.

34. Glenn LW, Teng SSK. In utero sonographic diagnosis of achondrogenesis. *J Clin Ultrasound.* 1985;13:195.

35. Chen H, Liu CT, Yang SS. Achondrogenesis: A review with special consideration of achondrogenesis type II (Langer–Saldino). *Am J Med Genet.* 1981;10:379.

36. Benacerraf B, Osathanondh R, Bieber FR. Achondrogenesis type I: Ultrasound diagnosis in utero. *J Clin Ultrasound.* 1984;12:357.

37. van der Harten JJ, Brons JTJ, Dijkstra PF, et al. Achondrogenesis, hypochondrogenesis, the spectrum of chondrogenesis imperfecta: A radiologic, ultrasonographic and histopathologic study of 23 cases. *Pediatr Pathol.* 1988; 8:571–597.

38. Kurtz AB, Filly RA, Wapner RJ, et al. In utero analysis of heterozygous achondroplasia: Variable time of onset as detected by femur length measurements. *J Ultrasound Med.* 1986;5:137.

39. Elejalde BR, de Elejalde MM, Hamilton PR, et al. Prenatal diagnosis in two pregnancies of an achondroplastic woman. *Am J Med Genet.* 1983;15:437.

40. Filly RA, Golbus MS, Carey JC, et al. Short-limbed dwarfism: Ultrasonographic diagnosis by mensuration of fetal femoral length. *Radiology.* 1981;138:653.

41. Sillence DO, Senn A, Danks DM. Genetic heterogeneity in osteogenesis imperfecta. *J Med Genet.* 1979;16:101–116.

42. Sillence DO, Barlow KK, Garber AP, et al. Osteogenesis imperfecta type II: Delineation of the phenotype with reference to genetic heterogeneity. *Am J Med Genet.* 1984;17:407–423.

43. Mertz E, Goldhofer W. Sonographic diagnosis of lethal osteogenesis imperfecta in the second trimester: Case report and review. *J Clin Ultrasound.* 1986;14: 380.

44. Brons JTJ, van der harten JJ, Wladimiroff JW. Prenatal ultrasonographic diagnosis of osteogenesis imperfecta. *Am J Obstet Gynecol.* 1988;159:176–181.

45. Elejalde BR, de Elejalde MM. Prenatal diagnosis of perinatally lethal osteogenesis imperfecta. *Am J Med Genet.* 1983;14:353.

46. Ghosh A, Woo JSK, Wan CW, et al. Simple ultrasonic diagnosis of osteogenesis imperfecta type II in early second trimester. *Prenat Diagn.* 1984;4:235.

47. Hobbins JC, Bracken MB, Mahoney MJ. Diagnosis of fetal skeletal dysplasias with ultrasound. *Am J Obstet Gynecol.* 1982;142:306.

48. Chervenak FA, Romero R, Berkowitz RL, et al. Antenatal sonographic findings of osteogenesis imperfecta. *Am J Obstet Gynecol.* 1982;143:228.

49. Aylsworth AS, Seeds JW, Bonner-Guilford W, et al. Prenatal diagnosis of a severe deforming type of osteogenesis imperfecta. *Am J Med Genet.* 1984;19:707.

50. Robinson LP, Worthen NJ, Lachman RS, et al. Prenatal

diagnosis of osteogenesis imperfecta type III. *Prenat Diagn.* 1987;7:7.

51. van der Harten JJ, Brons JTJ, Dijkstra PF. Perinatal lethal osteogenesis imperfecta: Radiologic and pathologic evaluation of seven prenatally diagnosed cases. *Pediatr Pathol.* 1988;8:233–252.

52. Kousseff BG, Mulivor RA. Prenatal diagnosis of second-trimester skeletal dysplasias: A prospective analysis in a high-risk population. *J Ultrasound Med.* 1983;2:99.

53. Wladimiroff JW, Niermeijen MF, van der Harten JJ, et al. Early prenatal diagnosis of congenital hypophosphatasia: Case report. *Prenat Diagn.* 1985;5:47–52.

54. Elejalde BR, de Elejalde MM, Pansch D. Prenatal diagnosis of Jeune syndrome. *Am J Med Genet.* 1985;21:433.

55. Lipson M, Waskey J, Rice J, et al. Prenatal diagnosis of asphyxiating thoracic dysplasia. *Am J Med Genet.* 1984; 18:273.

56. Schinzel A, Savoldelli G, Briner J, et al. Prenatal sonographic diagnosis of Jeune syndrome. *Radiology.* 1985; 154:777.

57. Skiptunas SM, Weiner S. Early prenatal diagnosis of asphyxiating thoracic dysplasia (Jeune's syndrome): Value of fetal thoracic measurement. *J Ultrasound Med.* 1987;6:41–43.

58. Kozlowski K, Masel J. Asphyxiating thoracic dystrophy without respiratory distress. Report of 2 cases of the latent form. *Pediatr Radiol.* 1976;5:30.

59. Friedman JM, Kaplan HG, Hall JG. The Jeune syndrome (asphyxiating thoracic dystrophy) in an adult. *Am J Med.* 1975;59:857.

60. Wladimiroff JW, Niermeijer MF, Laar J, et al. Prenatal diagnosis of skeletal dysplasia by real-time ultrasound. *Obstet Gynecol.* 1984;63:360.

61. Muller LM, Cremin BJ. Ultrasonic demonstration of fetal skeletal dysplasia. *S Afr Med J.* 1985;67:222–226.

62. Balcar I, Bieber FR. Sonographic and radiologic findings in campomelic dysplasia. *AJR.* 1983;141:481.

63. Fryns JP, van der Berghe K, van Assche A, et al. Prenatal diagnosis of campomelic dwarfism. *Clin Genet.* 1981; 19:199.

64. Winter R, Rosenkranz W, Hofmann H, et al. Prenatal diagnosis of campomelic dysplasia by ultrasonography. *Prenat Diagn.* 1985;5:1.

65. Slater CP, Ross J, Nelson MM, Coetzee EJ. The campomelic syndrome—prenatal ultrasound investigations: A case report. *SAMT.* 1985;67:863–866.

66. Beluffi G, Fraccaro M. Genetical and clinical aspects of campomelic dysplasia. *Prog Clin Biol Res.* 1982; 104:53.

67. Opitz JM. Comment to: Genetical and clinical aspects of campomelic dysplasia. Beluffi G, Fraccaro M. *Progr Clin Biol Res.* 1982;104:66.

68. Horton WA, Rimoin DL, Lachman RS, et al. The phenotypic variability of diastrophic dysplasia. *J Pediatr.* 1978;93:609.

69. Kaitila I, Ammala P, Karjalainen O, et al. Early prenatal detection of diastrophic dysplasia. *Prenat Diagn.* 1983; 3:237.

70. Mantagos S, Weiss RR, Mahoney M, et al. Prenatal diagnosis of diastrophic dwarfism. *Am J Obstet Gynecol.* 1981;139:1111.

71. Gembruch U, Niesen M, Kehrberg H, Hansmann M. Diastrophic dysplasia: A specific prenatal diagnosis by ultrasound. *Prenat Diagn.* 1988;8:539–545.

72. Gollop TR, Eigier A. Brief clinical report: Prenatal ultrasound diagnosis of diastrophic dysplasia at 16 weeks. *Am J Med Genet.* 1987;27:321–324.

73. Bod M, Creizel A, Lenz W. Incidence at birth of different types of limb reduction abnormalities in Hungary, 1975–1977. *Hum Genet.* 1983;65:27.

74. Goldberg MJ. *The Dysmorphic Child: An Orthopedic Perspective.* New York: Raven Press; 1987.

75. Pilarski RT, Pauli RM, Engber WD. Hand-reduction malformations: Genetic and syndrome analysis. *J Pediatr.* 1985;5:274.

76. Hecht JT, Scott CI Jr. Recurrent unilateral hand malformations in siblings. *Clin Genet.* 1981;20:225.

77. Tunobileck E, Yalcin C, Atasu M. Aglossia-adactylia syndrome (special emphasis on the inheritance pattern). *Clin Genet.* 1977;11:421.

78. Baraitser M. Genetics of Mobius syndrome. *J Med Genet.* 1977;14:415.

79. Sugarman GI, Stark HH. Mobius syndrome with Poland's anomaly. *J Med Genet.* 1973;10:192.

80. Happle R, Koch H, Lenz W. The CHILD syndrome: Congenital hemidysplasia with ichthyosiform erthyroderma and limb defects. *Eur J Pediatr.* 1980;134:27.

81. Martin Du Pan CH. Absence congenitale du perone sans deformation du tibia. *Revue D'Orthopedie.* 1924;3:227.

82. Pauli RM, Greenlaw A. Limb deficiency and splenogonadal fusion. *Am J Med Genet.* 1982;13:81.

83. Bonafede RP, Beighton P. Autosomal dominant inheritance of scalp defects with extrodactyly. *Am J Med Genet.* 1979;3:35.

84. Claus GH, Newman CGH. The thalidomide syndrome: Risks of exposure and spectrum of malformations. *Teratology.* 1986;13:555–573.

85. Waldenmaier C, Aldenhoff P, Klemm T. The Robert's syndrome. *Hum Genet.* 1978;40:345.

86. Romeo G, Zonana J, Lachman RS, et al. Grebe chondrodysplasia and similar forms of severe short-limbed dwarfism. *Birth Defects.* 1977;13:109.

87. Hamanishi C. Congenital short femur. *J Bone Joint Surg.* 1980;62:307.

88. Daentl DL, Smith DW, Scott C. Femoral hypoplasia—unusual facies syndrome. *J Pediatr.* 1975;86:107.

89. Burn J, Winter RJ, Baraitser M, Hall CM, et al. The femoral hypoplasia—unusual facies syndrome. *J Med Genet.* 1984;21:331–340.

90. Gupta DKS, Gupta SK. Familial bilateral femoral focal deficiency. *J Bone Joint Surg.* 1984;66A:1470–1472.

91. Tentamy S, McKusick V. *Birth Defects, National Foundation—March of Dimes.* New York: Alan R. Liss; 14(3):1978.

92. Miura T, Suzuki M. Clinical differences between typical and atypical cleft hand. *J Hand Surg.* 1984;9:311.

93. Barsky AJ. Cleft hand: Classification, incidence, and treatment. *J Bone Joint Surg.* 1964;46:1707.

94. Tada K, Yonenobu K, Swanson AB. Congenital central ray deficiency in the hand—a survey of 59 cases and subclassification. *J Hand Surg.* 1981;6:434.

95. Van den Berghe H, Dequeker J, Fryns JP, et al. Familial occurrence of severe ulnar aplasia and lobster claw feet: A new syndrome. *Hum Genet.* 1978;42:109.

96. Verma IC, Joseph R, Bhargava S, Mehta S. Split-hand and split-foot deformity inherited as an autosomal recessive trait. *Clin Genet.* 1976;9:8.

97. Rudiger RA, Haase W, Passarge E. Association of ectrodactyly, ectodermal dysplasia, and cleft lip palate. *Am J Dis Child.* 1970;120:160.

98. Leiter E, Lipson J. Genitourinary tract anomalies in lobster claw syndrome. *J Urol.* 1976;115:339–341.

99. Penchaszadeh VB, De Negrotti TC. Ectrodactyly-ectodermal dysplasia-clefting (EEC) syndrome: Dominant inheritance and variable expression. *J Med Genet.* 1976; 13:281–284.

100. Halal F, Homsy M, Perreault G. Acro-renal-ocular syndrome: Autosomal dominant thumb hypoplasia, renal ectopia, and eye defect. *Am J Med Genet.* 1984;17:753–762.

101. Chan KM, Lamb DW. Triphalangeal thumb and five-fingered hand. *Hand.* 1983;15:329–334.

102. Wood VE. Congenital thumb deformities. *Clin Orthop.* 1985;195:7–25.

103. Bujdoso G, Lenz W. Monodactylous splithand-splitfoot. *Eur J Pediatr.* 1980;133:207.

104. Carroll RE, Louis DS. Anomalies associated with radial dysplasia. *J Pediatr.* 1974;84:409–411.

105. Glanz A, Fraser FC. Spectrum of anomalies in Fanconi anaemia. *J Med Genet.* 1982;19:412–416.

106. Nilsson LR. Chronic pancytopenia with multiple congenital abnormalities (Fanconi's anaemia). *Acta Paediatrica.* 1960;49:518–529.

107. Auerbach AD, Sagi M, Adler B. Fanconi anemia: Prenatal diagnosis in 30 fetuses at risk. *Pediatrics.* 1985;76:794–800.

108. de Vries LS, Connell J, Bydder GM, et al. Recurrent intracranial haemorrhages in utero in an infant with alloimmune thrombocytopenia. Case report. *Br J Obstet Gynaecol.* 1988;95:299–302.

109. Higginbottom MC, Jones KL, Kung FH. The Aase syndrome in a female infant. *J Med Genet.* 1978;15:484–486.

110. Jones B, Thompson H. Triphalangeal thumbs associated with hypoplastic anemia. *Pediatrics.* 1973;52:609–612.

111. Zhang KZ, Sun QB, Tsung OC. Holt–Oram syndrome in China: A collective review of 18 cases. *Am Heart J.* 1986;111:573–577.

112. Muller LM, et al. The antenatal ultrasonographic detection of the Holt–Oram syndrome. *S Afr Med J.* 1985; 68:313–315.

113. Brons JTJ, van Geijn HP, Wladimiroff JW. Prenatal ultrasonographic diagnosis of the Holt–Oram Syndrome. *Prenat Diagn.* 1988;8:175–181.

114. Lewis KB, Bruce RA, Baum D, et al. The upper limb-cardiovascular syndrome. *JAMA.* 1965;193:1080–1086.

115. Uuspaa V. Upper extremity deformities associated with the orofacial clefts. *Scand J Plast Reconstr Surg.* 1978; 12:157–162.

116. Chemke J, Nisani R, Fischel RE. Absent ulna in the Klippel–Feil syndrome: An unusual associated malformation. *Clin Genet.* 1980;17:167–170.

117. Tentamy SA, Miller JD. Extending the scope of the VATER association: Definition of a VATER syndrome. *J Pediatr.* 1974;85:345.

118. Setzer ES, Reiz-Castaneda N, Severn C, et al. Etiologic heterogeneity in the oculoauriculo vertebral syndrome. *J Pediatr.* 1981;98:88–90.

119. Swanson AB, Tada K, Yonenubo K. Ulnar ray deficiency: Its various manifestations. *J Hand Surg.* 1984;9A:658–664.

120. Gausewitz SH, Meals RA, Setocuchi Y. Severe limb deficiency in Poland's syndrome. *Clin Orthop.* 1984;185:9–13.

121. David TJ. Preaxial polydactyly and the Poland complex. *Am J Med Genet.* 1982;13:333–334.

122. Lowry RB. Variability in the Smith–Lemli–Opitz syndrome: Overlap with the Meckel syndrome. *Am J Med Genet.* 1983;14:429–433.

123. Goodman RM, Sternberg M, Shem-Tob Y, et al. Acrocephalopolysyndactyly type IV: A new genetic syndrome in 3 sibs. *Clin Genet.* 1979;15:209–214.

124. Khaldi F, Bennaceur B, Hammou A, et al. An autosomal recessive disorder with retardation of growth, mental deficiency, ptosis, pectus excavatum and camptodactyly. *Pediatr Radiol.* 1988;18:432–435.

125. Christophorou MN, Nicolaidou P. Median cleft lip, polydactyly, syndactyly and toe anomalies in a non-Indian infant. *Br J Plast Surg.* 1983;36:447–448.

126. Hageman G, Willemse J. Arthrogryposis multiplexa congenita. Review with comments. *Neuroped.* 1983; 14:6.

127. Swinyard CA, Bleck EE. The etiology of arthrogryposis (multiple congenital contracture). *Clin Orthop.* 1985; 194:15.

128. Banker BQ. Neuropathologic aspects of arthrogryposis multiplex congenita. *Clin Orthop.* 1985;194:30.

129. Thompson GH, Bilenker RM. Comprehensive management of arthrogryposis multiplex congenita. *Clin Orthop.* 1985;194:6–14.

130. Gorczyca DP, McGahan JP, Kindfors KK, Ellis WG, Grix A. Arthrogryposis multiplex congenita: Prenatal ultrasonic diagnosis. J Clin Ultrasound. 1989;17:40.

131. Kirkinen P, Herva R, Leisti J. Early prenatal diagnosis of a lethal syndrome of multiple congenital contractures. *Prenat Diagn.* 1987;7:189–196.

132. Goldberg JD, Chervenak FA, Lipman RA, Berkowitz RL. Antenatal sonographic diagnosis of arthrogryposis multiplex congenita. *Prenat Diagn.* 1986;6:45.

133. Miskin M, Rothberg R, Rudd N, Benxie R, Shine J. Arthrogryposis multiplex congenita—prenatal assessment with diagnostic ultrasound and fetoscopy. *J Pediatr.* 1979;95:463.

134. Socol ML, Sabbagha RE, Elias S, et al. Prenatal diagnosis of congenital muscular dystrophy producing arthrogryposis. *N Engl J Med.* 1985;313:1230.

135. Hall JG. Genetic aspects of arthrogryposis. *Clin Orthop* 1985;194:44.

19 The Antenatal Sonographic Diagnosis of Syndromes

Beryl Benacerraf

Recent advances in ultrasound technology and sonography experience have permitted the detailed prenatal diagnosis of multiple congenital abnormalities involving almost all fetal organ systems (Fig. 19–1).[1-3] Prenatal diagnosis of various anomalies is highly accurate and appropriate counseling is now available to patients prior to the delivery of a malformed fetus.[4] It is not enough, however, to discover a fetal anomaly without seeking patterns of malformations that might fit into a syndrome.[5] Obstetric management may be quite different if the fetus is found to have multiple congenital abnormalities or a particular syndrome rather than a single finding involving only one organ system. Counseling the patients, as well as overall prognosis for morbidity and mortality, might differ if multiple congenital abnormalities are found. If these anomalies fit a pattern, and suggest that chromosomal studies are indicated, additional information would then be available which could be crucial in obstetrical management and outcome.[5,6] The sonologist must be aware of the patterns of malformation that comprise syndromes and must seek these patterns in every case where fetal abnormalities are suspected.

DOWN'S SYNDROME

The overall incidence of Down's syndrome (trisomy 21) is 1 in 660 newborns, which is the most common pattern of malformation in humans.[7] Until recently, very little has been accomplished in the morphologic sonographic diagnosis of fetuses with Down's syndrome. Cytogenic analysis has remained the only definitive method of diagnosis. Certainly many of the structural anomalies associated with Down's syndrome are not obvious enough to be detectable sonographically, such as hyperflexibility of joints, flat nasal profile, slanted palpebral fissures, anomalous auricles, dysplasia of pelvis, hypotonia, and brachycephaly.[7,8] There are, however, several morphologic signs that can now be identified sonographically in the second trimester that indicate fetuses at risk for Down's syndrome. These signs include a thickened nuchal fold,[9-13] shortened femurs,[13-20] and hypoplasia of the middle phalanx of the fifth digit.[7,8,21] Other, rarer

anomalies that are also associated with Down's syndrome include duodenal atresia and congenital heart disease, the atrio-ventricular (AV) canal in particular, which should prompt amniocentesis when encountered antenatally.

Abnormal thickening of the soft tissues at the back of the fetal occiput is present in 80% of neonates with Down's syndrome.[7,8] There is a thickened nuchal fold in approximately 42% of fetuses with Down's syndrome between 15 and 20 weeks, in a series of 3,825 fetuses that were studied sonographically at the time of amniocentesis.[11] Twenty-one of these fetuses had Down's syndrome by karyotype and nine (42%) had a thickened nuchal fold. In order to evaluate the nuchal soft tissues, a modified transverse view of the fetal head is used, which includes the cerebellum and occipital bone (Fig. 19–2). The nuchal fold is then measured from the outer edge of the occipital bone to the outer edge of the fetal skin. A measurement of 6 mm or more is considered abnormal. Nine of the 21 fetuses with Down's syndrome were found to have a nuchal fold measurement of 6 mm or more, and six of these had the abnormal nuchal fold as the only abnormal sonographic finding. The three remaining fetuses had generalized hydrops with cardiac malformation, multiple congenital abnormalities, and hydrocephalus, respectively (Fig. 19–3). Four of the remaining 3,816 fetuses had an abnormal or thickened nuchal fold but did not have Down's syndrome. Three of these had a normal karyotype, and the fourth had a 5P+ karyotype with multiple congenital abnormalities. This represented a 0.1% false-positive rate for the use of the nuchal fold in the diagnosis of Down's syndrome and a positive predictive value of 69% (9/13).

Fewer fetuses with Down's syndrome have a thickened nuchal fold at 16 weeks (42%) than in the neonatal period (80%). This represents a valuable finding, however, because it has a high positive predictive value and is an easy measurement to perform. Toi and associates[24] have reported a higher false-positive rate than ours. However, he studied fetuses between 19 and 26 weeks, which were older than those in our study, and his figure shows inclusion of the occipital bone in his measurement, unlike our technique. To establish the measurement, we demonstrated the normal nuchal fold in 303 consecutive nor-

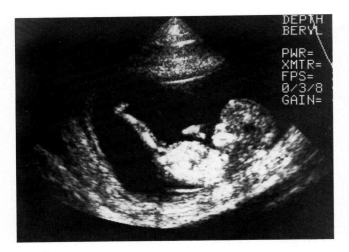

Fig. 19–1. Longitudinal view of a 12-week fetus showing normal anatomy of head, face and extremities.

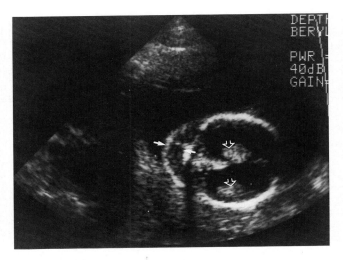

Fig. 19–3. Second trimester fetus with Down's syndrome who had hydrocephalus. The choroid plexus is compressed and displaced (*open arrows*) and there is a thickened nuchal fold (*solid arrows*).

mal fetuses undergoing genetic amniocentesis at 15 to 20 weeks, the age range at which this measurement is recommended.[25] There were no fetuses in our study who had a nuchal fold >6 mm, regardless of gestational age, although the numbers of fetuses aged 19 to 20 weeks were too small to be conclusive. We recommend the use of the nuchal fold measurement as described here for fetuses between 15 and 19 weeks, because this is the age group that has been extensively studied, and measurement norm has not been established for the older age groups. It must be stressed, however, that the measurement is taken from the outer edge of the occipital bone, not the inner edge, and that angling posteriorly beyond the occipital bone will yield a spuriously wide measurement.[25]

The majority of fetuses with Down's syndrome have a slightly shortened femur length compared to their normal counterparts of the same gestational age. This was evaluated in a collaborative study by Lockwood and colleagues[14] involving two different populations of fe-

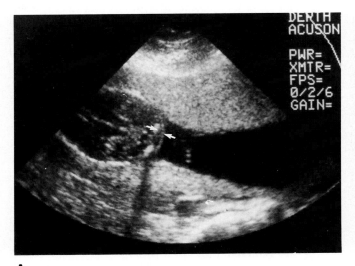

A

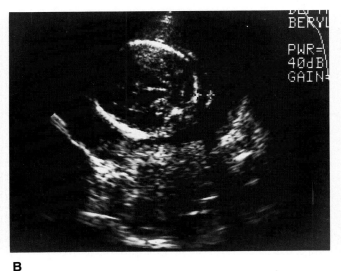

B

Fig. 19–2. **A.** Transverse view of the posterior fossa showing normal nuchal fold with no evidence of soft tissue thickening (*arrows*). **B.** Thickened nuchal fold indicated by caliper markers on 20-week fetus with Down's syndrome.

tuses between 15 and 23 weeks. A biparietal diameter (BPD):femur length ratio was consistently elevated in most fetuses with Down's syndrome compared to the control population throughout the second trimester. Using a cutoff value of 1.5 standard deviations above the normal population, the BPD:femur length ratio identified 50 to 70% of fetuses with Down's syndrome in 6% of the normal population. This study suggested that the BPD:femur length ratio would prove superior to current Down's syndrome screening methods.

We further evaluated 28 consecutive fetuses with Down's syndrome from a total of 5,500 fetuses scanned by a single sonologist at the time of amniocentesis, when they were between 15 and 20 weeks.[15] One hundred ninety-two (192) control fetuses between 15 and 20 weeks were used to establish the normal femur length for gestational age, and this was compared to the femur lengths of the 28 fetuses with Down's syndrome. A linear regression model of the normal femur length based on BPD was established for our control population. A ratio of measured femur length divided by expected femur length based on BPD could then be calculated, and a cutoff of 0.91 was used as the lower normal limit for the ratio. Specificity and sensitivity for the shortened femur was 98% and 69% respectively, indicating that 69% of Down's syndrome fetuses would be correctly identified using this method, subjecting 2% of normal fetuses to amniocentesis. The positive predictive value for the shortened femur varied according to the prevalence of the disease. For women at 1/250 risk of Down's syndrome, the positive predictive value was 12%; for those in the 1/500 risk group, it was 6.4%; and for those at low risk (1/1,000), the positive predictive value of a shortened femur length for detection of Down's syndrome was 3.3%.

It is important that the entire length of the femur be measured carefully, because only small changes in femur length can be misleading when this technique is used to screen for Down's syndrome. Several attempts must be made to obtain the longest possible femur length so as to ensure that the femur was not foreshortened inadvertently during the measurement. It is of note that the Yale group in the Lockwood study had a slightly different normal range for femur length according to gestational age than the Boston group;[14] however, within each population, the same relationship of shortened femurs in fetuses with Down's syndrome was present. This confirms that each center should establish its own norms and limits of confidence for the Down's syndrome risk assessment.

Recently, we studied an additional 20 consecutive second-trimester fetuses with Down's syndrome and compared them to 709 normal controls undergoing genetic amniocentesis. To standardize the use of the femur measurement for identifying fetuses at risk for having

Down's syndrome, all femur measurements in this study were performed by eight sonographers with varying levels of training. A regression analysis on the normal control fetuses comparing BPD to femur length yielded the following equation:

$$\text{Expected femur length} = -9.3105 + 0.9028 \times \text{BPD}$$

The ratio of measured to expected femur length of 0.91 or less identified 40% of fetuses with Down's Syndrome with a false-positive rate of 5%, with a positive predictive value of 3.1%. Eight of these 20 Down's syndrome fetuses (40%) had a thickened nuchal fold. Combining the nuchal fold with femur length raises the sensitivity of identifying affected fetuses to 45% and positive predictive value to 4.3% without significantly affecting the specificity.[13]

Our findings are in agreement with those of Brumfield,[13B] who studied 15 fetuses with trisomy 21. She found that a high BPD/femur ratio predicted Down's syndrome with a sensitivity of 40% and specificity of 97.8% (2.2% false positives). Perrella and associates[16] also found an association between trisomy 21 and the combination of short femurs and prominent nuchal fold (sensitivity 42%, specificity 88%). Hill and coworkers[20] found a sensitivity of 45% and specificity of 92.3% for the detection of fetuses with Down's syndrome using the femur length and nuchal fold; and Dicke and colleagues[19] also confirmed the association of slightly short femurs with second trimester fetuses with trisomy 21, although with a lower sensitivity. Grist and associates[18] reported that the measured to expected femur length ratio of 0.90 resulted in the sensitivity for identifying Down's syndrome fetuses of 50% with a false-positive rate of 6.5%. This yields a positive predictive value of 3%, similar to our recent experience.[13] Lynch and coworkers,[12] on the other hand, found that the nuchal fold was the most useful sonographic sign to distinguish Down's syndrome fetuses from their normal co-twin in a series of 11 twin pregnancies with one affected fetus in each pair.

Approximately 50% of fetuses with trisomy 21 have an associated heart defect, particularly ventriculoseptal defects (VSD) or endocardial cushion defects (Fig. 19–4).[23] In our series of 28 fetuses with Down's syndrome, only two had sonographic signs of congenital heart disease, having complete AV canal and hydrops. It is likely that the other fetuses in the remaining 26 had heart defects that were not detected sonographically in the second trimester, since 2 of 28 is a much smaller number than anticipated in fetuses with Down's syndrome.

It is well known that major congenital heart defects are detectable by prenatal sonography; however, less complex heart diseases, such as VSDs, are easily missed, particularly in fetuses who are not known to be at risk for congenital heart disease.[26] Several authors have reported that VSDs can be missed particularly in the second

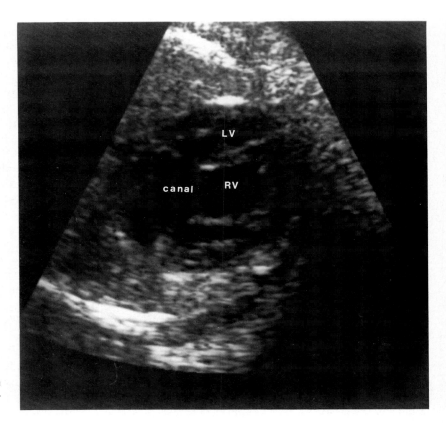

Fig. 19–4. Four-chamber view of the heart in a fetus with Down's syndrome, with an endocardial cushion defect or AV canal.

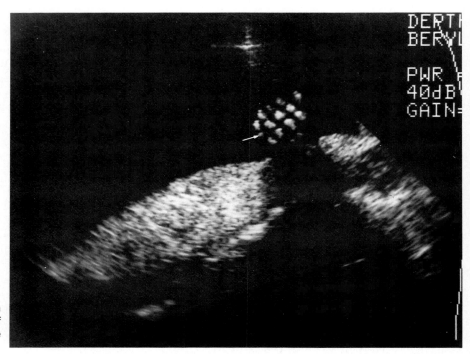

Fig. 19–5. Second trimester fetus with Down's syndrome showing evidence of hypoplasia of the middle phalanx of the fifth digit (*arrow*).

trimester.[27,28] Therefore, detection of congenital heart disease cannot be relied on in the second trimester to identify fetuses at risk for Down's syndrome. We studied 49 fetuses who were born with heart defects and who had undergone sonography at 18 weeks or more. Our study represented a mix of fetuses at high and low risk for heart defects, because all patients were included regardless of indication for the scan. Our findings indicated that detection of major heart defects was excellent, although minor or less life-threatening abnormalities of the heart were frequently missed. In particular, all nine fetuses with hypoplastic left or right heart were correctly identified; four of five fetuses with tetralogy of Fallot and two of three fetuses with transposition of the great arteries, as well as both fetuses with common AV canal, were correctly identified.[26] Fetuses with atrial septal defects (ASDs) and VSDs, aortic or pulmonic stenosis, or total anomalous pulmonary venous return, were not consistently identified sonographically, indicating room for improvement. We conclude that the identification of congenital heart defects by ultrasound in the second trimester cannot be relied on to identify fetuses at risk for chromosomal abnormalities.

Sixty percent of neonates with Down's syndrome are known to have hypoplasia of the middle phalanx of the fifth digit, with some inward curvature of that digit.[7,8] We have had the opportunity to examine five fetuses between 17 and 20 weeks, four of which were known to have Down's syndrome at the time of the sonographic examination, and one of which was strongly suspected to have it due to an AV canal defect, hydrops, and shortened femurs in a 40-year-old patient.[21] Four of these fetuses had an abnormal configuration with inward curvature of the fifth digit and a smaller than anticipated middle phalanx of that digit (Fig. 19–5). More work needs to be done to establish the normal appearance of the middle phalanx of the fifth digit and whether or not this sign has any potential in the antenatal detection of Down's syndrome.

Although other findings, such as duodenal atresia, can be helpful in suspecting that a fetus could have Down's syndrome, the classic double bubble appearance does not become apparent until after 22 to 24 weeks. Therefore, this abnormality is probably not detectable in the mid-second trimester when it most desirable to make the diagnosis (Fig. 19–6). Other abnormalities that occasionally have been seen with Down's syndrome, include two fetuses with clubfoot and two fetuses with hydrocephalus, unusual associations but ones that should prompt amniocentesis.

At present, amniocentesis is performed during the mid-trimester when the risk of giving birth to a live infant with Down's syndrome is 1 in 385 or 1 in 250 (0.4%) because of advanced maternal age or a low alphafetoprotein (AFP) level.[29-31] The positive predictive value of the sonographic signs described here is far superior than for advanced maternal age or low AFP. It may eventually be possible to combine the sonographic findings with AFP testing and age to better refine the risks of

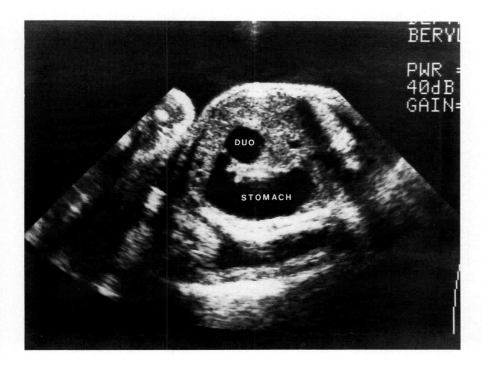

Fig. 19–6. Abdominal scan of a third-trimester fetus with Down's syndrome showing duodenal atresia. Note the polyhydramnios. DUO = duodenum.

women who may be carrying fetuses with Down's syndrome. It is known that 80% of fetuses with Down's syndrome are born to women who are younger than 35 years of age and who are not candidates for any cytogenetic evaluation.[29] Because only 20% of fetuses with Down's syndrome are born to older mothers and probably half of these women elect to undergo cytogenetic evaluation, 90% of fetuses with Down's syndrome are not detected antenatally by this screening method.[29,32,33] A low serum AFP currently identifies 20 to 30% of fetuses with Down's syndrome but, as a result, amniocentesis is offered to 5 to 11.6% of women with normal fetuses, a calculated positive predictive value as low as 0.7 to 1% for a population at risk of 1 in 250.[31,34,35] The positive predictive value for the abnormal nuchal fold and short femurs is 4.3% in our most recent study, which is equivalent to the chance of Down's syndrome incurred by a 44-year-old woman on the basis of age alone. Schoenfeld-DiMaio and associates[31] reported that 1/161 patients who had a low AFP had a fetus with Down's syndrome, yielding a positive predictive value far below that associated with the sonographic signs described here.

Only a small number of women are candidates for amniocentesis, whereas large numbers of pregnant women are now undergoing sonography without amniocentesis. If the signs described here were specifically looked for as a part of the fetal survey and amniocentesis was offered to women who carried fetuses with a thickened nuchal fold or shortened femur, potentially many more fetuses with Down's syndrome would be identified than is presently possible by maternal age and AFP testing alone.

TRISOMY 18

Trisomy 18 (Edward's syndrome) has an incidence of about 0.3 per 1,000 newborn babies and is one of the most common chromosomal defects associated with multiple congenital abnormalities.[7] The hallmark of trisomy 18 is polyhydramnios with intrauterine growth retardation and congenital abnormalities. Growth deficiency is a well-known part of this syndrome and, therefore, it is particularly important to make the antenatal diagnosis of trisomy 18 because of the universally poor prognosis.[37,38] These fetuses are often subject to premature delivery associated with fetal distress because of severe intrauterine growth retardation, and a cesarean section could be avoided if the presence of a lethal trisomy was known prior to delivery. The patient could also be saved from lengthy antenatal monitoring, hospitalizations, and so forth. The ultrasonographer, therefore, must be aware of the patterns and signs of malformations that suggest chromosome abnormalities so cytogenetic studies can be

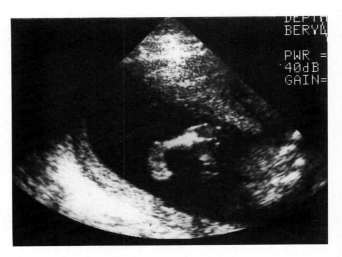

Fig. 19–7. Sixteen-week fetus with trisomy 18 showing clubbing of the foot.

offered. Particular abnormalities associated with trisomy 18 involve the hands and feet, with overlapping index finger over a clenched hand, clubfeet or rocker-bottom feet; also congenital heart disease; hernias, such as umbilical, diaphragmatic, or inguinal; and renal abnormalities such as horseshoe kidney.[38–44] The survival for fetuses with trisomy 18 is extremely poor and most infants with this syndrome will die within the first few hours or days of life.[45]

Sonographic identification of congenital clubfoot places the fetus at risk for trisomy 18, particularly when associated with polyhydramnios.[38,40–42,46] Between 10 and 50% of fetuses with trisomy 18 have congenital clubfoot or rocker-bottom foot (Fig. 19–7). In our series of 18 cases of congenital clubfoot, four had abnormal

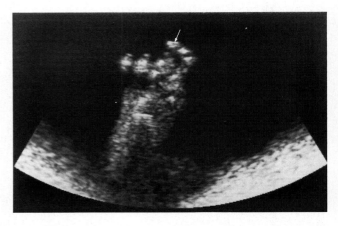

Fig. 19–8. Characteristic hand position of a fetus with trisomy 18. Hand is clenched in a fist with overlapping index finger (*arrow*).

The most common abnormal prenatal sonographic finding is posterior nuchal cystic hygromas, which can be very large and can be associated with generalized lymphedema of the fetus and hydrops (Fig. 19–23).[74–77] Fetuses with very large cystic hygromas associated with hydrops have a very poor prognosis. The cystic hygromas probably represent congenital lymphatic malformations resulting from obstruction of the lymphatics and absence of communication with the venous system in the neck.[77] These cysts are usually sonographically clear, although they often contain thin septations separating them into different compartments. They should not be confused with neural tube defects, because the spine is usually intact in cystic hygroma colli. Chervenak and associates[15] reported on 15 consecutive cases of nuchal hygroma, 13 of which were hydropic at the time of diagnosis. Nine died in utero, and one died a few hours after birth. There were 11 fetuses, or 73%, who had karyotypes of Turner's syndrome. Cystic hygroma can be associated with normal chromosomes, however, and Noonan's syndrome should be considered, particularly if the fetus is seen to be a male.[78,79] Noonan's syndrome is also associated with short stature, cubitus valgus, and congenital heart disease and is thought to be the male counterpart to Turner's syndrome but with a normal karyotype.[7] Patients with Noonan's syndrome, however, have mental retardation, which is not always a factor in Turner's syndrome. Nuchal cystic hygroma and congenital heart disease seen in the male fetus should suggest the diagnosis of Noonan's syn-

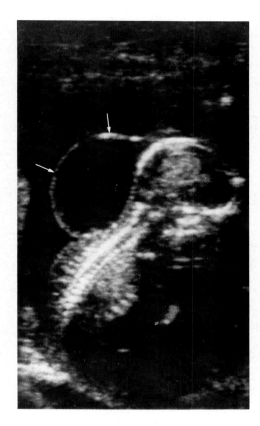

Fig. 19–23. Longitudinal view of the fetal neck showing a thick-walled cystic area that represents a cystic hygroma in a fetus with Turner's syndrome. Note the fetal spine is intact.

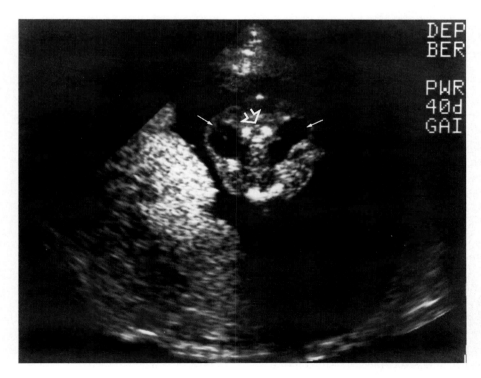

Fig. 19–24. Transverse view of the fetal neck in a fetus with Noonan's syndrome, showing lateral cystic hygromas on both sides. A cervical vertebra is shown by the *open arrow* and cystic hygromas are indicated by *small solid arrows.*

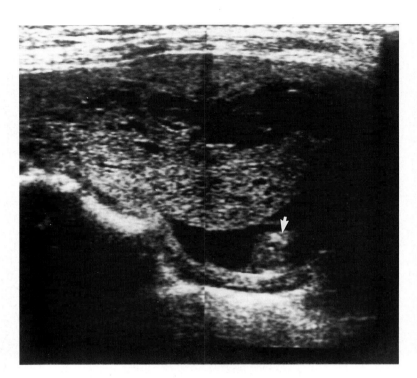

Fig. 19–25. Longitudinal view of the uterus showing a fetal pole (*arrow*) with markedly enlarged and hydropic placenta. This was a partial mole with triploidy.

drome (Fig. 19–24). Familial nuchal bleb can also mimic cystic hygromas and encephaloceles.[80]

Cystic hygromas do not always occur in the posterior nuchal area but can be present anywhere, including the chest, abdominal wall, and anterior neck. When congenital cystic hygroma occurs in an area other than the back of the neck, it is not usually associated with chromosomal abnormalities. It usually is an isolated finding with a relatively good prognosis after surgery.[81]

TRIPLOIDY

Triploidy represents a complete extra set of chromosomes and is estimated to occur in approximately 1% of conceptuses.[82] Most of these end in miscarriage, however, and triploidy accounts for 20% of chromosomal abnormalities identified in spontaneous abortions.[82] Progression of the pregnancy to birth is extremely rare, and when it does happen, death usually occurs within the first few hours of life. The longest survivor has been 10½ months; only a small number of these patients have lived a few days.[83] The most common ultrasound finding is severe symmetrical intrauterine growth retardation associated with oligohydramnios.[84]

Sonographic findings in triploidy are nonspecific and include abnormalities of almost every organ system, including meningomyelocele, holoprosencephaly, absence of the corpus callosum, cleft lip and palate, hydroceph-

alus, congenital heart disease such as ventriculoseptal defect and atrial septal defect, renal abnormalities such as hydronephrosis and multicystic kidney, and abnormalities of the hands and feet.[84–88] Although there are no salient features to suggest triploidy in particular, when any congenital abnormality is seen in association with severe intrauterine growth retardation, triploidy should be considered and karyotyping recommended.[87] Intrauterine growth retardation can occur as early as the second trimester and, in fact, we have seen it as early as the first trimester.[89] Abnormalities of the placenta may also be a clue to triploidy, particularly when a partial hyatidiform mole is present (Fig. 19–25).[90] Alternatively, the placenta can be very small and prematurely aged. It is crucial that the diagnosis be suspected sonographically so a karyotype can be done, because these fetuses are prone to fetal distress and early operative delivery secondary to their intrauterine growth retardation and placental insufficiency. Operative and early delivery does not improve the dismal prognosis and these patients can be spared lengthy antenatal monitoring and cesarean section if the correct diagnosis is known.

MECKEL–GRUBER SYNDROME

Meckel–Gruber syndrome is a severe disorder characterized by occipital encephalocele, polycystic kidneys, and postaxial polydactyly (Figs. 19–26, 19–27).[91] Meckel–

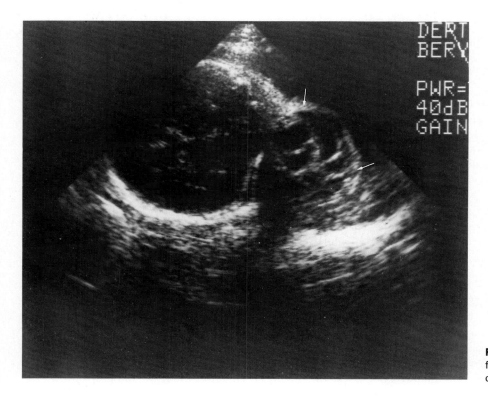

Fig. 19–26. Transverse view through the fetal head showing posterior encephalocele (*arrows*).

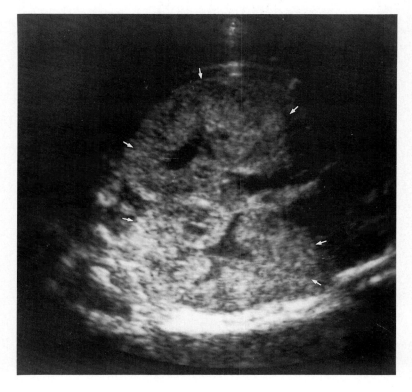

Fig. 19–27. Bilateral polycystic kidneys are shown longitudinally (*arrows*) in a fetus with Meckel–Gruber syndrome.

Gruber syndrome is an autosomal recessive disorder that carries a 25% risk of recurrence within families with a previously affected child.[92] Other associated abnormalities can include cleft lip and palate (30%), micrognathia, relatively short limbs, hepatic fibrosis and cysts, and occasionally hydrocephalus and omphalocele.[92,93] These fetuses have an exceedingly poor prognosis and seldom survive more than a few days or weeks.[7] The ultrasound findings of occipital encephalocele, microcephaly, homogeneously echogenic kidneys, oligohydramnios, and polydactyly should strongly suggest the diagnosis of Meckel–Gruber syndrome. Because this syndrome can mimic trisomy 13, however, karyotyping is indicated. Usually, the amniotic fluid will show marked elevations in AFP, a finding that is often used to screen mothers in families at risk for Meckel–Gruber syndrome.[7,94]

GOLDENHAR-GORLIN SYNDROME

Goldenhar-Gorlin syndrome is characterized by defects of the first and second branchial arches, which can be bilateral or unilateral, involving the face and cervical vertebrae.[7] When unilateral, it can be called hemifacial microsomia, which is thought to represent gradations in severity of Goldenhar-Gorlin syndrome.[95] The incidence

of Goldenhar-Gorlin syndrome is 1 in 3,000 to 1 in 5,000 births.[7] Other abnormalities that can be associated with the facial and cervical vertebral anomalies include ventriculoseptal defect and other congenital heart diseases, laryngeal abnormality, hypoplasia or aplasia of a lung, renal and limb abnormalities, occipital encephalocele and intrauterine growth retardation.[7] A recent case demonstrated unilateral abnormalities of the face, including hypoplasia of the right side of the mandible, agenesis of the right lung, hydroureter, and hydronephrosis of the right kidney (Figs. 19–28 and 19–29). All of this fetus's malformations were unilateral, which fit the pattern of the syndrome.

AMNIOTIC BAND SYNDROME

Amniotic band syndrome is thought to result from a partial rupture of the amnion. This results in mesodermic bands that form on the chorionic side of the amnion and become adherent to and entangled with the fetal body, causing defects of varying degrees of severity.[96,97] If the rupture occurs early, it can cause an extremely severe defect such as limb–body–wall complex abnormalities or severe cranio-facial defects.[96] If the amnion rupture occurs later in pregnancy, it may cause simply a limb or a digital constriction with amputations.[96] The incidence of

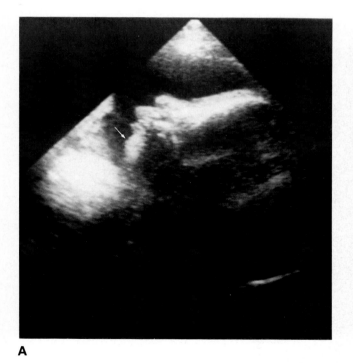

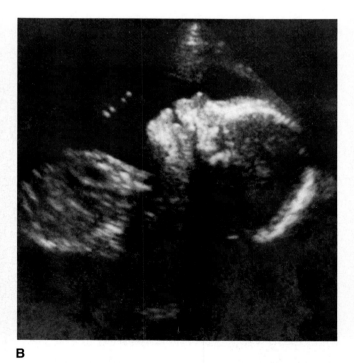

A   **B**

Fig. 19–28. A. Abnormal fetal profile with marked micrognathia (*arrow*) in a fetus with Goldenhar–Gorlin syndrome. **B.** Longitudinal view of the normal fetal profile showing relationship of the nose, mouth, and chin.

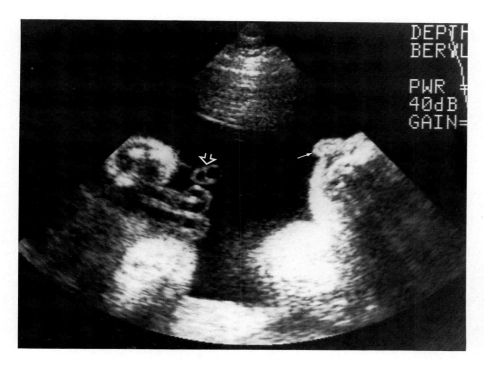

Fig. 19–29. Goldenhar-Gorlin syndrome. This view of the side of the fetal head shows a small skin tag in the region of the fetal ear (*small arrow*) and a two-vessel cord (*open arrow*). There was polyhydramnios. The micrognathia is shown in Fig. 19–28**A.**

amniotic band syndrome has been estimated at 1/5,000 to 1/10,000 pregnancies.[97] Amniotic bands are fibrous strands that extend from the outer surface of the chorion into the environment in which the fetus is developing. Mobile fetal extremities may become entangled and fetal parts can be trapped, constricted, and immobilized. The sonographic findings are varied, depending on the body part entangled or compressed.[96–98] The diagnosis can be made prepartum by identifying the bands sonographically.[98,99]

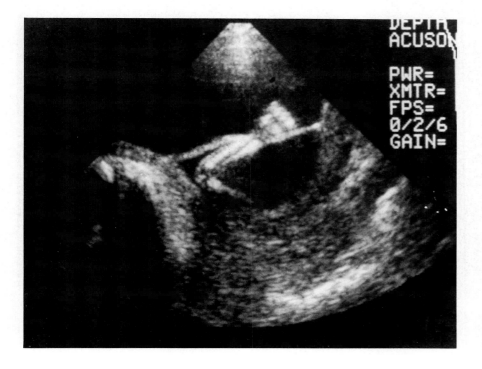

Fig. 19–30. Amniotic band in the vicinity of the fetal upper extremity. This fetus was born without abnormalities.

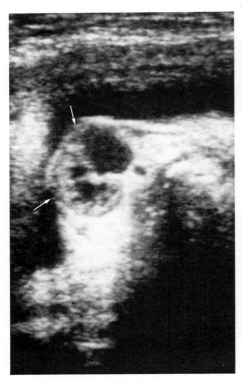

Fig. 19–31. Ectopia cordis in a fetus with amniotic band syndrome. Note that the heart protrudes into the amniotic fluid (*arrows*).

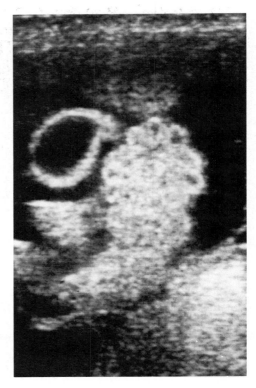

Fig. 19–33. View of fetal stomach and small bowel in the same fetus (Figs. 19–31 and 19–32) with amniotic band syndrome and complete limb–body–wall defect.

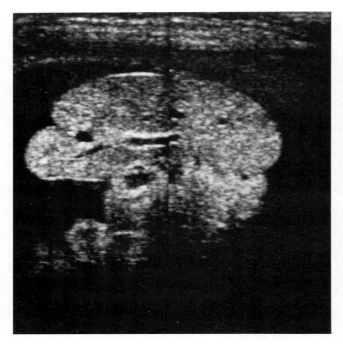

Fig. 19–32. Complete exteriorization of the fetal liver, almost entirely surrounded by amniotic fluid, in the same fetus as Fig. 19–31 with amniotic band syndrome.

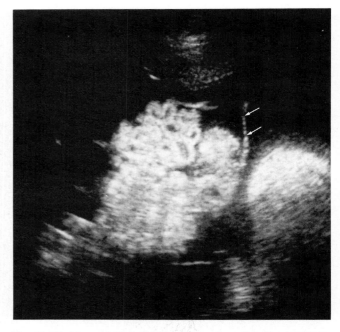

Fig. 19–34. View of the small and large bowel in the amniotic fluid with amniotic band syndrome and limb–body–wall defect. The band itself is shown by *arrows*. (Same case as Figs. 19–31 through 19–33.)

Clubbing of the feet is not an uncommon finding, as well as oligohydramnios. If the fetus swallows a fibrous strand, defects of the face and mandible will occur. It is known that amniotic bands can exist adjacent to a normal-appearing fetus without consequence to the fetus.[98] It is impossible to predict whether or not the fetus will become entangled with the bands as pregnancy continues, and no data are available regarding incidence of fetal involvement when amniotic bands are present (Fig. 19–30). Amniotic band syndrome has been reported in association with amniocentesis.[100]

Limb–body–wall complex is thought to be part of the spectrum of amniotic band syndrome.[96,101] Certainly, complete destruction of the body stalk can result from amniotic bands, as is shown in our case in which the bands were actually visualized both sonographically and pathologically (Figs. 19–31 through 19–34).

HOLT–ORAM SYNDROME

Holt–Oram syndrome was described in 1960, and consists of skeletal and cardiac abnormalities.[102] It is an autosomal dominant syndrome with different degrees of radial aplasia or hypoplasia, absence of hypoplasia of the thumb, and congenital heart disease, which consists mainly of ASD of the secundum type.[7] Ventriculoseptal defects as well as other types of congenital heart disease can occur less commonly. It is important to perform a good echocardiogram when hypoplasia or aplasia of the radius is present sonographically, and particularly to explore the patient's family history when looking for Holt–Oram syndrome (Fig. 19–35). Other syndromes associated with radial aplasia include trisomy 18, thrombocytopenia with absent radius, VATER association, and Robert's syndrome.[7] A search for other findings, such as those present in VATER association, is helpful when differentiating it from Holt–Oram syndrome. VATER association abnormalities include vertebral defects, anal atresia, tracheoesophageal fistula and esophageal atresia, renal anomalies, and radial dysplasia.[103]

CONCLUSION

Until recently the diagnosis of syndromes, both chromosomal and nonchromosomal, has been done by the geneticist and the dysmorphologist. With increasing user expertise in sonography and better equipment, it is possible to sonographically identify subtle morphologic fetal anomalies and fit them into patterns that would suggest particular syndromes or chromosomal abnormalities. Finding patterns of malformations suggestive of further evaluation by cytogenetics is crucial to those patients carrying fetuses with lethal malformations for whom obstetric management can be altered. It is also important to identify fetuses who have a particular syndrome with a known pattern of heredity such as Meckel–Gruber or Holt–Oram syndromes, because the parents would need special genetic counseling. It is also helpful for patients carrying fetuses with amniotic band syndrome to know that this is not known to be hereditary, and subsequent pregnancies are not thought to be at increased risk. Sonography can be very helpful in genetic counseling because patients may not be urged to have an autopsy on a demised fetus or abortus unless prompted by the sonologist. Knowledge of the syndromes, only a few of which have been outlined in this chapter, is vital to the sonologist.

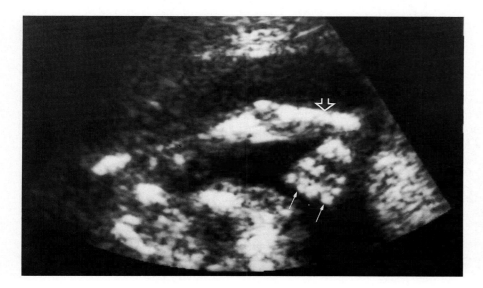

Fig. 19–35. Absent radius in a fetus with Holt–Oram syndrome. The patient herself had the syndrome and the fetus was at 50% risk. Note the absence of the radius and shortened ulnar (*open arrow*), as well as abnormal configuration of the hand with absent thumb (*small solid arrows*).

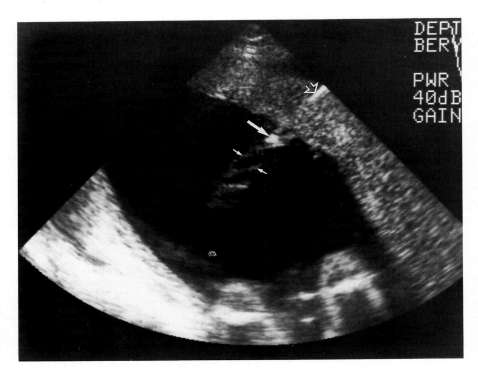

Fig. 19–36. Percutaneous umbilical blood sampling through an anterior placenta. The tip of the needle (*large solid arrow*) is seen within the umbilical vein, which is indicated distally by the *small arrows.* The *open arrow* shows the shaft of the needle.

Without such knowledge, the sonologist cannot piece together the patterns of malformations. We have found percutaneous umbilical blood sampling an excellent method of further evaluating fetuses at risk for chromosomal abnormalities, because a karyotype can be done in 48 hours (Fig. 19–36).[104] The majority of patients carrying fetuses with abnormal karyotypes are not likely to undergo amniocentesis or chorionic villus sampling unless the sonologist detects an anomaly that warrants it. It is therefore our duty to recognize these patterns of malformations and suggest further evaluation or genetic counseling.

REFERENCES

1. Dunne MG, Johnson ML. The ultrasonic demonstration of fetal abnormalities in utero. *J Reprod Med.* 1979;23:197.
2. Chervenak FA, Isaacson G, Mahoney MJ. Advances in the diagnosis of fetal defects. *N Eng J Med.* 1986;315:305.
3. Horger EO, Pai GS. Ultrasound in the diagnosis of fetal malformations: Implications for obstetrical management. *Am J Obstet Gynecol.* 1983;147:163.
4. Sabbagha RE, Sheikh Z, Tamura RK, et al. Predictive value, sensitivity, and specificity of ultrasonic targeted imaging for fetal anomalies in gravid women at high risk for birth defects. *Am J Obstet Gynecol.* 1985;152:822.
5. Vintzileos AM, Campbell WA, Nochimson DJ, et al. Antenatal evaluation and management of ultrasonically detected fetal anomalies. *Obstet Gynecol.* 1987;69:640.
6. Williamson RA, Weiner CP, Patil S, et al. Abnormal pregnancy sonogram: Selective indication for fetal karyotype. *Obstet Gynecol.* 1987;69:15.
7. Smith DW. Recognizable patterns of human malformation. In: *Major Problems in Clinical Pediatrics.* Philadelphia: W. B. Saunders; 1982;7:11–23, 30–31, 72–75.
8. Hall B. Mongolism in newborn infants. *Clin Pediatrics.* 1966;5:4.
9. Benacerraf BR, Barss VA, Laboda LA. A sonographic sign for the detection in the second trimester of the fetus with Down's syndrome. *Am J Obstet Gynecol.* 1985;151:1078.
10. Benacerraf BR, Frigoletto FD, Laboda LA. Sonographic diagnosis of Down syndrome in the second trimester. *Am J Obstet Gynecol.* 1985;153:49.
11. Benacerraf BR, Frigoletto FD, Cramer DW. Down syndrome: Sonographic sign for diagnosis in the second-trimester fetus. *Radiology.* 1987;163:811.
12. Lynch L, Berkowitz GS, Chitkara U, et al. Ultrasound detection of Down syndrome: Is it really possible? *Obstet Gynecol.* 1989;73:267–270.
13. Benacerraf BR, Cnaan A, Gelman R, Laboda LA, Frigoletto FD. Can sonographers reliably identify anatomy features associated with Down syndrome? *Radiology.* 1989;173:377–380.
14. Lockwood C, Benacerraf B, Krinsky A, et al. A sonographic screening method for Down syndrome. *Am J Obstet Gynecol.* 1987;157:803.
15. Benacerraf BR, Gelman R, Frigoletto FD. Sonographic identification of second trimester fetuses with Down syndrome. *N Engl J Med.* 1987;317:1371.

16. Perrella R, Duerinckx AJ, Grant EG, et al. Second-trimester sonographic diagnosis of Down syndrome: Role of femur-length shortening and nuchal-fold thickening. *AJR.* 1988;151:981–985.

17. Brumfield CG, Hauth JC, Cloud GA, et al. Sonographic measurements and ratios in fetuses with Down Syndrome. *Obstet Gynecol.* 1989;73:644–646.

18. Grist TM, Fuller RW, Albiez KL, Bowie JD. Femur length in ultrasound prediction of trisomy 21 and other chromosome abnormalities. (Abstr.) *Radiology.* 1989; 173(P):40.

19. Dicke JM, Gray DL, Songster GS, et al. Fetal biometry as a screening tool for the detection of chromosomally abnormal pregnancies. *Obstet Gynecol.* 1989;74:726–729.

20. Hill LM, Guzick D, Belfar HL, et al. The current role of sonography in the detection of Down syndrome. *Obstet Gynecol.* 1989;74:620–623.

21. Benacerraf BR, Osathanondh R, Frigoletto FD. Sonographic demonstration of hypoplasia of the middle phalanx of the fifth digit: A finding associated with Down syndrome. *Am J Obstet Gynecol.* In press.

22. Balcar I, Grant DC, Miller WA, et al. Antenatal detection of Down syndrome by sonography. *AJR.* 1984;143:29.

23. Copel JA, Pilu G, Kleinman CS. Congenital heart disease and extracardiac anomalies: Associations and indications for fetal echocardiography. *Am J Obstet Gynecol.* 1986; 154:1121.

24. Toi A, Simpson GF, Filley RA. Ultrasonically evident fetal nuchal skin thickening: Is it specific for Down syndrome? *Am J Obstet Gynecol.* 1987;156:150.

25. Benacerraf BR, Frigoletto FD. Soft tissue nuchal fold in the second trimester fetus: Standards for normal measurements compared to the fetus with Down syndrome. *Am J Obstet Gynecol.* In press.

26. Benacerraf BR, Pober BR, Sanders SP. Accuracy of fetal echocardiography. *Radiology.* 1987;165:847.

27. Sandor GGS, Farquarson D, Wittmann B, et al. Fetal echocardiography: Results in high-risk patients. *Obstet Gynecol.* 1986;67:358.

28. Allan LD, Crawford DC, Anderson RH, et al. Echocardiographic and anatomical correlations in fetal congenital heart disease. *Br Heart J.* 1984;52:542.

29. Adams MM, Erickson JD, Layde PM, et al. Down's syndrome: Recent trends in the United States. *JAMA.* 1981;246:758.

30. Hook EB, Cross PK, Schreinemachers DM. Chromosomal abnormality rates at amniocentesis and in live-born infants. *JAMA.* 1983;249:2034.

31. Schoenfeld-DiMaio M, Baumgarten A, Greenstein RM, et al. Screening for fetal Down's syndrome in pregnancy by measuring maternal serum alpha-fetoprotein levels. *N Eng J Med.* 1987;317:342.

32. Lippman-Hand A, Piper M. Prenatal diagnosis for the detection of Down syndrome: Why are so few eligible women tested? *Prenatal Diagnosis.* 1981;1:249.

33. Hook EB, Schreinemachers DM, Cross PK. Use of Prenatal Cytogenetic Diagnosis in New York State. *N Eng J Med.* 1981;305:1410.

34. Cuckle HS, Wald NJ, Lindenbaum RH. Maternal serum alpha-fetoprotein measurement: A screening test for Down syndrome. *Lancet.* 1984;1:926.

35. Spencer K, Carpenter P. Screening for Down's syndrome using serum a/fetoprotein: A retrospective study indicating caution. *Br Med J.* 1985;290:1940.

36. Palomaki GE, Haddow JE. Maternal serum a/fetoprotein, age, and Down syndrome risk. *Am J Obstet Gynecol.* 1987;156:460.

37. Kurjak A, Kirkinen P. Ultrasonic growth pattern of fetuses with chromosomal abberations. *Acta Obstet Gynecol Scand.* 1982;61:223.

38. Bundy AL, Saltzman DH, Pober B, et al. Antenatal sonographic findings in trisomy 18. *J Ultrasound Med.* 1986; 5:361.

39. Benacerraf BR, Frigoletto FD, Greene MF. Abnormal facial features and extremities in human trisomy syndromes: Prenatal US appearance. *Radiology.* 1986; 159:243.

40. Benacerraf BR. Antenatal sonographic diagnosis of congenital clubfoot: A possible indication for amniocentesis. *J Clin Ultrasound.* 1986;14:703.

41. Benacerraf BR, Miller WA, Frigoletto FD. Sonographic detection of fetuses with trisomy 13 and 18: Accuracy and limitations. *Am J Obstet Gynecol.* 1988;158:404.

42. Benacerraf BR, Frigoletto FD. Prenatal ultrasound diagnosis of clubfoot. *Radiology.* 1985;155:211.

43. Benacerraf BR, Adzick NS. Fetal diaphragmatic hernia: Ultrasound diagnosis and clinical outcome in 19 cases. *Am J Obstet Gynecol.* 1987;156:573.

44. Christianson AL, Nelson NM. Four cases of trisomy 18 syndrome with limb reduction malformation. *J Med Genetics.* 1984;21:293.

45. Carter PE, Pearn JH, Bell J, et al. Survival in trisomy 18: Life tables for use in genetic counseling and clinical pediatrics. *Clin Genetics.* 1985;27:59.

46. Jeanty P, Romero R, D'Alton M, et al. In utero sonographic detection of hand and foot deformities. *J Ultrasound Med.* 1985;4:595.

47. Shenker L, Reed K, Anderson C, et al. Syndrome of campodactyly, ankyloses, facial anomalies and pulmonary hypoplasia (Pena–Shokeir syndrome): Obstetric and ultrasound aspects. *Am J Obstet Gynecol.* 1985;152:303.

48. Robinow M, Johnson GF. The Gordon syndrome: Autosomal dominant cleft palate, camptodactyly and clubfeet. *Am J Med Genetics.* 1981;9:139.

49. Gilbert WM, Nicolaides KH. Fetal omphalocele: Associated malformations and chromosomal defects. *Obstet Gynecol.* 1987;70:633.

50. Benacerraf BR, Laboda L. Cyst of the fetal choroid plexus: A normal variant? *Am J Obstet Gynecol.* 1989;160:319.

51. Clark SL, DeVore GR, Sabey PL: Prenatal diagnosis of cysts of the fetal choroid plexus. *Obstet Gynecol.* 1988;72:585.

52. DeRoo TR, Harris RD, Sargent SK, et al. Fetal choroid plexus cysts: Prevalence, clinical significance, and sonographic appearance. *AJR.* 1988;151:1179.

53. Friday RO, Schwartz DB, Tuffli GA. Spontaneous intrauterine resolution of intraventricular cystic masses. *J Ultrasound Med.* 1985;4:385.

54. Chitkara U, Cogswell C, Norton K, et al. Choroid plexus cysts in the fetus: A benign anatomic variant or pathologic entity? Report of 41 cases and review of the literature. *Obstet Gynecol.* 1988;72:185.

55. Farhood AI, Morris JH, Bieber FR. Transient cysts of the fetal choroid plexus: Morphology and histogenesis. *Am J Med Genetics.* 1987;27:977.

56. Hertzberg BS, Kay HH, Bowie JD. Fetal choroid plexus lesions: Relationship of antenatal sonographic appearance to clinical outcome. *J Ultrasound Med.* 1989;8:77.

57. Nicolaides KH, Rodek CH, Gosden CM. Rapid karyotyping in non-lethal fetal malformation. *Lancet.* 1986; 1:283.

58. Bundy AL, Saltzman DH, Pober B, et al. Antenatal sonographic findings in trisomy 18. *J Ultrasound Med.* 1986;5:361.

59. Fitzsimmons J, Wilson D, Pascoe-Mason J, et al. Choroid plexus cysts in fetuses with trisomy 18. *Obstet Gynecol.* 1989;73:257.

60. Benacerraf BR, Harlow B, Frigoletto FD. Is genetic amniocentesis indicated for fetuses with choroid plexus cysts? *Am J Obstet Gynecol.* In press.

61. Patau K, Smith DW, Therman E, et al. Multiple congenital anomalies caused by an extra chromosome. *Lancet.* 1960;1:790.

62. Redheendran R, Neu RL, Bannerman RM. Long survival in trisomy 13 syndrome: 21 cases including prolonged survival in two patients 11 and 19 years old. *Am J Med Genetics.* 1981;8:167.

63. Saltzman DH, Benacerraf BR, Frigoletto FD. Diagnosis and management of fetal facial clefts. *Am J Obstet Gynecol.* 1986;155:377.

64. Greene MF, Benacerraf BR, Frigoletto FD. Reliable criteria for the prenatal sonographic diagnosis of alobar holoprosencephaly. *Am J Obstet Gynecol.* 1987;156:687.

65. Benacerraf BR, Frigoletto FD, Bieber FR. The fetal face ultrasound examination. *Radiology.* 1984;153:495.

66. Seeds JW, Cefalo RC. Technique for early sonographic diagnosis of bilateral cleft lip and palate. *Obstet Gynecol.* 1983;62:2(suppl).

67. Chervenak FA, Tortora M, Mayden K, et al. Antenatal diagnosis of median cleft face syndrome: Sonographic demonstration of cleft lip and hypotelorism. *Am J Obstet Gynecol.* 1984;149:94.

68. Salvoldelli G, Schmid W, Schinzel A. Prenatal diagnosis of cleft lip and palate by ultrasound. *Prenat Diagn.* 1982;2:313.

69. Christ JE, Meininger MG. Ultrasound diagnosis of cleft lip and cleft palate before birth. *Plast Reconstr Surg.* 1981;68:854.

70. Hegge FN, Prescott GH, Watson PT. Fetal facial abnormalities identified during obstetric sonography. *J Ultrasound Med.* 1986;5:679.

71. Pilu G, Reece EA, Romero R, et al. Prenatal diagnosis of cranio-facial malformations with ultrasonography. *Am J Obstet Gynecol.* 1986;155:45.

72. Jeanty P, Romero R, Staudach A, et al. Facial anatomy of the fetus. *J Ultrasound Med.* 1986;5:607.

73. Turner HH. A syndrome of infantilism, congenital web neck and cubitus valgus. *Endocrinology.* 1938;23:566.

74. O'Brien WF, Cefalo RC, Bair DG. Ultrasonographic diagnosis of fetal cystic hygroma. *Am J Obstet Gynecol.* 1980;138:464.

75. Garden AS, Benzie RJ, Miskin M, et al. Fetal cystic hygroma colli: Antenatal diagnosis, significance, and management. *Am J Obstet Gynecol.* 1986;154:221.

76. Robinow M, Spisso K, Buschi M, et al. Turner syndrome: Sonography showing fetal hydrops simulating hydramnios. *AJR.* 1980;135:846.

77. Chervenak FA, Isaacson G, Blakemore KJ, et al. Fetal cystic hygroma: Cause and natural history. *N Eng J Med.* 1983;309:822.

78. Zarabi M, Mieckowski GC, Mazer J. Cystic hygroma associated with Noonan's syndrome. *J Clin Ultrasound.* 1983;11:398.

79. Rahmani MR, Fong KW, Connor TP. The varied sonographic appearance of cystic hygromas in utero. *J Ultrasound Med.* 1986;5:165.

80. Bieber FR, Petres RE, McNamara R, et al. Prenatal detection of a familial nuchal bleb simulating encephalocele. The National Foundation Original Article Series. *Birth Defects.* 1979;15(5A):51.

81. Benacerraf BR, Frigoletto FD. Prenatal sonographic diagnosis of isolated congenital cystic hygroma, unassociated with lymphedema or other morphologic abnormality. *J Ultrasound Med.* 1987;6:63.

82. Boue J, Boue A, Lazar P. Retrospective and prospective epidemiological studies of 1,500 karyotyped spontaneous abortions. *Teratology.* 1975;12:11.

83. Sherard J, Bean C, Bove B, et al. Long survival in a 69, XXY triploid male. *Am J Med Genetics.* 1986;25:307.

84. Lockwood C, Scioscia A, Stiller R, et al. Sonographic features of the triploid fetus. *Am J Obstet Gynecol.* 1987;157:285.

85. Doshi N, Surti U, Szulman AE. Morphologic anomalies in triploid liveborn fetuses. *Human Pathology.* 1983; 14:716.

86. Wertelecki W, Graham JM, Sergovich FR. The clinical syndrome of triploidy. *Obstet Gynecol.* 1976;47:69.

87. Crane JJP, Beaver HA, Cheung SW. Antenatal ultrasound findings in fetal triploidy syndrome. *J Ultrasound Med.* 1985;4:519.

88. Edwards MT, Smith WL, Hanson J, et al. Prenatal sonographic diagnosis of triploidy. *J Ultrasound Med.* 1986; 5:279.

89. Benacerraf BR. First trimester intrauterine growth retardation: Associated with triploidy. *J Ultrasound Med.* In press.

90. Rubenstein JB, Swayne LC, Dise CA, et al. Placental changes in fetal triploidy syndrome. *J Ultrasound Med.* 1986;5:545.

91. Opitz JM, Howe JJ. The Meckel syndrome (dysencephalia splanchnocystica, the Gruber syndrome). *Birth Defects.* 1969;5:167.

92. Meckel S, Passarge E. Encephalocele, polycystic kidneys and polydactyly as an autosomal recessive trait simulating

widen as age advances. Therefore, the accuracy of a physical measurement parameter in predicting gestational age is inversely proportional to gestational age. This important clinical phenomenon has been observed for virtually every physical determinent of fetal age that can be measured by ultrasound. This observation is also of considerable importance in the recognition and classification of IUGR because it implies that with an intrinsic etiology (eg, aneuploidy), the disease process is evident early and uniformly, whereas with extrinsic disease the manifestation of clinical features is of later onset and more diverse in character.

The optimal method for ultrasound determination of fetal age varies with gestational age. In our clinical laboratory, a gestational sac, signaling intrauterine pregnancy, has been identified as early as the 25th day after the first day of the LNMP (conceptual age 10 days). The developing embryo has been visualized as early as the 34th day after LNMP (conceptual age 20 days), and fetal heart motion seen as early as the 38th day after LNMP (conceptual age 24 days). Although gestational sac volume can be used to estimate gestational age from as early as 4 weeks from LNMP, crown-rump length determination is the most practical early measure used. Crown-rump length can be determined from as early as 5 weeks' to 12 weeks' gestation, and remains one of the most accurate methods of fetal age determination. The range of error of estimate with crown-rump length is ± 3 days,[8] and is substantially more accurate than estimates based on menstrual history. From about the 12th week onward, crown-rump length determination becomes more difficult because of deflexion and variable position of the developing fetal head. From about 10 to 12 weeks, the fetal head may be well visualized and intracranial anatomical landmarks identified. The BPD can be measured from about 12 weeks on. Between the 12th and 20th weeks, this measurement yields an estimate error of less than 7 days.[9] In an ongoing study in our institution, we have been unable to show a significant difference in estimate error between crown-rump measurement done between 6 and 12 weeks and BPD measurements done between 12 and 20 weeks. Both yield estimate errors substantially less than those associated with dating by menstrual history. (Morrison I, Manning FA. 1988. Unpublished data.) Although fetal long bone structure (humerus and femur) is seen as early as 10 weeks' gestation, accurate measurement of length is difficult before about 14 weeks' gestation. Fetal long bone measurements are technically possible from about 14 to 16 weeks' gestation.

The technical error of measurement is relatively constant. The axial resolution of a given ultrasound line can be as high as 0.2 mm; this axial resolution does not vary with absolute target size. Therefore, assuming that the target insonation angle is appropriate and the guiding landmarks are seen, the error of estimate due to axial resolution is constant and minimal. However, as ultrasound resolution has increased, the selection of the start and end points for a given measurement has become more difficult. For example, BPD measurement by the older bistable B-mode methods was relatively simple because only the bone table of the calvarium produced a recognizable signal. With modern equipment, not only is the bone of the calvarium seen, but so are hair, skin, and subcutaneous tissue. It therefore becomes essential to assume that the beginning point of measurement is set at the calvarium surface and not the scalp surface.

The accuracy of gestational age estimates by ultrasound increases as more variables are measured. There is no doubt that a relationship exists between a growing fetal physical parameter and gestational age. In the early days of ultrasound determination of fetal age, dimensions of the fetal head were the only fetal landmarks that could be measured in a reproducible and certain manner. These dimensions, especially the BPD, became the mainstay of fetal age estimates. Now, using high-resolution ultrasound, we have a broad spectrum of fetal physical parameters that can be measured simply and accurately. To date, all such parameters have been shown to be subject to the vicissitudes of the inherent population variability that is characteristic of later pregnancy. No single variable has shown an appreciable advantage in predictive accuracy.

However, this inherent variability in a fetal population of equal age is not constant across physical variables; it changes for each individual parameter. This principle is of considerable clinical importance because the error of estimate for the mean of composite variables will always be less than the error for any single variable. For example, Hadlock and colleagues,[10] using a composite estimate of BPD, abdominal circumference, head circumference, and femur length, have shown 8% improvement in predictive accuracy in early pregnancy (12 to 18 weeks), and up to 28% improvement in late pregnancy (36 to 42 weeks). It seems reasonable therefore to conclude that all ultrasound estimates of fetal age beyond the crown-rump measurement stage should be based on several variables. Which variables, and how many should be included in the composite estimate, is currently an area of active research. It seems obvious that there will be a point of diminishing return at which the addition of further variables will no longer refine accuracy, but this point is still undefined. In our practice, we use a composite of BPD, femur length, and abdominal circumference to estimate fetal age. Estimates of fetal age based on a single variable, such as BPD, should and will disappear from clinical practice.

In late gestation, the accuracy of fetal age determination is enhanced by serial measurements. For reasons cited previously, determination of fetal age in late pregnancy (>20 weeks) based on a single ultrasound examination can be fraught with considerable error; the magnitude increases as gestational age advances (Fig. 20–1). The clinical dilemma this presents is common and usually occurs in the patient with an unknown or uncertain menstrual history who enters the medical system late in pregnancy. Because it is uncommon for dates to be underestimated by available menstrual data, patients such as these are frequently suspected to have IUGR.

The method of choice for evaluating such patients is the rate of fetal growth, as determined by serial estimates of fetal physical parameters, measured at time intervals spaced widely enough to account for inherent measurement error (usually >2 weeks). The concept is based on the curvilinear characteristics of the mean growth curve of the normal fetus and requires a composite estimate rather than one based on any single variable. Sabbagha and coworkers[11] have described a method, growth adjusted sonographic age, based on this principle. It uses estimates of BPD and abdominal circumference rate before 26 weeks, and some 10 to 12 weeks later, to calculate the slope of fetal growth.[12] When applied correctly, the method yields an estimate error of ± 1 week. Despite its theoretical appeal, the method is somewhat impractical because the first ultrasound scan must be done before 26 weeks. Therefore, it has not found widespread acceptance. An alternate method, depending on the same principle, involves serial composite measurements. Usually two and preferably three such measurements are spaced at least 2 weeks apart, and plotted against standard fetal growth curves. When applied between 24 and 32 weeks' gestation, this method yields an estimate error of ± 10 days. In our experience, fetal age estimates done after 32 weeks' gestation are subject to major error and are not of real clinical value. At that time, management is best based on assessment of fetal wellbeing and detection of ancillary signs of reduced fetal growth.

IUGR as a Diagnostic Tool

IUGR as defined by low weight percentile ranking does not invariably connote pathology, nor does a normal weight percentile exclude growth impairment. The IUGR population selected by ultrasound morphometric methods is a heterogenous population, the majority of whom (75 to 80%) are normal infants without extrinsic growth retardation. They merely manifest a genetic predisposition toward the lower end of the growth spectrum. Such fetuses are neither at increased perinatal risk, nor is there need of obstetric intervention for fetal indication.

Within a population of IUGR perinates, as defined by weight/age percentile rank, 20 to 25% will exhibit growth restraint due to pathologic influences. This ab-

normal subpopulation is mostly composed (approximately 75 to 80%) of perinates suffering from uteroplacental dysfunction of diverse etiology. As such this subset, representing some 15 to 20% of the entire IUGR population, are at very exaggerated risk for perinatal compromise and death. It is from this group that the large majority with complicated outcome is drawn. Accurate recognition of this subgroup via a barrage of ultrasound-based techniques, coupled with intensive monitoring of fetal growth and well-being and timely interventional strategies, has been the key to substantial reduction in morbid outcome. The remaining subgroup of IUGR fetuses, representing 5 to 10% of the total IUGR population, suffers growth restraint due to pathologic impairment of intrinsic growth potential. Impairment is either the result of chromosomal abberations (eg, trisomy 18, 21), intrinsic disruption of organ differentiation (eg, renal dygenesis) or development (eg, short limb dystrophies), or the result of severe insult of diverse nature (eg, rubella) in early embryonic and fetal stages. In such fetuses, because the prognosis is usually fixed by the time of diagnosis and is beyond a stage where effective therapies exist, the key ultrasound-based diagnostic steps are the recognition of etiology in order to avoid iatrogenic complications for the mother. The heterogeneity of the IUGR population dictates two loosely defined management schemes: timed intervention for the subset with extrinsic restraints on growth (15 to 20% of the population), and conservativism for the remainder (75 to 80% of the population). It follows that there must be a coupling of ultrasound-based diagnostic information to recognize the population at risk and to differentiate this subpopulation by etiology and specific risk. The failure to attend to this second component of the diagnostic process denigrates the value of ultrasound.

Adaptation and Compensation by the Fetus

It is becoming increasingly evident that the human fetus possesses inherent and remarkable reflex and adaptive processes by which it can compensate for the consequences of reduced growth potential. Such adaptation accounts for a myriad of ultrasound signs that may be used to determine the severity and possible etiology of the IUGR process, as well as provide crucial information about relative fetal risk. Included in methods of adaptation are hypoxemic reflex redistribution of cardiac output with selective reduction in perfusion of kidney and lung, manifested by diminished amniotic fluid production and ultimately oligohydramnios, and sustained cerebral blood flow manifested by increased carotid to aortic (umbilical artery) blood flow velocity ratio. Over a longer time span, these reflex redistributions in blood flow probably account for the "head sparing" phenomenon of extrinsic IUGR, which is manifested by an altered cranial-to-abdominal circumference.[14] Endocrine responses are complex, but include a rise in circulating arginene vaso-pressin, an aggravating factor in the development of oligohydramnios;[15] a rise in circulating catecholamines, resulting in loss of glycogen and thus reducing liver and muscle mass; and a reduction in fat stores. Central nervous system-mediated adaptive response includes a reduction in, and in extreme cases, cessation of skeletal muscle movement including respiratory movement, a response known to reduce oxygen consumption. The absence of breathing and movement over a sustained period of time in the growth-retarded fetus is suggestive of severe compromise and impending death.[16,17] Including these more indirect ultrasound-based signs with weight/age percentile estimates is very useful in refining diagnostic acuity, etiology, and prognostication for management strategies.

PRINCIPLES OF DIAGNOSIS OF IUGR

Because IUGR is a common condition (5 to 10% of pregnancies) and a common finding among stillbirths (26%), accurate prenatal recognition is of considerable clinical importance. The algorithm for ultrasound diagnosis of IUGR, and for plotting rational management rests on several key principles. These are:

1. The population of fetuses with growth impairment is heterogenous by etiology and by prognosis.
2. Accurate diagnosis depends on consideration of fetal morphometric, morphologic, and functional data as derived from ultrasound methods.
3. The accuracy of diagnosis and implementation of management strategies will vary directly with the certainty of the fetal age estimate.
4. Accurate diagnosis and selective management can result in significant reduction in mortality and morbidity associated with IUGR.

The most common entry mode of the patient with suspect IUGR into the ultrasound diagnostic schemata occurs as a result of a clinical diagnosis of a discrepancy between uterine size and gestational age. Uterine size can be measured objectively by symphysis to fundal height ratios or subjectively by an impression of reduced uterine volume. The predictive accuracy of clinical parameters for the diagnosis of IUGR is poor, both for positive and negative predictive accuracy. In our experience of more than 4,000 pregnancies referred with a clinical diagnosis of IUGR, the positive predictive accuracy, defined by delivery of an IUGR perinate, was only 16%. (F.A.M., unpublished data, 1988.) In contrast, almost 20% of IUGR fetuses delivered in our institution were not recognized by clinical examination (negative predic-

tive accuracy). Campbell and associates[18] have reported similar errors in diagnostic accuracy, although less extreme. These data would suggest that management of this condition by clinical examination only is fraught with so much error as to be relatively unreliable, except perhaps in extreme cases.

These parameters of clinical diagnostic accuracy become further compromised among patients in whom the menstrual history is unknown or uncertain or in whom clinical examination is difficult because of uterine anomaly, uterine fibroids, multiparity, or obesity. Among cases of multiple pregnancy, in which growth impairment of one or more of the fetuses is common, detection of IUGR by clinical assessment is inaccurate. It follows that a more precise and objective diagnostic measure must be employed to assess the fetus(es) with suspected IUGR. All existing evidence points to ultrasound as this objective modality.

Ultrasound methods are applied to the diagnosis of IUGR in two general ways. First, it is used to recognize a discrepancy between expected and observed fetal mass (volume) for a given gestational age. Second, it is employed to determine the etiology, severity, and prognosis for the observed discrepancy.

Recognition of Growth Impairment

The first step in diagnosis of IUGR involves calculation of fetal mass and gestational age, both of which may be estimated from discrete fetal measurements. Determination of fetal age from ultrasound-derived fetal morphometrics has been briefly referenced in this text and is described in detail elsewhere (see Chapter 7). Estimation of fetal mass (weight) is also derived from fetal morphometrics and is based on the assumption of a constant reproducible relationship between select fetal parameters and fetal volume. This method assumes a constant density of the fetus across a range of volume and among healthy and compromised fetuses. Several aspects of this presumed relationship warrant further comment, because the accuracy of diagnosis (and hence management) may depend critically on these assumptions.

Calculation of density (g per mL) using a water displacement method for calculation of volume indicates there is significant variation in density among the population of perinates and within different organ structures in the individual fetus (Fig. 20–2).[19] The average density of perinate is slightly less than water (0.919 ± 0.07 g/mL) but may vary from 0.833 to 1.012 g/mL (range of variation 21.5%). It may be calculated from these data that among a population of perinates of known volume the average error of weight (mass) estimate will be approximately 8%, but in some fetuses the average error may be as high as 21%. The density distribution among IUGR fetuses, a population in whom a reduction in body

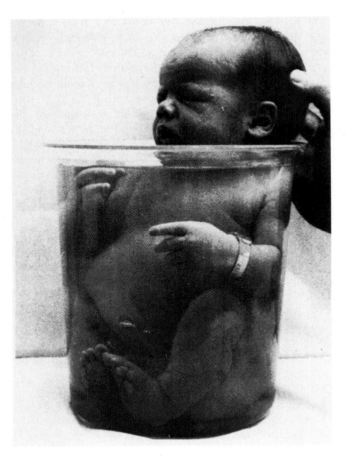

Fig. 20–2. A water displacement method for calculation of density (mass per volume) of the perinate. Calculation of density in the healthy neonate (shown here) is limited to estimate of all areas but the head, and is subject to error due to lung expansion. Total density is calculated in deceased perinates by comparable method. These studies indicate perinatal density is variable (0.866 to 1.021 g/mL) and may introduce unavoidable error in perinatal weight determination from volume estimates. (*Reproduced with permission from Thompson TE, Manning FA, Morrison I. J Ultrasound Med. 1983;2:113.*)

fat may be expected, is unknown and needs further study. Further, within the individual fetus the density of various structures is known to vary. For example, the mean density of the fetal head is 0.571 g/mL and of the body is 1.118 g/mL. Failure to consider these intrafetal variations can compound diagnostic error in fetuses with such conditions as dysmature IUGR, which in some instances are known to cause differential effects on organ growth (eg, head sparing).

The clinician ultrasonographer is presented with a number of formulae that use fetal morphometrics to calculate fetal mass. These methods are generally derived from an equation defining either a linear or exponential line of best fit of fetal morphometrics to recorded birth weight. Most formulae are derived from a relatively small population of uneven weight distribution, with variable interval between measurement and delivery, and do not account for change in relative density due to lung expansion. Considering these sources of error together with the potential error of mensuration of fetal parameter, it is not surprising there is considerable range of error between estimated (fetal) and measured (neonatal) weight. When volume is known with certainty (by water displacement method), the error of estimate is ± 7.2% (2 standard deviation).[19] Detailed, highly accurate measurement of neonatal physical dimension yields an estimate error of calculated weight of ± 8.2%, the slight increase in estimate error presumed due to measurement error.[19]

The most exact estimate of fetal volume is based on a static ultrasound method of serial cross-sectioned scan with computer reconstruction to calculate volume. This method, reported by McCallam and coworkers in 1979,[20] is time consuming and cumbersome but yields an estimate error comparable to direct displacement methods. Unfortunately, the method has not been reliably reproduced using dynamic ultrasound methods and hence is rarely employed. The most commonly used methods today are based on selective variables. Initially, fetal BPD was used to estimate fetal mass but because the fetal head represents only 20% of total fetal volume, it is not surprising this method proved so inaccurate as to be of no clinical value. Combining fetal head measurements (BPD or head circumference) with abdominal circumference measurements has been reported as a method for estimating fetal mass (Fig. 20–3.A,B). The initial formulae were described by Warsof and associates in 1977 and later modified by Shepard and colleagues in 1982.[21,22]

The method has several inherent disadvantages. Harman and coworkers[23] studied the method among 198 fetuses and outlined some of these disadvantages. They noted that in more than 20% (35 fetuses) the variance between estimated and observed weight exceeded 10%, that in 22% of cases BPD could not be reliably measured, and that the relationship between abdominal circumference and BPD in the growth-retarded fetus did not conform to the various equations derived by Warsof and Shepard. Hadlock and associates,[24,25] reported a method of fetal weight estimation based on composite measurements of head circumference, abdominal circumference, and femur length that yields an estimate of error of ± 15% (2 standard deviation).[24,25] Campbell's[26] report of abdominal circumference as a sole measure to estimate fetal weight has yielded interesting data demonstrating this method gives an estimate of error of ± 15%, comparable to more complex methods outlined previously. By such methods, IUGR is diagnosed when the estimated

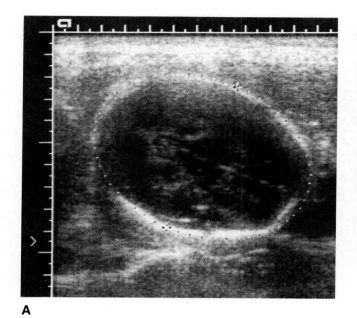

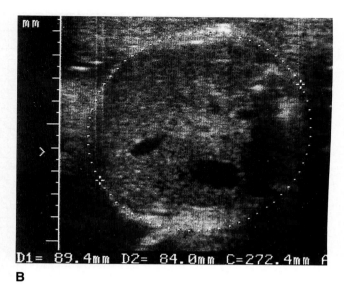

B

A

Fig. 20–3. A. Head circumference measured in the plane of the BPD. Head circumference is measured as outer diameter of skin surface, then combined with abdominal circumference to estimate fetal mass. The reliability of this method in fetuses with pathologic variance in head and abdominal circumference due to extrinsic growth restraint remains largely untested. **B.** Abdominal circumference measured in the plane of the upper abdomen in the region of maximal liver mass. Circumference may be measured directly, as illustrated here, or calculated from two perpendicular diameters. The latter method introduces a small error (± 1%) in calculation of true circumference.

weight falls below the 10th percentile for gestational age. Whereas the neonatal curves of weight-to-age include sex correction, described fetal curves usually do not consider sex differences due to potential error in sex assignment.

In our clinical laboratory, consideration of these diverse methods of fetal weight estimation has led us to an unexpected conclusion, that the usual criterion used to diagnose IUGR in the neonate, reduced mass relative to age, is not well suited to the diagnosis of the fetal condition. Despite the clinical attraction of using the fetal weight percentile, unavoidable errors of estimate introduced by density variation and measurement limitations may be of such proportion and variability as to introduce serious diagnostic error. Accordingly, we have abandoned using fetal weight estimates in the diagnosis of IUGR. We prefer instead to rely on the nonderived variables of measured abdominal and head circumferences to detect significant deviation in fetal growth (Fig. 20–4).

Serial assessment of fetal growth parameters, either derived (fetal weight estimates) or direct, are of considerable value in establishing the diagnosis of IUGR, in determining rate of progression, and often in determining etiology. With the exception of the fetus with extreme IUGR (<3rd percentile) or the fetus with overt functional signs of compromise (see the following discussion), serial

estimates of growth parameters are recommended for all fetuses with proven or suspected IUGR. The interval between examinations is not constant but may vary inversely with the gestational age at diagnosis, the presumed severity of disease at initial diagnosis, fetal well-being at diagnosis, maternal condition (eg, severity of hypertension), and with results of previous examination. The interval may vary directly with the uncertainty of menstrual dates and suspicion of a normal small fetus. Because the diagnosis and management of IUGR depends on other factors in addition to fetal growth parameters, it is essential to ensure confirmation of fetal well-being by antepartum testing in addition to such studies.

When fetal biophysical profile scoring is used for determination of well-being, growth parameters are usually measured weekly. When antepartum fetal heart rate testing methods are used to confirm fetal well-being, growth parameter determination may be extended to biweekly intervals. An interval of two weeks is recommended for comparison of growth parameters, because comparison at shorter intervals precludes differentiation of change because of measurement error. The potential for confusion is even greater when derived growth estimates (fetal weight) are used. Serial estimates done at biweekly intervals will generally yield one of the following

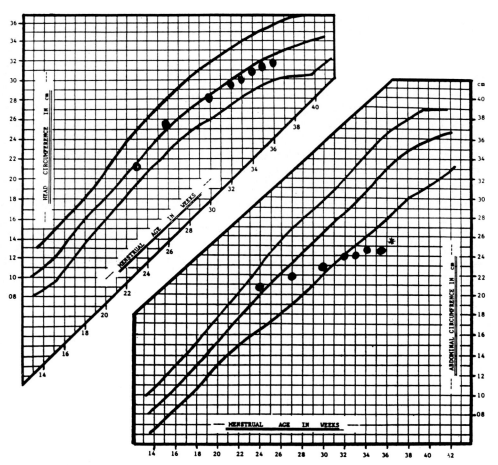

Fig. 20–4. Distribution plot of head circumference and abdominal circumference to gestational age, shown as the mean and 2 standard deviations of the mean. Data from fetal morphometrics are plotted as absolute values without reverting to weight conversion. Values recorded in an infant followed from 22 weeks' gestation are shown. Fetal head circumference growth remained essentially normal. In contrast, fetal abdominal circumference, initially normal, showed progressive decrease in growth velocity so that by 32 weeks it fell below 2 standard deviations of the mean. Functional signs remained normal until 36 weeks, at which time oligohydramnios had evolved, prompting delivery of a nonasphyxiated 2,300 g female neonate (5th percentile). The asterisk denotes the occurrence of an abnormal functional sign.

patterns. The growth velocity (change in measured parameters over time) may parallel the normal distribution curve, but remain below the 10th percentile. In such fetuses the diagnosis of a normal small fetus is most likely, although mistaken dates cannot be excluded with certainty. Such fetuses, in the absence of functional signs of compromise, require serial biweekly assessment to confirm continuing normal growth velocity. It is uncommon for such fetuses to develop subsequent aggravated growth restraint. The second pattern observed is a flattened growth velocity in which interval testing reveals a widening variance from expected growth velocity (Fig. 20–4). Such fetuses may be considered to have dysmature IUGR until proven otherwise and need intensive monitoring for functional signs of IUGR and a change in fetal condition. A variant may be observed in the fetus whose initial growth parameters are above the lower limit but subsequently fall through percentiles. Such fetuses can exhibit all the functional signs of dysmature IUGR and may die before the growth parameters ever fall below the lower limit of distribution.

Functional Evaluation of IUGR

Estimation of fetal growth parameters may be the method for initial recognition of IUGR, but it is ultrasound assessment of the functional signs that leads to the specific diagnosis, presumed etiology, and appropriate management. This evolution from recognition to specific assessment of fetal signs is a key step in reducing perinatal morbidity and mortality and iatrogenic complications for the mother.

The functional signs of IUGR may be loosely classified into hard signs and soft signs. The hard signs are measurable and reproducible and are of major value in assigning etiology and prognosis. Four hard signs are described below.

Assessment of Amniotic Fluid Volume. Amniotic fluid is readily visualized by ultrasound, and methods for semiquantitative determination of volume have proved useful in assessment of the IUGR fetus. Several methods for reporting amniotic fluid volume are used, including subjective assessment, a four-quadrant measurement score,[27] or measurement of the vertical diameter of the largest pocket.[28] The latter method is the one studied most extensively in the IUGR fetus, although the alternate methods may yield similar data. Oligohydramnios has been defined using the vertical diameter method as a pocket of fluid of <1 cm. This method was first applied in the diagnosis of IUGR by Manning and associates[28] in 120 patients referred with a clinical diagnosis of IUGR. Of these patients, 29 exhibited oligohydramnios of which 26 (89.9%) resulted in an IUGR fetus. In contrast, of 91 patients with normal amniotic fluid (>1.0 cm vertical pocket), five delivered an IUGR fetus (5.5%). These differences are highly significant. The association between oligohydramnios in fetuses with suspected IUGR and proven IUGR at delivery was confirmed by subsequent reports of Philipson and colleagues[29] (83% predictive accuracy), Patterson and coworkers,[30] Chamberlain and associates[31] (78.9% predictive accuracy), Gross and colleagues,[32] and Divon and associates[33] (100% predictive accuracy). Collectively these data suggest that, in the presence of intact membranes and a known functional genitourinary tract, the observation of oligohydramnios in the fetus with suspected growth failure confirms the diagnosis. Further, perinatal outcome in these fetuses, as well as larger populations of fetuses with oligohydramnios due to factors other than IUGR, indicates a sharp rise in perinatal mortality due to asphyxial complications. The corrected perinatal mortality (excluding congenital anomalies) between fetuses with normal fluid and fetuses with oligohydramnios is increased by more than 50-fold (1.97 per 1,000 to 194 per 1,000, respectively).[31] Aggressive intervention for oligohydramnios can virtually eliminate asphyxial perinatal deaths.[34] Therefore, the observation of oligohydramnios in the fetus with suspected growth failure should be considered a perinatal emergency and indication for intervention in the viable perinate.

The original report of the relationship of amniotic fluid volume and IUGR suggested that the presence of normal amniotic fluid volume conveyed a low risk of IUGR (5.5%).[28] Subsequent expanded studies have not borne out this conclusion. Reports by Hoddick,[35] Philipson,[29] and Chamberlain[31] all confirm that the presence of normal amniotic fluid volume cannot be used as a reliable method to exclude the diagnosis of IUGR. Because IUGR fetuses are a heterogeneous mix and include a preponderance of normal small fetuses, such poor negative predictive value of normal amniotic fluid volume estimate is not surprising.

The rate at which amniotic fluid volume may change in fetuses destined to develop oligohydramnios, including IUGR fetuses, is not well studied. In unpublished work

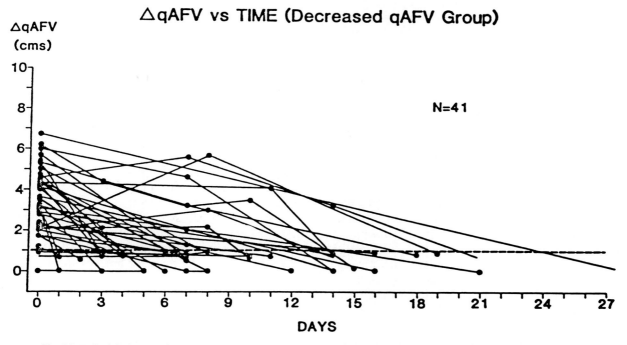

Fig. 20–5. Serial observations of amniotic fluid volume by largest vertical diameter among 41 fetuses destined to develop oligohydramnios, as defined by a maximal fluid pocket of <1 cm. The shortest transition from normal to decreased fluid was 1 day, the longest was 21 days, and the mean was 9l.2 days. (*Reproduced with permission from Chamberlain PF, Manning FA, unpublished data.*)

by Chamberlain and associates, in our clinical laboratory the transition from normal amniotic fluid to oligohydramnios (<1.0 cm) took an average of 9 days, but in some fetuses the transition was completed in as little as 1 day (Fig. 20–5).

The fetus with absent renal function due to primary bilateral parenchymal disease (agenesis or dysgenesis) presents a difficult diagnostic challenge. Such fetuses almost invariably present beyond 20 weeks' gestation with oligohydramnios and severe IUGR. Impaired visualization due to oligohydramnios can make recognition of renal parenchymal disorders extremely difficult. Differentiation from severe dysmature IUGR is of critical importance because the management strategies vary radically. The observation of urine within the fetal bladder and observed variation of bladder volume over time (hours) points directly to dysmature IUGR (assuming intact membranes). Administration of furosemide to the mother has been advocated in such circumstances with the expectation of transplacental passage and a fetal diuretic effect.[36] The theory, while intriguing, appears to be without substance because in the ovine fetus furosemide does not cross the placenta.[37] Administration to the dysmature fetus with subsequently proven intact renal function does not induce diuresis in utero.[38] The observation of a severely reduced thoracic-to-abdominal circumference ratio strongly suggests pulmonary hypoplasia,[39] a nearly uniform finding in fetuses with renal agenesis/dysgenesis. This diagnostic dilemma may be resolved by experimental methods such as instillation of normal saline into the amniotic cavity to enhance visualization of the renal fossae, direct injection (intramuscular or intravenous) of a diuretic to the fetus, or intravascular injection to improve an intrauterine fetal glomerular filtration rate.

Assessment of Fetal Well-Being. Knowing that the fetus under study is at minimal risk of asphyxial complications in the near future greatly reduces clinical anxiety surrounding the diagnosis of IUGR and reduces the need for immediate intervention for fetal indication. The myriad of fetal biophysic activities observed by real-time ultrasound examination can yield this critical information. This is discussed in detail in another chapter (see Chapter 25), but additional comments are warranted with specific reference to management of IUGR.

In its purest and most simplistic form, the management of IUGR depends on recognition and delivery of the fetus at risk of asphyxial complications, and observation and conservativism of the other fetuses. It may be argued that weight percentile ranking or growth velocity is of minimal significance provided the fetus is not exposed to conditions of asphyxia. The relationship between biophysical variables, as combined in a fetal biophysical profile score, and the risk of asphyxial complications has

been well described.[18] In the presence of normal variables, the risk of stillbirth within a week is less than 0.6 per 1,000, and as variables are lost, the risk rises so that when all variables are absent, the risk of asphyxial death reaches more than 600 per 1,000.[40] Similar trends are reported for perinatal morbidity.[41]

Application of these data to the management of IUGR has considerable clinical impact. In the immature IUGR fetus in whom the risk of prematurity-related mortality can be calculated and is known to be high, observation of a normal fetal biophysical profile score indicates the risks of sustained fetal life to be less than the risk of delivery. The balance may change until the neonatal risk becomes negligible and easy delivery can be accomplished. In contrast, in the fetus with a deteriorating score, intervention may be indicated even in the presence of considerable prematurity because the balance no longer favors continued fetal existence. This profile has been used in the management of more than 960 perinates in our center, yielding a corrected perinatal mortality of 12.5 per 1,000 (12 deaths). This death rate, while still clinically significant, is far below the expected rate for an untested similar population (100 per 1,000).

Direct measurement of fetal acid base and blood gas may be accomplished via ultrasound-guided percutaneous umbilical blood sampling. This involves identification of the placental insertion site of the umbilical vein into which a 20- or 22-gauge needle can be directed under dynamic ultrasound guidance (Fig. 20–6). Pure fetal blood samples are analyzed for pH, PO_2, PCO_2, and for karyotype. Blood gas and acid–base values have been studied in 53 small-for-gestational-age fetuses by Nicolaides and associates[42] and contrasted with values obtained in normal appropriate-for-gestational-age fetuses. The data demonstrated an umbilical vein PO_2 below 2 standard deviation of the mean for normals in 27 of 53 IUGR fetuses (50.9%).[42]

The risk of causing fetal death as a direct consequence of the sampling method, by causing fetal hemorrhage or initiation of chorioamnionitis, is significant. Nicolaides[42] reported a procedure-related loss rate of 1% (3 losses among 310 ongoing pregnancies), and Daffos[43] reported a loss rate of 1.2% (7 losses among 562 ongoing cases). At the time of writing, the clinical role of direct fetal blood sampling for investigation of IUGR, while intriguing, remains undetermined and is considered experimental.

Fetal Vessel Doppler Velocimetry. Mensuration of the spectrum of blood flow velocities in fetal vessels using pulsed or continuous-wave Doppler ultrasound methods is a relatively new and exciting development (see Chapter 12). Analysis of the flow velocity envelope of the umbilical artery and select major fetal vessels holds great promise

20–9). The patient enters the diagnostic point from a variety of routes, most notably by either clinical suspicion of IUGR or by recognition of suggestive signs in the course of ultrasound examination for other purposes. The multiple pregnancy represents a variant in entry to diagnosis because clinical detection of IUGR in one or both twins is very common.

At initial assessment, both morphometric and functional data are considered. The determination of IUGR at the outset is almost always based on fetal morphometric data. In the use of nonderived indices for morphometrics, usually abdominal circumference is recommended, although use of other indixes such as head and abdomen circumference, fetal mass estimation, or a ponderal index may be substituted. A normal distribution plot of abdominal circumference to gestational age and normal functional signs virtually excludes the diagnosis of IUGR in fetuses of known gestational age. Repeat assessment would only be indicated if the maternal condition changes or the clinical impression of IUGR persists or exacerbates. In the patient with unknown menstrual dates, repeat assessment at an interval sufficient to measure fetal growth (or absence thereof), usually 2 weeks, is indicated. If at repeat assessment the functional signs remain normal and normal growth parameters are demonstrated, the patient may be safely assumed to have mistaken data and discharged from the algorithm with the previously cited provisos. If the selected growth rate is below the lower limit ascribed (5th percentile) at first visit in a patient with known dates, or at repeat visits in a patient with unknown dates, a diagnosis of IUGR is established and efforts are then directed toward determining etiology, severity, and prognosis (Fig. 20–8). In such fetuses, ultrasound assessment should be done at least weekly and conservative management continued, provided fetal growth is demonstrated and functional signs remain normal (Fig. 20–9). Intervention in such fetuses may take place when fetal maturity is affirmed and delivery can be instituted with minimal difficulty.

In the fetus with a proven major anomaly, a decision toward total conservative management with a view to absolute minimization of maternal risk is the usual rule. In our center, a prompt delivery is indicated in an IUGR fetus regardless of gestational age by either a confirmed abnormal biophysic profile score, isolated observation of oligohydramnios by defined criteria (<1 cm largest vertical pocket), or both in an IUGR fetus of at least 25 weeks gestation. Umbilical artery velocimetry and intrafetal proportion are not used to precipitate intervention, but rather to guide the frequency of fetal surveillance. In the presence of a distinctly abnormal pulsatility index or absent diastolic flow, fetal surveillance should be intensified. The finding of reverse diastolic flow to prompt delivery in the IUGR fetus remains inconclusive at present,

but it seems likely that with further experience this finding will also be a signal to precipitate immediate delivery. In the dysmature IUGR fetus, as well as in other types, it has been our policy to continue conservative management only until fetal maturity is affirmed and delivery can be accomplished with minimal maternal risk. This method of management has been applied to more than 1,200 proven IUGR fetuses, yielding a corrected perinatal mortality (excluding fetuses with anomalies) of 12.5 per 1,000. This represents a significant reduction from the expected rate among IUGR fetuses (60 to 80 deaths per 1,000).

REFERENCES

1. Morrison I, Olson J. Weight specific stillbirths and associated causes of death: An analysis of 765 consecutive stillbirths. *Am J Obstet Gynecol*. 1985;152:975.
2. Streeter H, Manning FA. Classification of neonatal morbidity and mortality by birth weight percentile in IUGR neonates. *Proc Soc Obstet Gynecol Canada*. 1980. (Abstract).
3. Lubchenco LO, Hansman C, Dressler M, et al. Intrauterine growth as estimated from liveborn birthweight data at 24–42 weeks of gestation. *Pediatrics*. 1963;32:793.
4. Grennert L, Persson P, Gerrser G, et al. Benefits of ultrasound screening of a pregnant population. *Acta Obstet Gynecol Scand*. 1978;78(suppl):5.
5. Usher RH, Boyd ME, McLean FH, et al. Assessment of fetal risk in postdates pregnancies. *Am J Obstet Gynecol*. 1988;158:259.
6. Maternal physiology in pregnancy: Duration of pregnancy. In: Eastman WJ, Hellman LM, eds. *Williams Obstetrics*, New York: Appleton-Century-Crofts; 1966:218.
7. Campbell S. Fetal growth. *Clin Obstet Gynecol*. 1974;1:41.
8. Robinson HP. Sonar measurement of fetal crown-rump length as a means of assessing maturity in the first trimester of pregnancy. *Br Med J*. 1973;4:28.
9. Hadlock FP, Deter R, Harrist R, et al. Fetal biparietal diameter: A critical re-evaluation of the relation to menstrual age by means of realtime ultrasound. *J Ultrasound Med*. 1982;1:97.
10. Hadlock FP, Deter R, Harrist R, et al. Computer assisted analysis of fetal age in the third trimester using multiple fetal growth parameters. *J Clin Ultrasound*. 1983;11:313.
11. Sabbagha RE, Hughey M, Depp R. The assignment of growth-adjusted sonographic age (GASA): A simplified method. *Obstet Gynecol*. 1978;51:383.
12. Tamura RK, Sabbagha RE. Percentile ratios of sonar fetal abdominal circumference measurements. *Am J Obstet Gynecol*. 1980;138:475.
13. Librach CT, Hogdall CK, Doran TA. Weights of fetuses with autosomal trisomies at termination of pregnancy: An investigation of etiological factors of low serum alpha-fetoprotein levels. *Am J Obstet Gynecol*. 1988;158:290.
14. Campbell S. Ultrasound measurement of the fetal head to abdomen circumference ratio in assessment of growth re-

tardation. *Br J Obstet Gynaecol.* 1977;84:165.

15. Towell ME, Figueroa J, Markowitz S, et al. The effect of mild hypoxemia maintained for 24 hours on maternal and fetal glucose, lactate, cortisol, and anginene vasopressin in pregnant sheep at 122 to 139 days' gestation. *Am J Obstet Gynecol.* 1987;157:1550.

16. Manning FA, Platt LD, Sipos L. Antepartum fetal evaluation: Development of a fetal biophysical profile. *Am J Obstet Gynecol.* 1980;136:787.

17. Manning FA, Morrison I, Lange IR, et al. Fetal assessment based on fetal biophysical profile scoring: Experience in 12,620 referred high risk pregnancies. I: Perinatal mortality by frequency and etiology. *Am J Obstet Gynecol.* 1985; 151:343–50.

18. Campbell S. The assessment of fetal growth by diagnostic ultrasound. *Clin Perinatol.* 1974;1:507.

19. Thompson TE, Manning FA, Morrison I. Determination of fetal volume in utero by an ultrasound method correlation with neonatal birth weight. *J Ultrasound Med.* 1983;2:113.

20. McCallum WD, Brinkley TF. Estimation of fetal weight from ultrasound measurement. *Am J Obstet Gynecol.* 1979;133:195.

21. Warsof SL, Gohari P, Berkowitz RL, et al. The estimation of fetal weight by computer assisted analysis. *Am J Obstet Gynecol.* 1977;128:881.

22. Shepard MJ, Richards VA, Berkowitz RL, et al. An evaluation of two equations for predicting fetal weight by ultrasound. *Am J Obstet Gynecol.* 1982;152:47.

23. Harman CR, Holme S, Gardiner R, et al. Ultrasonic weight estimation in the "clinically small" fetus: A prospective comparison of two methods. *Proc Soc Obstet Gynecol Canada.* Annual Meeting. Abstract. 1984.

24. Hadlock FP, Deter R, Harrist R, et al. Fetal abdominal circumference: Relation to menstrual age. *AJR.* 1982; 139:367.

25. Hadlock FP, Deter R, Harrist R, et al. A date-independent predictor of intrauterine growth retardation: Femur length/abdominal circumference ratio. *AJR.* 1983;141:979.

26. Campbell S, Wilkin P. Ultrasonic measurement of fetal abdominal circumference in the estimation of fetal weight. *Br J Obstet Gynaecol.* 1975;82:689.

27. Phelan JP, Platt LD, Yeh S. The role of ultrasound assessment of amniotic fluid volume in the management of the postdate pregnancy. *Am J Obstet Gynecol.* 1985; 151:304.

28. Manning FA, Hill LM, Platt LD. Qualitative amniotic fluid volume determination by ultrasound: Antepartum detection of intrauterine growth retardation. *Am J Obstet Gynecol.* 1981;139:254–258.

29. Philipson EH, Sokol RJ, Williams T, et al. Oligohydramnios: Clinical associations and predictive value for intrauterine growth retardation. *Am J Obstet Gynecol.* 1983;146:271.

30. Patterson RM, Prihoda, TJ, Pouliot MR. Sonographic amniotic fluid measurement and IUGR: A reappraisal. *Am J Obstet Gynecol.* 1984;157:4406.

31. Chamberlain PF, Manning FA, Morrison I, et al. Ultrasound evaluation of amniotic fluid. I: The relationship of marginal and decreased amniotic fluid volume to perinatal outcome. *Am J Obstet Gynecol.* 1984;150:245.

32. Gross TL, Sokol RJ, Wilson M, et al. Using ultrasound and amniotic fluid determinations to diagnose IUGR before birth: A clinical model. *Am J Obstet Gynecol.* 1982;143:265.

33. Divon MY, Chamberlain PF, Sipos L, et al. Identification of the small for gestational age fetus with the use of gestational age—independent indices of fetal growth. *Am J Obstet Gynecol.* 1986;155:1197.

34. Bastide A, Manning FA, Harman CR, et al. Ultrasound evaluation of amniotic fluid: Outcome of pregnancies with severe oligohydramnios. *Am J Obstet Gynecol.* In press.

35. Hoddick WK, Callen, PW, Filly RA, et al. Ultrasonographic determination of qualitative amniotic fluid volume in intrauterine growth retardation: Reassessment of the 1 cm rule. *Am J Obstet Gynecol.* 1984;149:758.

36. Barrett RJ, Rayburn WF, Barr MJ Jr. Furosemide (Lasix) challenge test in assessment bilateral fetal hydronephrosis. *Am J Obstet Gynecol.* 1983;147:846.

37. Chamberlain PF, Cumming M, Torchia M, et al. Ovine fetal urine production following maternal intravenous furosemide administration. *Am J Obstet Gynecol.* 1985; 151:815.

38. Harman CR. Maternal furosemide may not provoke urine production in the compromised fetus. *Am J Obstet Gynecol.* 1984;150:322.

39. Nimrod C, Nicholson S, Davies D, et al. Pulmonary hypoplasia testing in clinical obstetrics. *Am J Obstet Gynecol.* 1988;158:277.

40. Manning FA, Morrison I, Harman CR, et al. Fetal assessment by fetal BPS: Experience in 19,221 referred high risk pregnancies. II: The false negative rate by frequency and etiology. *Am J Obstet Gynecol.* 1987;154:880.

41. Manning FA, Morrison I, Harman CR, et al. Fetal Assessment by fetal biophysical profile score. III. Positive predictive accuracy of the abnormal test. *Am J Obstet Gynecol.* In press. 1989.

42. Nicolaides KH. Cordocentesis. *Clin Obstet Gynecol.* 1988;31:123.

43. Daffos F, Capella-Pavlovsky M, Forestier F. Fetal blood sampling during pregnancy with use of a needle guided by ultrasound: A study of 606 consecutive cases. *Am J Obstet Gynecol.* 1985;153:655.

44. McCowan LM, Erskine LA, Richie K. Umbilical artery Doppler flow studies in the preterm small for gestational age fetus. *Am J Obstet Gynecol.* 1987;156:644.

45. Reuwer PJ, Rietman EA, Sijmour MW, et al. Intrauterine growth retardation: Prediction of perinatal distress by Doppler ultrasound. *Lancet.* 1987;2:415.

46. Marsal K, Presson P. Ultrasonic measurement of fetal blood wave velocity forms as a secondary diagnostic test in screening for intrauterine growth retardation. *J Clin Ultrasound.* 1988;16:239.

47. Wladimiroff JW, Tonge HM, Stewart AA. Doppler ultrasound assessment of cerebral blood flow in the human fetus. *Br J Obstet Gynaecol.* 1986;93:471.

48. Grannum PAT, Berkowitz RL, Hobbins JC. The ultrasound changes in the maturing placenta and their relationship to fetal pulmonic maturity. *Am J Obstet Gynecol.* 1979; 133:915.

49. Harman CR, Holmes S, Gardiner G, et al. Ultrasound placental grading and IUGR—Is there a connection? *Proc Soc Obstet Gynecol Canada.* Abstract. June 1984.

50. Deter RL, Hadlock FP, Harrist R, et al. Evaluation of normal fetal growth and the detection of IUGR. In: Callen PW, ed. *Ultrasonography in Obstetrics and Gynecology.* Philadelphia: Saunders; 1983:128–131.

51. Nicolaides K, Bradley RJ, Soothill P, et al. Maternal oxygen therapy for intrauterine growth retardation. *Lancet.* 1987; 1:942.

21 Sonography in Diabetic Pregnancies

Dinesh M. Shah

Before the availability of insulin, pregnancy among women with type I diabetes mellitus (insulin-dependent) was rare, due to the high incidence of amenorrhea. When pregnancy did occur in these women in the pre-insulin era, it was generally associated with disastrous consequences. Maternal mortality was as high as 25%, primarily due to ketoacidosis, and perinatal mortality was close to 50%. Even with the advent of insulin therapy, maternal mortality remained significantly high in the 1920s and 1930s. After the reduction in overall maternal mortality that took place in the 1940s, increasing attention was paid to the high perinatal mortality (20%) still remaining in diabetic pregnancies. Recent advances in perinatal care have significantly reduced perinatal morbidity and mortality in these women.[1-4]

Despite these improvements, diabetic gravidas are still at high risk for adverse perinatal outcome. Maternal diabetes adversely affects the fetus in several ways. Ultrasonography can make significant contributions to the clinical management of a number of features of diabetic fetopathy, including the following.

1. Congenital malformations, which occur much more frequently in fetuses of women with diabetes
2. Fetal macrosomia, which occurs more commonly in such fetuses
3. Fetal death rate, which is significantly higher compared to the general population
4. Higher risk of respiratory distress in infants of diabetic mothers
5. Fetal growth retardation in diabetic women with vasculopathy

This chapter will address the role of ultrasonography in the perinatal management of diabetic pregnancies, including the following areas.

1. Estimation of gestational age
2. Evaluation for congenital malformations
3. Evaluation of fetal growth
4. Assessment of fetal status

ESTIMATION OF GESTATIONAL AGE

Although the need for an accurate determination of gestational age is self-evident, it is all the more critical in diabetic pregnancies for (1) interpretation of alpha-fetoprotein levels, (2) evaluation of fetal growth patterns, and (3) the timing of amniocentesis and delivery. The clinical estimation of gestational age may be unsatisfactory in a significantly large number of cases, even with a reliable menstrual history, and may thus be inadequate for critical management decisions in a diabetic pregnancy.[5]

The two most widely used ultrasound measurements for gestational age assessment are crown-rump length (CRL) in the first trimester, and biparietal diameter (BPD) in the second.[6,7] Estimates based on CRL measured at up to 12 weeks' gestation are highly accurate, and will predict delivery date to within 5 days.[8] The standard BPD measurement is also useful when carried out before 24 weeks of gestation.[9,10] Increasing fetal size and flexion toward the end of the first trimester make estimates of CRL more difficult and less accurate, while the slower rate of head growth and larger biologic variation make BPD of less use in the third trimester of pregnancy. Femur length is also a valuable predictor of gestational age, and is almost as reliable as BPD.[11] It is especially useful when it is technically not possible to measure BPD. The biocular distance may also be used to estimate gestation when the BPD cannot be obtained.[12]

In a sonographer-oriented routine ultrasound program, the value of screening an entire obstetric population for prediction of gestational age based on a single measurement of CRL and BPD was evaluated.[13] Ultrasound cephalometry before 18 weeks was found to be the single best dating parameter. The first sonographic examination to determine dates should be performed in the second trimester, prior to 20 weeks' gestation whenever possible. Such early examination would also assist in interpretation of alpha-fetoprotein levels, as well as in early detection of major fetal malformations. If the first ultrasound examination determining gestational dating differs significantly from clinical dating, it is generally necessary to repeat the ultrasound examination with at least 3 weeks' interval between the two examinations. The second examination should be performed well before 28 weeks' gestation. Gestational age can then be determined by the methods of either mean projected gestational age or growth-adjusted sonographic age.[14]

There is some evidence to suggest that early fetal

growth delay detected by ultrasound may be a marker for increased risk of congenital malformations in diabetic pregnancy.[15] Crown-rump length measurement may be useful in accurate interpretation of gestational age-correlated biochemical data such as glycosylated hemoglobin and alpha-fetoprotein, but it is important to recognize that such interpretations may be limited by early fetal growth delay.

EVALUATION FOR CONGENITAL MALFORMATIONS

An association between diabetes mellitus and congenital malformations has been suspected since the nineteenth century.[16,17] As early as 1885, it was reported that congenital anomalies occurred in the infants of diabetic mothers. Pederson, Tygstrup, and Pederson published the first study identifying a higher incidence of congenital anomalies among infants of mothers with longstanding insulin-dependent diabetes than among a general control population.[18] In their study of 853 infants of diabetic mothers (IDM) born between 1926 and 1963, 6.4% had major congenital anomalies, compared to 2.1% of 1,265 control newborns. Since that time, multiple studies have confirmed threefold to fourfold higher rates of malformations among IDM than among newborns of nondiabetic mothers.[19,20]

The exact etiology leading to increased incidence of congenital anomalies among IDM remains unknown. Maternal insulin does not cross the placenta and therefore exerts no direct influence upon the fetus. Animal studies of insulin-induced hypoglycemia treated by supplemental feeding did not reveal increased congenital anomaly formation.[21] In addition, the Collaborative Perinatal Project, a prospective study of 48,437 subjects from 14 institutions, revealed that neither diabetic men nor women with pregnancy-induced glucose intolerance were at increased risk for producing children with congenital anomalies, thus questioning the possibility of a gene-linked factor.[20]

However, diabetes mellitus is characterized by alterations of carbohydrate metabolism, and evidence does exist to support a concept of teratogenecity of byproducts of aberrant metabolism. Animal studies have suggested that untreated hypoglycemia during organogenesis may be teratogenic.[22,23] Excessive ketone body exposure has been shown to cause neural tube defects in mouse embroyos.[24] Several retrospective clinical studies have reported an association between poor diabetic control, ie, hyperglycemia, in early pregnancy, and congenital malformation.[25,26] The most convincing evidence suggesting teratogenic effects of hyperglycemia comes from Miller and colleagues.[25] They examined the relationship between maternal glycosylated hemoglobin (HbA_{1c}—a re-

flection of the preceding 6 to 8 week's glycemic control) levels before 14 weeks of gestation and congenital anomalies of birth. They found a 22% incidence of congenital anomalies among IDM if maternal HbA_{1c} was greater than 8.5% and a 3% incidence if HbA_{1c} was less than 8.5%. However, a recent study by Mills and associates[27] did not find a correlation of hyperglycemia and HbA_{1c} with malformation. These data suggest that more sensitive measures are needed to identify teratogenic mechanisms or that only some malformations may be preventable by early good glycemic control. The authors further stated that more favorable outcomes in the early entry group, including lower incidence of congenital malformations, justify the attempt to good metabolic control around the time of conception.

Mills and coworkers[28] identified the time of embryonic development using a morphologic approach. Their findings determined the gestational age at which the more common anomalies afflicting IDM are formed, and revealed that by the end of the sixth gestational week the affected systems are completed. The effect of diabetes on pregnancy in terms of malformations is not to produce a specific phenotype or syndrome, but to affect multiple organ systems.[29] A range of malformations in these systems occurs with increased incidence in IDM. Based on the literature and on state-wide data collected from Washington, it has been possible to estimate the relative risk of these malformations (see Table 21–1).[29] Many of the defects that are common in the general population (eg, neural tube defects and cardiac anomalies) occur at an increased rate in IDM, and, therefore, even though the relative risk of sacral dysgenesis is high, the most common malformations in IDM are neural tube defects and cardiac anomalies.

Sonographic detection of recognizable congenital malformations that occur more frequently in fetuses of

TABLE 21–1. MALFORMATIONS IN IDM IN ORDER OF RELATIVE RISK

Malformation	Relative Risk	Incidence in IDM (%)
Sacral dysgenesis	200–600	0.2–0.5
Holoprosencephaly	40–400	0.8
Situs inversus	84	
Ureter duplex	23	
Renal agenesis	6	
Cardiac anomalies	4	3.2
Anencephalus	3	0.57

Note: Even though the relative risk of sacral dysgenesis is high, the most common malformations in IDM are neural tube defects and cardiac anomalies.
(*Modified with permission from Mills JL. In: Gabbe SG, Oh W, eds.* Infant of the Diabetic Mother. *Report of the 93 Ross Conference on Pediatric Research. Columbus, Oh: Ross Laboratories, 1987:12–19.*)

TABLE 21–2. SYSTEMIC CLASSIFICATION OF DETECTABLE MALFORMATIONS OF INFANTS OF DIABETIC MOTHERS

Central Nervous System
Open neural tube defects
Anencephaly
Neural tube defects other than anencephaly
Closed neural tube defects
Holoprosencephaly

Cardiovascular System
Transpositions of great vessels
Ventricular septal defects
Coarctation of aorta
Atrial septal defect

Renal and Urologic System
Ureteral duplication
Renal agenesis
Hydronephrosis

Skeletal System
Caudal regression syndrome
Arthrogryposis (multiple flexion contractures)

Other
Situs inversus
Single umbilical artery

diabetic mothers is an important aspect of management of diabetic pregnancy. Table 21–2 provides a systemic classification of these detectable malformations and forms the basis of a systematic sonographic approach for their diagnosis.

Central Nervous System Malformations

The increased incidence of central nervous system mal-

formations among IDM is well recognized. Four of the 13 malformations in Miller's study of 116 infants of insulin-dependent diabetic women involved the central nervous system.[25] Kucera[19] noted anencephaly as one of the ten anomalies more likely to be present among offspring of diabetic mothers. In light of the seriousness of these malformations, and the widespread use of maternal serum alpha-fetoprotein screening programs, it is important to review relevant aspects of the role of maternal serum alpha-fetoprotein testing in clinical management.

MATERNAL SERUM ALPHA-FETOPROTEIN

Human alpha-fetoprotein (AFP) was recognized as a fetal-specific globulin in 1956.[30,31] A glycoprotein, AFP is synthesized by the yolk sac, gastrointestinal tract, and fetal liver, but the latter dominates the synthesis.[32] The level of AFP in fetal plasma peaks between 10 and 13 weeks' gestation at about 3,000 mg/mL. Alpha-fetoprotein enters the fetal urine and from there is passed into amniotic fluid.[33]

The level of AFP in amniotic fluid varies according to gestational age, with the highest concentration being found between 14 and 16 weeks' gestation and then steadily decreasing. (See Fig. 21–1.) Maternal serum AFP concentrations are highest between 28 and 32 weeks' gestation. Because AFP from amniotic fluid enters the maternal circulation, Brock and Sutcliffe first suggested serum AFP determination as a basis for screening for neural tube defects (NTD).[34] In a large collaborative study

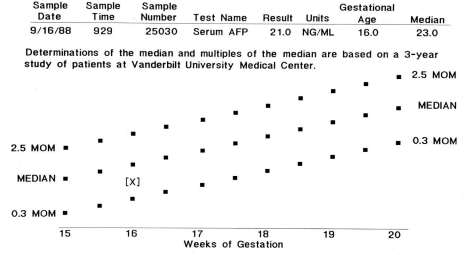

Sample Date	Sample Time	Sample Number	Test Name	Result	Units	Gestational Age	Median
9/16/88	929	25030	Serum AFP	21.0	NG/ML	16.0	23.0

Determinations of the median and multiples of the median are based on a 3-year study of patients at Vanderbilt University Medical Center.

Conclusion: The serum AFP quantitates within the reference range for this gestational age. A neural tube defect or other fetal developmental abnormalities associated abnormal AFP values are unlikely.

Fig. 21–1. Graphic reporting of maternal serum alpha-fetoprotein.

in the United Kingdom, 18,684 singleton and 163 twin pregnancies without NTD and 301 singleton pregnancies with NTD from 19 centers underwent AFP screening between 16 and 18 weeks' gestation.[35] At this gestation period, a 2.5 multiples-of-the-median (MOM) level of AFP was associated with a detection rate of 88% for anencephaly and 79% for open spina bifida, with a 3.3% false positive rate (ie, no NTD but elevated MSAFP). Similar results were obtained in the Swedish study of 7,158 MSAFP determinations between 14 and 20 weeks gestation.[36] Several other studies have confirmed these results, and the case for offering AFP screening in all pregnancies is sound. Because infants of diabetic mothers are at higher risk for NTD, a case can be made for routine AFP screening in these gravidas. It is critical that a backup service of perinatal consultation, intensive ultrasound evaluation, and genetic counseling be provided to all patients with elevated MSAFP.[37]

Maternal serum alpha-fetoprotein screening is generally performed between 16 and 18 weeks' gestation. Individual laboratories may have specific gestational age ranges for determining AFP testing, depending on their own data (15 to 20 weeks for our laboratory). The cutoff value for diagnosis of abnormal AFP levels may also vary (2.5 versus 3 versus 5 MOM) among individual laboratories. Levels of MSAFP are higher in patients with twin gestation and fetal demise and are affected by maternal weight and race. It is preferable, then, that appropriate corrections be applied by the laboratory in reporting results. (See Fig. 21–1.) After ruling out these two most obvious causes, wrong gestational age is the most common reason for abnormally elevated MSAFP because the AFP level changes with gestational age. Thus, ultrasound-based pregnancy dating will assist in correct interpretation of MSAFP.

After applying the above clinical correlations, less than 2% of patients will be diagnosed to have a "confirmed" elevated AFP level. The risk of neural tube defect for infants of these individuals is on the order of 10 to 15%. They should receive counseling and be offered amniocentesis for definitive diagnosis. Pregnancy loss rate with amniocentesis is stated to be 0.5%.[37] The purpose of amniocentesis in these patients is to obtain the amniotic fluid AFP level and, if this is elevated, to obtain the acetylcholinesterase (ACE) level. Acetylcholinesterase is a neural-tissue-specific enzyme. If both ACE and AFP are elevated in amniotic fluid, the chance of neural tube defect is virtually 100%. However, levels of AFP or ACE in amniotic fluid do not determine the severity of the defect. Amniotic fluid in these patients should also be processed for fetal karyotype after appropriately counseling the patient regarding its implications.

Patients with high amniotic fluid AFP but normal levels of ACE may have an anomaly other than neural tube defect (eg, omphalocele), and they should be eval-

uated for it by intensive sonographic examination. The condition of the majority of patients with high MSAFP but normal amniotic fluid AFP can be explained on the basis of feto-maternal bleeding. A few may have sonographically recognizable retrochorionic hematomas.[38] In patients with elevated MSAFP and normal sonogram, the risk of neural tube defect is substantially lower (0.28%) than the risk (10 to 15%) derived from MSAFP alone, and patients may have to be counseled both before and after sonography is performed.[39]

Regardless of MSAFP level, all diabetic pregnancies should be sonographically evaluated for detection of neural tube defects. Central nervous system anomalies commonly recognized as occurring more frequently in infants of diabetic mothers are listed in Table 21–2. Closure of the neural tube normally begins in the cervical region of the cord and proceeds in both the cephalad and caudal directions with the anterior and posterior neuropore finally closing around 38 to 40 days of the gestation. Thus, all open neural tube defects occur prior to the sixth week of gestation. Specific anomalies are discussed below.

Anencephaly

This is the most common anomaly affecting the central nervous system, with an increased incidence of 0.57% in the fetus in a diabetic pregnancy. This represents a threefold increase over that expected in the normal population (0.19%).[40] Anencephaly results from a failure of the neural tube to close at the cranial pole. The cerebral hemisphere (telencephalon) may be affected alone, or along with the diencephalon and midbrain or the spinal cord.[41] Secondary degenerative changes occur, resulting in the absence of cerebral hemispheres. The frontal bones above

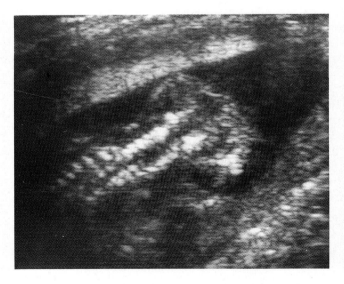

Fig. 21–2. A case of anencephaly. Absence of cranial vault is clearly recognizable in this view.

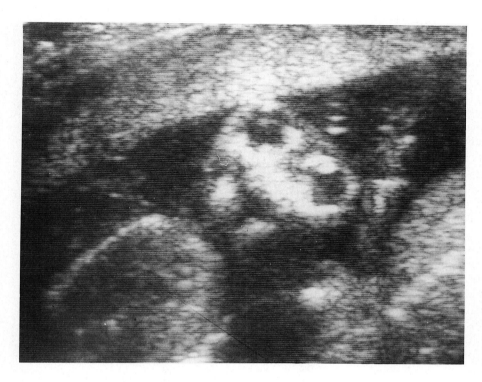

Fig. 21–3. Typical frog-face appearance on sonogram of the fetus in Fig. 21–2 with anencephaly. Again, note absence of cranial vault. A loop of umbilical cord and fetal hand are visualized instead in the normal location of the cranial vault.

the supraciliary ridge, the parietal bone and the squamous part of the occipital bone, which make up the cranial vault, are usually absent.

Diagnosis of anencephaly therefore depends on recognition of the absence of cerebral hemispheres and cranial vault. Cranial meninges are generally flat against the remainder of the brain and do not form a protruding cystic mass. Anencephalic neonates have a short neck and protrusion of the eyeballs, giving them a frog-face appearance. The sonographic features of this are quite typical as shown in Figures 21–2 and 21–3. Diagnosis in the second or third trimester of pregnancy is relatively easily made, but rarely a fetal head deeply engaged in the pelvis or severe microcephaly may pose some difficulty. Sector scanning in the longitudinal plane may allow better visualization in the retro and infrapubic region, and occasionally transperineal scanning may assist in the recognition of a deeply engaged fetal head. The prognosis for these infants is uniformly fatal and termination of pregnancy at any time in gestation is considered an ethically acceptable option.[42,43]

Holoprosencephaly

Maternal diabetes is thought to increase the risk of this holoprosencephaly, the result from failure of cleavage of the prosencephalon. Median facial structures normally induced by prechordal mesenchyma generally show defects in association with holoprosencephaly. These facial defects include cyclopia, hypotelorism, median or bilateral cleft lip, and flat nose. The cerebral anomalies also

vary depending on degree of the failure of midline cleavage. These include the most severe form: alobar, the intermediate form; semilobar; and the least severe form, lobar holoprosencephaly. Sonographic diagnostic features depend to some degree on the severity of the defects. In the alobar and semilobar varieties, identification of a single sickle-shaped ventricle in the axial plane is most suggestive of holoprosencephaly.[44] Diagnosis of the lobar form is difficult because the lateral ventricles appear separated due to the interhemispheric fissure, except in the frontal portion. Facial defects are a further clue and indicate the need for intensified evaluation of cerebral hemisphere cleavage. The prognosis of holoprosencephaly depends on its severity and associated chromosomal abnormalities, if present. Obstetric management depends on gestational age at diagnosis, severity of the condition, and parental wishes, and must include extensive counseling. For further details on this condition, refer to the chapter on intracranial and facial abnormalities.

Cardiovascular Anomalies

Cardiovascular malformations that occur with increased frequency in infants of diabetic mothers have been listed in Table 21–2. These defects are by far the most common defects of such infants. Patients with higher levels of first trimester HbA$_{1c}$ are at highest risk and should receive intensified cardiac evaluation during second trimester ultrasonography with specific attention to the malformations listed in Table 21–2. For details on ultrasonic diagnosis of these anomalies and their implication and management, refer to Chapter 8 on fetal cardiac sonography.

Caudal Regression Syndrome

Lenz and Maier first suggested that hypoplasia of the sacrum and lower extremities (primary features of the syndrome) was more common in offspring of diabetic mothers.[45] This has been suggested by subsequent investigators, and caudal regression syndrome is said to occur at the rate of 0.2% to 0.5% in IDM. The primary defect is in the midposterior axis mesoderm and in its most severe form is presumably the consequence of a wedge-shaped early deficit of the caudal blastema.[46] All degrees of severity may occur, and primarily depend on the relative length and width of early caudal deficit.[45] Associated anomalies, depending on the severity of the syndrome, may include imperforate anus, absence of external genitalia, renal agenesis, absence of internal genitalia except gonads, a single umbilical artery, absence of bladder, and fusion of the lower limbs (sirenomelia).

Prenatal diagnosis of the syndrome by sonography has been reported. Such a case example is shown in Figures 21–4 and 21–5. The principal findings of caudal regression syndrome as diagnosed by sonography are the interruption of the lower distal lumbar spine and abnormality of limb position or movement. The lumbar spine interruption may appear as a deficit in the alignment

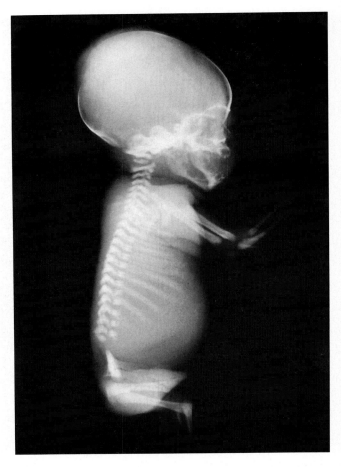

Fig. 21–5. Postnatal lateral radiograph of fetus in Fig. 21–4 at 26 weeks. Fetal death occurred in association with diabetic coma and adult respiratory distress syndrome.

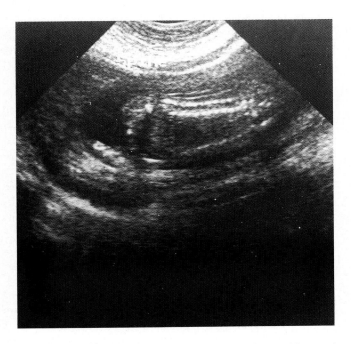

Fig. 21–4. Sonogram of a 23 weeks' gestation fetus with sacral agenesis. Compare this "lateral" view of fetus to radiographic features.

of the vertebra with a "hole" or a step between two levels, with the distal-most level being collapsed closer to the proximal level. This may also present as angulation of the spine with the apex of the angulation pointing towards the back of the fetus.

Limb contracture and absence of movement is also typical. There may be some webbing at the knee or at the hip, and deformity of the foot, with talipes equinovarus being the most common. Rocker-bottom foot is also a possibility. Dislocation of the hip or, worse, approximation of the two femoral heads with agenesis of the sacrum is another finding (Fig. 21–6).

Prognosis depends on the associated anomalies and severity of the syndrome. Obstetric management would depend on the above features, gestational age, and parental wishes, and must include extensive counseling.

Renal and Urologic Anomalies

Defects involving this system that show preponderance

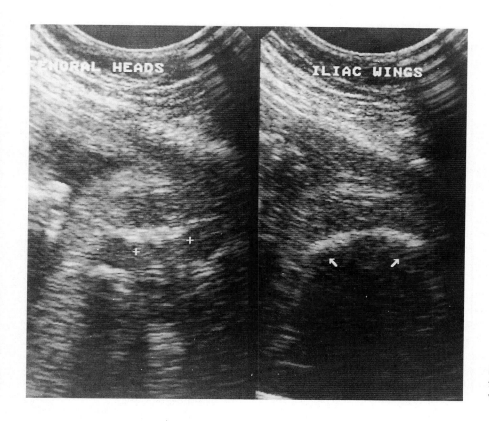

Fig. 21–6. Case of sacral agenesis shows femoral heads close to each other; iliac wings are not normally separated.

in IDM are listed in Table 21–2. These include ureteral duplication, renal agenesis, and hydronephrosis. Serious genito-urinary (GU) anomalies are frequently associated with significant oligohydramnios. Therefore, the presence of oligohydramnios in a fetus of a diabetic woman should prompt systematic evaluation, especially for urinary abnormalities. The most severe of these, renal agenesis, may be either unilateral or bilateral. When it affects both sides (bilateral), severe oligohydramnios, essentially anhydramnios, (ie, total absence of amniotic fluid) is present. A representative case of renal agenesis is shown in Figure 21–7. Ureteral duplication, if associated with ureteropelvic junctional obstruction, may show hydronephrosis, and duplicated ureters may be visible on ultrasound. Hydronephrosis with normal bladder may occur due to obstruction or reflex phenomenon above the level of urinary bladder. These abnormalities require systematic evaluation by an experienced sonographer. For details on ultrasonic diagnosis, progress, and management of GU abnormalities, refer to Chapter 18.

Other Anomalies

Other anomalies include situs inversus and a single umbilical artery. Sonographic diagnosis of fetal situs is discussed in Chapters 9 and 17 as part of the discussion of cardiac and gastrointestinal abnormalities.

EVALUATION OF FETAL GROWTH

Infants of diabetic mothers are primarily at risk for macrosomia and they may be at risk for fetal growth

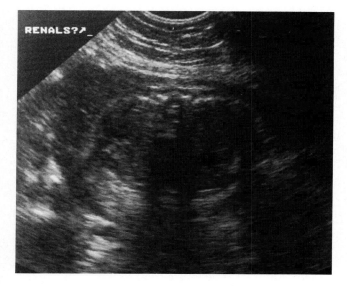

Fig. 21–7. A case of renal agenesis with anhydramnios, ie, total absence of amniotic fluid.

retardation in the presence of severe vascular disease. Sonographic evaluation in intrauterine growth retardation is addressed in Chapter 21, and this section will discuss macrosomia in IDM.

Macrosomia is clinically defined as birth weight in excess of 4,000 g, or above the 90th percentile for a given gestational age.[47,48] The etiology of hypersomatism or macrosomia is thought to be secondary to fetal hyperinsulinemia resulting from maternal hyperglycemia.[49] Maternal glucose is readily transferred to the fetus across the placenta, resulting in fetal hyperglycemia. This stimulates the fetal pancreas to increase its production and release of insulin. Pedersen has proposed that the concomitant presence of excessive substrate and insulin enhances fetal glycogen synthesis, lipogenesis, and protein synthesis. Experimental data exist supporting insulin as a growth hormone. The administration of insulin to fetal rats and lambs has resulted in increased size of the newborn and deposition of fat in adipose tissue.[50–54] Experimental diabetes in rhesus monkeys noted findings consistent with some of the clinical observations made in humans.[55] There was no change in brain weight, while visceral organs and adipose tissue were significantly enlarged. Increase in fetal levels of deoxyribonucleic acid (DNA) and proteins has been demonstrated in animal models, indicating cellular hyperplasia and hypertrophy in some organs and body areas.[56]

Fetal macrosomia in IDM is characterized by a disparity in growth rates of various tissues. The brain is insulin-insensitive tissue and does not show the accelerated growth of the fetal trunk. The fetal trunk tends to be larger due to both visceral growth and deposition of adipose tissue. The extremities are also noted to have increased deposition of adipose tissue. These clinical features form the basis for sonographic detection of fetal macrosomia.

Murata and Martin[57] have reported no difference in BPD between IDM and fetuses of nondiabetic controls during the 13th through 37th weeks of gestation. Most authors do agree that the BPD is not significantly larger in the infant of the diabetic mother compared to those of nondiabetic controls. Therefore, sonographic measurements of fetal BPD alone is of little value in the detection of fetal macrosomia.[58] Use of sonographic fetal abdominal transverse diameter has been suggested in antepartum diagnosis of macrosomia.[58] In approximately 50% of IDM, the abdominal circumference at the level of the ductus venosus exceeded 2 standard deviations above the mean for 28 to 32 weeks' gestation, suggesting a diagnosis of accelerated fetal trunk growth. Neonatal evidence of macrosomia corroborated the sonographic findings in that study.

Campbell and Thomas,[59] and Jeanty and Romero[60] have constructed a nomogram of head-to-abdominal circumference ratio with mean, 5th, and 95th percentile ranks for the 13th through 42nd week gestational range, which may be useful in assessing head-to-body proportions. The nomogram of Jeanty and Romero is shown in Chapter 7. Wladimiroff and associates[61] obtained chest size measurements by a cross-sectional dimension immediately caudal to the fetal heart pulsation. This measurement is likely to be significantly influenced by accelerated growth of the fetal liver and therefore reflective of macrosomia. Using this single determination, they reported a detection rate of fetal macrosomia of 80% in relation to the 90th percentile of the birth-weight-for-gestational-age, and 47% in relation to the 95th percentile for given gestational age.[62] Houchang and colleagues[62] have used a chest-circumference ratio to head size in identifying macrosomic infants at high risk for traumatic delivery.

ASSESSMENT OF FETAL STATUS

Sonographic Guidance for Amniocentesis

Determination of fetal pulmonary maturity by testing for phospholipids in amniotic fluid is an important aspect of the management of diabetic pregnancies. These tests generally include lecithin: sphingomyelin ratio (L:S) and phosphotidyl glycerol concentration. Amniocentesis for this purpose is timed according to gestational age, past obstetric history, and current clinical events.

Sonography has proved valuable in needle guidance for amniocentesis.[63,64] Sonography greatly improves the feasibility of the procedure and reduces the number of "unable to tap" cases to close to zero. In addition, sonographic guidance can significantly improve the procedure's safety.

Biophysical Profile

The use of fetal events (movement and breathing), detected by real-time sonography, for assessment of fetal well-being has been extensively reported. Manning and coworkers were the first to demonstrate the clinical utility of real-time assessment along with fetal heart rate evaluation in the management of high risk pregnancies. A modified scheme using exclusive real-time-detected fetal events has also been shown to be a useful tool in fetal assessment.[65,66]

REFERENCES

1. Molsted-Pedersen L. Pregnancy and diabetes: A survey. *Acta Endocrinol (Copenh).* 1980;94:13.
2. Larsson J, Ludvigsson J. Perinatal dodelighet ved diabetes graviditet. *Lakartidningen.* 1974;71:155.

3. White P. Pregnancy complicating diabetes. *Am J Med.* 1949; 7:609.

4. Gabbe SG, Mestman JH, Freeman RK, et al. Management and outcome of pregnancy in diabetes mellitus, classes B to R. *Am J Obstet Gynecol.* 1977;129:723.

5. Callen PW. *Ultrasonography in Obstetrics and Gynecology.* Philadelphia: WB Saunders; 1983;21–37.

6. Robinson HP. Sonar measurement of the fetal crown-rump length as a means of assessing maturity in first trimester pregnancy. *Br. Med J.* 1973;4:28.

7. Campbell S, Newman GB. Growth of the fetal biparietal diameter during pregnancy. *J Obstet Gynaecol Br Commonw.* 1971;78:513.

8. Robinson HP, Fleming JEE. A critical evaluation of sonar crown-rump length measurements. *Br J Obstet Gynaecol.* 1975;82:702.

9. Hadlock FP, Deter RL, Harrist RB, Park SK. Fetal biparietal diameter. A critical re-evaluation of the relation to menstrual age by means of real-time ultrasound. *J Ultrasound Med.* 1982;1:97.

10. Bennett MJ. Real-time ultrasound in the second and third trimesters of pregnancy. In: Bennett MJ, Campbell S, eds. *Real-time Ultrasound in Obstetrics.* Oxford, England: Blackwell; 1980;49–61.

11. O'Brien GD, Queenan JT, Campbell S. Assessment of gestational age in the second trimester by real-time ultrasound measurement of the femur length. *Am J Obstet Gynecol.* 1981;139:540.

12. Jeanty P, Dramaix-Wilmot M, Van Gansbeke D, et al. Fetal ocular biometry by ultrasound. *Radiology.* 1982;143:513.

13. Campbell S, Warsof SL, Little D, Cooper DJ. Routine ultrasound screening for the prediction of gestational age. *Obstet Gynecol.* 1985;65:613.

14. Kopta MM, Tomich PG, Crane JP. Ultrasonic methods of predicting the estimated date of confinement. *Obstet Gynecol.* 1981;57:657.

15. Pedersen JF, Molsted-Pedersen L. Early fetal growth delay detected by ultrasound marks increased risk of congenital malformation in diabetic pregnancy. *Br Med J.* 1981; 283:80.

16. Mills JL. Malformations in infants of diabetic mothers. *Teratology.* 1982;25:385.

17. Mills JL, Baker L, Goldman AS. Malformations in infants of diabetic mothers occur before the seventh gestational week: Implications for treatment. *Diabetes.* 1979;28:292.

18. Pedersen IM, Tygstrup I, Pedersen J. Congenital malformations in newborn infants of diabetic women. Correlation with maternal diabetic vascular complications. *Lancet.* 1964;1:1124.

19. Kucera J. Rate and type of congenital anomalies among offspring of diabetic women. *J Reprod Med.* 1971;7:61.

20. Chung CS, Myrianthopoulos NC. Factors affecting risks of congenital malformations: Report from the Collaborative Perinatal Project. *Birth Defects.* 1975;11:23. Original Article Series.

21. Horii N, Watanabe G, Ingalls TH. Experimental diabetes in pregnant mice. Prevention of congenital malformations in offspring by insulin. *Diabetes.* 1966;15:194.

22. Kalter H, Warkany J. Experimental production of congenital malformation in mammals by metabolic procedure. *Physiology Review.* 1959;39:69.

23. Smithberg M, Rummer MN. Teratogenic effects of hypoglycemic treatments in inbred strains of mice. *Am J Anatomy.* 1963;113:479.

24. Horton WE, Sadler TW. Effects of maternal diabetes on early embryogenesis. Alterations in morphogenesis produced by the ketone body, B-hydroxybuterate. *Diabetes.* 1983;32:610.

25. Miller E, Hare JW, Cloherty JP, et al. Elevated maternal hemoglobin A_{1c} in early pregnancy and major congenital anomalies in infants of diabetic mothers. *N Engl J Med.* 1981;304:1331.

26. Leslie RDG, John PN, Pyke DA, White JM. Haemoglobin A_1 in diabetic pregnancy. *Lancet.* 1978;2:958.

27. Mills JL, Knopp RH, Simpson JL, et al. Lack of relation of increased malformation rates in infants of diabetic mothers to glycemic control during organogenesis. *N Engl J Med.* 1988;318:671.

28. Mills JL, Baker L, Goldman AS. Malformations in infants of diabetic mothers occur before the seventh gestational week. *Diabetes.* 1979;28:292.

29. Mills JL. Congenital malformations in diabetes. In: Gabbe SG, Oh W, eds. *Infant of the Diabetic Mother.* Report of the 93rd Ross Conference on Pediatric Research. Columbus, Ohio: Ross Laboratories, 1987;12–19.

30. Bergstrand CG, Czar B. Demonstration of a new protein fraction in serum from the human fetus. *Scand J Clin Lab Invest.* 1956;8:174.

31. Halbrecht I, Klibanski C. Identification of a new normal embryonic haemoglobin. *Nature.* 1956;178:794.

32. Gitlin D, Perricelli A, Gitlin GM. Synthesis of alpha fetoprotein by liver, yolk sac, and gastrointestinal tract of the human conceptus. *Cancer Res.* 1972;32:979.

33. Gitlin D, Boesman M. Serum alpha feto-protein, albumin, and gamma globulin in the human conceptus. *J Clin Invest.* 1966;45:1826.

34. Brock DJH, Sutcliffe RG. Alpha-fetoprotein in the antenatal diagnosis of anencephaly and spina bifida. *Lancet.* 1972; 2:197.

35. U.K. collaborative study on alpha-fetoprotein in relation to neural-tube defects: Maternal serum-alpha-fetoprotein measurement in antenatal screening for anencephaly and spina bifida in early pregnancy. *Lancet.* 1977;1:1324.

36. Kjessler B, Johansson SGO, Lidbjork G, et al. Alpha-fetoprotein (AFP) levels in maternal serum in relation to pregnancy outcome in 7158 pregnant women prospectively investigated during their 14th-20th week post last menstrual period. *Acta Obstet Gynecol Scand.* 1977;69:25.

37. Main DM, Mennuti MT. Neural tube defects: Issues in prenatal diagnosis and counseling. *Obstet Gynecol.* 1986; 67:1.

38. Fleischer AC, Kurtz AB, Wapner RJ, et al. Elevated alpha-fetoprotein and a normal fetal sonogram: Association with placental abnormalities. *AJR.* 1988;150:881.

39. Richards DS, Seeds JW, Katz VL, et al. Elevated maternal serum alpha-fetoprotein with normal ultrasound: Is amniocentesis always appropriate? A review of 26,069 screened patients. *Obstet Gynecol.* 1988;71:203.

40. Soler NG, Walsh CH, Malins JM. Congenital malformations in infants of diabetic mothers. *J Med.* 1976;178:303.

41. Norman RM. Malformations of the nervous system, birth injury and diseases of early life. In: Blackwood W, McMenemy WH, Meyer A, et al, eds. *Greenfield's Neuropathology.* Baltimore: Williams & Wilkins; 1967;324–440.

42. Chervenak FA, Farley MA, Walters L, et al. When is termination of pregnancy during the third trimester morally justifiable? *N Engl J Med.* 1984;310:501.

43. Boehm FH. Management of the unanticipated neural tube defect in late pregnancy. *Clin Obstet Gynecol.* 1984;27:78.

44. Romero R, Pilu G, Jeanty P, et al. *Prenatal Diagnosis of Congenital Anomalies.* Norwalk, Conn: Appleton & Lange; 1988;59–65.

45. Lenz W, Maier E. Congenital malformations and maternal diabetes. *Lancet.* 1964;2:1124.

46. Smith DW, Jones KL. *Recognizable Patterns of Human Malformation.* Philadelphia: WB Saunders; 1982;486.

47. Elliott JP, Garite TJ, Freeman RK, et al. Ultrasonic prediction of fetal macrosomia in diabetic patients. *Obstet Gynecol.* 1982;60:159.

48. Golditch IM, Kirkman K. The large fetus: Management and outcome. *Obstet Gynecol.* 1978;52:285.

49. Freinkel N, Dooley SL, Metzger BE. Care of the pregnant woman with insulin-dependent diabetes mellitus. *N Engl J Med.* 1985;313:96.

50. Pedersen IM, Tygstrup I, Pedersen J. Congenital malformations in newborn infants of diabetic women. Correlation with maternal diabetic vascular complications. *Lancet.* 1964;1:1124.

51. Ylinen K, Raivio K, Teramo K. Hemoglobin A_{1c} predicts the perinatal outcome in insulin-dependent diabetic pregnancies. *Br J Obstet Gynaecol.* 1981;88:961.

52. Vohr BR, Lipsitt LP, Oh W. Somatic growth of children of diabetic mothers with reference to birth size. *J Pediatr.* 1980;97:196.

53. Kim YS, Young K. A new animal model for fetal macrosomia in diabetic pregnancy. *Exp Molec Pathol.* 1981;35:388.

54. Kim YS, Yoon YJ, Jatoi I, et al. Fetal macrosomia in diabetic multiparous animals. *Diabetologgia.* 1981;20:213.

55. Merkatz IR, Adam PAJ. *The Diabetic Pregnancy. A Perinatal Perspective.* New York: Grune & Stratton; 1979.

56. Kim YS, Yoon YJ, Jatoi I, et al. Fetal macrosomia in experimental maternal diabetes. *Am J Obstet Gynecol.* 1981;139:27.

57. Murata Y, Martin CB. Growth of the biparietal diameter of the fetal head in diabetic pregnancy. *Am J Obstet Gynecol.* 1973;115:252.

58. Ogata ES, Sabbagha R, Metzger BE, et al. Serial ultrasonography to assess evolving fetal macrosomia. *JAMA.* 1980;243:2405.

59. Campbell S, Thomas A. Ultrasound measurement of the fetal head to abdomen circumference ratio in the assessment of growth retardation. *Br J Obstet Gynaecol.* 1977;84:165.

60. Jeanty P, Romero R. *Ultrasonography in Obstetrics.* New York: McGraw-Hill; 1984.

61. Wladimiroff JW, Bloesma CA, Wallenburg HCS. Ultrasonic diagnosis of the large-for-dates infant. *Obstet Gynecol.* 1978;52:285.

62. Houchang D, Modanlou HD, Komatsu G, et al. Large-for-gestational age neonates: Anthropometric reasons for shoulder dystocia. *Obstet Gynecol.* 1982;60:417.

63. Romero R, Jeanty P, Reece EA, et al. Sonographically monitored amniocentesis to decrease intraoperative complications. *Obstet Gynecol.* 1985;65:426.

64. Jeanty P, Rodesch R, Romero R, et al. How to improve your amniocentesis technique. *Am J Obstet Gynecol.* 1983;146:593.

65. Shah DM, Brown JE, Salyer SL, et al. Modified scheme for biophysical profile. *Am J Obstet Gynecol.* 1989;160:586–591.

66. Dicker D, Feldberg D, Yeshaya A, et al. Fetal surveillance in insulin-dependent diabetic pregnancy: Predictive value of the biophysical profile. *Am J Obstet Gynecol.* 1988;159:800.

22 The Sonographic Evaluation of Multiple Gestation Pregnancy

Clifford S. Levi • Edward A. Lyons • Daniel J. Lindsay • Dennis Gratton

Although multiple gestation pregnancies account for approximately 1% of all births,[1,2] they represent a disproportionately large percentage of perinatal deaths.[1-4] The perinatal mortality rate among twins is 10 to 14%, which is five to ten times the expected rate for singletons.[1-4] As a result, all multifetal pregnancies are considered to be high-risk.

In order to positively impact the clinical management of multiple gestation pregnancy, the role of sonography must be to:

1. Identify the number of embryos/fetuses
2. Characterize the amnionicity and chorionicity
3. Identify the fetuses with risk factors (ie, intrauterine growth retardation [IUGR]) that increase perinatal morbidity and mortality
4. Detect congenital malformations

In the process, the management of the pregnancy may be altered.

INCIDENCE OF TWINNING

Dizygotic Twins
Dizygotic or fraternal twins arise from two separate fertilized ova and always produce dichorionic, diamniotic pregnancies.[1,5] This form of twinning accounts for approximately 70%[1,2,5] of all twin pregnancies, with an incidence of approximately 1 in 90 live births. The incidence of dizygotic twinning is variable and is increased by many factors including:

1. *Maternal age and parity.*[1,2] The incidence of twinning increases with advancing maternal age and with increases in parity, peaking in the 35- to 40-year age group.
2. *Ethnic origin.*[1,2] In North America, caucasians have an incidence of 1 in 100 whereas blacks have an incidence of 1 in 79. In Japan the incidence is less, approximately 1 in 155 live births.
3. *Heredity.*[1,2] A maternal family history of dizygotic twinning is associated with a higher incidence of twins.

In a study by White and Wyshak,[6] the incidence of dizygotic twin births in women who themselves were dizygotic twins was 1 in 58.

4. *Ovulation induction agents.*[1,2,7] Clomiphene is associated with a 7% to 9% incidence of multifetal gestation, while hMG (human menopausal gonadotrophin) is associated with an 18% incidence. The ratio of multiple gestation pregnancies to twin pregnancies increases with the use of ovulation-induction agents.
5. *In vitro fertilization.* In vitro fertilization is associated with an increased incidence of multifetal pregnancies, related to the number of fertilized ova implanted. With ovulation induction and in vitro fertilization, the incidence of heterotopic pregnancy is also increased (infra vide).

It has been postulated that the common element resulting in increased incidence of dizygotic twinning is increased maternal serum follicle stimulating hormone, either from endogenous or exogenous sources.[7]

Monozygotic Twinning
Monozygotic twins arise from a single fertilized ovum. They are less common than dizygotic twins and represent approximately 1 in 250 births.[1,2,5,7] This rate of twinning is constant and is not influenced by factors affecting the incidence of dizygotic twinning. When compared to dizygotic twins, monozygotic twins are at higher risk for perinatal mortality and for congenital malformations. In a multicenter study by Naeye and associates,[3] the perinatal mortality rate was 2.7 times greater than that for dizygotic twins.

Polyzygous Gestation
Multiple gestation with more than two fetuses may occur with combinations of monozygous and polyzygous embryos. The presence of polyzygous embryos may enhance the occurrence of monozygotic division.[6] The incidence of triplets is approximately 1 in 8,100 pregnancies.[5] Expressing the incidence exponentially, it has been estimated that triplets occur once in 90^2 pregnancies, quad-

ruplets once in 90[3] pregnancies, and quintuplets once in 90.[45]

PERINATAL MORTALITY

The leading cause of perinatal mortality in multiple gestation pregnancies is premature delivery and the resultant complications of immaturity. In a multicenter study, Naeye and colleagues[3] identified amniotic fluid infection syndrome with intact membranes as the etiology of 60% of perinatal deaths and as the leading cause of premature labor. They postulated that overdistension of the uterus in twin pregnancy, with resultant greater exposure of fetal membranes to the bacterial flora of the vagina at the cervical os, may be the etiology of amniotic-fluid infection syndrome. The ratio between fetal and neonatal demise caused by amniotic-fluid infection syndrome was 1.0 to 1.6 in Naeye's series.[3] Other causes of death included premature rupture of the membranes in 11%, monovular twin transfusion syndrome in 8%, and congenital anomalies in 7%. Other complications included maternal hypertension, maternal anemia, postpartum hemorrhage, uterine atony, placental abruption, infarcts and previa, as well as cord abnormalities of prolapse, intertwinement, vasa previa, and velamentous insertion. Other complications are polyhydramnios and complications of labor including dystocia and those related to position and lie.[1,3,7]

DIAGNOSIS

Physical Examination
The history and physical examination may be helpful in raising the physician's index of suspicion of a twin pregnancy. With clinical skills alone, up to 50% of twin gestations may be unsuspected until delivery.[1,8]

In the second trimester, the physical examination may reveal a uterus that is large for the fetus' age. The diagnosis of twins can be made by palpation of more than one fetal head or auscultation of two fetal hearts. This becomes difficult in the obese patient, in the presence of polyhydramnios, or with a large anterior placenta.

The differential diagnosis of "large-for-dates" uterus includes normal gestation with an inaccurate menstrual history, fibroids, polyhydramnios, and hydatidiform mole. An adnexal mass or elevation of the uterus by a distended urinary bladder can mimic a large-for-dates uterus. The most common outcome of a patient referred with a large-for-dates uterus on clinical evaluation, in our experience using sonography, is a singleton fetus, entirely normal uterus, placenta, and amniotic fluid volume.

Sonographic Findings
Early clinical diagnosis of twins in the first and second trimesters may be difficult. Perhaps the most important role of sonography is in early detection of the multifetal pregnancy. In a study by Persson in 1983, the routine use of ultrasound in obstetrics was associated with the reduction of the mean gestation age of twin detection from 35 to 20 weeks.[9] Early diagnosis is crucial because approximately 70% of perinatal deaths occur prior to 30 weeks' gestation.[4] With current equipment, multifetal pregnancy should be detectable within the first 7 weeks of gestation. The ease with which the diagnosis of multifetal pregnancy can be made has led some groups to suggest that routine sonography be performed in the second trimester as a screening procedure, and again at approximately 31 weeks (if multiple gestation is found) to detect other complications related to twinning.[9]

Hormonal Assay
Attempts have been made to identify a hormonal assay that can be used to differentiate a singleton fetus from a multiple gestation pregnancy. Maternal serum levels of human chorionic gonadotropin (hCG) and human placenta lactogen (hPL) are related to the placental mass and are statistically higher in multiple-gestation pregnancies than in single pregnancies.[10–12]

A maternal serum hPL level that is greater than 1 standard deviation above the mean in the second or third trimester suggests the presence of a twin pregnancy. If the pregnancy is complicated by fetoplacental dysfunction, the hPL level may not be elevated and the diagnosis of twins may be missed. Knight and coworkers[12] demonstrated twin detection rate of only 45.9% when the 90th percentile of the hPL level for singletons was used as a cutoff point.

In a study by Thiery and colleagues,[10] maternal serum hCG levels were elevated significantly in 5 of 9 twin pregnancies in the first trimester, and in 72% of 39 twin pregnancies in the second and third trimester. Knight and associates[12] demonstrated a twin detection rate of 78.3% of 37 pregnancies using the 90th percentile of maternal serum alpha-fetoprotein (AFP) in singletons as a cutoff point.

The combined use of hPL and AFP assays in the study by Knight and coworkers[12] raised the twin detection rate to only 80%. Thiery and colleagues[10] demonstrated a twin detection rate of 95% when either or both of the maternal serum levels of hPL or hCG were elevated greater than 1 standard deviation above the mean for single pregnancies. They felt that hormonal levels were too inconsistent throughout pregnancy to be useful as a screening test, but elevated levels of either hCG or hPL should alert the obstetrician to the possibility of a twin pregnancy. Because of the inherent inaccuracies in hormonal tests in predicting the presence of a twin gestation, their use is very limited in this area.

Maternal serum AFP (MSAFP) levels are currently used as a screening test for fetal neural tube defects (NTD). Twin pregnancies act as a false-positive in these NTD screening programs. The mean AFP level for twins is approximately 2.5 multiples-of-the-mean (MOM) calculated for normal singleton pregnancies.[13] In a twin pregnancy when the MSAFP level is greater than 5 MOM, the outcome is significantly worse than for those with levels below 5 MOM. In a study by Ghosh and associates,[13] over 50% of those twin pregnancies with a MSAFP level greater than 5 MOM ended in abortion, stillbirth, or fetus papyraceous, or were associated with either concordant or discordant neural tube defects.[14]

EMBRYOLOGY

Dizygotic twins arise from two separate fertilized ova and always produce dichorionic, diamniotic twin pregnancies (Fig. 22–1). If implantations of the two blastocysts are in close proximity to one another, the two placentae may fuse.[5]

Monozygotic twins arise from division of a single fertilized ovum (Fig. 22–1). The results of this division depend on the stage at which division occurs and can be divided into three types.[1,5]

1. *Dichorionic, diamniotic* (less than 4 days post fertilization). Division of the zygote between the two-cell (blastomere) and morula stages, prior to formation of the inner cell mass (approximately three days postfertilization), will result in a dichorionic, diamniotic twin pregnancy. This type represents 18 to 36% of monozygotic twinning.[1,5] As with dizygotic twins, the placentae and chorions may fuse.
2. *Monochorionic, diamniotic* (4 to 8 days). The most common form of monozygotic twinning results from division of the inner cell mass, usually at 4 to 8 days postfertilization. The cells destined to become the chorion have already formed, resulting in a pregnancy with two embryos, a single chorion, and two amnions (a diamniotic, monochorionic twin pregnancy).
3. *Monochorionic, monoamniotic* (more than 8 days). If division occurs after formation of the amnion (approximately day 8) a monochorionic, monoamniotic twin pregnancy will result. This represents approximately 4% of monozygotic twins.[5] Incomplete division occurring after formation of the embryonic disc (after day 13) results in conjoined twins. It has been estimated that conjoined twins represent approximately 2.5% of all monozygotic twins.[5]

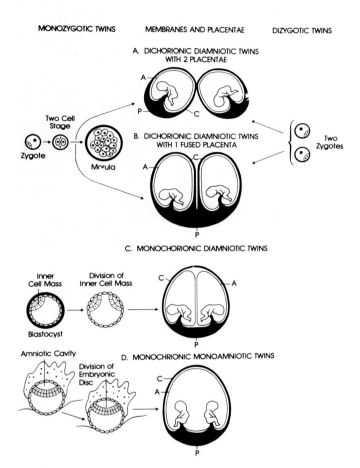

Fig. 22–1. Dichorionic diamniotic twins with two placentae or one fused placenta may be formed either by two separate zygotes or by the division of a single zygote at less than 4 days postfertilization between the two-cell stage and the morula stage. Monochorionic diamniotic twins are formed by division of the inner cell mass during the blastocyst stage from 4 to 8 days postfertilization. Monochorionic monoamniotic twins are formed by division of embryonic disc during the blastocyst stage after the formation of the amniotic cavity at 8 days postfertilization. A = amniotic membrane; C = chorionic membrane; P = placenta.

SONOGRAPHIC EVALUATION

First Trimester

Early articles describing ultrasound in twins dealt mainly with the sensitivity of ultrasound in the diagnosis of twin pregnancy. With high-resolution real-time equipment and the advent of endovaginal sonography, the diagnosis of multifetal gestation should be consistently made after 6 to 7 weeks' menstrual age. Identification of the amnion is now commonplace, allowing for reliable determination of amnioticity and chorionicity in multifetal pregnancies.

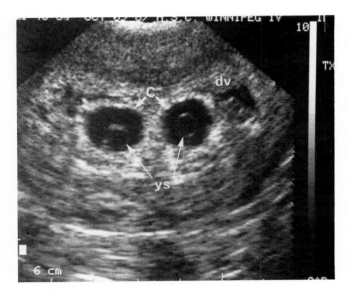

Fig. 22–2. Endovaginal sonogram in the coronal plane of a dichorionic diamniotic gestation at 6.5 weeks' menstrual age. A yolk sac is seen within each chorionic sac. ys = yolk sac; C = chorion; dv = decidua vera.

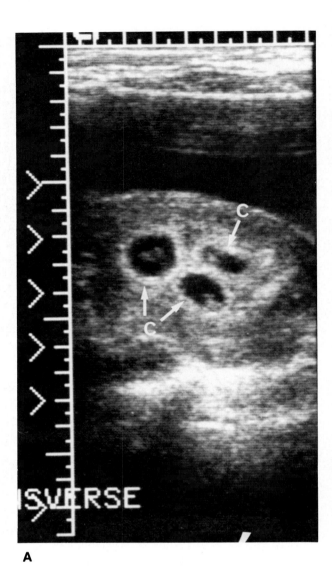

A

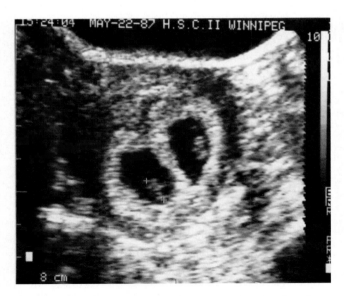

Fig. 22–3. Transvesicle scan in the transverse plane showing a dichorionic diamniotic gestation at approximately 6.5 weeks' menstrual age.

B

Fig. 22–4. Transvesicle sonogram is the transverse plane at 7 weeks' (**A**) and 13 weeks' (**B**) menstrual age in a triplet pregnancy resulting from in vitro fertilization. Three separate chorionic sacs are present, indicative of a trichorionic triamniotic triplet pregnancy. C = chorion.

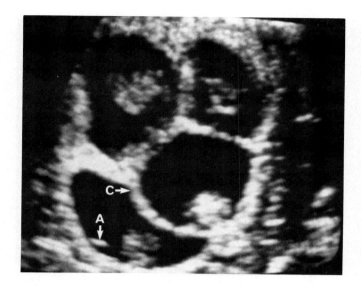

The diagnosis of twin gestation in the first trimester depends on the following observations:

1. *Dichorionic, diamniotic:* Two chorions seen as two separate echogenic rings (Figs. 22–2 through 22–5)
2. *Monochorionic, diamniotic:* A single echogenic chorionic ring with two well-defined yolk sacs and embryos, separated by the amniotic membrane(s). Very

Fig. 22–5. Quadruplets. Four gestational sacs and embryos are demonstrated at 9 weeks' menstrual age following hMG stimulation. Four separate chorionic cavities are present. C = chorion; A = amnion. (*Courtesy of M. Gillieson, MD, Ottawa General Hospital. Reprinted from Lyons EA, Levi CS. Ultrasound in the first trimester of pregnancy. Radiol Clin North Am. 1982;20:2–12, with permission.*)

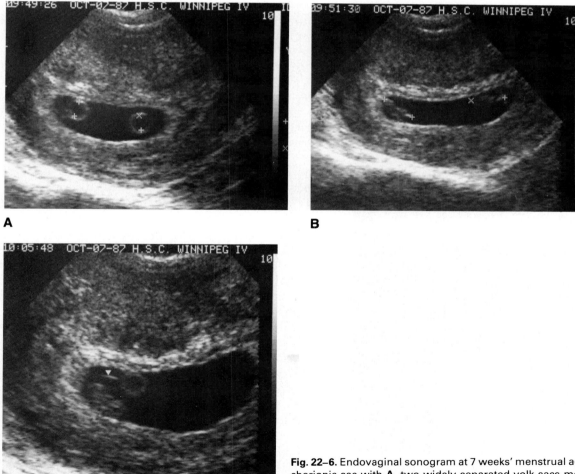

Fig. 22–6. Endovaginal sonogram at 7 weeks' menstrual age showing a single chorionic sac with **A.** two widely separated yolk sacs measuring 3.6 mm in diameter; **B.** two live embryos with crown–rump lengths of 8.3 and 8.8 mm; and **C.** an amniotic membrane (*arrowhead*) around one of the embryos.

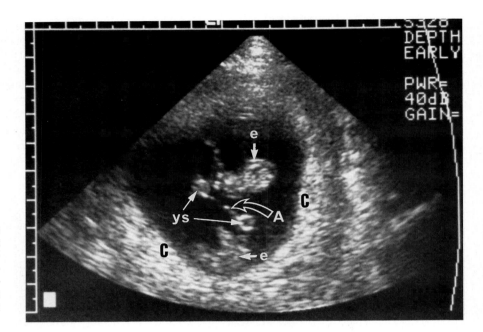

Fig. 22–7. A transabdominal scan in the sagittal plane through the gravid uterus at 9.5 weeks' menstrual age. A single chorionic sac is present. The amniotic membrane of the posterior embryo is seen separating the two embryos. e = embryo; ys = yolk sac; A = amniotic membrane; C = chorion.

early in development, only the yolk sacs will be seen before the embryos are visible (Figs. 22–6 and 22–7)

3. *Monochorionic, monoamniotic:* A single echogenic chorionic sac with two well-defined embryos without any identifiable intervening amnion (Fig. 22–8)

Using transvesical sonography, twin sacs should be identifiable within the uterus by 6 weeks' menstrual age

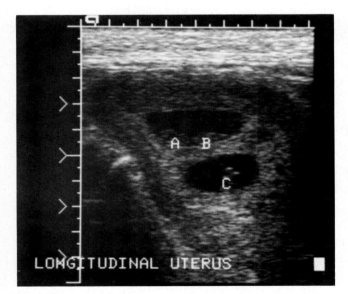

Fig. 22–8. Transvesicle scan of a triplet gestation. The posterior sac contains one embryo (C) of a dichorionic triplet pregnancy, whereas the anterior sac has two distinct embryos (A,B) and represents a monochorionic monoamniotic sac.

(MA). At this stage one would expect to see two distinct chorionic sacs as two echogenic rings within the endometrium. Using an endovaginal transducer with a high frequency crystal, one should be able to visualize the yolk sac even at 38 to 40 days (5.5 to 6 weeks MA), when the mean sac diameter is 8 mm.[15]

In the first trimester the chorion is seen as a thick hyperechoic ring density whereas the amnion is a thin filamentous membrane. The chorion has been seen as early as the beginning of the 5th week MA (29+ days), and routinely seen by 5.5 to 6 weeks' MA using the endovaginal approach. The amnion is not normally identified until after visualization of the yolk sac and fetus, usually by 6 to 6.5 weeks. In the first trimester, a dichorionic twin pregnancy will be identified as two separate hyperechoic rings in the endometrium. In order to be certain of the diagnosis of twins a yolk sac *and fetus* must be visualized in each chorionic sac. As discussed previously, monozygotic and dizygotic dichorionic twin pregnancies are sonographically indistinguishable.

A monochorionic diamniotic twin pregnancy will be demonstrated as a single chorionic cavity containing two yolk sacs, and later as two embryos, each with cardiac activity. Monochorionic twins always arise from a single fertilized ovum (ie, monozygotic).

Second and Third Trimesters

Diagnosis of a twin gestation after 13 weeks' MA has been possible sonographically for the past 20 years. By this time the fetus has a crown-rump length of at least 6.5 cm, is fully developed, active, and surrounded by copious amounts of amniotic fluid. The real breakthroughs in sonographic evaluation of twin gestations have been in early identification of fetal membranes and fetal anomalies.

Membranes and Placentae

Because of the poorer prognosis[1] and higher incidence of congenital anomalies and fetal wastage[1] in monoamniotic twins, it is critical to visualize the amniotic membrane.[16] In an article by Mahoney and coworkers,[16] identification of an amniotic membrane separating two fetuses had a 100% positive predictive value for diamniotic twin pregnancies. The amniotic membrane was identifiable in only 85% of diamniotic twin pregnancies (sensitivity). We feel it is important to perform serial studies until the amnionicity can be determined sonographically. When the condition is present, sonographic visualization of cord entanglement, a complication of monochorionic monoamniotic twin pregnancies, can be used to distinguish between monoamniotic and diamniotic twins.

In the second trimester, documentation of two placental sites is indicative of a dichorionic pregnancy (Fig.

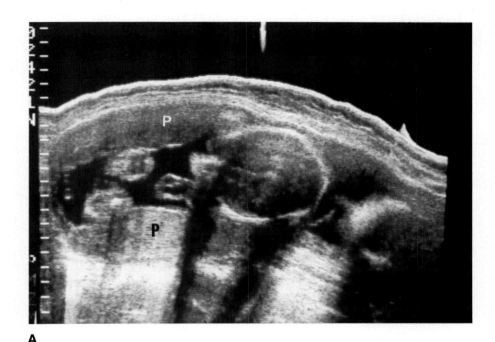

A

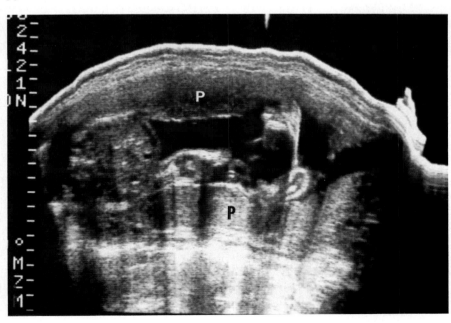

B

Fig. 22–9. A. Longitudinal and **B.** transverse B-scans of a twin pregnancy at 27 weeks' menstrual age. Two placentae (P) are present, indicative of a dichorionic diamniotic twin pregnancy.

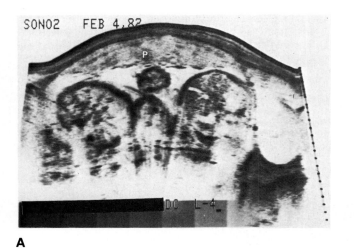

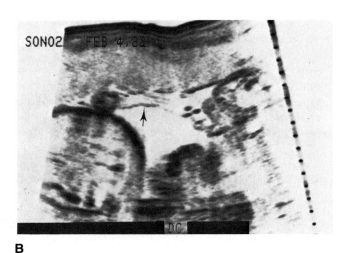

A   **B**

Fig. 22–10. A. Twins at 34 weeks' menstrual age. Longitudinal scan demonstrating a single anterior placenta in a twin pregnancy. P = placenta. **B.** The arrow points to a membrane separating the two fetuses.

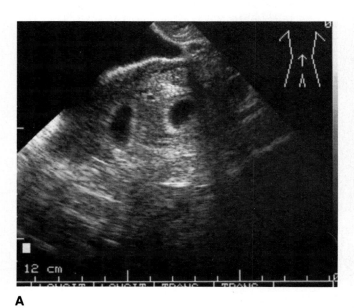

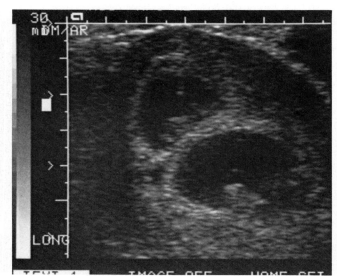

A   **B**

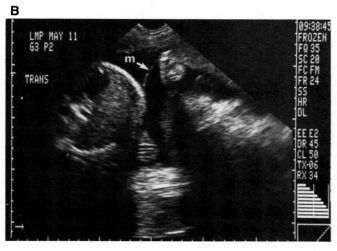

Fig. 22–11. Sonograms on the same patient of a dichorionic diamniotic gestation at **A.** 6.5, **B.** 7.5 and **C.** 35 weeks' menstrual age. **A.** Clearly shows the widely separated gestational sacs. **B.** Shows a thick membrane separating the chorionic cavities. **C.** The third trimester scan at 35 weeks shows only a thin membrane, which is in fact comprised of the four layers of amnion and chorion. It would be difficult to differentiate this from a monochorionic diamniotic pregnancy on the basis of the membrane separating the fetuses in the third trimester. M = membrane.

C

22–9). In the series by Mahoney and associates,[16] sonographic demonstration of two placentae was predictive of a dichorionic pregnancy in 100% of cases but the sensitivity of this finding was only 32%. Conversely, a single placenta (Fig. 22–10) was identified in all monochorionic pregnancies but the accuracy of prediction of a monochorionic pregnancy when only one placenta was seen was only 49%. These findings indicate that it is not always easy to identify the presence of two separate placentae when they are present, and that the two placentae may occasionally fuse in dichorionic pregnancies.

Differentiation between monochorionic and dichorionic twins on the basis of the membrane separating the two fetuses, is generally not possible after fusion of the amnion and chorion at 16 weeks.[17] In monochorionic diamniotic twins this membrane is composed of two layers of amnion, whereas in dichorionic twins it is composed of four layers, two chorion and two amnion. In both cases the membrane may appear as only a thin specular reflector (Fig. 22–11). If only one placenta is seen it may not be possible to determine the chorionicity unless stigmata of monovular twin-transfusion syndrome are present, or unless the twins are of different gender. Monovular twin-transfusion syndrome is seen only in monochorionic twin pregnancies, which are by definition monozygotic.

Mahoney and associates describe a characteristic appearance of the chorionic/amniotic membrane that can be used to distinguish it from other "membranes of pregnancy" such as synechiae, uterine septations, and amniotic bands.[16] When two placentae are present, the chorionic/amniotic membrane extends obliquely from the edge of one placenta to the contralateral edge of the other placenta (Fig. 22–12). In the case of a single placenta, the chorionic/amniotic membrane arises from the central portion of the placental site.[16] (See Fig. 22–10.)

The relationship of the chorionic/amniotic membrane to the fetus includes these factors:

• The fetus frequently touches the membrane but does not cross it
• The membrane does not entrap any portion of the fetus
• The membrane does not adhere to the fetus[16]
• No free edge of the membrane is demonstrated

Growth

Most authors agree that the growth pattern in the first and second trimesters is the same for twins as for singletons.[18–20] Studies using birth weight data have suggested a drop-off in growth curves in twins, as compared to singletons beginning at 27 to 35 weeks MA.[21] A decrease in the weight of fetal organs can be demonstrated for twins from about 30 weeks on.[22]

Although some sonographic studies maintain that biometry for twins is the same as that for singletons,[2]

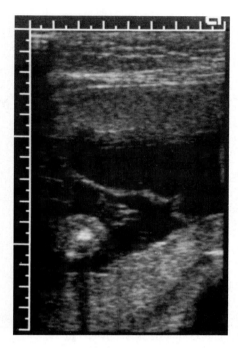

Fig. 22–12. Transvesical sonogram of a dichorionic diamniotic gestation at 20.5 weeks' menstrual age showing the membrane extending from one placenta anteriorly and obliquely to the contralateral corner of the posterior placenta.

other studies have demonstrated a decrease in growth parameters in the third trimester in accordance with non-ultrasound data.[18–20] A recent study by Grumbach and associates[18] demonstrated a decrease in twin biparietal diameter growth after 31 to 32 weeks, abdominal circumference growth after 32 to 33 weeks, but no alteration of the femoral length growth pattern compared to its growth in singletons. The growth curves and charts from the study by Grumbach and associates are shown in Figs. 22–13 through 22–15.

The importance of serial measurement of growth parameters in twins in the second and third trimesters is to enable the early identification of IUGR.

COMPLICATIONS

Abortion

In the mid 1970s several reports were published describing a high incidence of concomitant blighted ovum and normal intrauterine gestation.[23–25] Based on these data, the incidence of twins was thought to be 1 in 50[25] with 71% of twin gestations that were diagnosed by ultrasound resulting in singletons at the time of delivery. This phenomenon was labeled the "disappearing fetus." With the advent of high-resolution equipment, it became apparent that in most cases the second sac was a normal

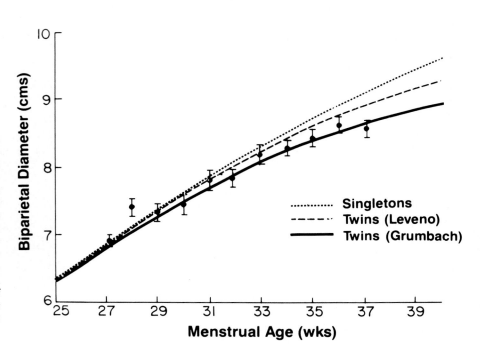

Fig. 22–13. Comparison of regression curves for twin BPD in the study by Grumbach and associates, twin BPD derived from the study by Leveno and colleagues,[53] and singleton BPD derived from the study by Kurtz and coworkers.[54] Solid dots represent mean observed twin BPD for each week of gestation from the data of Grumbach and associates and error bars represent ±1 standard deviation for each mean value. (*Reprinted with permission from Grumbach K, Coleman BG, Arger PH, Mintz MC, Gabbe SV, Mennuti MR. Twin and singleton growth patterns compared using US.* Radiology. *1986; 158:237–241.*)

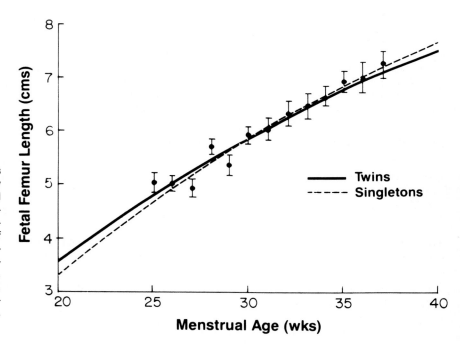

Fig. 22–14. Comparison of regression curves for twin fetal femoral lengths in the study by Grumbach and associates and singleton fetal femoral length derived from Hadlock and coworkers.[55] Solid dots represent mean observed fetal femoral lengths for each week of gestation, and error bars represent ±1 standard deviation for each mean value. (*Reprinted with permission from Grumbach K, Coleman BG, Arger PH, Mintz MC, Gabbe SV, Mennuti MR. Twin and singleton growth patterns compared using US.* Radiology. *1986;158:237–241.*)

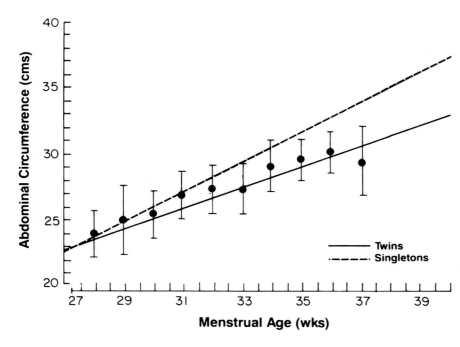

Fig. 22–15. Comparison of regression curves for twin AC from the data of Grumbach and associates and singleton AC derived from the study by Deter and colleagues.[56] Solid dots represent mean observed twin AC for each week of gestation, and error bars represent ±1 standard deviation for each mean value. (*Reprinted with permission from Grumbach K, Coleman BG, Arger PH, Mintz MC, Gabbe SV, Mennuti MR. Twin and singleton growth patterns compared using US. Radiology. 1986;158:237–241.*)

phenomenon: either blood in the endometrial canal related to implantation hemorrhage or a prominent hypoechoic decidua vera, but not a true gestational sac (Fig. 22–16). There is no doubt, therefore, that the early reports on the disappearing fetus were incorrect and based on a faulty premise. Twin gestational sacs with two embryos have indeed been recorded and with subsequent reabsorption of one of the embryos (Figs. 22–17 and 22–18).

The incidence of this occurrence has recently been described by Barzilai and coworkers (unpublished data). In their study, in only one twin pregnancy did one embryo die and the other progress to term. In 4 of the 22 twin pregnancies seen within the first trimester, both embryos died, two sets before 12 weeks and two at near 20 weeks. This represented an overall fetal loss of 30% in pregnancies seen from 5 to 10 weeks MA, and less than 4% when seen after 11 weeks.

A recent case report has been published describing patients with two gestational sacs, both with live embryos demonstrated by sonography in the first trimester in which one gestational sac was completely resorbed while the other survived to term.[26] This is a rare phenomenon and should not be confused with the early reports of the disappearing fetus.

Intrauterine Growth Retardation

Intrauterine growth retardation is one of the major factors leading to high perinatal mortality in twins. The prevalence of IUGR in twins is 25%,[18,19,27,28] which is ten times greater than the prevalance in singleton pregnancies.[27] Twins represent 17% of all growth-retarded fetuses.

Discordant fetal growth is defined as an intrapair *birth weight discrepancy* of 20 to 25% and, if present, places the twins in a high-risk group, predominantly due

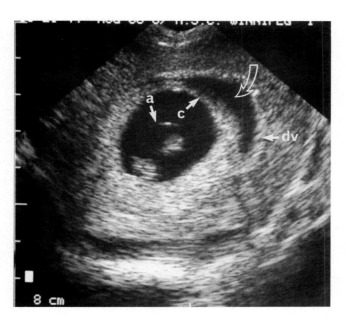

Fig. 22–16. Endovaginal sonogram of singleton pregnancy at 8 weeks' menstrual age. An implantation hemorrhage is present within the endometrial canal adjacent to the gestational sac. Curved open arrow = implantation hemorrhage; dv = decidua vera; c = chorion laeve-decidua capsularis; a = amnion.

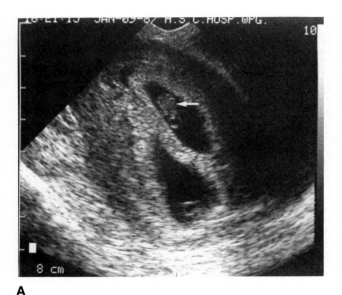

A

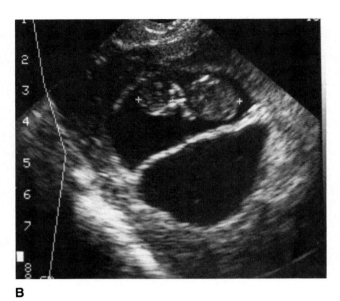

B

Fig. 22–17. A. Endovaginal sonogram in the sagittal plane of a dichorionic diamniotic twin pregnancy at 7.5 weeks' menstrual age with the death and re-absorption of one embryo (twin b). Twin A (*arrow*) was well visualized and embryonic cardiac activity was noted at real time. Only a yolk sac was identified in the second gestational sac. Presumably the embryo was reabsorbed following early embryonic demise. **B.** Subsequent endovaginal sonogram at 15 weeks' menstrual age. Twin A has demonstrated inadequate growth in the interval. No cardiac activity is seen in this dead fetus. No evidence of twin B or its yolk sac is now identified.

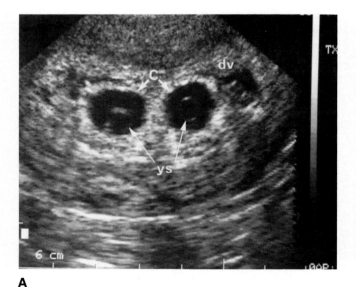

A

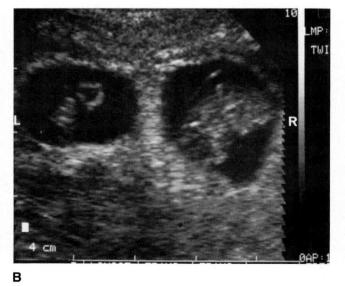

B

Fig. 22–18. A. A twin dichorionic gestation at 6 weeks menstrual age with well-defined yolk sacs demonstrated. **B.** At 8 weeks, the sac on the right contains a large embryo and yolk sac while the sac on the left has only the remnants of an embryo with no cardiac activity and a yolk sac. At delivery only one normal fetus was present. R = right; L = left.

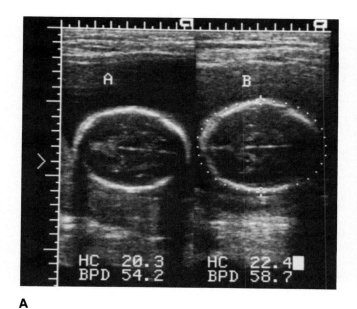

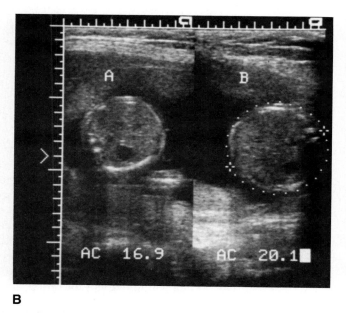

A

B

Fig. 22–19. Sonograms of the **A.** fetal heads and **B.** abdomens in a twin gestation with discordant growth. The head and abdomen of twin A are smaller than the head and abdomen of twin B. At birth twin A weighed 3,250 g and twin B weighed 3,010 g.

to IUGR (Fig. 22–19). If discordant growth is present, the risk of perinatal death (usually of the smaller twin) is 20%, which is 6.5 times greater than in twins with concordant growth.[28]

Leveno and colleagues[29] stated that a difference between twins in biparietal diameter (BPD) of 5 mm or greater after 28 weeks is suggestive of discordant fetal growth, and if greater than 7 mm, it was associated with fetal death in 20% of cases. More recent studies have shown that the BPD is an insensitive and nonspecific indicator of discordancy.[28,30] This finding is attributed to three major causes:

1. Inability to obtain satisfactory BPD measurements late in pregnancy
2. When the discordancy is based on placental insufficiency with nutritional asymmetry (ie, significantly different delivery of nutrients to each fetus), changes in BPD occur late in the course of IUGR[18,28,30,31]
3. Discrepancies in head shape between the fetus (ie, dolichocephaly in breech fetuses)

In a study by Storlazzi and coworkers,[28] the *estimated fetal weight* was predictive of discordancy in 100% of cases when discordancy was defined as a birth weight difference of $\geqq$ 25%. With a birth weight difference of $\geqq$ 20%, the estimated fetal weight and abdominal circumference (AC) had similar sensitivities (80%) and negative predictive values (93%). Storlazzi suggested that a difference in AC of 20 mm or more could be used as a screen for discordancy. If the AC difference is 20 mm or greater, fetal weight measurements should be obtained; however, if the AC difference is less than 20 mm, weight estimation is unnecessary because the negative predictive value for discordancy is 93%.[28]

Although IUGR more commonly affects one twin, IUGR in both fetuses (concordant IUGR) does occur.[19] As a result, fetal measurements are most effective in predicting IUGR when an earlier study is available that can be used as a baseline indicator of gestational age. As with IUGR in singletons, the biophysical profile is a more reliable indicator of outcome than fetal measurement. As a result, although it is important to monitor fetal growth in the second and third trimesters, assessment of the biophysical profile of the fetus serially after 28 weeks is critical.

Gerson and associates used pulsed Doppler to evaluate IUGR and discordancy in twins.[31] They sampled umbilical venous blood flow using published data for singletons as normal values (110 to 120 mL/min/kg).[32] They also evaluated umbilical arterial systolic/diastolic ratios, using singleton data as normal values (Table 22–1).[33]

TABLE 22–1. NORMAL SINGLETON DATA UMBILICAL ARTERY FLOW

Systolic/Diastolic Ratio	Gestational Age
<5	<28 weeks
<4	28–33 weeks
<3.5	>34 weeks

Used by permission from reference 33.

The data of Gerson and associates confirmed normal growth in 44 of 45 normal fetuses. Discordancy was predicted with a sensitivity of 81.8%, a positive predictive value of 90%, and a negative predictive value of 95.6%.

Nimrod and colleagues[34] studied the systolic/diastolic ratios and pulsatility index in the fetal thoracic aorta and umbilical artery in 30 sets of twins, and correlated their findings to fetal outcome. In addition, the Doppler data included aortic peak and end-diastolic velocity, and aortic flow volume. When combined with the BPD, the sensitivity was 82% and specificity was 30% in predicting outcome.

Monovular Twin Transfusion Syndrome

According to Brennan,[35] the sonographic diagnosis of monovular twin transfusion syndrome (Fig. 22–20) is based on the following criteria:

1. Disparity of fetal size in fetuses of the same sex
2. Disparity in size of the two amniotic sacs
3. Two cords with disparity in size or number of vessels
4. A single placenta with areas of varying echogenicity of the cotyledons supplying the two cords
5. Hydrops in either fetus or findings of congestive failure in the recipient fetus[35]

The monovular twin-transfusion syndrome is usually associated with placental arteriovenous anastomoses. While anastomotic channels are rare in dichorionic placentae, the majority of monochorionic (monozygotic or monovular) twins have some form of an anastomosis. Anastomotic channels may be artery-to-artery, vein-to-vein or artery-to-vein, with the artery-to-artery type being the most common.[7]

Arteriovenous anastomoses usually proceed through a placental cotyledonary capillary bed and result in direct shunting of blood from the circulation of one fetus to the other. Some degree of twin-to-twin transfusion is seen in 15 to 30% of all monozygotic twins.[2,36]

The donor twin is usually growth-retarded and has a marked reduction of amniotic fluid volume. If the growth-retarded (donor) fetus survives to the neonatal period, then hypotension, hypovolemia, hypoglycemia, and hypothermia may complicate the clinical course. In contrast, the recipient fetus may suffer complications of overperfusion in utero (ie, cardiomegaly, fetal hydrops and polyhydramnios. In the neonatal period, the complications of hypervolemia and hyperviscosity, including

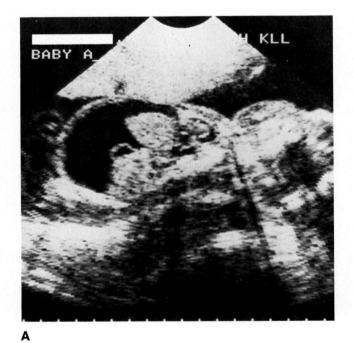

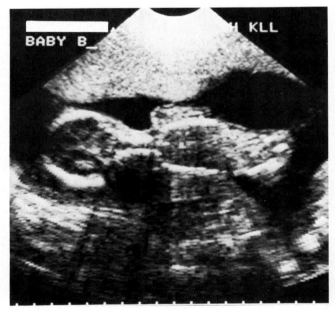

A   **B**

Fig. 22–20. Twin-to-twin transfusion syndrome. **A.** Fetus shows evidence of severe fetal ascites (A) and skin thickening (*arrow*). This fetus subsequently died. **B.** Fetus is small and does not show fetal ascites. Fetus B survived.

hyperbilirubinemia, cardiac failure, and occlusive thrombosis may occur.[1,2]

In the second trimester, discordant growth is more commonly caused by monovular twin-transfusion syndrome than by relative placental insufficiency with IUGR. Placental insufficiency occurs more commonly in the third trimester. Premature labor in the second trimester is common in the monovular twin-transfusion syndrome, resulting in a high perinatal mortality rate.

Using real-time pulsed Doppler, Pretorius and coworkers[37] evaluated the systolic/diastolic ratios in eight twin pregnancies with monovular twin-transfusion syndrome. An abnormal ratio, as defined by Giles and coworkers,[36] was seen in at least one fetus in five of the eight twin pregnancies. Previous data suggested that an intrapair difference in the systolic/diastolic ratio of 0.4 or greater is predictive of a significant difference in birth weight (350 g).[38] In the study by Pretorius and co-

workers,[37] Doppler ratios were unable to differentiate between the donor and recipient fetuses and could not provide prognostic data regarding outcome.

The amniotic membrane may be difficult to identify because it is so closely applied to the donor fetus (Fig. 22–21). This finding has been termed "the stuck twin" by Mahoney and colleagues.[16] In the stuck-twin syndrome, the donor fetus will usually die and macerate. This fetus will appear much smaller than the recipient and will have profound oligohydramnios, whereas the recipient usually has marked polyhydramnios.

In extreme cases of twin transfusion where arterial-arterial and venous-venous anastomosis exist, the blood flow in the donor fetus may be completely reversed, resulting in an "acardiac monster."[2] Anomalous development results in absence of the heart and upper limbs, and in deformity of the lower limbs, cranium, brain, and face, which may present in a variety of forms.

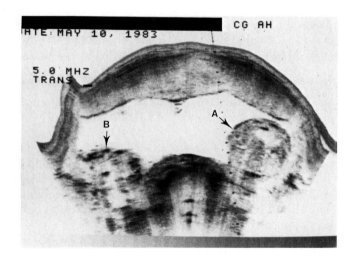

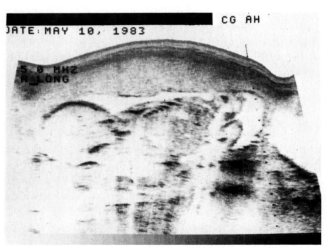

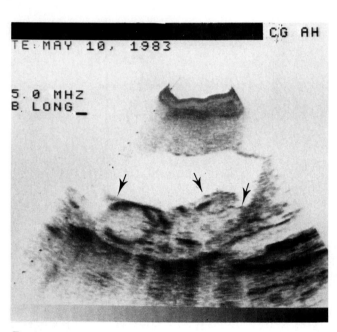

B

C

Fig. 22–21. A. Transverse scan through the maternal abdomen of a 23-year-old female with twins at 24 weeks' menstrual age. No evidence of fetal cardiac pulsation or fetal movement could be demonstrated in the twin to the maternal right (twin B). Twin A is a normal appearing fetus with associated polyhydramnios. B. Longitudinal scan through twin B demonstrating a small compressed fetus and oligohydramnios consistent with a "stuck twin." The arrows point to the membrane separating the two gestational sacs. C. Longitudinal scan through twin A.

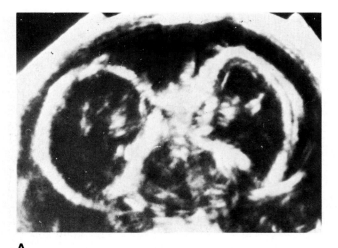

A

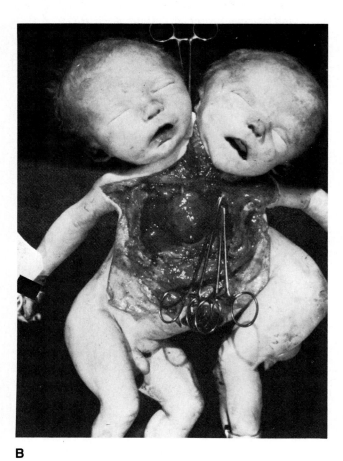

B

Fig. 22–22. A. Two fetal heads are present immediately adjacent to one another with both fetuses facing posteriorly. Serial scan planes through the fetus revealed a single thorax diagnostic of conjoined twins. **B.** The conjoined twins at postmortem.

Conjoined Twins

As discussed in the section on embryology, a division of the embryonic disc at least 13 days after fertilization results in conjoined twins (Fig. 22–22). By definition, they must always be monozygotic, monochorionic, and monoamniotic. When no amniotic membrane is identified by ultrasound, a high index of suspicion should be maintained for a monoamniotic gestation. If the twins face each other, there is a strong possibility of conjoined twins. However, absence of this finding does not rule out the diagnosis. When both twins are nearly completely formed, the joined area is most commonly the thorax anteriorly (thoracopagus). Less common sites of junction include abdominal (omphalopagus), posterior (pyopagus), cephalic (craniopagus), or caudal (ischiopagus).[1,5] When the duplication is less complete, the attachment is often lateral.[1]

Heterotopic Pregnancy

Heterotopic pregnancy is defined as a coexistent intrauterine and extrauterine (ectopic) gestation. The incidence of heterotopic pregnancy was originally estimated to be 1 in 30,000[39]; however, the true incidence is probably closer to 1 in 7,000.[40,41] The incidence is increased in ovulation induction, specifically, in vitro fertilization, as well as in patients who have conditions associated with an increased incidence of ectopic pregnancy. An example of the latter is a past history of pelvic inflammatory disease.

The diagnosis of heterotopic pregnancy is difficult. Sonographic findings are largely nonspecific and include adnexal mass, free fluid in the posterior cul de sac, and an intrauterine gestational sac (Fig. 22–23). These findings may also be seen with rupture of any ovarian cyst, commonly a corpus luteum cyst.

As with simple ectopic pregnancies, it is important that a decidual cast not be mistaken for an intrauterine pregnancy. A clear double decidual sign must be present to differentiate between an intrauterine pregnancy and a decidual cast prior to visualization of the yolk sac or embryo. Endovaginal sonography is particularly helpful in assessing the early chorionic sac, in that one can visualize the yolk sac at an earlier stage than with transvesical scanning.[15]

The diagnosis of heterotopic pregnancy may be made with certainty when an intrauterine gestational sac with a yolk sac or fetus is seen at the same time as a gestational sac and fetus in the adnexa. Of interest is that twin ectopic pregnancies have previously been described as a rare phenomenon. Since the introduction of endovaginal sonography, our department has identified twin ectopics in two patients in the last 2 years, suggesting that the incidence may be higher than previously reported (Fig. 22–24).

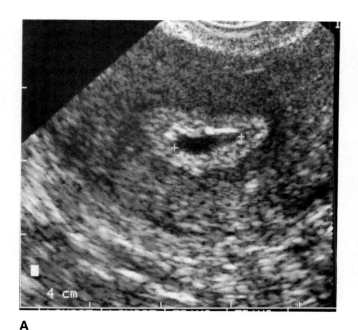

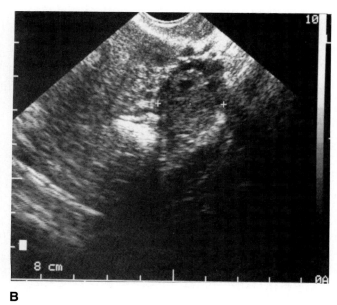

B

A

Fig. 22–23. Heterotopic pregnancy. **A.** Endovaginal coronal sonogram of the uterus demonstrating an intrauterine gestational sac (proven at D&C). **B.** The endovaginal coronal sonogram of the left adnexa demonstrating a 2.03 cm mass proved to be a left tubal pregnancy and hematoma at laparotomy.

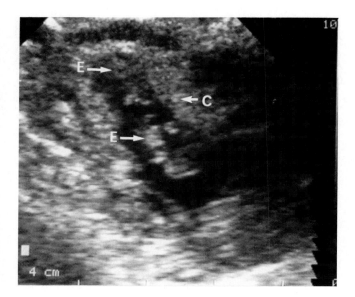

Fig. 22–24. Endovaginal sonogram at 7 weeks' menstrual age demonstrating a live monochorionic diamniotic twin pregnancy in the left fallopian tube. E = embryo; C = chorion.

Hydatidiform Mole Associated with Pregnancy

Hydatidiform mole associated with pregnancy may occur in one of two forms: complete and partial.

A complete mole is a dizygotic twin pregnancy is which one of the twins has developed normally while the other has become a mole (Fig. 22–25). The malignant potential and local invasiveness of these moles is the same as for a hydatidiform mole alone.

Partial moles arise from the placenta of the fetus and are not considered part of a twin pregnancy.[42,43] (See Figure 22–26.) The fetus most often has an abnormal karyotype, usually triploid with multiple congenital abnormalities.[42,44,45] Although malignancy has been reported, the malignant potential is very low. Partial moles are almost always benign.[46]

Sonographically, a complete mole may be seen as a discrete echogenic mass separate from the placenta of a normal coexistent fetus. Molar tissue adjacent to the placenta, however, may represent either a complete or partial mole. A similar sonographic appearance may be seen with a hematoma adjacent to the placenta, a partially necrotic leiomyoma,[46–48] or hydropic degeneration of the

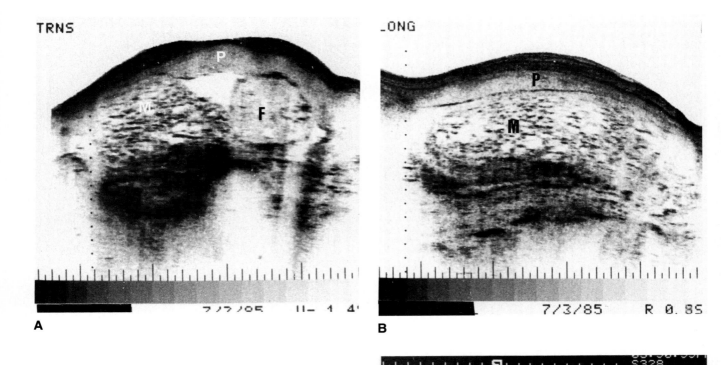

Fig. 22–25. Complete molar pregnancy associated with a normal fetus. **A.** Transverse and **B.** longitudinal B-scans showing hydatidiform mole (M) associated with the fetus (F). **C.** Transverse real-time sonogram shows that the hydatidiform mole is separate from the placenta (P).

placenta. The pulsed Doppler demonstration of high-velocity low-resistance flow which is characteristic of molar pregnancy will help to differentiate it from hematomas or leiomyomata.

Congenital Anomalies

The incidence of congenital anomalies appears to be twice as common in the infants of a twin gestation as in a singleton. One study showed that major malformations occur in approximately 2.12% of infants of a twin gestation as opposed to 1.05% of singletons. Minor malformations occur in 4.13% of twins as opposed to 2.45% of singletons.[1] Most, but not all, studies have shown similar findings.

The incidence of malformations in monozygotic twins is higher than in dizygotic twins. It has been suggested that the etiology for monozygotic twinning may also be the cause of errors in early morphogenesis, resulting in an associated congenital anomaly.[3,49,50]

The concordance rate for anomalies is higher in monozygotic twins than in dizygotic twins. The rate of concordance of most congenital anomalies in monozygotic twins is 5 to 50%; the majority of these have a rate of 10 to 20%.[49] Of particular interest, anencephaly and hydrocephaly are rarely concordant.[51] Congenital cardiac malformations were originally described as being rarely concordant; however, recent studies suggest a rate of 23%

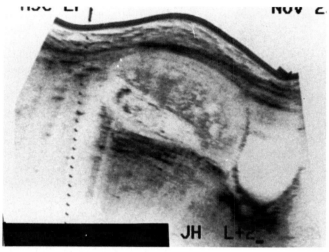

A

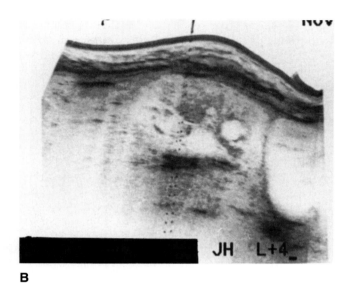

B

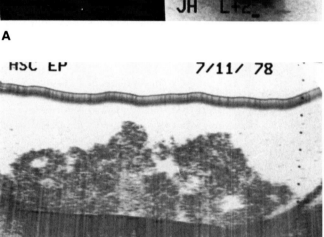

C

Fig. 22–26. Partial mole. Longitudinal B-scans **A.** 2 cm and **B.** 4 cm to the right of the mid-line showing a hydatidiform mole arising from the placenta associated with a dead fetus. **C.** Sonographic examination of the placenta in a water bath demonstrates vesicular tissue typical of a hydatidiform mole.

in monozygotic and 4.9% in dizygotic twins. The lack of concordance in many anomalies emphasizes the necessity for careful sonographic examination of each fetus in a multifetal pregnancy. When genetic amniocentesis is necessary regardless of the zygocity, it is critical that each amniotic cavity be sampled. The use of dilute indigo carmine dye during amniocentesis has been suggested to ensure sampling of each amniotic cavity.[1]

Fetus Papyraceous

Fetus papyraceous represents a dead fetus that is compressed by the expanding amniotic cavity of the other twin. It is surrounded by its own fetal membranes but little or no amniotic fluid. The water content of the fetus is gradually reabsorbed, further decreasing its size. Fetus papyraceous may occur in either monozygotic or dizygotic twinning, with the exception of the monochorionic, monoamniotic type.

Fetus in Fetu

Fetus in fetu is a very rare anomaly in which a "parasitic" twin is included in the retroperitoneum of the upper abdomen of the "bearer" fetus. The "included" fetus has a well-developed vertebral axial skeleton, which has been used to differentiate it radiographically and pathologically from a teratoma.[52]

SUMMARY

Twin pregnancies continue to present a challenge in modern obstetric practice. The identification of multiple gestation pregnancies can now be reliably made by ultrasound in virtually all cases. With the advent of high-resolution sonography, and in particular the introduction of endovaginal sonography, earlier diagnosis of chorionicity, amnionicity, and complications related to multiple-gestation pregnancy can be made. Fetal growth patterns, a presence of discordant growth, and the biophysical profile remain important in monitoring fetal well-being. The role of pulsed Doppler examination of the umbilical artery in twin pregnancies remains to be established.

REFERENCES

1. Multifetal pregnancy. In: Pritchard JA, MacDonald PC, Gant NF, eds. *Williams Obstetrics.* 17th ed. Norwalk, Conn: Appleton-Century-Crofts; 1985;503–524.
2. Crane JP. Sonographic evaluation of multiple pregnancy. *Seminars in US CT MR.* 1984;5:144–156.
3. Naeye RL, Tafari N, Judge D, Marboe CC. Twins: Causes of perinatal death in twelve United States cities and one African city. *Am J Obstet Gynecol.* 1978;131:267–272.
4. Hawrylyshyn PA, Barkin M, Bernstein A, Papsin FR. Twin pregnancies—a continuing perinatal challenge. *Obstet Gynecol.* 1982;59:463–466.
5. Moore KL. The fetal membranes placenta. In: Moore KL. *The Developing Human.* 3rd ed. Philadelphia: WB Saunders; 1982;111–139.
6. White C, Wyshak G. Inheritance in human dizygotic twinning. *New Eng J Med.* 1964;271:1003–1005.
7. Benirschke K, Kim CK. Multiple pregnancy: Part I. *N Engl J Med.* 1973;288:1276–1284.
8. Persson P-H, Grennert L, Gennser G, Kullander S. On improved outcome of twin pregnancies. *Acta Obstet Gynecol Scand.* 1979;58:3–7.
9. Persson P-H, Kullander S. Long-term experience of general ultrasound screening in pregnancy. *Am J Obstet Gynecol.* 1983;146:942–947.
10. Thiery M, Dhont C, Vandekerekhove D. hCG & hPL in twin pregnancies. *Acta Obstet Gynecol Scand.* 1976; 56:495–497.
11. Gennser G, Grennert L, Kullander S, Persson P-H, Wingerup L. Human placental lactogen in screening for multiple pregnancies. *Lancet.* 1975;274.
12. Knight GJ, Kloza EM, Smith DE, Haddow JE. Efficiency of human placental lactogen and alpha-fetoprotein measurement in twin pregnancy detection. *Am J Obstet Gynecol.* 1981;141:585–586.
13. Ghosh A, Woo JSK, Rawlinson HA, et al. Prognostic significance of raised serum alpha-fetoprotein levels in twin pregnancies. *Br J Obstet Gynaecol.* 1982;89:817.
14. Finlay D, Dillon A, Heslip M. Ultrasound screening in a twin pregnancy with high serum alpha-fetoprotein. *J Clin Ultrasound.* 1981;9:514–515.
15. Levi CS, Lyons EA, Lindsay DJ. Early diagnosis of nonviable pregnancy with endovaginal US. *Radiology.* 1988;167:383–385.
16. Mahony BS, Filly RA, Callen PW. Amnioticity and chorionicity in twin pregnancies: Prediction using ultrasound. *Radiology.* 1985;155:205–209.
17. Burrows PE, Lyons EA, Phillips HJ, Oates I. Intrauterine membranes: Sonographic findings and clinical significance. *J Clin Ultrasound.* 1982;10:1–8.
18. Grumbach K, Coleman BG, Arger PH, Mintz MC, Gabbe SV, Mennuti MT. Twin and singleton growth patterns compared using US. *Radiology.* 1986;158:237–241.
19. Secher NJ, Kaern J, Hansen PK. Intrauterine growth in twin pregnancies: Prediction of fetal growth retardation. *Obstet Gynecol.* 1985;66:63–68.
20. Houlton MCC, Marivate M, Philpott RH. The prediction of fetal growth retardation in twin pregnancy. *Br J Obstet Gynaecol.* 1981;88:264–273.
21. Divers WA Jr, Hemsell DL. The use of ultrasound in multiple gestations. *Obstet Gynecol.* 1979;53:500–504.
22. Naeye RL. Organ composition in newborn parabiotic twins with speculation regarding neonatal hypoglycemia. *Pediatrics.* 1964;34:415–418.
23. Levi S. Ultrasonic assessment of the high rate of human multiple pregnancy in the first trimester. *J Clin Ultrasound.* 1976;4:3–5.
24. Varma TR. Ultrasound evidence of early pregnancy failure in patients with multiple conceptions. *Br J Obstet Gynaecol.* 1979;86:290–292.
25. Robinson HP, Caines JS. Sonar evidence of early pregnancy failure in patients with twin conceptions. *Br J Obstet Gynaecol.* 1977;84:22–25.
26. St J Brown B. Disappearance of one gestational sac in the first trimester of multiple pregnancies—ultrasonographic findings. *J Can Assoc Radiol.* 1982;33:273–275.
27. Manlan G, Scott KE. Contribution of twin pregnancy to perinatal mortality and fetal growth retardation: Reversal of growth retardation after birth. *Can Med Assoc J.* 1978;118:365–368.
28. Storlazzi E, Vintzileos AM, Campbell WA, Nochimson BJ, Weinbaum PJ. Ultrasound diagnosis of discordant fetal growth in twin gestations. *Obstet Gynecol.* 1987;69:363–367.
29. Leveno KJ, Santos-Ramos R, Duenhoelter JH, Reisch JS, Whalley PJ. Sonar cephalometry in twin pregnancy: Discordancy of the biparietal diameter after 28 weeks' gestation. *Am J Obstet Gynecol.* 1980;138:615–619.
30. Erkkola R, Ala-mello S, Piiroinen O, Kero P, Sillanpaa M. Growth discordancy in twin pregnancies: A risk factor not detected by measurements of biparietal diameter. *Obstet Gynecol.* 1985;66:203–206.
31. Gerson AG, Wallace DM, Bridgens NK, Ashmead GG, Weiner S, Bolognese RJ. Duplex Doppler ultrasound in the evaluation of growth in twin pregnancies. *Obstet Gynecol.* 1987;70:419–423.
32. Gill RW, Kossoff G, Warren PS, Garrett WJ. Umbilical venous flow in normal and complicated pregnancy. *Ultrasound Med Biol.* 1984;10:349–363.
33. Trudinger BJ, Giles WB, Cook CM, Bombardieri J, Collins L. Fetal umbilical artery flow velocity waveforms and placental resistance: clinical significance. *Br J Obstet Gynaecol.* 1985;92:23–30.
34. Nimrod C, Davies D, Harder J, et al. Doppler ultrasound prediction of fetal outcome in twin pregnancies. *Am J Obstet Gynecol.* 1987;156:402–406.

35. Brennan JN, Diwan RV, Rosen MG, Bellon EM. Fetofetal transfusion syndrome: Prenatal ultrasonographic diagnosis. *Radiology.* 1982;143:535–536.

36. Giles WB, Trudinger BJ, Cook CM. Fetal umbilical artery flow velocity—time waveforms in twin pregnancies. *Br J Obstet Gynaecol.* 1985;92:490–497.

37. Pretorius DH, Manchester D, Barkin S, Parker S, Nelson TR. Doppler ultrasound of twin transfusion syndrome. *J Ultrasound Med.* 1988;7:117–124.

38. Farmakides G, Schulman H, Saldana LR, Bracero LA, Fleischer A, Rochelson B. Surveillance of twin pregnancy with umbilical arterial velocimetry. *Am J Obstet Gynecol.* 1985;153:789–792.

39. DeVoe RW, Pratt JH. Simultaneous intrauterine and extrauterine pregnancy. *Am J Obstet Gynecol.* 1948;56:1119–1126.

40. Hann LE, Bachman DM, McArdle CR. Coexistent intrauterine and ectopic pregnancy: A re-evaluation. *Radiology.* 1984;152:151–154.

41. Richards SR, Stempel LE, Carlton BD. Heterotopic pregnancy. Reappraisal of incidence. *Am J Obstet Gynecol.* 1982;142:928–930.

42. Block MF, Merrill JA. Hydatidiform mole with coexistent fetus. *Obstet Gynecol.* 1982;60:129–134.

43. Fisher RA, Sheppard DM, Lawler SD. Twin pregnancy with complete hydatidiform mole (46,XX) and fetus (46,XY): Genetic origin proved by analysis of chromosome polymorphisms. *Br Med J.* 1982;284:1218–1220.

44. Czernobilsky B, Barash A, Lancet M. Partial moles: A clinicopathologic study of 25 cases. *Obstet Gynecol.* 1982;59:75–77.

45. Szulman AE, Surti U. The clinicopathologic profile of the partial hydatidiform mole. *Obstet Gynecol.* 1982;59:597–602.

46. Fleischer AC, Jones HW III, James AE Jr. Sonography of trophoblastic diseases. In: Sanders RC, James AE Jr, eds. *The Principles and Practice of Ultrasonography in Obstetrics and Gynecology.* 3rd ed. Norwalk, Conn: Appleton-Century-Crofts. 1985:387–398.

47. Sauerbrei EE, Salem S, Fayle B. Coexistent hydatidiform mole and live fetus in the second trimester. An ultrasound study. *Radiology.* 1980;135:415–417.

48. Callen PW. Ultrasonography in evaluation of gestational trophoblastic disease. In: Callen PW, ed. *Ultrasonography in Obstetrics and Gynecology.* 1st ed. Philadelphia: WB Saunders; 1983;259–270.

49. Schinzel AAGL, Smith DW, Miller JR. Monozygotic twinning and structural defects. *J Pediatr.* 1979;95:921–930.

50. Benirschke K, Kim CK. Multiple pregnancy: Part II. *N Engl J Med.* 1973;288:1329–1336.

51. Hay S, Wehrung DA. Congenital malformations in twins. *Am J Hum Genet.* 1970;22:662–678.

52. Broghammer BJ, Wolf RS, Geppert CH. The included twin or fetus in fetu. *Radiology.* 1963;80:844–846.

53. Leveno KJ, Santos-Ramos R, Duenhoelter JH, Reisch JS, Whalley PJ. Sonar cephalometry in twins: a table of biparietal diameters for normal twin fetuses and a comparison with singletons. *Am J Obstet Gynecol.* 1979;135:727–730.

54. Kurtz AB, Wapner RJ, Kurtz RJ, et al. Analysis of biparietal diameter as an indicator of gestational age. *J Clin Ultrasound.* 1980;8:319–326.

55. Hadlock FP, Harrist RB, Deter RL, Park SK. Fetal femur length as a predictor of menstrual age: Sonographically measured. *AJR* 1982;138:875–878.

56. Deter RL, Harrist RB, Hadlock FP, Carpenter RJ. Fetal head and abdominal circumferences. II: A critical re-evaluation of the relationship to menstrual age. *J Clin Ultrasound.* 1982;10:365–372.

23 Sonography of Nonimmune Hydrops Fetalis

Arthur C. Fleischer • Philippe Jeanty • Dinesh M. Shah • Frank H. Boehm

Hydrops fetalis refers to a variety of conditions which are associated with a markedly swollen and edematous fetus. The severely affected fetus usually has effusions into the peritoneal, pleural, and/or pericardial spaces.

Hydrops fetalis is divided into those causes that are associated with isoimmunization to an erythrocyte antigen [isoimmune hydrops (IIH)], and those that are not [nonimmune hydrops (NIH)]. Each of these types has a relatively specific cause and predictable prognosis. With the more widespread use of Rh immune globulin (RhIG) prophylaxis over the last several years, the relative incidence of nonimmune to isoimmune hydrops has significantly changed. Although the actual incidence of NIH to IIH varies, depending upon the screened population, the incidence of NIH at most medical centers is far greater than IIH.

Isoimmunization to a particular erythrocyte antigen usually results in severe hemolytic anemia in the fetus. With the advent of RhIG prophylaxis, the incidence of hemolytic disease in newborns declined from 40.5/10,000 live births to 14.3/10,000 between 1970 and 1979.[1] Despite the widespread use of RhIG prophylaxis for non-sensitized Rh mothers, approximately 1.5% of all pregnancies are complicated by isoimmunization. The use of both antepartum and postpartum RhIG has further reduced the incidence of isoimmunization from 0.1 to 0.3%. Even though the incidence is low, IIH is associated with a perinatal mortality rate between 25 and 30%.[12]

As opposed to IIH, nonimmune hydrops results from a variety of anatomic and/or functional disorders not related to any immunologic cause.[2] It has been estimated that 3% of all fetal mortality is related to NIH.[3] Unfortunately, anywhere from 70% to 90% of fetuses affected by NIH die in the perinatal period.[1]

This chapter reviews new developments in sonographic detection, evaluation, and sonographically-guided procedures of the hydropic fetus related to nonimmunologic causes. In particular, the role of percutaneous umbilical cord blood sampling for fetal karyotyping is emphasized. The importance of a detailed sonographic evaluation of the fetus in determining the spe-cific cause and severity of nonimmune hydrops is described. Assessment of the fetal condition of the NIH fetus through the expanded role of real-time observations by sonography is also discussed.

NONIMMUNE HYDROPS (NIH)

The sonographic findings which are common to both severe nonimmune and immune hydrops include peritoneal, pleural, or pericardial effusions and/or skin thickening due to edema (anasarca).[3] The specific anomalies which can be associated with NIH are related to the underlying structural and functional defect. Table 23–1 lists the various conditions associated with nonimmune hydrops. These are classified into fetal, placental, and maternal abnormalities.

Even though NIH is associated with specific fetal structural and functional anomalies, in approximately 30 to 40% of cases, an exact etiology cannot be found.[1] Although dependent upon the population studied, two of the most common disorders associated with NIH are probably congenital heart disease and arrhythmias.[6] The next most common cause of NIH is probably chromosomal abnormalities. Nonimmunologic hematologic abnormalities such as thalassemia probably account for the other cause of NIH that is most common worldwide. As in the case of isoimmune hydrops, structural abnormalities of the heart are common in fetuses with a chromosomal disorder.

Although it is extremely rare, there have been reports of spontaneous resolution of fetal ascites in a hydropic fetus.[4] We have documented a case of spontaneous resolution of a left-sided pleural effusion, and there have been reports of resolution of a chylothorax after repeated sonographically-guided thorocenteses between 20 and 23 weeks.[8]

Sonographic evaluation for evidence of hydrops should initially focus on the presence or absence of peritoneal, pleural, or pericardial fluid. Because the living fetus does not remain stationary in utero, the exact lo-

TABLE 23–1. CONDITIONS ASSOCIATED WITH NONIMMUNE HYDROPS

Condition	Figures	Condition	Figures
I. Fetal		E. *Multisystem Disorders*	
A. *Cranial*		1. Chromosomal	23–4A,B,C,
Hydrocephalus		Trisomy 21	5A,B
Vein of Galen aneurysm		Turner's syndrome 45X0	
B. *Cardiovascular*		Other trisomies	
Severe congenital heart disease:	23–1A–C	Triploidy Mosaicism	
ASD, VSD, hypoplastic left heart,		2. Intrauterine infections	23–2F
pulmonary valve insufficiency,	23–2G,H,I,J	Syphilis	
Ebstein's anomaly, subaortic		Toxoplasmosis	
stenosis		Cytomegalovirus	
Premature closure of foramen ovale		Leptospirosis	
Myocarditis		Chagas disease	
Large arteriovenous malformation		Congenital hepatitis	
Tachyarrhythmias: atrial flutter,		Herpes simplex	
supraventricular tachycardia		3. Hematologic	
Bradyarrhythmias, especially those		Homozygous α-thalassemia	
associated with complete heart		Chronic fetomaternal transfusion	23–3A,B,C
block		F. *Miscellaneous Congenital Anomalies*	
Fibroelastosis		Meconium peritonitis	23–7H
Intrapericardial teratoma		Tuberous sclerosis	
C. *Pulmonary*		Small-bowel volvulus	
Cystic adenomatoid malformation of	23–2A,B,C,	Twin-to-twin transfusion	23–7A,B,C
lung	23–6B	Cystic hygroma	23–7C,D,E
Pulmonary lymphangiectasia		Sacrococcygeal teratoma	
Pulmonary hypoplasia		**II. Placental/Umbilical Cord Dwarfism**	
Congenital chylothorax	23–7F,G	Umbilical vein thrombosis	
Mediastinal teratoma		Chorioangioma	23–1E
Extralobar pulmonary sequestration		Umbilical cord knots	
D. *Renal/Retroperitoneal*		**III. Maternal Disease**	
Congenital nephrosis		Diabetes mellitus	
Renal vein thrombosis		Toxemia	
Neuroblastomatosis		Severe anemia	
Posterior urethral values (urinary asci-		**IV. Idiopathic**	
tes)	23–7B		

cation of these collections will vary. Small intraperitoneal collections usually begin to gather within the peritoneum surrounding the liver or spleen. Be aware that the abdominal wall musculature can appear as a hypoechoic band near the umbilical cord insertion on the ventral abdominal wall. One way of determining whether or not a hypoechoic area represents fluid is by closely examining the area of the abdomen near the site that the umbilical cord enters the body. If both sides of the umbilical vein can be seen clearly as it traverses the anterior abdominal wall, then intraperitoneal fluid is probably present.[5] Abnormal thickening of the skin is usually first recognized around the calvarium. Do not mistake excessive fat in the subcutaneous layer (macrosomia) of the fetus of a diabetic mother with diffuse edema of the skin (anascara) seen in the hydropic fetus.

Identifying Abnormalities

Once the hydropic fetus is identified, the sonographer should systematically examine the fetus for anatomic and/or functional abnormalities that may be associated with NIH.

In the head, it is possible to detect a dilated lateral ventricle secondary to a viral encephalopathy, or associated with a chromosomal anomaly. Rarely, a vein of Galen aneurysm may produce sufficient arteriovenous shunting to result in a hydropic fetus.

Cardiac arrhythmias and malformations are the most common causes of NIH.[6] One should examine the heart closely for structural malformations such as hypoplastic left ventricle, as well as evaluate the cardiac rate and rhythm by M-mode (Fig. 23–1). Supraventricular tachyarrhythmias can be treated in utero and are among the more common arrhythmias associated with hydrops.[6]

Thoracic lesions that result in obstruction to venous return, such as a mediastinal teratoma or cystic adenomatoid malformation, should be excluded by a detailed sonographic evaluation of the thorax and its contents (Fig. 23–2A). The presence of large pleural effusions usually portends pulmonary hypoplasia.

Renal disorders that have been associated with NIH include congenital nephrosis, which may cause NIH due to urinary protein loss. To date, no definite sonographic anatomic abnormalities of the kidney have been reported

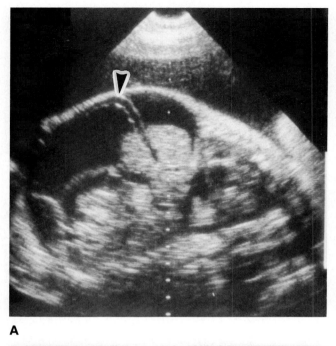

A

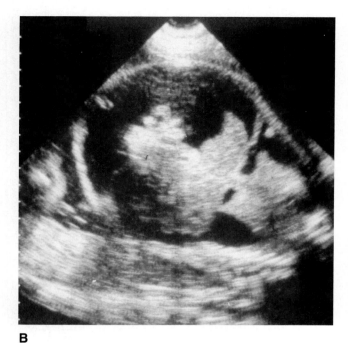

B

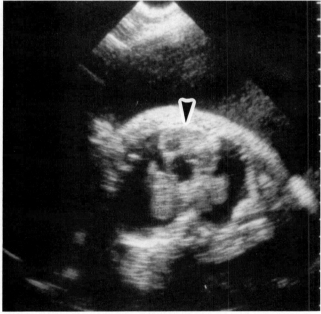

C

Fig. 23–1. NIH associated with severe bradycardia and multiple cardiac defects. **A.** Massive ascites and pleural effusions. Umbilical vein (*arrow*) is surrounded by ascites. **B.** Another long-axis imaging showing pleural effusions that surround the lungs. **C.** Short-axis view of heart showing its midline location and thickened myocardium (*arrowhead*).

associated with this disorder. Neuroblastomatosis may result in NIH secondary to obstruction of venous return in the inferior vena cava.

There are several multisystem disorders that may result in NIH. These include conditions associated with systemic infections, hematologic abnormalities, and syndromes associated with abnormal chromosomal composition. Percutaneous umbilical vein sampling is useful in detecting hematologic disorders such as α-thalassemia, which may result in NIH. Rarely, NIH is associated with

placental or umbilical cord abnormalities (Fig. 23–2B). Hydrops fetalis associated with a placental chorioangioma can be attributed to excessive arteriovenous shunting that occurs within the tumor. This, perhaps, results in reduced blood flow to the fetus. The plethoric twin affected by twin-to-twin transfusions also can become hydropic because of high output failure (Fig. 23–3).

Thus, there is a large variety of disorders which may result in NIH. In general, the hydropic fetus should be considered a severely compromised fetus, one that may

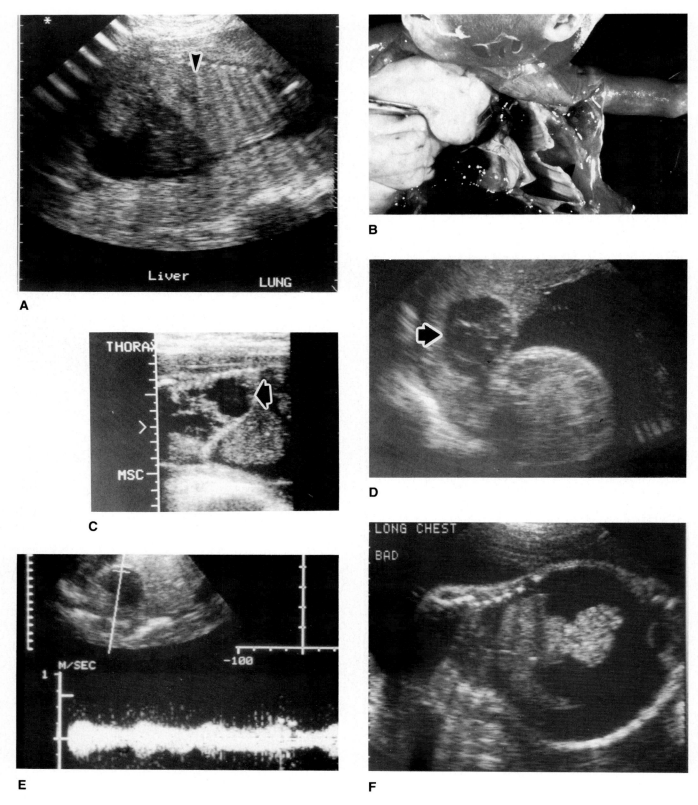

Fig. 23–2. Miscellaneous causes of NIH. **A.** Cystic adenomatoid malformation (microcystic type) appearing as solid mass (*arrowhead*) enlarging right lung. **B.** Gross specimen of **A** at autopsy. **C.** Cystic adenomatoid malformation (*arrow*) containing several cystic spaces. **D.** Chorioangioma appearing as hypoechoic mass (*arrow*) near cord origin. **E.** Turbulent arterial and venous flow was detected on duplex Doppler exam of chorioangioma in **D. F.** Massive hydrops secondary to CMV infection in 27-week fetus. No liver or brain calcification was seen. (*Figure continued.*)

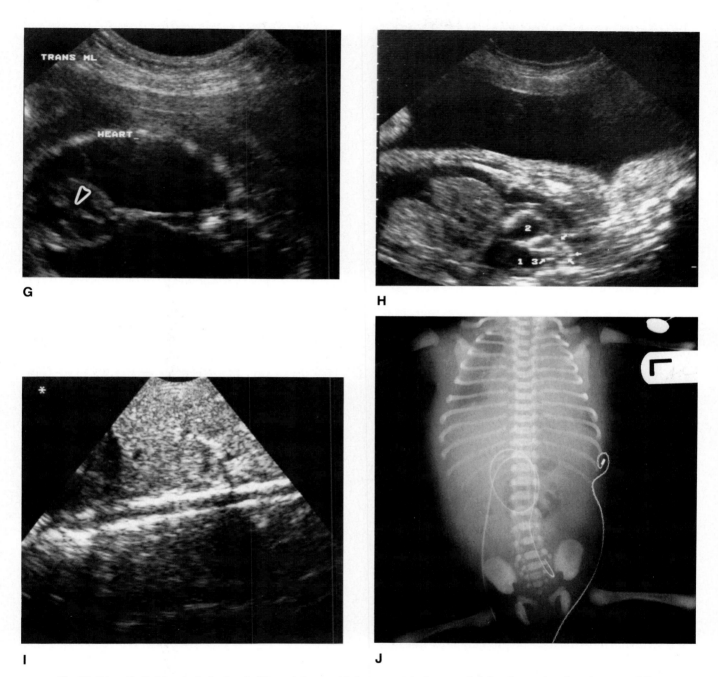

Fig. 23–2 (cont). G. Massively hydropic 22-week fetus with large ventricular septal defect (*arrowhead*) and an overriding aorta. **H.** Hydrops associated with arterial calcinosis. Aortic arch (*arrows*) is calcified. 1 = left ventricle; 2 = right ventricle; 3 = mitral valve. **I.** Long axis of calcified aorta (*arrow*) in neonate shown in **H. J.** Radiograph of neonate in **H,I** showing calcified distal abdominal aorta and common iliac artery (*arrow*).

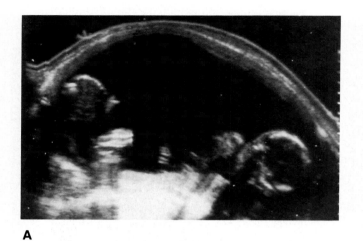

A

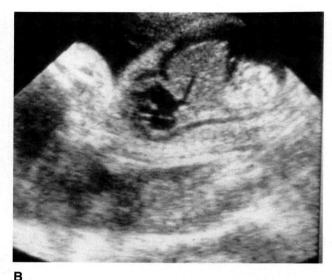

B

Fig. 23–3. Nonimmune hydrops associated with twin-to-twin trans-fusion. **A.** Static sonogram showing twins and hydramnios (*curved arrow*). **B.** Long axis of hydropic twin showing enlarged heart and liver floating within ascites. **C.** Short axis through heart of hydropic twin adjacent to the cojoined twin's head.

C

be agonal (near death). Therefore, serial biophysical pro-file testing and non-stress testing should be used to assess its condition.

Other abnormalities which may be encountered with a hydropic fetus include hydramnios, oligohydramnios, and an abnormally-thickened placenta. Hydramnios may be secondary to a lack of fetal swallowing due to a com-promised fetal condition. Oligohydramnios usually por-tends a poor prognosis and may indicate poor fetal renal function. A thickened placenta may result from vascular engorgement secondary to increased resistance to for-ward flow to the fetus. It is postulated that this might be detected with continuous wave Doppler as high sys-tolic peak of the umbilical artery flow.

Management of NIH

Sonography has an important role in the management of nonimmune hydrops which is not associated with a spe-cific anatomic or functional abnormality. Because there is a high incidence of chromosomal abnormalities with nonimmune hydrops, amniocentesis or percutaneous cordocentesis is indicated to determine whether or not the condition is related to an abnormal karyotype[7] (Figs. 23–4 through 23–6). Amniocentesis can be performed if hydrops is detected before 20 to 22 weeks since 2 to 4 weeks are required for cell culture. The technique of percutaneous cordocentesis has been described in detail in several papers.[7] As reported by Daffos, the compli-cation of this procedure is low, with a fetal death rate of

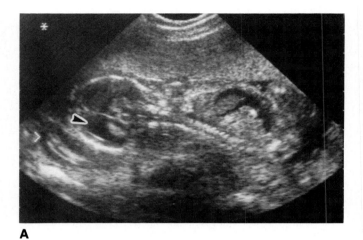

A

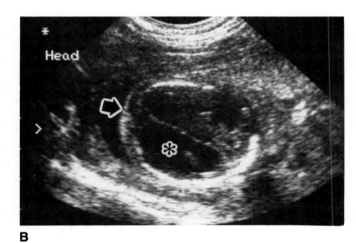

B

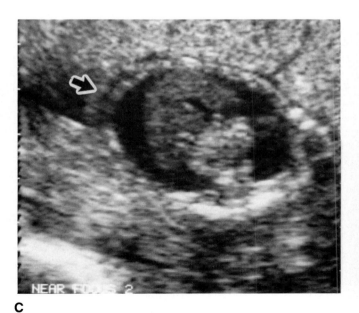

C

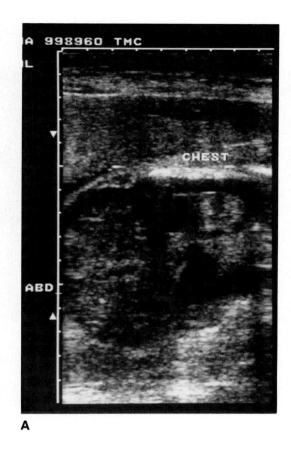

A

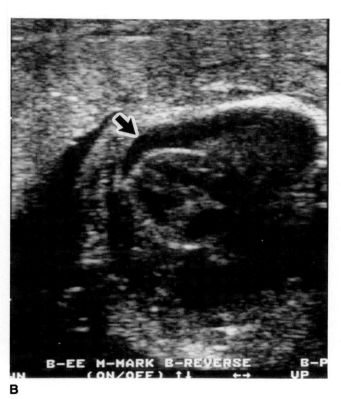

B

Fig. 23–4. NIH associated with trisomy in 17-week fetus. **A.** Long axis of 16-week fetus showing ascites and dilated lateral ventricles (*arrowhead*). **B.** Axial sonogram through head showing dilated lateral ventricle (*) and skin edema (*arrow*). **C.** Anasarca of abdominal wall (*arrow*) and ascites.

Fig. 23–5. NIH associated with trisomy 21 in 26-week fetus proven by PUBS. **A.** Massive ascites and pleural effusions. **B.** Long axis of heart showing pericardial effusion (*arrow*).

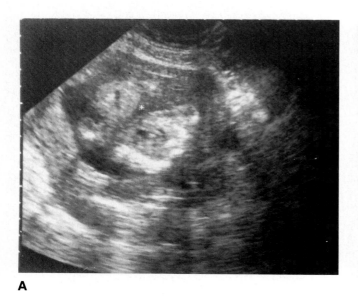

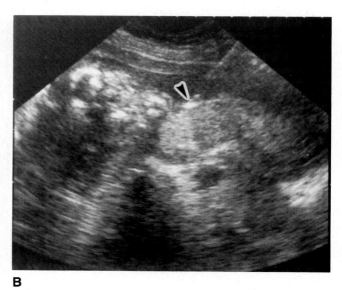

Fig. 23–6. Sonographically-guided procedures. **A.** 17-week fetus with omphalocele. PUBS performed for karyotyping. **B.** Percutaneous umbilical vein blood sampling (PUBS). The tip of needle (*arrowhead*) is lodged within umbilical vein.

1.1% and a spontaneous abortion rate of 0.8%.[7] The data obtained from this procedure on the karyotype of the fetus allow coherent and coordinated management of the fetus affected by nonimmune hydrops. This is especially true of one which does not exhibit a recognizable structural anomaly.

SONOGRAPHIC MIMICS OF FETAL HYDROPS

There are certain conditions which may be associated with sonographic findings that mimic that of a hydropic fetus. In most cases, these disorders involve excess fluid in a particular body cavity such as the peritoneum or pleural spaces. Rarely, the excessive body fat of a macrosomic fetus may mimic the anasarca seen in a severely hydropic fetus (Fig. 23–7).

Specifically, conditions which can mimic the findings of hydrops include: urinary ascites, secondary to bladder or renal collecting system rupture; intraperitoneal fluid associated with or resulting from a rupture of a viscus; chylothorax resulting in an accumulation of lymphatic fluid, secondary to thoracic duct rupture; and intraperitoneal and pleural effusions seen with cystic hygromas (Fig. 23–8). Although it may not be possible to differentiate these disorders from those associated with true hydrops via sonography, there are certain features which may suggest the difference. These include: distension of the bladder and/or renal collecting systems associated with urinary ascites, secondary to posterior urethral

valves in a male fetus; abnormally distended loops of bowel associated with meconium peritonitis; and unilateral hydrothorax on the left with thoracic duct rupture. The redundant skin covering a shrunken thorax of a thantotrophic dwarf may mimic a hydropic fetus, but the fetal limbs are significantly shortened. A cystic mass arising from the back of the neck can usually be recognized in a fetus with cystic hygroma. The intraperitoneal and pleural effusions occasionally seen with cystic hygromas are associated with disruption in lymphatic return. Thickening of the skin secondary to lymphangiectasia can also be seen. Cystic hygromas in females are frequently associated with Turner's syndrome.

PROGNOSIS FOR THE NIH FETUS

Even with accurate sonographic diagnoses and aggressive treatment, the hydropic fetus has, in general, a poor prognosis. In nonimmune hydrops, the prognosis is related to the underlying anatomic, chromosomal, or structural abnormalities. In one series of severely hydropic fetuses with NIH, only 32% of fetuses survived the neonatal period, with five of the nine survivors having an uncertain or poor prognosis.[9] The best prognosis in the NIH group usually involves the fetus that has a potentially-correctable arrythmia.

Rarely, hydrops resolves spontaneously. We have observed a left-sided effusion detected at 16 weeks resolve before 21 weeks (Figs. 23–7F,G). There are several isolated case reports documenting transitory fetal ascites.

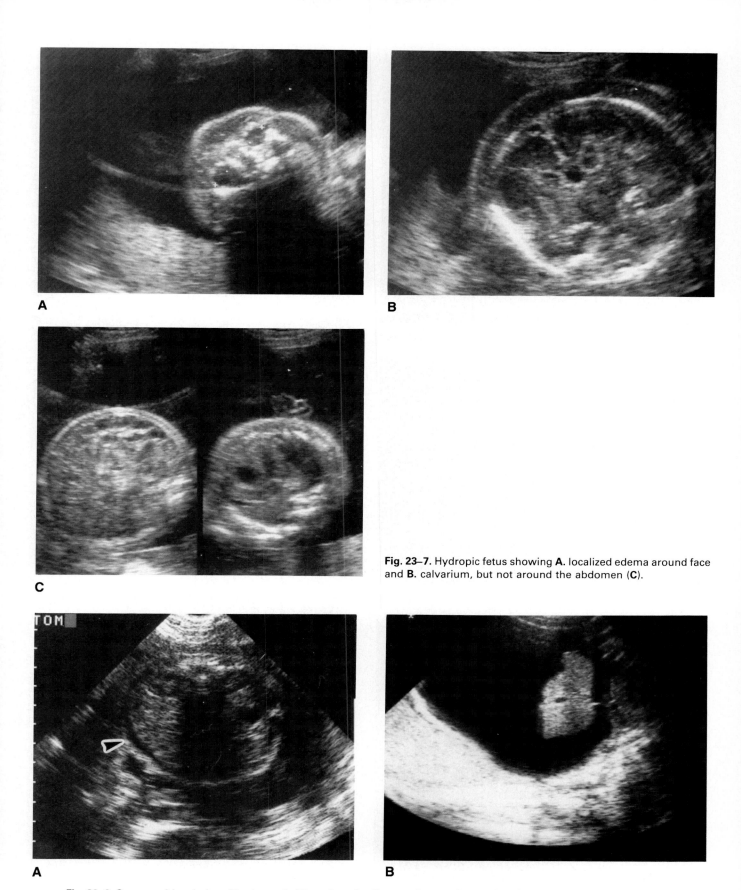

Fig. 23–7. Hydropic fetus showing **A.** localized edema around face and **B.** calvarium, but not around the abdomen (**C**).

Fig. 23–8. Sonographic mimics of hydrops. **A.** ''Pseudoascites'' appearing as a hypoechoic band along anterior abdominal wall. **B.** Massive urinary ascites secondary to ruptured renal collecting systems associated with posterior urethral valves. Liver is surrounded by ascites. (*Figure continued.*)

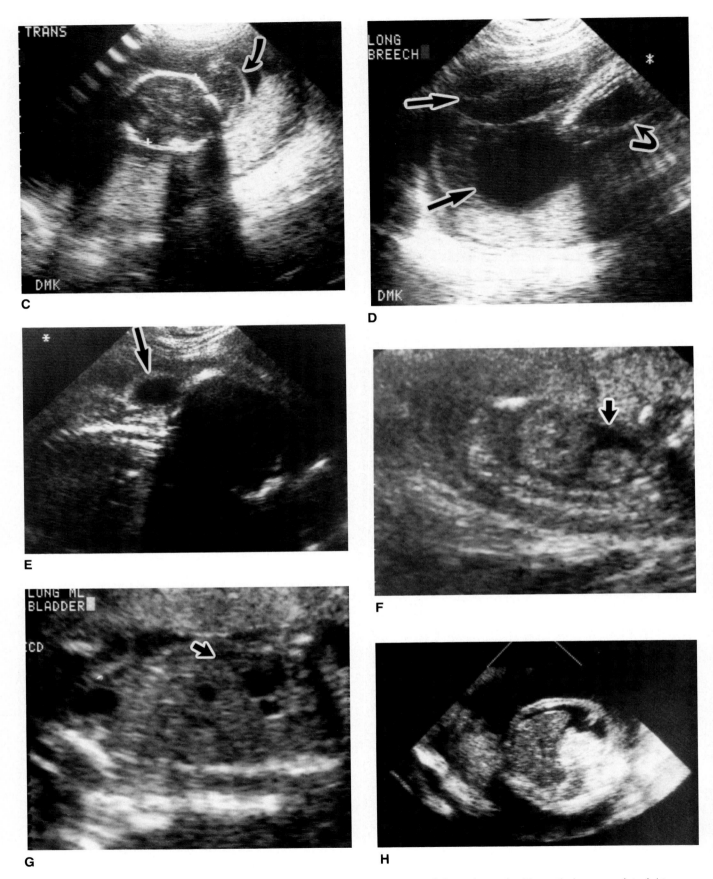

Fig. 23–8 (cont). C. Masssive facial edema. **D.** Pleural effusion in 16-week fetus (*arrow*) with cystic hygroma (*straight arrows*). **E.** Same patient as in **D** showing cystic hygroma arising from posterior aspect of neck. **F.** Left-sided hydrothorax (*arrow*) in 16-week fetus. **G.** One month later, left-sided effusion has spontaneously resolved (*arrow*). **H.** Intraperitoneal fluid secondary to bowel perforation from meconium peritonitis.

One case of transitory fetal ascites was attributed to a sequalae of twin-to-twin transfusion.[10] In general, cases of spontaneous regression are extremely rare and, once hydrops is present, it rarely resolves except after successful therapeutic intervention.[11]

SUMMARY

Sonography has a major role in identification, evaluation, and treatment of the hydropic fetus. Although the prognosis of the NIH fetus is in general poor, sonographic evaluation is important for determining proper management. In addition, the technique of sonographically-guided percutaneous umbilical vein sampling affords an accurate assessment of chromosome etiology of NIH by enabling rapid karyotyping of the fetal blood.

Acknowledgments
The authors thank Joan Johnson and John Bobbitt for their assistance in manuscript preparation.

REFERENCES

1. Warsof SL, Nicolaides KH, Rodeck C. Immune and non-immune hydrops. *Clin Obstet Gynecol.* 1986; 29:533–541.
2. Etches PC, Lemons JA. Nonimmune hydrops fetalis: report of 22 cases including three siblings. *Pediatrics.* 1979; 64:326–332.
3. Fleischer AC, Killam AP, Boehm FH, et al. Hydrops fetalis: sonographic evaluation and clinical implications. *Radiology.* 1981; 141:163–168.
4. Platt LD, Collea JV, Joseph DM. Transitory fetal ascites: an ultrasound diagnosis. *Am J Obstet Gynecol.* 1978; 132:906–908.
5. Hashimoto BE, Filly RA, Callen PW. Fetal pseudoascites: further anatomic observations. *J Ultrasound Med.* 1986; 5:151–152.
6. Kleinman CS, Donnerstein RL, DeVore GR, et al. Fetal echocardiography for evaluation of in utero congestive heart failure. *N Engl J Med.* 1982; 306:568–575.
7. Daffos F, Capella-Pavlovsky M, Forestier F. Fetal blood sampling during pregnancy with use of a needle guided by ultrasound: a study of 606 consecutive cases. *Am J Obstet Gynecol.* 1985; 153:655–660.
8. Nicolaides KH, Rodeck CH, Lange I, et al. Fetoscopy in the assessment of unexplained fetal hydrops. *Br J Obstet Gynaecol.* 1985; 92:671–679.
9. Mahony BS, Filly RA, Callen PW, Chinn DH, Golbus MS. Severe nonimmune hydrops fetalis: sonographic evaluation. *Radiology.* 1984; 151:757–761.
10. Lubinsky M, Rapoport P. Transient fetal hydrops and "prone belly" in one identical female twin. *N Engl J Med.* 1983; 308:256–258.
11. Benacerraf B, Frigoletso F, Wilson M. Successful mid trimester thorocentesis with analysis of the lymphocyte population in pleural effusion. *Am J Obstet Gynecol.* 1986; 155:398–399.
12. Cyr DR, Guntheroth WG, Nyberg DA, Smith JR, Nudelman SR, Ek M. Prenatal diagnosis of an intrapericardial teratoma: a cause of nonimmune hydrops. *J Ultrasound Med.* 1988; 7:87–90.

24 Ultrasound in the Management of the Alloimmunized Pregnancy

Christopher R. Harman

This chapter reflects what has happened throughout the field of perinatal medicine in recent years—a revolution. Developments facilitated by high-resolution ultrasound, in some cases possible only because of ultrasound, have changed the management of significant blood group sensitization. High-resolution fetal imaging has led to highly specific, detailed physical examination. Invasive testing guided by real-time ultrasound yields direct biochemical, hematologic, and respiratory measurements that quantify fetal disease. Ultrasound-guided transfusion procedures allow treatment of even the most severely ill, with the expectation of excellent results at virtually all levels of alloimmune disease.

Ultrasound-facilitated management of the patient with alloimmune disease is an ideal model for assessment of the practice of perinatal medicine. It demonstrates the mature integration of an understanding of the disease process, the etiology, pathologic changes, mechanisms for investigation, mechanisms for treatment and, perhaps most importantly, the means of prevention. As such, no better model exists to illustrate the fundamental role of ultrasonic fetal evaluation in the new obstetrics.

BASIC PATHOPHYSIOLOGY

While "atypical" blood group antigens are assuming a larger role in etiology of alloimmune disease, anti-D sensitization (Rh disease) remains the cause of 80 to 90% of clinical hemolytic disease of the fetus and newborn (HDFN).[1-4] The mortality of serious HDFN has continued to fall with ongoing improvements in neonatal care. An equally important factor in the overall decline of this disease entity is a lower incidence (Table 24–1). As the ultimate result of better management of those who are sick combined with fewer sick babies, perinatal death due to alloimmunization is seldom encountered in the general population (5 to 8 per 10,000 live births). The significance of these statistics is that Rh disease is now an unusual category of fetal disease. In addition, it is virtually totally treatable, readily detectable, and readily monitored. Survival at the 100% level is within our grasp. Even though HDFN may be seen with decreasing frequency and, therefore, be more difficult for the general

ultrasonographer to recognize, it remains a correctable cause of perinatal mortality and neonatal morbidity, which deserves careful attention.

In any pregnancy where mother and fetus have differing blood types (therefore, in virtually all pregnancies where mother and father have different blood types), maternal sensitization can occur.[5] In order to effect a mature antibody response, the mother must have been sensitized at some prior point, perhaps even as remote as the mother's time as a fetus (Fig. 24–1). With prior immune exposure to a given antigen, the second exposure to that antigen results in the mature response. A "sensitized" woman is one with a detectable antibody; when this antibody is immunoglobulin G it can cause fetal disease. Immunoglobulin G readily crosses the placenta. The exact gestational age at which this begins is not certain; it may be as early as 8 to 10 weeks.

The pathophysiology of the fetal aspects of this disease is well understood (Fig. 24–1). The fetus expresses Rh antigens on his red blood cells, virtually as these are present. Once exposed, the mother mounts a competent antibody response against the fetal red cell antigens. As the antibody binds fetal circulation, it triggers fetal reticuloendothelial system digestion of fetal red blood cells. Deformed cells are removed from circulation, mainly in the spleen, and disposed of ultimately by hemolysis and phagocytosis.

With worsening anemia, the fetus compensates by maximizing red cell production in liver, spleen, intestinal wall, and other sites to a minor extent, probably mediated by fetal erythropoietin. In the liver, the erythropoietic islands of cells enlarge and, when subjected to further demands, coalesce and occupy the majority of hepatic structure, causing displacement of hepatic cellular function, occlusion of transport pathways, and disruption of enzyme systems on a cellular basis.[6] The ultimate result of this "hepatotoxic" hematopoiesis is liver failure. Hemolysis continues, so the anemia remains uncorrected, and worsens. Physically, this amounts to the ultimate form of fetal disease, hydrops fetalis: hepatosplenomegaly, hypoproteinemia, hypoalbuminemia, ascites, complete anasarca, pericardial effusions, pleural effusions, cardiac failure, impaired placental circulation and function, and ultimately intrauterine death.

TABLE 24–1. FACTORS IN THE DECLINING FREQUENCY OF HDFN

Reduced Exposure to Rh+ Blood
    Later first pregnancy
    Lower parity
    Detailed cross-matching
    ? Lower rate of TPH
Reduced Sensitization with TPH
    Postpartum prophylaxis (90%)
    Antepartum/event prophylaxis (9%)
    Therapeutic IgG for massive exposure

TPH = transplacental hemorrhage

In the newborn, hydrops fetalis presents many management problems, including difficulties in ventilation, enormous tissue edema, metabolic acidosis, cardiac instability, pulmonary immaturity, and abnormal chest wall compliance. Even the nonhydropic infant is at substantial risk of bilirubin toxicity, which in its most serious form (kernicterus) can cause death or severe cerebral damage.

The ultimate goals of the management of alloimmunization are to reduce even further the sensitization of women at risk, to facilitate timely diagnosis and investigation of fetuses affected with disease, and to provide treatment when disease is severe enough to pose a threat to intrauterine survival. The essential role of ultrasound in all three processes will become clear to the reader.

PREVENTION OF ALLOIMMUNIZATION

Ultrasound has a critical role in preventing alloimmunization. Sensitization of the woman to her fetus' blood, in almost all instances, depends on transmission of fetal blood to the maternal circulation. This may happen spontaneously, as a result of transplacental hemorrhage (TPH) or several other factors (Table 24–2). At least 75% of all

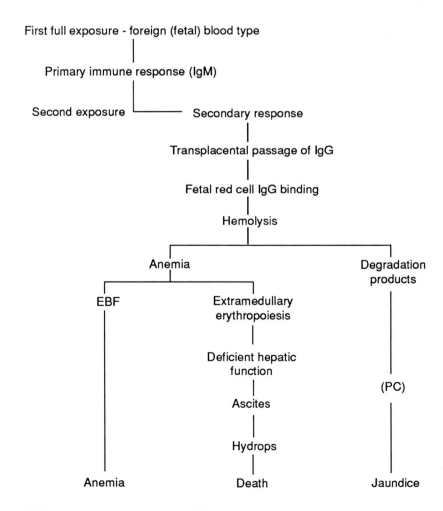

Fig. 24–1. Development and impact of maternal sensitization.

EBF = erythroblastosis fetalis;   PC = placental clearance.

TABLE 24–2. MATERNAL EXPOSURE TO RH+ BLOOD

Spontaneous Transplacental Hemorrhage
    At delivery
    Abruptio placentae
    Antepartum
    Miscarriage
    Fetal death
Traumatic TPH
    Chorion villus sampling
    Amniocentesis
    Therapeutic abortion
    Dilatation and currettage
    Fetal blood sampling
    Intrauterine fetal transfusion
    External version
    Obstetric manipulation

TPHs occur at delivery, but up to 10% happen by 28 weeks' gestation.

Obstetric interference adds substantially to the risk of TPH before term. Procedures such as genetic amniocentesis, chorion villus sampling, percutaneous umbilical blood sampling, and external version are all associated with increased risk of TPH and, therefore, of maternal sensitization. Whereas many protective influences can help moderate the frequency of sensitization associated with transplacental hemorrhage, the usual cause of severe fetal disease is that at some point the mother was exposed to fetal blood bearing the incompatible antigen. Although the detailed application of Rh-immune globulin (Winrho intravenously, Rhogam intramuscularly) will prevent sensitization in many such cases, it is simplistic to believe that TPH is an inconsequential side effect. The primary approach in controlling sensitization, therefore, is to reduce the frequency of transplacental hemorrhage.

There is no doubt that ultrasound-guided procedures are less likely to generate transplacental hemorrhages and, therefore, are less dangerous. For example, genetic amniocentesis with ultrasound direction produces only one tenth the TPHs of those done without ultrasound guidance.[7] Current studies show no patients becoming sensitized when use of ultrasound and immune prophylaxis are combined for genetic amniocentesis. Adequate ultrasound guidance for any procedure includes identification of the origin of the cord at the placenta, the entire course of the free umbilical cord, and accurate placental localization. Placental abnormalities, including succenturiate lobes, vasa previa, and so forth, are clearly within the definition of "placental localization." Renewed emphasis on choosing a route that does not traverse the placenta has undoubtedly reduced the frequency of TPH. At the same time, diligent application of Rh-immune prophylaxis with the procedure, as well as Kleihauer

testing to detect any fetal–maternal hemorrhage following the procedure, can produce the ideal result: no woman is sensitized as a result of the intervention.

In the sensitized pregnant woman, however, different levels of concern need to be applied. The pregnant woman who is already sensitized cannot be protected by any amount of Rh immunoglobulin, nor by carefully selecting a "thin" area of the placenta to transverse. Maximum effort is indicated in avoiding the placenta completely. It is our firm policy to defer genetic amniocentesis, for example, when the pregnant woman is seriously sensitized, and the placenta is completely anterior.

INVESTIGATION OF THE ALLOIMMUNIZED PREGNANCY

So-called "critical levels" of maternal antibody are applied on an institutional basis. Once the mother has significant sensitization, further calibration of her antibody level will not accurately reflect the likelihood of fetal disease. A mother with a titer of 1:128 in albumin is just as likely to have severe disease if her titer remains stable as another patient whose antibody titer rises from 1:64 to 1:256 at the same gestational age. In women so sensitized, the target of investigation must be the fetus.

Amniocentesis for Amniotic Fluid Bilirubin

Bilirubin is the end product of fetal disposal of the waste products of hemolysis. In fetal life, the primary biochemical product of hemolysis is unconjugated (indirect) bilirubin, most of which is transferred across the placenta into the maternal circulation. A minor amount is circulated in the enterohepatic loop within the fetus, ultimately excreted via the fetal lung into the amniotic fluid. Transvascular passage from intramembranous fetal vessels to amniotic fluid may be significant, but has not been quantified. Amniotic fluid spectrophotometry, (the ΔOD 450, a measure of the fluid's "yellowness"), correlates with the amount of bilirubin present. Indications for amniocentesis are summarized in Table 24–3.

Amniocentesis provides ongoing reassurance that

TABLE 24–3. INDICATIONS FOR AMNIOCENTESIS FOR ΔOD 450

- Previous intrauterine death related to Rh disease.
- Neonatal disease requiring exchange transfusion.
- Significant antibody titer rise.[a]
- "Suggestive" ultrasound findings but no hydrops, when serial data are not available, cordocentesis not available.

[a] Specific to the lab concerned. In the Manitoba program, 1:16 albumin titer, or absolute level of >1.0 μg/l.

more invasive fetal testing is not yet necessary. Rarely, such testing provides false reassurance.[8] Detailed physical examination, described later in this chapter, must be added to amniocentesis to determine the extent of fetal disease.[9] If there is evidence of accelerated fetal disease, the amniocentesis may be properly deferred in favor of fetal blood sampling. Clearly, amniocentesis in the face of obvious hydropic fetal disease is superfluous. Having been scanned to determine the extent and severity of hydropic fetal disease, such a patient should be referred promptly to a center capable of intravascular fetal transfusion.

Amniocentesis is done under ultrasound direction, although direct visualization of the needle entering the

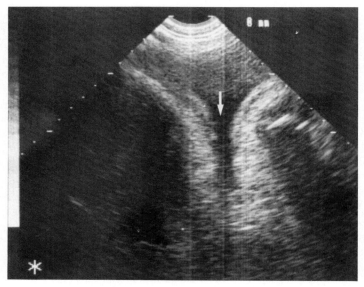

A

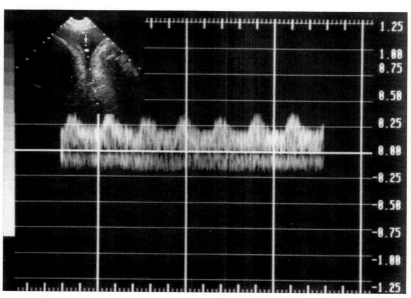

Fig. 24–2. Doppler ultrasound in amniocentesis. **A.** An apparently clear pocket of fluid (*arrow*). **B.** It contains an arterial pulse! A different site was chosen.

B

amniotic fluid cavity may not always be necessary. When the placenta is posterior, or when a clear path (at least 1 cm × 1 cm) is visible lateral to an anterior placenta, real-time observation of needle placement at amniocentesis is not used. If transplacental amniocentesis is absolutely necessary, a 22-gauge or smaller needle is used rather than the 20-gauge spinal needle normally used, and great care is taken to identify and avoid fetal vessels on the surface of the placenta. In most cases, however, the necessity of such a procedure is becoming increasingly infrequent. Where transplacental insertion is necessary, fetal blood sampling is the superior choice. Some authors believe that amniocentesis should occupy an extremely minor role in the management of such patients.[8-10] The arguments on both sides of this issue have not yet been resolved.[11,12] At the University of Manitoba, amniocentesis remains a valuable component of our ability to investigate fetal disease at an early stage of pregnancy.

Careful note is taken of the location of the cord and, if at all possible, the target pocket of amniotic fluid should contain no loops of cord, close to the surface or otherwise. If there is any doubt whatsoever about the quality of the image, Doppler ultrasound can be valuable in certifying a cord-free pocket (Fig. 24–2).[13] In order to achieve these criteria, the ultrasonographer must have an open mind as to the angle of approach. Anywhere the needle can be placed can be considered for an approach to the amniotic cavity. This includes the extreme lateral approach which may or may not necessitate passage of the needle close to maternal structures even though one might not otherwise consider it eligible for needle puncture. In such cases, continuous real-time ultrasound imaging of the needle as it advances is preferable. A 10-mL aliquot is obtained and rapidly decanted into a light-proof container. Unless the fluid is grossly contaminated with particulate matter such as blood or vernix, or deeply stained with heme pigment (green) or denatured blood (brown or red), the fluid should be analyzed directly and not centrifuged.

Following removal of the amniocentesis needle, careful observation is made to detect any intraamniotic bleeding. Bleeding of maternal origin may persist for some time, tends to be "gentle" in its appearance ("falling leaves"), and does not produce a "plume" or a "jet" within the amniotic fluid.[14] Very small amounts of fetal blood under pressure can produce these ultrasound appearances (Fig. 24–3). In all cases, a maternal blood sample for Kleihauer investigation is drawn 2 to 5 minutes after the procedure. Fetal cells present in the maternal circulation may be cleared extremely rapidly and not be detected if the Kleihauer is drawn more than 10 minutes after the procedure. If blood is accidentally obtained at

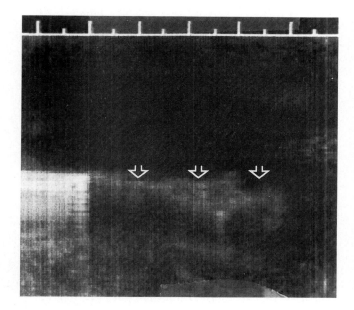

Fig. 24–3. Waterbath image of infusion of only 0.025 mL of blood through a 25-gauge needle (bright linear echoes at left), producing turbulence (*arrows*).

the time of amniocentesis, this should also be sent for Kleihauer examination, and blood typing if fetal.

Maternal Kleihauer testing is the standard for changing timing of serial tests. Significant amounts of fetal blood in the maternal circulation call for more frequent testing. Maternal antibody titer measurements may also be important in advancing the date of any investigation. It is clear that amniocentesis, and the role of the ultrasonographer in providing the eyes for this procedure, cannot be performed in isolation from the other clinical factors.

PHYSICAL US EXAMINATION OF THE ALLOIMMUNIZED FETUS

The reasons for performing a detailed obstetric ultrasound examination in the alloimmunized pregnancy are basically the same as the reasons for initiating testing (either amniocentesis or fetal blood sampling). Thus, the sonographer examining a fetus in an alloimmunized pregnancy should be aware of mode of sensitization, antibody quantification and qualification, and a firm gestational age on which to base a competent appraisal of the fetus. The specific observations of subtle signs of incipient disease are able to be accomplished within the context of a normal obstetric scan, but a formatted exam ("data sheet") is helpful in assuring consistency.

The purpose of this ultrasound examination is manifold. Objective data are necessary because the physical examination has limited sensitivity in the nonhydropic fetus,[15] but laboratory data in isolation are not sufficient in formulating prognosis and management plans. Physical examination is quite subjective, is highly variable from fetus to fetus, and may change rapidly in a given individual.[16] The examination, however, is an important part of the investigative process of the alloimmunized pregnancy, and part of the effort to define the extent of fetal disease. (While maternal antibody titration assesses the risk of fetal disease, and amniocentesis suggests the cumulative rate of hemolysis [the "range" of disease], physical examination defines the extent of fetal disease.) Fetal anemia per se can only be measured using direct means, fetal blood sampling by cordocentesis (see following discussion), but examination demonstrates the extremes of compromise to which the fetus has gone in trying to alleviate the anemia. Comprehensive examination includes the fetus, cord, placenta, and amniotic fluid.

Fetal Examination

Anemia does not appear to bear any pathognomonic signs. Increased cardiac work, high velocity/flow situations, or small pericardial effusions have been suggested as accurate signs of the need for intervention transfusion, but as yet no controlled studies of these techniques have been reported.[17,18]

A serious degree of fetal anemia may be present without frank hydrops.[19] Many fetuses tolerate low hemoglobin concentrations without major hepatic compromise due to overwhelming hematopoiesis; this may well be dependent on tissue oxygenation, normal to very low hematocrit levels. In other situations, hemolysis may be so rapid, in the form of a fetal hemolytic crisis, that fetal physical changes do not have time to evolve to the full-blown picture that "ought to" accompany profound fetal anemia.[20] There is much additional variability even when hydrops is concerned, with hemoglobin values ranging from seriously low to profoundly low among fetuses with very similar physical appearances. It is clear, then, that hemoglobin levels cannot be specifically predicted by physical examination, with or without ΔOD 450 results.

It is also clear, however, that the best assessment of the fetal problem, and of the need and urgency of intrauterine treatment, is based on a comprehensive evaluation that includes history, physical examination, and laboratory data.[21,22] Fetal examination when the fetus is not yet hydropic is relatively straightforward.[5,14] Routine biometry is performed to ascertain the skeletal basis for gestational age, using the mean of multiple gestational age parameters (head circumference, biparietal diameter, femur length, abdominal circumference, and foot length).[23] This aids in interpreting ΔOD 450 values, es-

tablishes where on the gestationally-dependent slope the mean hemoglobin should lie, and helps predict lung maturity in terms of intrauterine versus extrauterine management. A careful screen of possible anomalies is performed, and detailed examination of fetal anatomy is carried out. The example of a fetus with trisomy 21 with thickened occipital region, moderate ascites, and elevated ΔOD 450 (secondary to gastrointestinal obstruction, not hemolysis), reinforces the need to consider a differential ultrasound diagnosis even when lab data seem obvious.

Subtle signs of impending ascites include: double outlining of hollow organs such as stomach, gall bladder, urinary bladder (Fig. 24–4), and later in gestation, fluid separating loops of small bowel.[24] Male fetuses may show expanding hydroceles (Fig. 24–5).

The few milliliters of fluid normally present in the abdomen may be detected by modern high-resolution ultrasound instruments. Further, the concept of "pseudo-ascites" deserves some mention.[25] This is the appearance noted in fetal cross section at the level of the dome of the diaphragm descending to the anterior abdominal wall, at which the abdominal wall musculature and the diaphragm may lie in apposition. Because both of these skeletal muscle structures are echo-poor, an apparent fluid rim may appear at this level (Fig. 24–6). Ascites does not usually accumulate at this level. If it is

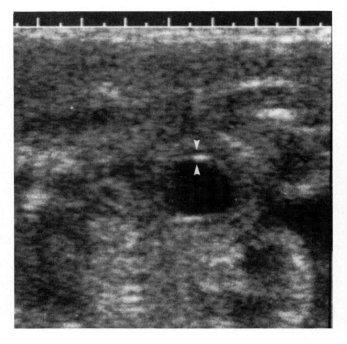

Fig. 24–4. Impending ascites. The fetal bladder wall outlined (*arrows*) on both sides, by urine inside and a small amount of ascites on the peritoneal surface.

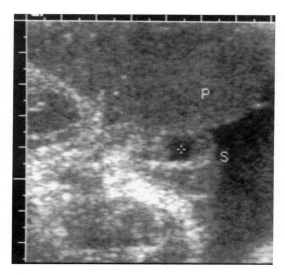

Fig. 24–5. Male fetus with serious anti-D hemolysis, 30 weeks' gestation. First sign of progression to hydropic disease was a small hydrocele (*asterisk*). S = scrotum; P = placenta, which is bulging.

not continuous with the same fluid rim at the dome of the diaphragm, or situated in the fetal pelvis, it is probably pseudo-ascites. Such a fluid rim also should be clearly visible in both longitudinal and transverse planes.

This appearance associated with a rising titer or sus-

picious amniotic fluid value may produce a recommendation for intrauterine therapy. In such circumstances, placing the observation in context with serial fetal abdominal circumference measurements, trends in amniotic fluid values, and past history may help in deferring the procedure. The use of fetal umbilical blood sampling, without transfusion, can be pivotal in such situations. Once again, this emphasizes the necessity for integration of information rather than simply reporting ultrasound findings.

In the absence of overt ascites, other generalized signs of fetal edema/anasarca are seldom present. In our experience, it is of little value to carry out systematic measurements of abdominal wall thickness, scalp thickness, or assessment of other areas of the integument. Without ascites, significant peripheral edema is usually a combination of artifact and wishful thinking, or may be associated with other abnormalities of the fetus independent of the alloimmune process. Similar comments can be made for pleural effusions, which are seldom present in the absence of ascites.

The same may not be true of pericardial effusions. De Vore and colleagues rely on the presence of pericardial effusions detected by M-mode ultrasound examination to initiate invasive therapy.[18,26] Such monitoring in sensitized patients may detect minor pericardial effusions as small as 2 to 3 mm in size. Our experience does not agree with theirs. In our laboratory, high-resolution ultrasound instruments such as the Acu-

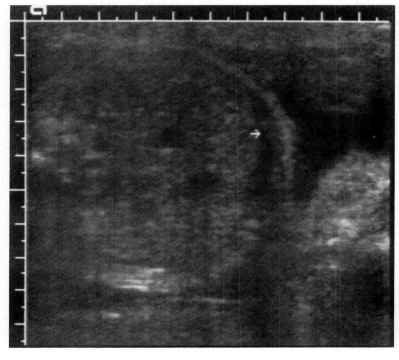

Fig. 24–6. Pseudo-ascites. The apparent "fluid rim" (*arrow*) was not seen in the fetal pelvis or at the top of the liver, and disappeared when the fetus changed position.

son 128 are sometimes able to demonstrate small amounts of pericardial fluid in the healthiest, nonaffected fetuses. At the time of publication, no randomized study of such fetuses has been published. The expertise to perform such detailed M-mode echocardiography may not be widely disseminated. We do not rely on this subtle finding to initiate investigation. It is our experience that large pericardial effusions (>4 mm) are usually associated with other obvious signs of fetal disease. Large effusions, such as in Fig. 24–13, are prognostically significant and may alter some aspects of management (eg, the total volume of blood administered at a single intravascular transfusion [IVT], being aware of the possibility of cardiac tamponade with hypervolemia).

Changes in the abdominal circumference may be one of the most valuable ultrasound signs of impending disease in the nonhydropic fetus. Special care must be taken in performing this measurement in sensitized pregnancies, to observe the landmarks (bifurcation of the

portal vein within the liver and a smooth oval cross-section). Measurement should be taken from skin to skin, using an elliptical calliper when possible (see Fig. 24–26).[13] Sudden increases in percentile ranking of the fetal abdominal circumference suggest significant hepatomegaly secondary to advancing hepatopoiesis (Fig. 24–7).[27,28] Changes in fetal position may produce artifactual rises in percentile ranking, as demonstrated in Fig. 24–7.B, but one should not ignore significant changes in established percentile ranking. If a sharp rise in abdominal circumference growth is shown in association with an antibody titer that could potentially cause severe disease, serial amniocenteses or fetal blood sampling, depending on placental localization, should be initiated. In the fetus already being followed by amniocentesis, a sudden rise in abdominal circumference calls for confirmation of the "benign" amniotic fluid results by fetal blood sampling. Because the ultrasound examination may well be pivotal in these situations, and

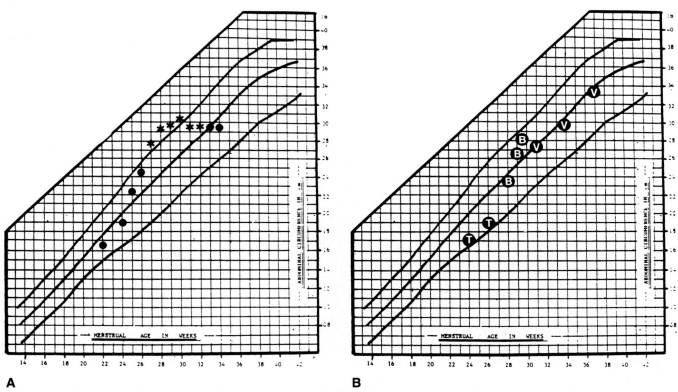

A   **B**

Fig. 24–7. A. "Growth Chart." Serial abdominal circumference measurements in a fetus who developed severe anti-D alloimmune disease. Starting at 22 weeks, four measurements show acceleration in abdominal circumference (accompanied by rising amniotic fluid bilirubin). At 26 weeks, intravascular fetal transfusions were begun, three procedures over 6 1/2 weeks, with weekly AC measurements (*). Measurements taken at 33 and 34 weeks' gestation, after the transfusions were complete, showed fetal AC at previously established level (40th percentile) with corresponding decrease in liver size. **B.** Serial abdominal circumference in a fetus who switched from transverse lie, to breech, to vertex. Mother had stable 1:8 titer anti-Kell, but the rise in AC was troubling. A single amniocentesis at 30 weeks demonstrated a low zone I fluid.

because the ultrasonographer is frequently not the person deciding management plans, meticulous attention to measurement techniques is necessary.

Subjective signs of hepatosplenomegaly, such as the bottom edge of the liver lying as low as the fetal right iliac crest, or splenomegaly with the spleen extended >2 cm below the left costal margin, may suggest accelerating disease. Especially when the same observer does the serial examinations, these findings should give rise to detailed investigation. On the other hand, if "suspicious" findings are present in the initial examination, and are not supported by definite findings in maternal titers or amniotic fluid results, careful consultation should precede any dangerously invasive investigations. This is particularly true of "possible hepatosplenomegaly" and of the subjective placental signs of disease described below.

Hydrops Fetalis

The original descriptions of hydrops fetalis, of course, refer to the appearance of stillborn infants who had suffered the ultimate consequence of intrauterine alloimmune disease. In most centers, the neonatologist is not often confronted by this awful appearance, but the intrauterine ultrasound correlates of this appearance may still present antenatally (Figs. 24–8 through 24–13). The classic findings of the most severe form of disease, preceding fetal death by only days, are illustrated here.

Ascites. As noted above, modest collections of fluid may exist prior to ultrasound being able to delineate them. The threshold for ascites being visualized is not certain, but based on serial observations of intraperitoneal transfusion, estimates can be made. At 30 mL, the double-

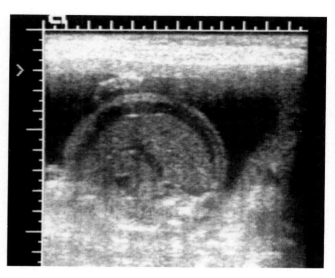

Fig. 24–8. "Early" ascites. Small rim of intraperitoneal fluid, not associated with significant fetal edema or other effusions. Fetal hemoglobin 66 g/L at 26 weeks' gestation.

outlining (Fig. 24–4) and an increased contrast of the abdominal contents first appear. At 50 mL, a distinct fluid rim (such as in Fig. 24–8) begins to be visible. At 100 mL, a classic picture of ascites is clear.[14] (See Fig. 24–9.)

At the other end of the scale, changes in large volumes of ascites may be difficult to monitor, as abdominal wall tension and intraabdominal organs will cause the fluid to appear in fairly consistent fashion over a wide range of volumes. In our experience, serial measurement

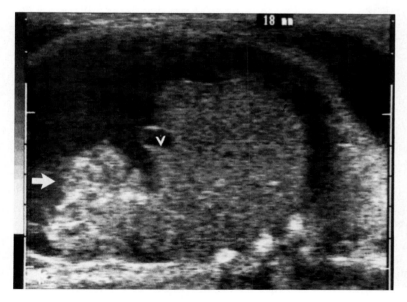

Fig. 24–9. Massive fetal ascites. Longitudinal view of abdomen of hydropic fetus at 24 weeks. The chest is to the right, with lower three ribs seen at lower right. Ascites outlines the liver, with umbilical vein entering at V. The more echogenic small bowel (*arrow*) hangs freely in the fluid. The abdominal circumference was >97.5 percentile; the abdominal wall was not thicker than normal.

of fetal ascites is a poor way of documenting response to therapy. Prior to onset of any therapy, the ascites is bright yellow and crystal clear. If intraperitoneal transfusions (IPT) are used in managing such fetuses, the blood introduced into the peritoneal cavity produces changes notable by ultrasound. Turbidity of the fluid, both when the fetus moves and in more or less static views, can be observed, but is not a reliable indicator of amount of blood absorption. It may well be that the same examiner following the patient will produce the best evidence of improvement following transfusion.

Fetal Edema. Figure 24–10 demonstrates the most severe form of fetal facial edema, the so-called Buddha face. In this case, the forehead and cheeks are so waterlogged with edema that the eye sockets are lost in contour. Head size and body size can be grossly overestimated due to intense tissue swelling (Fig. 24–11). In some cases, abdominal wall edema can be noted prior to the extreme of facial edema, but serial measurements of abdominal wall thickness are not helpful in predicting severity or rate of deterioration in fetuses with accelerated disease. Expression of abdominal wall edema varies greatly with gestational age and fetal position, and may be reduced as tension rises with further deterioration. In addition, the acuity of current high-resolution instruments makes

it quite possible to overemphasize the nature of edema. Especially in the occipital region, normal scalp thickness may be exaggerated simply by fetal posture, creating an impression of scalp edema. It is most helpful, therefore, to obtain serial examinations by the same observer, using each available area to monitor edema. A careful review of the following structures will illustrate fetal edema if present: face, including eyelids, nostrils, lips, and ears; scalp, frontal as well as occipital; abdominal wall thickness; and hands and feet. Particularly helpful in evaluation of hands and feet, and in some areas of the face, is to observe the fetus while it moves. The edematous hand cannot close properly, and although movements may be seen, these are stiff and limited in range (Fig. 24–12).

Pericardial and Pleural Effusions. When present in the severely hydropic fetus, these effusions are very obvious. Pericardial effusions may reach large dimensions (Fig. 24–13), and interfere with myocardial contractility. Such observations are important in the occasional fetus in whom cardiac output is impaired and call for reduced volumes at the initial intravascular transfusions.[28] Pleural effusions are seen with less frequency and should be regarded with some suspicion when the fetus is responding to therapy, especially if they persist longer than pericardial effusions and ascites. Invasive testing will provide adequate fetal samples of either amniotic fluid or blood for genetic studies to exclude the unusual but definite possibility of alloimmunization that exists in conjunction with serious fetal anomalies that lead to effusions, ascites, or both. Pleural effusions usually resolve quite rapidly with therapy, although pericardial effusions in a number of infants treated in our center have been the last thing to resolve while the fetus was improving. It is not uncommon for pericardial effusion to last 3 to 4 weeks after fetal hemoglobin has been restored to a normal level.

Fetal Behavior. Fetal well-being is assessed using the biophysical profile score (BPS).[29,30] Behavioral indices monitored by ultrasound, including fetal body and limb movement, fetal tone, fetal breathing movements, and amniotic fluid volume, are assessed in the same fashion as for other high-risk pregnancies. Cardiotocography is frequently used in completing the antenatal assessment of such fetuses, especially in observations immediately before and after intrauterine procedures. The BPS is usually normal (8 to 10/10) through a wide range of fetal disease. This demonstrates the functional evidence that the fetus is able to maintain homeostasis despite severe impairment of hematologic function. A BPS of 4/10 or less (the moribund fetus) is almost exclusively found in fetuses with the most severe structural evidence of hydrops fetalis, and is a severe prognostic sign.[9,16,31] The complete absence of fetal behavior in a fetus illustrating

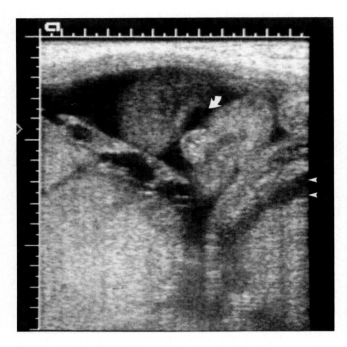

Fig. 24–10. "The Buddha face." The forehead is at upper center, with the swollen face angled down to the right. The left eye (*arrow*) is closed by edema. The chin rests on the chest, which shows a pleural effusion (*double arrow*).

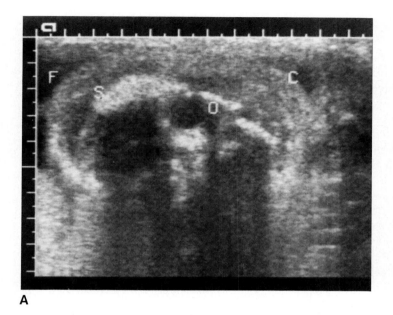

A

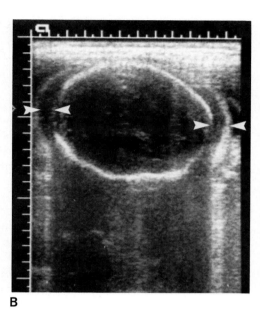

B

Fig. 24–11. Scalp edema. **A.** The fetus is surrounded by a 2-cm thick mass of edema. The face, identified by (0) (left orbit) and (S) (top of skull) is dwarfed by edema shown by (C) (surface of left cheek) and (F) (forehead). This fetus survived intact, after seven IVT. **B.** In axial plane, the "halo" of edema is best seen anteriorly and posteriorly (*between arrows*).

typical signs of hydrops fetalis constitutes a fetal emergency for which the only means of rescue is direct vascular access, either intrauterine or following emergency cesarean section. Such fetuses do not respond to series of intraperitoneal fetal transfusion, perhaps on the basis of absent fetal breathing movements.[32]

Intravascular fetal data available suggest that these fetuses are indeed acidotic, hypoxic, and have serious perfusion problems. Where this extent of disease was lethal with IPT, with fetal intravascular transfusion (IVT), even these fetuses may be rescued.

In such situations, the return of normal fetal be-

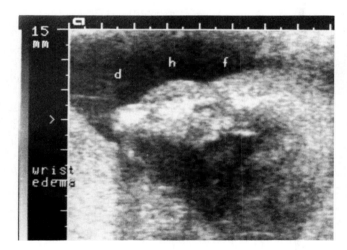

Fig. 24–12. Skin edema. Scan shows fetal arm in longitudinal view. Distorted by edema, the forearm (f), hand and wrist (h), and digits (d) remained in a fixed position for several days after hemoglobin and pH were restored to normal by a series of IVT. The fetus regained normal movement before normal anatomy, resulting in limbs that moved "like paddles."

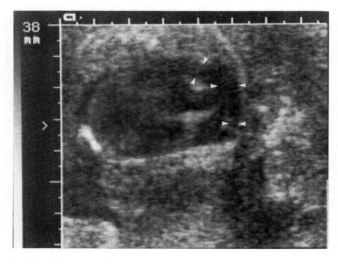

Fig. 24–13. Pericardial effusions. This fetus at 23 weeks had striking ascites, placental edema, and severe facial and scalp edema. The large pericardial effusion (*arrows*) was the last sign of extravascular fluid displacement to resolve, 3 weeks following restoration of normal hemoglobin levels.

havior, shown by rapid increase in fetal movements with normal tone, and soon after that the return of regular, cyclic, fetal breathing movements, demonstrates the value of BPS in the posttransfusion phase. In several instances, restoration of hemoglobin to a normal range, associated with a rise in PO_2 and correction of acidotic pH, along with resumption of normal behavior, has been demonstrated within 30 minutes of transfusion.[16,31] The survival of 5/6 fetuses in this condition demonstrates the maxim that no fetus with a heartbeat is beyond treatment.

Amniotic Fluid

Fetuses with early stages of disease tend to have increased amniotic fluid. This may not always exceed the ultrasound threshold for hydramnios (>8.0 cm in maximum vertical amniotic-fluid pocket depth), but it certainly meets subjective impressions of increased fluid. Although some have found this to be a reliable first indicator of the onset of fetal disease,[33] it may not be a reliable enough sign on which to base management.[15] Reduced amniotic fluid volume is an ominous sign. A maximum pocket depth of less than 2 cm signifies reduced production of amniotic fluid, as can be seen in end-stage disease or when intrauterine growth retardation (IUGR) is associated with alloimmunization. Umbilical cord access should be sought urgently when such a finding is associated with hydropic fetal disease.

Qualitative examination of the amniotic fluid includes documentation of backbleeding after vascular access, approximation of volumes lost at the end of the transfusion, and noting of the presence of any intraamniotic clot (Fig. 24–14). In the case illustrated, fetal thrombocytopenia was so severe that backbleeding of greater volume than had been given at the first transfusion occurred rapidly after withdrawal of the needle.[34] The intraamniotic clot formed quickly after the backbleeding, and rapidly contracted to grasp the cord and fetal limbs firmly, and lie adherent to the fetal abdomen. An increase in the amount of free-floating particles after transfusion correlates with a small amount of backbleeding, and normal hemostasis. Masses of such particles (evident as a snowstorm) when the fetus moves a limb vigorously are of little significance when detailed fetal hematology is known. Such particles may persist for several weeks after the last fetal transfusion.

Umbilical Cord

Detailed identification of the umbilical cord at its two ends is an integral part of prepration for a fetal IVT. The placental end of the cord is the target of first choice in IVT, and is identified in maximum detail. With the anterior placenta, or with the posterior placenta and generous amniotic fluid, this identification is not difficult (see Fig. 24–20). In the more mature fetus with a posterior cord insertion, the area of the placenta where the cord is anchored may be completely obscured. Similarly, the anterior cord insertion may not be ideally visualized when the fetus is large, the fluid is reduced, and when the cord is wrapped around a fetal limb, neck, or torso. In experience with over 300 cord procedures, the lesson we learned has been to take as much time as necessary, to use maternal repositioning, fetal manipulation, or simply to defer the procedure to another time in order to obtain optimal visualization.

Serial fetal umbilical vein diameter does not correlate at all with onset or extent of fetal disease.[35-37] In addition to its lack of correlation, this measurement itself varies significantly with fetal position, tension on the cord, nuchal or other loops, and with advancing gestational age.

Placenta

This may be the earliest site of manifestations of accelerated fetal alloimmune hemolysis. As disease progresses, placental architecture is lost, with gradual assumption of the "ground glass" appearance (Fig. 24–15). The placenta becomes more erect and stiffer, and the presence of maternal "lakes," as seen in the more relaxed placenta, is lost. Eventually, the placenta as-

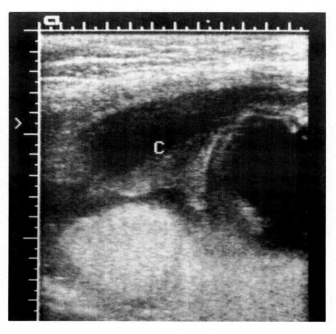

Fig. 24–14. Large intraamniotic clot, following thrombocytopenic hemorrhage after intravascular fetal transfusion. This image was obtained approximately 30 minutes after needle was removed from posterior cord insertion, as the clot (C) gradually contracted up against the abdominal wall. Retransfusion was necessary due to extensive backbleeding.

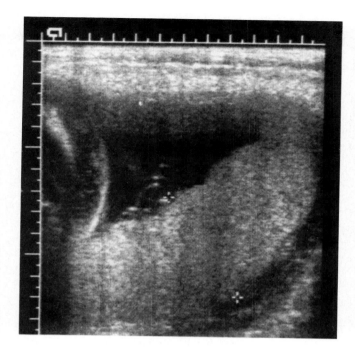

Fig. 24–15. Typical "ground glass" placenta found in serious alloimmune disease. The placenta has lost much of its architecture and shows a generally uniform position with ablation of maternal intervillous spaces. Maximum thickness >6 cm (calipers), grossly thickened for 22 weeks' gestation. Cord insertion lies to the immediate left of upper caliper.

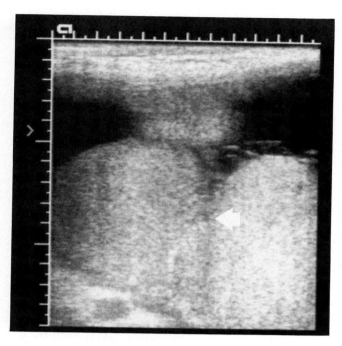

Fig. 24–16. Hydropic placenta. In this case the edema has proceeded even further, with the placenta grossly enlarged, rigid, very thickened, and distended so that the true cord insertion (*arrow*) lies >2 cm below buckled surface of the placenta.

sumes a rigid, spherical appearance with a puckered chorionic surface. In the most severe forms of placental edema, the placenta may reach thicknesses of 8 to 10 cm and weigh as much as 2.0 kg at the time of delivery. One such example is depicted in Fig. 24–16, which demonstrates the cord insertion puckered as much as 3 cm below the amniotic/membrane interface. This most severe form of placental distortion may not resolve even over a successful course of intrauterine fetal therapy.

ULTRASOUND CLASSIFICATION OF DISEASE STATE

Based on the rather straightforward findings described, the physical extent of fetal disease can be classified as shown in Fig. 24–17.[9] The reader should be careful not to infer that fetal disease proceeds in a regular, step-by-step fashion, or that disease neatly segregates into these classifications. Nicolaides and associates[15] have demonstrated in convincing fashion that morphometrics, whatever the object measured, are probably not of much use in quantifying fetal anemia. The purpose of the classifications shown here is not to refute that argument, but simply to illustrate the levels of compromise that are

associated with different depths of anemia. The classification assists in standardization of results for comparison, and helps formulate prognosis. The classes are briefly described as follows:

Class 0 fetuses underwent cordocentesis due to suspected alloimmune disease, based on historical data, or marginal or suspicious ΔOD 450 values, and/or suspicious ultrasound findings. In all cases, a pure fetal blood sample was obtained, but no transfusion was performed. All of these fetuses ($n = 14$) were delivered with normal hemoglobin levels, at mature gestation, without fetal or neonatal transfusion. In the majority of cases, the fetus was proven not to have the antigen in question, while in five cases the fetus was antigen-positive but did not require transfusion. None of these fetuses had any of the serious findings of accelerated alloimmune disease on serial examination.

Class 1 fetuses were all shown to have elevated ΔOD 450 on amniocentesis, in most cases in several samples. All fetuses in class 1 required treatment by IVT. All fetuses in this class were antigen-positive, Coombs' complete in <1 minute, had elevated serum bilirubin, and demonstrated progressive, accelerated loss of fetal hemoglobin on serial sampling. In six of these fetuses, initial cordocentesis values showed a normal hemoglobin con-

Class	Ultrasound Appearance				Abnormal BPS < 4/10
	Placenta	Ascites	Effusion	Anasarca	
0	−	−	−	−	−
1	+	−	−	−	−
2	+	+	−	−	−
3	+	+	+	+	−
4	+	+	+	+	+

Fig. 24–17. Ultrasound classification of alloimmune disease.

centration, with subsequent cordocenteses at intervals of 7 to 14 days demonstrating the need for initiation of therapy. None of these fetuses demonstrated fetal signs of accelerated disease, but almost all demonstrated increased amniotic fluid (>8.0 cm maximum vertical amniotic-fluid pocket depth) and loss of detailed placental architecture. Fetal hemoglobin in these fetuses ranged from 120 g/L, the threshold for initiating transfusion, to as low as 52 g/L in a fetus at 31 6/7th weeks. In that particular patient, the placenta was grossly edematous, but the fetus demonstrated no other signs of accelerated disease. For this class, the mean hemoglobin at first sampling was 96 g/L. In cases where serial fetal abdominal circumference measurements were available, two thirds showed a rise in percentile rank of 20 or more. Subjective evidence of hepatomegaly was cited in one half.

Class 2 fetuses have been described as "mild hydrops." The findings include hydramnios and loss of placental architecture, with a trend toward an increased placental thickness, a homogeneous placental appearance, and a uterine shape which is spherical as opposed to oval in cross-section, signifying an increase in uterine tone. The fetus demonstrates ascites of varying extent, the minimum threshold for diagnosis of ascites being 5 mm of transverse fluid rim width. Fetuses in this group do not have generalized body edema, with maximum occipital scalp thickness <7 mm. Fetal behavior is normal, with a BPS of 8/8 or 10/10. Fetal hemoglobin in these fetuses ranges from 32 to 66 g/L at first sample. In all cases of class 2 disease, the ascites reversed promptly (mean 11 days) and fetal appearance did not deteriorate into class 3 or 4, once IVT was initiated. As seen in Fig. 24–18, there is significant overlap with class 1 disease and classes 3 and 4 (as discussed below). Peripheral smears of blood from these fetuses contain few if any erythroblasts.

Class 3 fetuses have very severe-appearing fetal disease. This includes massive fetal ascites, scalp edema, skin edema, digital and facial edema, of the extent illustrated in Figs. 24–8 through 24–13. Despite this accelerated disease, and very low hemoglobins ranging from 22 g/L at 20 weeks to 56 g/L at 30 weeks, these

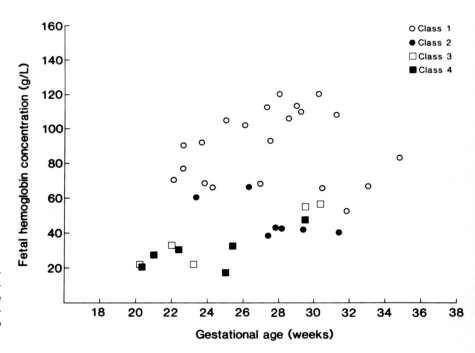

Fig. 24–18. Distribution plot of fetal hemoglobin concentration at time of first fetal blood sampling. Note the wide range covered by class 1 (nonhydropic) fetal disease. There is also significant overlap among classes 2, 3 and 4.

fetuses maintained normal PO_2 and normal pH, evidenced by normal BPSs. In all cases where serial IVT was carried out, normal BPS was maintained and intact survival was achieved. In one case, traumatic exsanguination occurred during the first IVT, and intracardiac fetal transfusion failed to resuscitate the fetus. Class 3 disease tends to occur earlier, and therefore requires an increased number of procedures compared with class 2. As experience accumulates, the differentiation of class 2 from class 3 disease may become less distinct.

Class 4 is clearly differentiated from any of the other classes by the absence of fetal behavior. The fetus hangs completely limp, although posture may be stiffened to some extent by the extreme nature of peripheral edema. These fetuses constitute a fetal emergency. Delay of even a few hours may result in an irretrievable level of acidosis and hypoxemia. In fact, the only fetal death among these class 4 infants was a fetus whose pH was 6.95 in the umbilical vein on first entry of the needle. Despite pH as low as 7.11, and fetal hemoglobin levels as low as 17 g/L, the majority of these fetuses can be salvaged.

This above classification is presented not in the hope of imposing a rigid categorization of fetal disease on the reader, but to illustrate that certain appearances may correlate reasonably well with the more "objective data." It is obvious that there is significant overlap among fetuses with similar classifications of disease, and that one could not by any means predict fetal hemoglobin on the basis of ultrasound appearance. It is a clinical reality that more severe disease correlates with a poorer prognosis. Taken from another point of view, fetal hemoglobin does not necessarily indicate the depth of disease to which the fetus has dropped.

The considerable overlap between classes of disease, groups of hemoglobin measurements, or depictions of fetal blood smear evaluation, simply emphasizes the importance of gathering all available data before assigning prognosis, determining management plans, or electing delivery over intrauterine management.

DOPPLER ULTRASOUND

As with many issues in fetal monitoring, the use of Doppler ultrasound is rapidly expanding in alloimmune disease. At the present time, much research is being carried out, and reports are relatively few.[17,38,39] In this area, the reader may well be advised to undertake a current review, rather than to rely on this chapter to give complete information. Detailed comment on some aspects, however, is possible. Several reviews have demonstrated a correlation with higher-than-usual velocities in umbilical arteries when the fetus is anemic. These higher velocities in systole and, in some studies diastole as well,

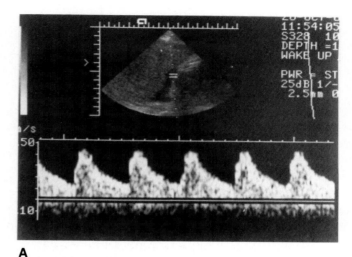

A

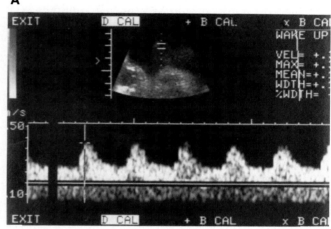

B

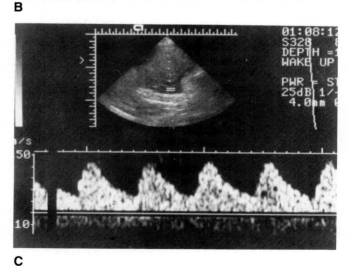

C

Fig. 24–19. Umbilical vein velocity waveforms from 30-week fetu at time of IVT No. 4. **A.** Pretransfusion. Hemoglobin 96 g/L. **B.** A the 90-mL mark of the transfusion. **C.** 18 hours posttransfusior Hemoglobin 190 g/L. There are significant changes in **B**, probabl related to the large volume expansion given over only 20 minute: Despite doubling of the hematocrit, the pretransfusion and pos transfusion waveforms are virtually identical.

are evidenced in elevated velocity waveform indices such as the Porcelot ratio (PR) and the systolic:diastolic ratio (SDR).

In our experience, neither ratio is of much use in predicting hemoglobin levels posttransfusion or at any time in the subsequent course of fetal management. The correlations are too vague to rely on Doppler patterns to defer therapy, or to reschedule a transfusion at an earlier time, with the present level of data. The lack of correlation between blood viscosity (as largely determined by particle density or hematocrit) and PR or SDR is striking.[40] Nearly half the fetuses transfused with large quantities of densely-packed donor blood showed no change whatsoever in Doppler velocity waveform indices. Both PR and SDR remained unchanged in 45% of infants who received additions of 40 to 60% to their blood volume over a period of as little as 5 1/2 minutes, and on average, 14 minutes. This volume load, taken in context of donor blood which measured 255 to 310 g/L in concentration, meant that the thickness of fetal blood was increased on average 100%. Even in the face of these serious volume and viscosity challenges, fetal blood flow varied little (Fig. 24–19).

This does not refute the use of Doppler ultrasound, of course, but suggests that the cardiovascular status of fetuses in all but the most moribund state is able to accept such changes without significant disruption.

Doppler ultrasound is an invaluable tool in identifying the course of fetal vessels, in excluding the presence of loops of fetal cord within amniotic fluid spaces, and in surveillance of the occasional fetus with a cord hematoma at the time of IVT. A growing conviction that Doppler ultrasound identifies fetuses at risk for IUGR/hypoxemic intrauterine compromise means its addition to the regime for fetal monitoring described under the heading, "Biophysical Profile Scoring," above.[41,42]

The normal Doppler velocity waveform pattern illustrated in Fig. 24–19.A. might be reassuring, but we have yet to observe a critical role for Doppler in observation or management of fetuses severely affected by alloimmune disease. Absent end-diastolic velocities (pathognomonic of abnormal blood flow in other groups of fetuses) have not been seen in association with the acidosis and profound anemia of class 3 and 4 disease. Because the technique is still in the process of development, it would be foolish to make rigid statements at the time of writing.

INVASIVE FETAL PROCEDURES

Indications
Mandatory indications for fetal blood sampling include confirmation of a therapeutic-range ∆OD 450 (either a single high zone III fluid or an inevitable progression of serial measurements >80% of zone II) or any hydropic class of fetal disease. Relative indications for cordocentesis can be summarized to reflect any situation in which (1) there may be a large discrepancy between ∆OD 450 and fetal hemoglobin, or (2) cordocentesis may be safer than amniocentesis. Situation (1) includes any mother with historically demonstrated virulent antibody, or when there is a recent dramatic rise in titer, suggesting the possibility of fetal hemolytic crisis.[43] If a placenta-free route for the amniocentesis is not available, cordocentesis should be considered at any gestation (situation 2). This will frequently be up to the ultrasonographer to decide.

Cordocentesis
Fetal blood sampling by cordocentesis is always diagnostic in nature, but in many cases, the need for immediate transfusion will be quite evident. All cases of hydropic disease, for example, should be transfused at the same time the initial fetal blood sample is obtained. Thus, a team approach is essential in organizing these procedures. If it is likely that the fetus will require transfusion immediately (all hydropic disease, highly suggestive ∆OD 450s, very aggressive history, and so forth), then the procedure is done in tandem with an initial fetal transfusion. With nonhydropic disease, cordocentesis is generally done as a solitary procedure with transfusion to follow later as indicated. For cordocentesis as a solitary procedure, light maternal sedation is used only if the placenta is posterior and prophylactic antibiotics are not routinely employed.

The cord insertion is identified meticulously, as shown in Fig. 24–20, making full use of the "zoom" feature on the ultrasound instrument. Although the experience of the operators is key, there is no substitute for a high-resolution ultrasound machine. The curvilinear array is particularly popular in Europe and in some centers in North America.[44,45] It would appear from close review of the literature that no particular scan head offers distinct advantages over another. Location of the insertion of the cord into the placenta may include manipulation of the mother or the fetus to obtain better views (Fig. 24–21). Doppler ultrasound may be effective in distinguishing maternal vascular spaces from fetal vessels along the placental surface. In general, however, insistence on an "ideal" cord insertion, 0.5 to 1.0 cm above the surface, will resolve this problem.

The technique described is that used at the University of Manitoba for all cordocenteses, as well as intrauterine transfusion procedures. There are many variations.[10,44–46] This routine has been applied to more than 300 intrauterine procedures over the past 2 years. Two operators perform the procedure, one manipulating

many of them associated with ultrasound-facilitated care, deserves further attention.

REFERENCES

1. Bowman JM. Maternal blood group immunization. In: Creasy RK, Resnik R, eds. *Maternal—Fetal Medicine: Principles and Practice.* 2nd ed. Philadelphia: WB Saunders; 1989:613–649.

2. Wenk RE, Goldstein P, Felix JK. Kell alloimmunization, hemolytic disease of the newborn, and perinatal management. *Obstet and Gynecol.* 1985;66:473–476.

3. Bowell PJ, Brown SE, Inskip MJ. The significance of anti-c alloimmunization in pregnancy. *Br J Obstet Gynecol.* 1986;93:1044–1048.

4. Bowman JM, Harman CR, Manning FA, Pollock JM. Severe erythroblastosis fetalis produced by anti-cellano. *Vox Sang.* 1989;56:187–189.

5. Harman CR, Manning FA. Alloimmune disease. In: Pauerstein CJ, ed. *Clinical Obstetrics.* New York: John Wiley: 1987;441–469.

6. Bowman JM. Blood group immunization in obstetric practice. *Curr Probl Obstet Gynecol.* 1983;7:1.

7. Bowman JM, Pollock JM. Transplacental fetal hemorrhage after amniocentesis. *Obstet Gynecol.* 1985;66:749–754.

8. Nicolaides KH, Rodeck CH, Mibashan RS, Kemp JR: Have Liley charts outlived their usefulness? *Am J Obstet Gynecol.* 1986;155:90.

9. Harman CR, Bowman JM, Menticoglou SM, Manning FA. Ultrasound classification of fetal alloimmune disease. Correlation with fetal hematology. *Proc Soc Perinat Obstet.* Abstract 19. New Orleans: Feb, 1989.

10. Reece EA, Copel JA, Scioscia AL, Grannum PAT, DeGennaro N, Hobbins JC. Diagnostic fetal umbilical blood sampling in the management of isoimmunization. *Am J Obstet Gynecol.* 1988;159:1057–1062.

11. Harman CR, Bowman JM, Pollock JM, Lewis M. Maternal antibody responses to invasive intrauterine fetal procedures. *Vox Sang.* In press.

12. Bowell PJ, Selinger M, Ferguson J, Giles J, MacKenzie IZ. Antenatal fetal blood sampling for the management of alloimmunized pregnancies: Effect upon maternal anti-D potency levels. *Br J Obstet Gynecol.* 1988;95:759–764.

13. Harman CR. Comprehensive examination of the human fetus. *Fet Med Rev.* In press.

14. Harman CR. Specialized applications of obstetric ultrasound: Management of the alloimmunized pregnancy. *Seminars in Perinatology.* 1985;9:184.

15. Nicolaides KH, Fontanarosa M, Gabbe SG, Rodeck CH. Failure of ultrasonographic parameters to predict the severity of fetal anemia in rhesus isoimmunization. *Am J Obstet Gynecol.* 1988;158:920.

16. Harman CR, Bowman JM, Manning FA, Lange IR, Menticoglou S, Johnson J. Moribund alloimmune hydrops: Intravascular fetal transfusion is the only hope. Vancouver, BC: June, 1988. *Proc Soc Obstet Gynecol.*

17. Copel JA, Grannum PA, Belanger K, Green J, Hobbins JC. Pulsed Doppler flow-velocity waveforms before and after intrauterine intravascular transfusion for severe erythroblastosis fetalis. *Am J Obstet Gynecol.* 1988;158:768–774.

18. DeVore GR. The prenatal diagnosis of congenital heart disease: A practical approach for the fetal sonographer. *J Clin Ultrasound.* 1985;13:229–245.

19. Nicolaides KH, Warenski JC, Rodeck CH. The relationship of fetal plasma protein concentration and hemoglobin level to the development of hydrops in rhesus isoimmunization. *Am J Obstet Gynecol.* 1985;152:341–344.

20. Harman CR, Bowman JM, Manning FA, Lange IR, Menticoglou S, Johnson J. Intravascular fetal transfusion: Integration into a successful Rh program. Vancouver, BC: June, 1988. *Proc Soc Obstet Gynecol.*

21. Harman CR. Fetal monitoring in the alloimmunized pregnancy. In: Smith MK, ed. *Clinics in Perinatology.* Philadelphia: WB Saunders; 1989.

22. Frigoletto FD, Greene MF, Benacerraf BR, Barss VA, Saltzman DH. Ultrasonographic fetal surveillance in the management of the isoimmunized pregnancy. *N Engl J Med.* 1986;430:432.

23. Hadlock FP, Deter RL, Harrist RB, Park SK. Estimating fetal age: Computer-assisted analysis of multiple fetal growth parameters. *Radiology.* 1984;152:497–501.

24. Benacerraf BR, Frigoletto FD. Sonographic sign for the detection of early fetal ascites in the management of severe isoimmune disease without intrauterine transfusion. *Am J Obstet Gynecol.* 1985;152:1039–1041.

25. Hashimoto BE, Filly RA, Callen PW. Fetal pseudoascites: Further anatomic observations. *J Ultrasound Med.* 1986; 5:151.

26. DeVore GR, Donnerstein RI, Kleinman CS, et al. Fetal echocardiography. II. The diagnosis and significance of a pericardial effusion in the fetus using real-time–directed M-mode ultrasound. *Am J Obstet Gynecol.* 1982;144:693–701.

27. Harman CR, Bowman JM. Intraperitoneal fetal transfusion. In: Chervenak F, Isaacson G, Campbell S, eds. *Textbook of Ultrasound in Obstetrics and Gynecology.* Boston: Little, Brown; 1988.

28. Vintzileos AM, Campbell WA, Storlazzi E, Mirochnick MH, Escoto DT, Nochimson DJ. Fetal liver ultrasound measurements in isoimmunized pregnancies. *Obstet Gynecol.* 1986;68:162–167.

29. Manning FA, Menticoglou S, Harman CR, Morrison I, Lange IR. Antepartum fetal risk assessment: The role of the fetal biophysical profile score. *Bailliere's Clin Obstet Gynecol.* 1987;1:55–72.

30. Manning FA, Morrison IR, Harman CR, Lange I, Menticoglou S. The fetal biophysical profile score: Functional practical aspects. *Contemp Issues Obstet Gynecol.* 1988; 3:83–92.

31. Harman CR, Manning FA, Bowman JM, Lange IR, Menticoglou SM. Use of intravascular transfusion to treat hydrops fetalis in a moribund fetus. *Can Med Assoc J.* 1988; 138:827–830.

32. Menticoglou SM, Harman CR, Manning FA, Bowman JM. Intraperitoneal fetal transfusion: Paralysis inhibits red cell absorption. *Fetal Therapy.* In press.

33. Chitkara U, Wilkins I, Lynch L, Mehalek K, Berkowitz RL. The role of sonography in assessing severity of fetal anemia in Rh- and Kell-isoimmunized pregnancies. *Obstet Gynecol.* 1988;71:393–398.

34. Harman CR, Bowman JM, Menticoglou SM, Pollock JM, Manning FA. Profound fetal thrombocytopenia in Rhesus disease: Serious hazard at intravascular transfusion. *Lancet.* 1988;2:741–742.

35. DeVore GR, Mayden K, Tortora M, Berkowitz R, Hobbins JC. Dilatation of the fetal umbilical vein in rhesus hemolytic anemia: A predictor of severe disease. *Am J Obstet Gynecol.* 1981;141:464.

36. Witter FR, Graham D. The utility of ultrasonically measured umbilical vein diameters in isoimmunized pregnancies. *Am J Obstet Gynecol.* 1983;146:225.

37. Reece EA, Gabrielli S, Abdalla M, O'Connor TZ, Hobbins JC. Reassessment of the utility of fetal umbilical vein diameter in the management of isoimmunization. *Am J Obstet Gynecol.* 1988;159:937–938.

38. Rightmire DA, Nicolaides KH, Rodeck CH, Campbell S. Fetal blood velocities in Rh isoimmunization: Relationship to gestational age and to fetal hematocrit. *Obstet Gynecol.* 1986;68:233–236.

39. Fairlie F, Lang GD, Lowe G, Walker JJ, Sibai BM. Blood viscosity and umbilical artery flow velocity waveform pulsatility index. New Orleans: Feb. 1989. *Proc Soc Perinat Obstet.* Abstract 286.

40. Harman CR. Doppler velocity waveform analysis before and after intravascular fetal transfusion. Quebec, Canada: 1989. *Proc Soc Obstet Gynecol.*

41. Trudinger BJ, Giles WB, Cook CM, Bombardieri J, Collins L. Fetal umbilical artery flow velocity waveforms and placental resistance: Clinical significance. *Br J Obstet Gynecol.* 1985;92:23–30.

42. Trudinger B. Doppler ultrasound assessment of blood flow. In: Creasy RK, Resnik R, eds. *Maternal–Fetal Medicine: Principles and Practice.* 2nd ed. Philadelphia: WB Saunders; 1989:254–267.

43. Pollock JM, Bowman JM, Manning FA, Harman CR. Fetal blood sampling in Rh hemolytic disease. *Vox Sang.* 1987; 53:139–142.

44. Daffos F, Capella-Pavlovsky M, Forestier F. Fetal blood sampling during pregnancy with use of a needle guided by ultrasound: A study of 606 consecutive cases. *Am J Obstet Gynecol.* 1985;153:655–660.

45. Nicolaides KH. Cordocentesis. *Clin Obstet Gynecol.* 1988; 31:123–135.

46. Weiner CP. Cordocentesis. *Obstet Gynecol Clin N Am.* 1988;15:283–301.

47. deCrespigny LCh, Robinson HP, Quinn M, Doyle L, Ross A, Cauchi M. Ultrasound-guided fetal blood transfusion for severe rhesus isoimmunization. *Obstet Gynecol.* 1985; 66:529.

48. Nicolaides KH, Soothill PW, Clewell W, Rodeck CH, Campbell S. Rh disease: Intravascular fetal blood transfusion by cordocentesis. *Fetal Therapy.* 1986;1:185.

49. Westgren M, Selbing A, Stangenberg M. Fetal intracardiac transfusions in patients with severe rhesus isoimmunization. *Br Med J.* 1988;296:885–886.

50. Harman CR, Manning FA, Bowman JM, Lange IR, Menticoglou S, Johnson J. Intravascular fetal transfusion: Technical aspects. Vancouver, BC: June 1988. *Proc Soc Obstet Gynecol.*

51. Harman CR, Bowman JM, Manning FA, Menticoglou SM. Intrauterine fetal transfusion. Intraperitoneal versus intravascular approaches: A case-controlled comparison. Quebec, Canada: June, 1989. *Proc Soc Obstet Gynecol.*

52. Watts DH, Lathy DA, Benedetti TJ, Cyr DA, Easterling TR, Hickok D. Intraperitoneal fetal transfusion under direct ultrasound guidance. *Obstet Gynecol.* 1988;71:84.

53. Moise KH, Carpenter RJ Jr, Kirshon B, et al. Comparison of four types of intrauterine transfusion technique for the treatment of red cell alloimmunization. New Orleans: Feb, 1989. *Proc Soc Perinat Obstet.* Abstract 187.

54. Barss VA, Benacerraf BR, Greene MF, Frigoletto FD: Use of a small-gauge needle for intrauterine fetal transfusions. *Am J Obstet Gynecol.* 1986;155:1057–1058.

55. Harman CR, Manning FA, Bowman JM, Lange IR: Severe Rh disease—poor outcome is not inevitable. *Am J Obstet Gynecol.* 1983;145:823–829.

56. Poissonnier M-H, Brossard Y, Demedeiros N, et al. Two hundred intrauterine exchange transfusions in severe blood incompatibilities. *Am J Obstet Gynecol.* 1989;161:709–713.

57. Grannum PAT, Copel JA, Moya FR, et al. The reversal of hydrops fetalis by intravascular intrauterine transfusion in severe isoimmune fetal anemia. *Am J Obstet Gynecol.* 1988; 158:914–919.

25 Dynamic Ultrasound-Based Fetal Assessment: The Fetal Biophysical Profile Score

Frank A. Manning

The development and perfection of specific and accurate diagnostic tests for identification of the fetus at risk for death or damage in utero has long been a major challenge and elusive goal for obstetricians and perinatologists. In recent years, several parallel and cogent developments within the obstetric community and the community at large have added further impetus to research in methods of fetal risk assessment. In general, the practice of obstetrics, and fetal medicine in particular, has shifted away from reliance on nonspecific maternal clinical markers of potential fetal disease such as fundal height measurements and subjective or perceived measurement of fetal activity, toward more specific and direct examination of the fetus per se. The evolution of diagnostic ultrasound from single-line display through composite B-mode display, and to high-resolution real-time B-mode display, and the concomitant development of Doppler ultrasound from instruments that detect only gross movement to highly specialized instruments creates a technologic base on which knowledge of fetal medicine may be expanded.

Medical and surgical advances in the care of maternal diseases such as hypertension and diabetes during pregnancy have led to a greater understanding of the influence of disease processes on the developing fetus. In turn, this created the need for better discrimination of the fetus at risk. The great advances in neonatal care in recent years have continued to lower the gestational age at which premature birth can result in a viable neonate. The well-recognized phenomenon that perinatal asphyxia greatly reduces the probability of neonatal survival at any age, and that this effect is greatest in the immature neonate, calls for a highly accurate determination of fetal condition. Finally, societal and consumer demands and expectations have served to spur the development of accurate diagnostic tests to determine immediate fetal health and future risk. Currently, small family size and higher maternal age at first pregnancy may increase anxiety about the well-being of progeny. This and other factors may also encourage research efforts toward development of diagnostic tests of fetal condition.

Historically, early attempts at identification of markers of fetal disease were based on biochemical analysis of maternal biologic fluids. A variety of compounds were measured, including peptide hormones such as human placental lactogen; enzymes such as placental alkaline phosphatase and leucine aminopeptidase (oxytocinase); steroids such as progesterone, estriol, estrone, estetral, and total estrogen; and specific proteins such as alpha fetoprotein. The concentrations of each and the variation over time were related to clinical outcome. With time and cumulative clinical experience, these tests, at least as markers of fetal asphyxia, have been abandoned and replaced by more specific and direct fetal biophysical indices of fetal condition. The major reason for this shift has been because the association between changes in the given substance and outcome, although apparent in population statistics, became very difficult to interpret in the individual case. Explained another way, the specificity and sensitivity of the earlier biochemical markers pale when compared to those reported with biophysical indices. The extent of shift in technologies has been dramatic and profound. Prior to the introduction of fetal biophysical profile scoring at the University of Manitoba, over 10,000 estriol determinations were done yearly. By the second year of the program using fetal biophysic indices, estriol measurement fell to less than 100 per year. Currently, virtually no estriol analyses are done. This shift from maternal biochemical to fetal biophysical testing was associated with a substantial and sustained fall in perinatal mortality of up to 60%.[1]

The impact of high-resolution dynamic ultrasound imaging on the development of the science of fetology cannot be overestimated. A principal tenet of the author is that the ability to "see" the fetus and its environment, and to monitor fetal activities and responses to intrinsic and extrinsic stimuli, shifts the factual and psychologic basis of the practice of fetal medicine profoundly. With this technologic advance comes greater recognition of disease and the opportunity to effect treatment, and in some cases, to cure. The ability to visualize the fetus and its activities allows for application of the time-honored principle of physical examination, albeit indirect, creating the emerging concept of the "fetus as a patient." A second major tenet is that on a wider scale, the growing ability to accurately catalogue fetal responses to potentially detrimental maternal disease states (such as hypertension) expands our understanding of the mechanisms by which maternal condition influences fetal health. It then becomes possible to specifically identify and accurately differentiate fetal risk from maternal risk. This allows the abandonment of a universal or generalized management approach to obstetric problems, that of routine delivery of all fetuses after 42 weeks' gestation. A more selective approach can be taken based on fetal risk such as delivery of all postmature fetuses when signs of compromise (such as oligohydramnios) are observed.[2,3] The potential impact of such a management scheme on reducing iatrogenic maternal and fetal disease is both obvious and substantiated.[2,3]

As a result of advances in dynamic ultrasound imaging, the number of fetal biophysical variables that may be studied and monitored in the human fetus is enormous. They range from monitoring such gross activities as fetal body and breathing movements[4-6] to estimation of sleep state by monitoring lens motion in the fetal eye,[7] and from such simple measurements as recording fetal heart rate[8] to such complex measurements as flow determination in umbilical vessels.[9] Monitoring specific organ system function, such as the frequency and character of peristalsis, or urine production rates and micturition is now possible.[10] Assessment is now routinely possible of the intrauterine environment including qualitative amniotic fluid volume determination,[3,11,12] placental architecture and pathology,[13,14] and cord position.[15] In general, it may be stated that the limitations in obtaining direct and indirect information about the fetus and its environment are more the result of practical clinical time constraints than of technical ability. This burgeoning source of fetal information, although exciting, requires some degree of pragmatic organization in order to be of clinical value. Whereas it seems obvious that reliance on any simple test (ie, antepartum heart rate testing) to detect a myriad of potential fetal diseases is inappropriate in the light of current development, monitoring of all possible variables is so time-consuming as to be prohibitive. It seems likely that by cumulative experience, a battery of simultaneous observations producing results falling within accepted limits of accuracy and clinical testing time will evolve. Fetal biophysical profile scoring, as described herein, is one such attempt.[16] The sound principle on which this method is based is that the greatest accuracy in differentiation of the normal from the compromised fetus is achieved when multiple fetal and environmental parameters are considered in concert.

FETAL DISEASE PROCESSES: BASIC CONSIDERATIONS

In general, serious fetal disease, although of diverse etiologies, may be categorized into three main groupings according to pathophysiologic process. These are: (1) fetal asphyxial states (either acute or chronic), (2) developmental or functional anomalies, or both, and (3) acquired disease due to exposure to noxious agents such as maternal antibody (isoimmunization syndromes), infectious organism (eg, cytomegalic inclusion disease), or alteration in the uterine environment (eg, transplacental hemorrhage, rupture of membranes). In the untested population, fetal asphyxial states are the most common cause of fetal death or damage (50 to 60%), followed by developmental anomalies (25 to 30%) and acquired diseases (15 to 20%).[17] The relative proportion of fetal death or damage attributed to any of these general categories can be expected to change in accordance with the extent and degree of sophistication of fetal surveillance methods. Recognition of fetal asphyxia may permit intervention and prevention of fetal death, whereas prenatal recognition of developmental anomalies presents fewer opportunities for therapeutic intervention. This phenomenon was observed in a study of 12,620 high-risk pregnancies monitored by fetal biophysical profile scoring.[1] In this study population, the overall fetal death rate fell significantly as did the asphyxial fetal death rate, whereas the relative proportion of death due to anomaly more than doubled. Specific testing methods, including dynamic ultrasound, may be used in the identification of the major disease category and may also be used to monitor the extent and progression of the disease process. In the fetus with developmental anomalies, classification of disease in accordance with prognosis, progression, fetal maturity, and the availability of treatment has proven useful in devising management strategies (Table 25–1).[18]

Monitoring of fetal biophysical activities plays a critical role in the identification of the asphyxiated fetus. Fetal asphyxial states define a spectrum of conditions ranging from transient episodes of hypoxemia without associated acidosis to sustained hypoxemia with associated metabolic or respiratory acidosis. Asphyxia in the fetus, as in the extrauterine patient, produces effects on multiple organ systems and, therefore, the signs of asphyxia are multiple and diverse. The degree of manifestation of these signs will vary with the extent, duration, and chronicity of the asphyxial insult. Fetal hypoxemia and acidosis, either alone or in combination, produce reflex changes in distribution of cardiac output, the extent and duration of which will vary with the nature of the insult. The fetus retains a unique ability to redistribute its cardiac output away from organ systems nonvital to fetal life (lung, kidney, gut, skeleton) toward vital organs

TABLE 25–1. CLASSIFICATION OF CONGENITAL ANOMALIES BY MANAGEMENT PRINCIPLES

Class	Prognosis	Progressive	Pulmonary Maturity	Recommended Management	Examples[a]
I	Good	No	Not applicable	Expectant; intervene for obstetric indication	Arrested hydrocephalus, intermittent cardiac arrhythmia
II	Survival with treatment	Yes	Yes	Deliver; neonatal treatment	Uretero-pyloric obstructive disease, arrhythmia with failure, chylothorax, nonimmune hydrops, hydrocephalus
III	Survival with treatment	Yes	Immature	R/O other anomalies; intrauterine treatment	Distal obstructive uropathy, arrhythmia with failure, hydrocephalus (aqueduct stenosis)
IV	Hopeless	Not applicable	Not applicable	Observation only; no intervention for fetal indications	Anencephaly, hypoplastic left ventricle, E-trisomy, D-trisomy, renal agenesis

[a] A partial list.

(the fetal heart, brain, adrenals, and placenta) (Fig. 25–1). This protective redistribution of cardiac output is reflex in origin, resulting from hypoxemic or acidemic stimulation of aortic body chemoreceptors.[19,20] With sustained or strong stimulus, the extent of this redistribution may be profound, resulting in near total cessation of perfusion of the fetal lung and kidney, while brain and placental flow increase substantially. Prolonged or repetitive stimuli initiating the redistribution reflex may result in diminished amniotic fluid production due to decreased urine production and lung liquid flow. Clinical correlates of oligohydramnios and fetal asphyxia are described elsewhere.[11] Asphyxial-induced oligohydramnios may further compound the extent of fetal asphyxia by rendering the umbilical cord more vulnerable to compression forces.

The pathologic and pathophysiologic sequelae of intrauterine asphyxia in the fetal brain depend on the nature and duration of the asphyxial insult. The effect of acute total asphyxia and partial prolonged asphyxia on the fetal brain has been studied extensively in the subhuman primate fetus (*Macaca mulatta*) by Myers.[21]

In the human fetus, asphyxia commonly results from a chronic reduction in uteroplacental perfusion, aggravated by acute reduction in perfusion during uterine contractions including Braxton-Hicks contractions. Human fetal asphyxia may then be best viewed as a chronic progressive disease, the extent and rate of progression being

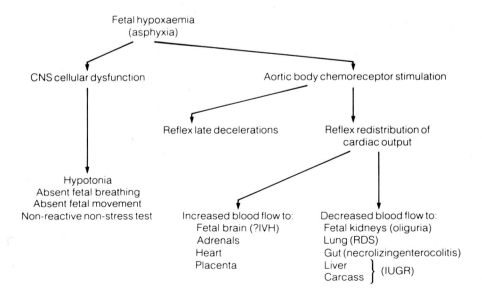

Fig. 25–1. A schematic representation of fetal responses to hypoxemia. Not included in this figure are endocrine responses, such as release of ADH from the posterior pituitary and catecholamine release from the adrenal medulla and other chromaffin tissue. Such endocrine responses may potentiate the reflex cardiovascular responses to hypoxemia.

variable and protean in nature. In this context, the monkey model of partial prolonged asphyxia closely approximates the human condition.[21] In the monkey fetus, partial prolonged asphyxia produces an initial increase in brain blood flow followed by a selective redistribution of cerebral flow such that cortical basal ganglia and thalamic blood flow decrease while brain stem perfusion remains unaltered or increases. Cerebral edema develops as a presumed result of translocation of brain fluid into the intracellular space. Carbon[14]-labeled antipyrine studies demonstrate focal and generalized reduction in perfusion of the cerebral cortex and basal ganglion.

Biophysical functional correlates of these pathologic processes can be observed in the human and animal fetus. Central nervous system hypoxemia or asphyxia, or both, even of a relatively minor degree, produce profound alterations in the frequency and patterning of biophysical activities and responses. Fetal hypoxemia in sheep, produced by administration of a hypoxic gas mixture to the ewe, consistently produces fetal apnea, which usually persists for some time after blood gas homeostasis of the fetus has been restored.[22] Human fetal correlates of this phenomenon have been observed. Maternal hypoxemia has been reported associated with prolonged fetal apnea.[23] Under some experimental conditions, maternal cigarette smoking has been shown to cause a fall in the incidence of fetal breathing movements[24,25] although this was not confirmed in other studies.[26] In the pregnant rhesus monkey model, cigarette smoke exposure produced a fall in fetal PO_2.[27] In fetal lambs, hypoxemia has been shown to produce a significant and sustained reduction in forelimb movement; once more, the persistence of this effect exceeded the duration of the hypoxic insult.[28] In fetal lambs and monkeys, hypoxemia results in loss of heart rate variability.[29,30] The effect of fetal hypoxia on biophysical coupling of heart rate acceleration with fetal movement has not been studied in animals, but a prolonged loss of the association has been noted in human fetuses exhibiting profound depression at birth.[31]

In summary, these observations in animal and human fetuses suggest that asphyxia may result in significant alteration in central nervous system (CNS) function and that this loss of function may be manifested by absence of normal biophysical variables. Because central nervous tissue is known to be among the tissues most sensitive to oxygen supply, it follows that observation of this organ's function and output may be an important indirect indicator of the state of fetal oxygenation. The temporal and functional characteristics of fetal CNS function after recovery from asphyxia are not well studied. It does appear, however, that recovery of function may be delayed relative to restoration of normal blood gases.[22,28] In contrast, in animal models the observation of return of normal biophysical activities after an asphyxial insult almost always indicates normal blood gas values.[22,28] Variations, if any, in sensitivity to hypoxemia/asphyxia of specific areas of brain tissue responsible for initiation of biophysical activities are largely unexplored, but are of major clinical interest. It is known, for example, that a fall in fetal PO_2 of as little as 6 mm Hg can induce apnea in fetal lambs and monkeys.[22,32,33] However, whether or not the same degree of hypoxemia alters other biophysical activities (eg, fetal tone or body movements), and to what extent, has not been studied in detail. Therefore, it is uncertain whether increasing degrees of hypoxemia result in progressive loss of given biophysical functions or whether, at a critical level of hypoxemia, all such functions are lost at or near the same time. Clinical observation in the human fetus suggests that a gradient response exists. For example, fetal breathing movements disappear early in the course of progressive hypoxemia, whereas fetal movements disappear with more advanced disease.[1,16]

The biophysical signs of fetal asphyxia may be grouped into two main categories according to their temporal relationships to the asphyxial insult. Changes in biophysical activities occurring during the insult and for some variable time afterward may be termed acute, or immediate, effects and include such changes as loss of breathing movements, tone, movement, heart rate reactivity, and variability. With continued experience it is likely that other changes such as alteration in state as reflected by eye movements, alteration in peristaltic patterns, loss of purposeful movements, and loss of evoked fetal reflex responses may be included in the assessment of the acute effects of hypoxemia. The changes in amniotic fluid volume related to the asphyxial insult take some time to develop and, therefore, may be termed chronic, or delayed, signs of fetal asphyxia.

The concept of multiple fetal biophysical variables monitoring to detect the presence or absence of fetal asphyxia is based on observation of these acute and chronic effects of asphyxia or organ function. By surveying the end result of specific organ function, the presence, extent, and duration (chronicity) of the insult may be approximated. A wide spectrum of results may be predicted depending on the severity and duration of the insult and the extent of recovery, if any, and the relationship between the time of insult and the time of observation. Initially, asphyxia will cause a loss of acute variables (breathing, movement, tone, heart rate reactivity) while amniotic fluid volume may be normal. Repeated episodes of hypoxemia with recovery between episodes may cause oligohydramnios while acute variables may be normal. Progressive and severe asphyxia will produce both oligohydramnios and absent acute biophysical variables. Such combined monitoring of biophysical variables has both theoretic and proven advantages over any single variable assessment technique.

BIORHYTHMS AND FETAL BIOPHYSICAL ACTIVITIES

Central nervous system energy output and activity are not constant events but vary in a nonrandom pattern. Fetal brain electrical activity, as measured by electrocortical leads, exhibits rhythmic variations in both frequency and intensity.[34] In general, an inverse relationship between the frequency and intensity of discharge is observed, resulting in two main patterns: (1) low-frequency–high-voltage pattern (quiet sleep pattern) and (2) high-frequency–low-voltage pattern (active sleep, rapid-eye-movement sleep). In the fetus, an alternative pattern of these sleep states over a 20- to 40-minute period is usually observed. These patterns of CNS energy are coupled with alterations in biophysical activities. For example, in quiet sleep, fetal breathing movements tend to be absent or infrequent, isolated, and of large amplitude (fetal sighing). During active sleep, bursts of fetal breathing movements of varying frequency and amplitude are observed.[34] Similarly, rapid fetal eye movements are infrequent during quiet sleep and are usually observed only during active sleep (hence the designation rapid-eye-movement sleep).[35]

The influence of sleep state on fetal biophysical activities is of major importance in the interpretation of fetal biophysical variable data. The observation of normal biophysical activities is indicative of a functional and therefore nonasphyxiated fetal CNS, rendering consideration of fetal sleep state unnecessary. In contrast, failure to recognize the presence of normal biophysical activities requires consideration of fetal sleep state. Both quiet sleep, a normal periodic fetal event, and fetal asphyxia, a pathologic fetal condition, can result in depression or absence of fetal biophysical activities. The clinical significance of each cause is vastly different. Differentiation of these effects is achieved by extending the observation period beyond the minimal expected time for pattern shift (20 minutes) or repeating the observation at some later point. In either case, subsequent observation of normal activities confirms normality, whereas persistent absence of activities suggests an asphyxial etiology.

Fetal biophysical activities, as a reflection of CNS activity and energy, provide a direct window to nervous tissue function as well as an important indirect clinical window to the state of fetal oxygenation. In the course of monitoring these variables, either alone or in combination, it becomes theoretically possible to detect the presence or absence of intrinsic and extrinsic factors that depress nervous activity, including fetal asphyxia, and to determine the duration and progression of these influences. Detection of asphyxia is for the most part done by exclusion, after ruling out absence of variables due to normal (intrinsic) CNS rhythms,[35] the presence of circulating CNS depressant agents acquired from the mother (eg, tranquilizers),[36] or major fetal CNS trauma. Loss of fetal biophysical activities, although the most common, is not the only expression of perinatal CNS response to injury. In the asphyxiated newborn, depressed or absent biophysical activities (such as spontaneous movement, generalized hypotonia, and failure to establish spontaneous respiration) are an initial response, frequently followed by increased abnormal movements (seizures) and hypertonia. The effect of long-term asphyxia on fetal biophysical activities remains conjectural. Seizure activity in the human fetus resulting from either severe asphyxia or in utero opiate withdrawal and characterized by repetitive episodes of clonic movement of all limbs has been observed.[37] Further, extreme degrees of fetal tachypnea (rate >140 breaths per minute) preceding fetal death have been observed in poorly controlled pregnant diabetic patients.[38] Prompt intervention in human fetuses with profound tachypnea may result in intact survival.[39] To date, prenatal recognition of postinjury hypertonia or loss of reflex activity has not been reported. Finally, it seems important to re-emphasize that, because the etiologies of fetal death and damage in utero are diverse, monitoring of only one system, the CNS, cannot predict all pathophysiologic processes. Prenatal screening for other serious disease processes such as developmental anomalies is a necessary adjunct to monitoring of biophysical activities.

This new information resource is beginning to create important changes in the practical and philosophical basis of the practice of perinatal medicine. Among these changes are the ones discussed below.

The presence of fetal disease is determined more accurately. The clinical significance of such determination for the affected fetus is obvious; the corollary of the statement may be of even greater clinical importance. Improved discrimination of the fetus who is *not* at immediate risk, even in the presence of risk factors in the mother, permits selective conservative management, thereby avoiding potential maternal and perinatal iatrogenic complication.

The progressive pathophysiology of fetal disease is defined with greater accuracy. Balancing of fetal versus neonatal risks remains an intrinsic part of perinatal management decisions. By knowing with considerable assurance the rate at which a perinatal disease process is progressing in a given fetus, a rational decision regarding the need for and timing of perinatal intervention can be reached. Consider for example the severely growth-retarded but immature fetus that exhibits functional biophysical signs of impending fetal death. In our center, we have intervened on behalf of such fetuses with birthweights of less than 600 g with intact perinatal survival. The alternate corollary is equally important clinically. In the immature growth-retarded fetus without any functional biophysical signs of immediate compromise, conservative management based on close fetal surveillance may permit continued maturation in utero, thereby reducing the risk of neonatal immaturity-related complications.

In some fetal disease states fetal prognosis may be assigned with certainty. The risks of perinatal management decisions must always be compared with maternal risks. For some fetal pathologic conditions, usually those involving developmental anomalies, a hopeless prognosis may be assigned with certainty. Consider for example the fetus with renal agenesis (Potter's syndrome). Classically, such fetuses present with early-onset severe intrauterine growth retardation and exhibit a high frequency of intrapartum fetal distress. In the absence of accurate forewarning, operative intervention with its attendant maternal risks may occur without any real or potential benefit for the fetus. The high incidence of fetal distress during labor in this and other anomalous fetal conditions is well described.[40] Further forewarning of fetal disease and expected prognosis can aid in decisions regarding where and when delivery should take place. In the fetus with a developmental anomaly for which either in utero or neonatal therapy is an option, referral to a center capable of providing the needed care may be lifesaving.

Disease specific testing schemes are becoming a practical reality. Until recently, the method selected for antepartum fetal surveillance and the frequency of testing have been determined by arbitrary criteria. Fitting such an arbitrary model to the spectrum of fetal disease and fetal disease progression has never been satisfactory. The reason some centers advocate weekly testing for the fetus whose mother is hypertensive remains unclear because the effect of this disease state on both mother and fetus is widely variable. A more rational approach would involve initial testing to determine fetal condition, then tailoring subsequent testing according to the change, if any, in maternal and fetal condition. Similarly, the application of one testing modality (eg, antepartum fetal cardiotachography) to all fetal diseases is not easily understood. In some conditions (eg, the postdate fetus), assessment of other biophysical markers of impending fetal trouble may yield superior information.[2,3] The concept of disease-specific testing, applicable to all forms of antepartum testing but best achieved with dynamic fetal ultrasound evaluation, implies consideration of both pathophysiologic characteristics and progression in selecting the method and frequency of antepartum testing. Consider again the postdate fetus (>42 completed weeks) in whom induction is difficult because of an unfavorable cervix. Frequent evaluation of amniotic fluid volume at least twice weekly may be the preferable method of man-

agement. The fetus severely affected by the alloimmunization syndrome is another example of this principle. In the isoimmunized fetus, except in extreme circumstance, antepartum fetal heart rate monitoring offers little insight into fetal condition and prognosis. In contrast, daily assessment by dynamic ultrasound allows determination of rate of change of physical signs (eg, ascites) of the disease process long before the fetal heart rate is affected.

Fetal biophysical profile scoring is a method of fetal risk surveillance based on a composite assessment of both acute and chronic markers of fetal disease. Because the method uses dynamic ultrasound monitoring, it also yields fetal morphologic and morphometric data as well as information on the contiguous fetal structures (placenta and umbilical cord). This envelope of fetal information is then interpreted within the clinical context to arrive at a management decision. The method may be viewed as performing a physical examination of the fetus, including determination of vital signs. Specific details of criteria for performing the test, interpretation of test results, and impact of this method on reducing perinatal mortality and morbidity in the at risk population are described below.

FETAL BIOPHYSICAL PROFILE SCORING

Method

In this center, fetal biophysical profile scoring is only used in referred patients with recognized high-risk factors. The gestational age at which testing is begun has been arbitrarily set at the minimal gestational age at which intervention would be considered should an abnormal result be encountered. Over the years since the inception of the program, the lower limit of age for testing has fallen as the probability of intact premature birth at lower gestational ages has improved. At the time of writing, the minimal gestational age for testing at this center is 25 weeks.

At each testing, in addition to the fetal biophysical profile score, fetal morphometric data are obtained (biparietal diameter, femur length, abdominal circumference), an anatomical screen for structural or functional anomaly is done, and the placenta and umbilical cord are assessed. The fetal biophysical profile score is obtained by components. First, variables recorded by dynamic ultrasound methods are assessed and coded numerically using a binary approach to variable recognition. Variables are coded as normal or abnormal according to fixed criteria, then assigned an arbitrary score of 2 if normal and 0 if abnormal (Table 25–2). The variable is coded as normal whenever the set criteria are reached, regardless of the duration of observation. However, in view of the well-

TABLE 25–2. BIOPHYSICAL PROFILE SCORING: TECHNIQUE AND INTERPRETATION

Biophysical Variable	Normal (Score = 2)	Abnormal (Score = 0)
Fetal breathing movements	At least 1 episode of FBM of at least 30 sec duration in 30-min observation	Absent FBM or no episode of >30 sec in 30 min
Gross body movements	At least 3 discrete body/limb movements in 30 min (episodes of active continuous movement considered as single movement)	2 or fewer episodes of body/limb movements in 30 min
Fetal tone	At least 1 episode of active extension with return to flexion of fetal limb(s) or trunk. Opening and closing of hand considered normal tone	Either slow extension with return to partial flexion or movement of limb in full extension. Absent fetal movement
Reactive fetal heart rate (FHR)	At least 2 episodes of FHR acceleration of >15 beats/min and of at least 15-sec duration associated with fetal movement in 30 min	Less than 2 episodes of acceleration of FHR or acceleration of >15 beats/min in 30 min
Qualitative amniotic fluid volume (AFV)	At least 1 pocket of AF that measures at least 2 cm in 2 perpendicular planes	Either no AF pockets or a pocket <2 cm in 2 perpendicular planes

FBM = fetal breathing movement; FHR = fetal heart rate; AFV = amniotic fluid volume; AF = amniotic fluid.

recognized variation in distribution of fetal biophysical activities,[41] a given dynamic variable must fall below set criteria for at least 30 minutes before being coded as abnormal.

Amniotic fluid volume is assessed using a semi-quantitative method: amniotic fluid volume is considered abnormal when the largest pocket of fluid measures less than 2 cm in two perpendicular axes. This represents a change from the previously used more stringent definition of oligohydramnios (vertical pocket <1 cm), and is based on an analysis of our ongoing experience (Fig. 25–2).

In the original method of fetal biophysical profile scoring, the presence or absence of fetal heart rate acceleration with fetal movements (a nonstress test [NST]) was done regardless of results obtained by dynamic ultrasound monitoring.[16] However, in a recent review of 26,257 tests among 12,620 referred high-risk patients, we noted the predictive accuracy of the four ultrasound-monitored variables, when normal, to be equal to that achieved by addition of the NST component.[16] This observation prompted a prospective study in which the NST was used only when one or more ultrasound variables were abnormal.[42] Because the results confirmed our hypothesis, we modified the profile scoring method so that the NST is used only when one or more of the ultrasound-monitored variables are abnormal. It remains our impression that in the presence of one or more abnormal

variables the NST adds valuable information to the decision-making process. Further, the additional information contained in the heart-rate record, such as the presence or absence of normal long-term variability and the presence or absence of periodic decelerations, may help in determining fetal condition and risk.

Clinical Interpretation

Antepartum fetal assessment by biophysical profile scoring is limited at present to referred patients with recognized maternal or fetal high-risk factors. Our working rule has been to begin the testing scheme when the results may be reasonably expected to influence clinical management. As a result of this policy, the gestational age at initial entry is progressively decreasing as improvements in neonatal survival increase. As mentioned, we accept patients from 25 weeks' gestation onward. The frequency of repeat testing is somewhat fluid, depending on initial and subsequent maternal and fetal condition. In general, however, we schedule repeat testing on a weekly basis for all except postdates, diabetic, and alloimmunized patients. The latter high-risk groups are seen at least twice weekly and, in some cases (severe Rh disease), are seen daily. Clinical management is based on the test score as interpreted, along with obstetric factors (eg, favorability of the cervix for induction), maternal condition and, if morbid, the extent and progression of maternal disease, and other fetal factors including

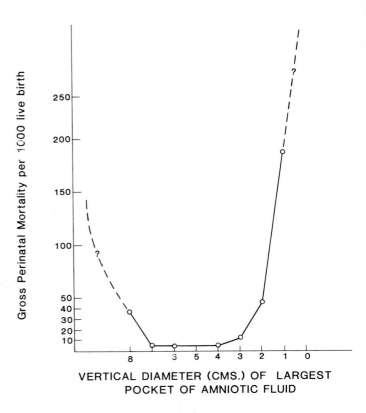

Fig. 25–2. Distribution among 7,562 high-risk patients of gross (uncorrected) perinatal mortality relative to the largest pocket of amniotic fluid recorded before delivery. Because perinatal mortality increases sharply at the 2-cm pocket level, we have modified the criteria for interpretation of decreased amniotic fluid volume accordingly. The rise in PNM with increased fluid (pocket >8 cm) is mostly due to associated anomalies whereas the PNM with decreased fluid (pocket <2 cm) is largely due to asphyxial complications. (*Reproduced with permission from Creasy R, Resnick P, eds.* Maternal-Fetal Medicine. *Philadelphia: 1984;203.*)

the presence or absence of anomalies and in selected cases confirmation of pulmonary maturity by amniotic fluid phospholipid profile (Table 25–3).

The fetal biophysical profile score provides an accurate estimate of the risk of fetal death in the immediate future. When this risk is low, as with a normal score, intervention is indicated only for obstetric or maternal factors. Thus, for example, in the postdate pregnancy with a favorable cervix (obstetric factor), we would induce labor regardless of the test score. In contrast, in the postdate fetus with a normal score whose mother had an unfavorable cervix, we would not induce labor but rely on serial fetal assessment. When an abnormal score, oligohydramnios, or both are encountered, we would induce labor regardless of the cervical favorability. With serious maternal disease (eg, preeclampsia), we would intervene despite a normal fetal biophysical score if the maternal condition were deteriorating. However, in the same patient with severe but stable disease, we would use a normal test score result to delay intervention until fetal maturity was certain and the cervix was favorable for induction. The presence of oligohydramnios in a normal fetus with functioning renal tissue, as evidenced by fetal bladder emptying and filling and with intact membranes, is always considered an indication for induction despite the presence of normal movement, breathing, tone, and heart-rate reactivity. This approach is based on an ex-

tensive review of the relationship of ultrasound-defined oligohydramnios to perinatal mortality,[11] and subsequent prospective study indicating intervention for oligohydramnios can improve perinatal outcome.[43] In the fetus with an equivocal test but normal fluid (score: 6 of 10), we advocate delivery of a mature fetus when the cervix is favorable. However, in the immature fetus or when the cervix is not favorable for induction, repeat testing is undertaken within 24 hours. If subsequent testing is normal, as will occur in 75% of instances, no intervention for fetal indication is contemplated. If the repeat test remains equivocal or becomes abnormal, intervention is indicated. In the fetus with abnormal score (<4 of 10), we would advocate immediate intervention unless there are recognized correctable compounding factors. Such factors might include a history of fetal trauma, an intrauterine condition for which treatment is possible (eg, Rh isoimmunization), maternal drug effects on the fetus (eg, recent narcotic or sedative administration), or when extreme fetal immaturity is certain (gestational age <25 weeks). The potential error for misinterpretation of the biophysical profile score has been outlined by Vintzileos and colleagues.[44]

Clinical Results

Clinical testing of the concept of fetal biophysical profile scoring began with a prospective blind clinical study in

TABLE 25–3. INTERPRETATION OF FETAL BIOPHYSICAL PROFILE SCORE RESULTS AND RECOMMENDED CLINICAL MANAGEMENT

Test Score Result	Interpretation	PNM[1] Within 1 wk Without Intervention	Management
10 of 10 8 of 10 (normal fluid) 8 of 8 (NST not done)	Risk of fetal asphyxia extremely rare	<1 per 1000	Intervention only for obstetric and maternal factors. No indication for intervention for fetal disease
8 of 10 (abnormal fluid)	Probable chronic fetal compromise	89 per 1000[11]	Determine that there is functioning renal tissue and intact membranes. If so, deliver for fetal indications
6 of 10 (normal fluid)	Equivocal test, possible fetal asphyxia	Variable	If the fetus is mature, deliver. In the immature fetus, repeat test within 24 hr. If <6/10 deliver.
6 of 10 (abnormal fluid)	Probable fetal asphyxia	89 per 1000[11]	Deliver for fetal indications
4 of 10	High probability of fetal asphyxia	91 per 1000[1]	Deliver for fetal indications
2 of 10	Fetal asphyxia almost certain	125 per 1000[1]	Deliver for fetal indications
0 of 10	Fetal asphyxia certain	600 per 1000[1]	Deliver for fetal indications

216 high-risk patients[16] and continues today with reported prospective studies involving more than 65,000 tests in more than 26,000 high-risk patients.[43–48] In the original blind study, the five components of the score were recorded serially and the relationship between the last test result and perinatal outcome was determined. Each variable of the score was also considered independently and related to outcome. The overall perinatal mortality for the study group was 50.9 per 1,000; the corrected mortality (achieved by exclusion of anomalous fetuses) was 32.4 per 1,000.[16] The false-negative rate (that is, stillbirth of a structurally normal fetus within 1 week of last normal test result) was lowest with normal fetal tone (6.9 per 1,000) and highest with a reactive NST (12.8 per 1,000). The positive predictive accuracy (that is, stillbirth within 1 week of last abnormal test result) was highest when fetal breathing movements were absent (115.5 per 1,000), and lowest when the NST was abnormal (58.5 per 1,000). Combining variables always improved all measures of test accuracy, which reached a maximum when all five variables were considered. In this blind study, the perinatal mortality ranged from nil when all variables were normal to 60% when all were abnormal. Intermediate score values yielded intermediate perinatal loss rates. This initial study, although confirming the clear relationship between test score and outcome, could not, by the nature of the blind study design, offer any insight

into whether or not intervention based on score results could reduce perinatal loss. Recent research efforts in our and other clinical testing laboratories have been directed to answering this critical question.

We began a prospective open study at our center in which test scores were used to guide management in referred high-risk pregnancies. The principal guidelines for score-based interventions are outlined in Table 25–3. We have used historic nonrandomized controls drawn from the same population, but not subjected to testing, with which the study group was compared. Within this control population, the perinatal mortality is 14.3 per 1,000, rising to 65 per 1,000 in the high-risk subsegment. In our initial prospective study of 1,184 high-risk patients, the observed perinatal mortality was 5.06 per 1,000.[45] In a larger subsequent published series, we reported outcome in 12,620 high-risk patients (26,257 tests). The gross perinatal mortality was 7.37 per 1,000; the corrected perinatal mortality rate (excluding lethal anomalies and severe isoimmunization syndromes) was 1.9 per 1,000.[11] The series is now expanded to include 19,212 patients (44,828 tests) and the gross perinatal mortality remains at less than 7 per 1,000; the corrected perinatal mortality is less than 2 per 1,000.[48] In a separate and independent study of the method, Baskett and associates[1] reported experience with 5,034 pregnancies (11,532 tests); the gross perinatal mortality rate was 7.6 per 1,000, the corrected rate was 3.1 per 1,000.[46] The stillbirth rate may be considered a more sensitive measure of test accuracy because it is not influenced by fetal age and maturity. In our series, the corrected stillbirth rate is 1.18 per 1,000, whereas in Baskett's series the corrected stillbirth rate was 0.95 per 1,000. Thus, this method of fetal assessment has produced a significant fall in perinatal mortality.

Combining series, the incidence of normal test score results in high-risk patients is 97.5% (43,707 of 44,828 tests), the incidence of equivocal results is 1.68% (735 of 44,828 tests) and of abnormal results is 0.82% (367 of 44,828 tests).[1,45] Because the expected death rate is approximately 14 per 1,000 (1.4%), this distribution of test scores approximates the actual incidence of disease. This improved fit of distribution of test scores to expected disease incidence (natural history) is achieved while maintaining a remarkably low false-negative rate (fetal death within one week of a normal score) (Fig. 25–3). In combined studies, 16 stillbirths of structurally normal fetuses with normal last score are reported among 23,396 patients, yielding a false-negative rate of 0.68 per 1,000.[46,48] This low rate of failure to identify the fetus at risk of dying has major clinical significance because it permits conservative management in the individual fetus, thereby reducing interventions with their attendant perinatal and

maternal risks. We consider the low-false negative rate with fetal biophysical profile scoring to be among its most significant advantages.

A comparison of the distribution of perinatal death by etiology among tested and nontested patients also lends support to the value of fetal biophysical profile scoring. In the study population in which management decisions were based on fetal biophysical profile score results, the distribution of the fewer deaths changed; 66.7% of deaths were due to lethal anomaly, 7.5% were due to alloimmunization syndrome, and 25.8% were due to asphyxia. In the untested population, 10% of deaths were due to lethal anomaly and 64% due to asphyxia-related causes. We interpret these differences to indicate that the relative rise in deaths attributed to lethal anomaly between the tested and untested groups (66.7% versus 10% respectively) is due to a reduction of asphyxial deaths in the tested population.

More recently we have studied the relationship of the last fetal biophysical profile score before delivery and the incidence of perinatal morbidity, defined collectively by the presence of any combination of a 5-minute Apgar score <7, intrauterine growth retardation (<3rd percentile for age and sex), operative delivery for fetal distress in labor, and an umbilical vein pH (at delivery) equal to or less than 7.20.[49] As shown in Fig. 25–4, perinatal morbidity as well as mortality rise progressively and in significant increments as the score decreases.

The concept of disease-specific testing by fetal biophysical profile scoring is new and just now undergoing clinical testing. Preliminary results are encouraging. Johnson and coworkers have studied the role of fetal biophysical profile scoring in the management of the post-date pregnancy and, more recently, in the pregnant diabetic. In each study, mortality and morbidity were sharply reduced from that expected.[2,50] Disease-specific testing using modified biophysical profile scoring is reported in patients with premature rupture of membranes[51] and twin pregnancies,[52] yielding good results. In ongoing studies, Harman and colleagues (unpublished data, 1988) have used fetal biophysical profile scoring as an adjunctive method for determining the timing of intrauterine treatment and delivery in the isoimmunized fetus. Although preliminary at present, the results are most encouraging. Anecdotally, in one case an Rh-isoimmunized mother with three previous hydropic fetal deaths presented, at 24 weeks, with repeat early fetal hydrops. Despite fetal intraperitoneal transfusion, the fetus continued to deteriorate. The fetal biophysical profile score, which was initially normal, became progressively more abnormal despite treatment, finally reaching a score of 2 of 10 (normal fluid only). An ultrasound-guided direct fetal umbilical vein sample revealed a hemoglobin of 4 g, of which 97% was donor. An immediate intravascular transfusion

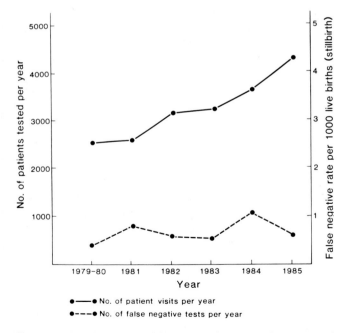

Fig. 25–3. The frequency of fetal death (corrected for anomaly) within 1 week of last normal fetal biophysical profile score, as recorded on an annual basis since 1979 in the fetal assessment program at the University of Manitoba. Despite an increase in case load and complexity, the negative predictive accuracy of the normal test remains relatively consistent and remarkably low (mean 0.68 deaths per 1,000 fetuses with a normal score).[48]

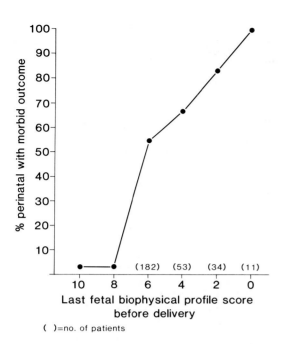

Fig. 25–4. The incidence of morbid perinatal outcome relative to the last fetal biophysical profile score recorded before delivery. Management was based on principles outlined in Table 25–3.

resulted in a rapid recovery in the profile score, reaching normal values within 1 day and remaining normal throughout the course of the pregnancy. Although we realize that any conclusion based on a single case can be fraught with error, this single experience does help to underscore the potential significance of the clinical testing method in the fetus with serious unstable disease.

SUMMARY

The advent of ultrasound fetal imaging and the evolution of dynamic imaging (real-time) methods have opened great new vistas in which fetal responses in health and disease may be monitored with remarkable precision and clarity. Contained within this new wealth of information may lie the key to direct determination of the fetus at risk for death or damage in utero. Consideration of fetal activities so plainly recognized by conventional dynamic ultrasound methods and an assessment of fetal environment appear to be integral parts of this process. We predict that although modification of the original concept of fetal biophysical profile scoring, most likely by addition of new variables, will occur, the fundamental principle

of the testing method will remain an essential aspect of fetal assessment.

REFERENCES

1. Manning FA, Morrison I, Lange IR, et al. Fetal assessment based on fetal biophysical profile scoring: Experience in 12,620 referred high risk pregnancies. I: Perinatal mortality by frequency and etiology. *Am J Obstet Gynecol.* 1985;151:343.

2. Johnson J, Harman CR, Lange IR, et al. Fetal biophysical profile scoring in the management of post-dates pregnancy: A prospective study. *Am J Obstet Gynecol.* In press.

3. Phelan JP, Platt LD, Yeh S. The role of ultrasound assessment of amniotic fluid volume in the management of the postdate pregnancy. *Am J Obstet Gynecol.* 1985;151:304.

4. Sanders RC, James AE Jr. Ultrasound: Fetal movements and fetal condition. In: Chamberlain PF, Manning FA. *Principles and Practice in Obstetrics and Gynecology.* 3rd ed. Norwalk, Conn: Appleton-Century-Crofts; 1984: 175–188.

5. Platt LD, Manning FA. Fetal breathing movements: An update. *Clin Perinat.* 1980;7:425.

6. Patrick JE, Challis JRG. Measurement of human fetal breathing in healthy pregnancies using realtime ultrasound. *Semin Perinatol.* 1980;4:275.

7. Martin CB Jr. On behavioural states in the human fetus. *J Reprod Med.* 1981;26:425.

8. Nochimson DJ, Turbeville JS, Terry JE, et al. The nonstress test. *Obstet Gynecol.* 1978;51:419.

9. Campbell S, Griffin DR, Pearce JM, et al. New Doppler technique for assessing uteroplacental blood flow. *Lancet.* 1983;1:675.

10. Chamberlain PFC, Manning FA, Morrison I, et al. Circadian rhythm in bladder volumes in the term human fetus. *Obstet Gynecol.* 1984;674:657.

11. Chamberlain PFC, Manning FA, Morrison I, et al. Ultrasound evaluation of amniotic fluid. I: The relationship of marginal and decreased amnioic fluid volumes to perinatal outcome. *Am J Obstet Gynecol.* 1984;150:245.

12. Chamberlain PFC, Manning FA, Morrison I, et al. Ultrasound evaluation of amniotic fluid. II: The relationship of increased amniotic fluid to perinatal outcome. *Am J Obstet Gynecol.* 1984;150:250.

13. Grannum PAT, Berkowitz RL, Hobbins JC. The ultrasonic changes in the maturing placenta and their relationship to fetal pulmonic maturity. *Am J Obstet Gynecol.* 1979;133:915.

14. Kaufman AJ, Fleischer AC, Thieme G, et al. Separated chorioamnion and elevated chorion: Sonographic features and clinical significance. *J Ultrasound Med.* 1985;4:119.

15. Lange IR, Manning FA, Morrison I, et al. Prenatal diagnosis of cord prolapse. *Am J Obstet Gynecol.* 1985;151:1083.

16. Manning FA, Platt LD, Sipos L. Antepartum fetal eval-

uation: Development of a fetal biophysical profile score. *Am J Obstet Gynecol.* 1980;136:787.

17. Morrison I. Perinatal mortality. *Seminar Perinatol.* 1985;9:144.

18. Manning FA, Lange IR, Morrison I, et al. Treatment of the fetus in utero: Evolving concepts. *Clin Obstet Gynecol.* 1984;27:378.

19. Dawes GS, Duncan SLB, Lewis BV, et al. Cyanide stimulation of the systemic arterial chemoreceptors in fetal lambs. *J Physiol.* 1969;201:117.

20. Cohn HE, Sacks ET, Heyman MA, et al. Cardiovascular responses to hypoxemia and acidemia in fetal lambs. *Am J Obstet Gynecol.* 1974;120:817.

21. Myers RE. Experimental models of perinatal brain damage: Relevance to human pathology. In: Gluck L, ed. *Intrauterine Asphyxia and the Developing Brain.* Yearbook Medical Publishers; 1977:378.

22. Boddy K, Dawes GS, Fisher R, et al. Foetal respiratory movements, electrocortical and cardiovascular responses to hypoxemia and hypercapnia in sheep. *J Physiol.* (London), 1974;243:599.

23. Manning FA, Platt LD. Maternal hypoxemia and fetal breathing movements. *Obstet Gynecol.* 1979;53:758.

24. Manning FA, Wyn-Pugh E, Boddy K. Effect of cigarette smoking on fetal breathing movements in normal pregnancies. *Brit Med J.* 1975;1:552.

25. Gennsar G, Marsand K, Brantmark B. Maternal smoking and fetal breathing movements. *Am J Obstet Gynecol.* 1975;123:861.

26. Thalar I, Goodman JD, Dawes GS. Effect of cigarette smoking on fetal breathing movements. *Am J Obstet Gynecol.* 1980;138:282.

27. Socol ML, Manning FA, Murata Y, et al. Maternal smoking causes fetal hypoxia: Experimental evidence. *Am J Obstet Gynecol.* 1982;142:214.

28. Natale R, Clewlow F, Dawes GS. Measurement of fetal forelimb movements in the lamb in utero. *Am J Obstet Gynecol.* 1981;140:545.

29. Dalton KJ, Dawes GS, Patrick JE. Diurnal, respiratory and other rhythms of fetal heart rate in lambs. *Am J Obstet Gynecol.* 1977;127:414.

30. Murata Y, Martin CB, Ikenoue KT. Fetal heart rate accelerations and late decelerations during the course of intrauterine death in chronically catheterized fetal monkeys. 1981; Proc. Society for Gynecological Investigation. Abstract 253.

31. Brown R, Patrick JE. The non-stress test: How long is enough? *Am J Obstet Gynecol.* 1981;141:645.

32. Harding R, Poore ER, Cohen GL. The effect of brief episodes of diminished uterine blood flow on breathing movements, sleep states and heart rate in fetal sheep. *J Develop Physiol.* 1981;3:231.

33. Martin CB Jr, Murata Y, Petrie RH, et al. Respiratory movements in fetal rhesus monkeys. *Am J Obstet Gynecol.* 1974;119:939.

34. Dawes GS, Fox HE, Leduc BM, et al. Respiratory movements and rapid eye movement sleep in the foetal lamb.

J Physiol. (London), 1972;220:119.

35. Ruckebusch Y, Gaujoux M, Eghbali B. Sleep cycles and kinesis in the fetal lamb. Electroencephalog. *Clin Neurophysiol.* 1977;42:226.

36. Piercy WN, Day MN, Weins AH, et al. Alteration of ovine respiratory-like behavior by diazepam, caffeine and doxapram. *Am J Obstet Gynecol.* 1977;127:43.

37. Unsars JG, Szeto HH. Precipitated opiate abstinence in utero. *Am J Obstet Gynecol.* 1985;151:441.

38. Boddy K, Dawes GS. Fetal breathing. *Br Med Bull.* 1975;31:1.

39. Manning FA, Heaman M, Boyce D, et al. Intrauterine fetal tachypnea. *Obstet Gynecol.* 1981;58:398.

40. Powell-Phillips WP, Towel M. Abnormal fetal heart rate associated with congenital anomalies. *Br J Obstet Gynecol.* 1980;87:270.

41. Patrick JE, Campbell K, Carmichael L. Patterns of human fetal breathing during the last 10 weeks of pregnancy. *Obstet Gynecol.* 1980;56:24.

42. Manning FA, Harman CR, Lange IR, et al. Modified fetal biophysical profile scoring by selective use of the non-stress test. *Am J Obstet Gynecol.* In press.

43. Bastide A, Manning FA, Harman CR, et al. Ultrasound evaluation of amniotic fluid: Outcome of pregnancies with severe oligohydramnios. *Am J Obstet Gynecol.* In press.

44. Vintzileos AM, Campbell WA, Ingardia CJ, et al. The fetal biophysical profile score and its predictive value. *Obstet Gynecol.* 1983;62:271.

45. Manning FA, Baskett TF, Morrison I, et al. Fetal biophysical profile scoring: A prospective study in 1184 high risk patients. *Am J Obstet Gynecol.* 1981;140:289.

46. Baskett TF, Allen AC, Gray JH, et al. Fetal biophysical profile scoring and prenatal death. *Obstet Gynecol.* 1987;70:357.

47. Platt LD, Eglington GS, Sipos L. Further experience with the fetal biophysical profile score. *Obstet Gynecol.* 1983;61:480.

48. Manning FA, Morrison I, Harman CR, et al. Fetal assessment based on fetal biophysical profile scoring: Experience in 19,221 referred high risk pregnancies. II: An analysis of false negative fetal death. *Am J Obstet Gynecol.* In press.

49. Manning FA, Morrison I, Harman CR, et al. Fetal assessment based on fetal biophysical profile scoring: Positive predictive accuracy of perinatal morbidity by the abnormal score. Vancouver, BC: June 1988; Proc. Society of Obstetricians and Gynecologists of Canada. Abstract.

50. Johnson J, Lange I, Harman CR, et al. Management of the pregnant diabetic using fetal biophysical profile scoring. *Obstet Gynecol.* 1988;72:841–846.

51. Vintzileos AM, Feinstein SJ, Lodeiro J, et al. Fetal biophysical profile and the effect of premature rupture of membranes. *Obstet Gynecol.* 1986;67:818.

52. Lodeiro JG, Vintzileos AM, Feinstein S, et al. Fetal biophysical profile in twin gestation. *Obstet Gynecol.* 1986;67:824.

26 Sonographically Guided Chorionic Villus Sampling

James P. Crane

Sonographically guided chorionic villus sampling (CVS) has been performed in the United States since approximately 1984. The major advantage of CVS is early and rapid prenatal diagnosis. The procedure can be performed as early as 9 weeks' menstrual age, with cytogenetic results available within 48 to 96 hours. In contrast, genetic amniocentesis typically is not performed until 15 to 17 weeks' menstrual age, with an additional 2 to 3 weeks required to culture the amniotic fluid cells. Pregnancy is therefore nearly half completed before a definitive diagnosis can be established. If a significant fetal abnormality is identified, the prospective parents must make a difficult choice: whether to carry or terminate the pregnancy. Postponing this decision until the midtrimester is even more difficult for two reasons. First, fetal movement has been perceived and significant parental–fetal bonding has typically occurred by this time. Second, the pregnancy is generally public knowledge by the midtrimester, raising concerns about what others may think should pregnancy termination be elected. In contrast, first trimester prenatal diagnosis offers the opportunity for private and early decision making.

This chapter includes a discussion of the concept, history, and techniques for CVS. Indications, risks, and potential sources of diagnostic error will also be addressed.

CONCEPT AND INDICATIONS FOR CVS

Genetically, the placenta is considered a fetal organ. Cytogenetic, DNA, and biochemical studies of chorionic villi, therefore, indirectly reflect fetal genetic constitution. In addition, the cytotrophoblast is an active, rapidly dividing tissue containing many spontaneous mitoses for direct chromosome analysis. In contrast, amniotic fluid cells have desquamated from fetal skin and mucosal surfaces. Only 20% of these cells are viable at the time of collection.[1] Consequently, amniotic fluid cells must be cultured in the laboratory for 7 to 14 days before chromosome studies can be performed.

Major indications for CVS are listed in Table 26–1. Advanced maternal age is most common, accounting for nearly 90% of procedures. Interest in first-trimester pre-

natal diagnosis is often dictated by prior reproductive experiences. For example, parents with a previous chromosomally abnormal child are more likely to request early prenatal diagnosis than are couples who are carriers of autosomal recessive biochemical diseases. First-trimester prenatal diagnosis is also often requested by women who are carriers for sex-linked diseases because of the high recurrence risk (50%) in male offspring.

HISTORY OF CVS

First-trimester prenatal diagnosis is not a new concept. In 1969, Hahnemann and Mohr[2] attempted blind transcervical trophoblast biopsy in 12 patients using a 6-mm diameter instrument. While successful tissue culture was possible, half of these subjects subsequently aborted spontaneously. In 1973, Kullander and Sandahl[3] used a 5-mm diameter fiberoptic endocerviscope with biopsy forceps to perform transcervical chorionic villus sampling in 39 patients requesting pregnancy termination. While tissue culture was successful in 49% of cases, two of the subjects subsequently became septic.

In 1974, Hahnemann[4] described his further experience with first-trimester prenatal diagnosis using a 2.5-mm hysteroscope and cylindrical biopsy knife. Once again, significant complications, including inadvertent rupture of the amniotic sac, were encountered. By this time, the safety of midtrimester genetic amniocentesis had become established and further attempts at first-trimester prenatal diagnosis were abandoned in the western hemisphere.

Two technologic advances occurred to allow reintroduction of CVS in the early 1980s. The first of these was the development of real-time sonography, making sonographic guidance of trophoblast sampling possible. At the same time, sampling instruments were miniaturized and refined. In 1982, Kazy and associates[5] reported first-trimester transcervical CVS using either a 1.7-mm diameter hysteroscope with biopsy forceps or a flexible 2-mm biopsy forceps with real-time sonographic guidance. In 39 cases, pregnancy was electively terminated 5 to 10 days after the biopsy. Repeat sonographic evaluation immediately prior to termination confirmed con-

TABLE 26–1. MAJOR INDICATIONS FOR CVS

Maternal age 35 or greater at delivery
Previous child with nondisjunctional chromosome abnormality
Parent carrier of balanced translocation or other chromosome disorder
Both parents carriers of autosomal recessive biochemical disease
Women who are carriers for a sex-linked disease

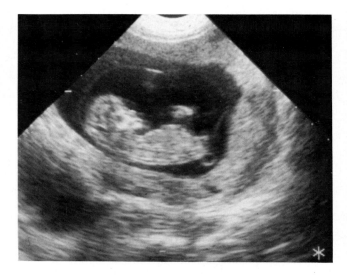

Fig. 26–2. Sonogram at 10.8 weeks' gestation (menstrual age).

tinued fetal cardiac motion in all instances. An additional 13 patients elected to continue their pregnancies after CVS had excluded a genetic abnormality. No fetal losses occurred in this group.

In 1982, Old and colleagues[6] reported first-trimester diagnosis of beta thalassemia major using DNA from chorionic villi obtained by sonographically guided transcervical aspiration biopsy with a 1.5-mm diameter polyethylene catheter. Using a similar technique, Brambati[7] diagnosed trisomy 21 at 11 weeks' gestation. Several CVS programs were subsequently established both in Europe and the United States. More than 60,000 procedures have now been performed worldwide.[8]

CVS SAMPLING TECHNIQUES

Chorionic villi cover the entire surface of the gestational sac until 9 weeks' menstrual age. As sac growth continues, the villi regress except at the implantation site where they are associated with the decidua basalis (Fig. 26–1).

Villi in this area rapidly proliferate to form the chorion frondosum or fetal component of the placenta. The chorion frondosum can be readily visualized sonographically after 9 weeks' menstrual age (Fig. 26–2).

Chorionic villus sampling can be performed either transcervically or transabdominally. Fetal loss rates associated with various techniques are provided in Table 26–2. Transcervical catheter aspiration under real-time sonographic guidance is most commonly employed. Fiberoptic instrumentation has been associated with higher

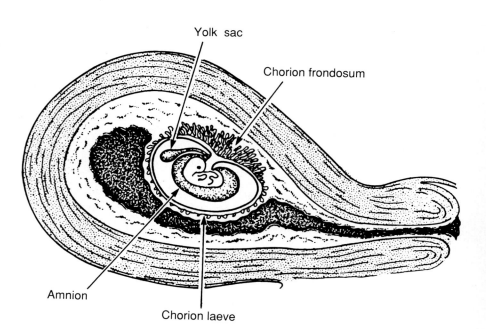

Fig. 26–1. Diagram of first-trimester pregnancy illustrating relevant anatomic landmarks.

TABLE 26–2. CVS TECHNIQUE VERSUS FETAL LOSS RATE[a]

Technique	Number of Patients	Fetal Loss
Ultrasound-guided aspiration	15,341	3.4%
Transcervical biopsy forceps	549	7.7%
Transabdominal needle aspiration	851	3.5%

[a] All pregnancies completed.
Adapted with permission from: Jackson L. CVS Registry Newsletter. *1988;24:1.*

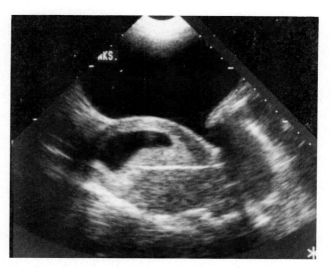

Fig. 26–4. Sonogram illustrating sonographically guided chorionic villus sampling at 10.5 weeks' menstrual age. The catheter can be identified beneath the posteriorly implanted placenta.

postprocedure loss rates and therefore abandoned by most centers.

Transabdominal CVS may be particularly useful when the placenta is implanted in a fundal or high anterior location because transcervical access may be limited in these situations. Theoretically, the transabdominal approach may also carry less risk of infection because the genital tract has a normal bacterial flora and may also harbor pathologic organisms. The relative risk of infection with transcervical versus transabdominal CVS will ultimately be established as more data are collected.

Sonographically guided transcervical CVS is best performed at 9 to 12 weeks' menstrual age. The chorion frondosum is not well developed prior to 9 weeks and is therefore difficult to image sonographically. Access may be limited after 12 weeks' menstrual age, due to the increasing distance between the cervix and placental site as uterine growth continues.

The procedure is performed in the lithotomy position using a standard examination table with foot stirrups. The maternal bladder should be moderately full to provide an acoustic window through which the vagina, cervix, and uterus can be imaged (Fig. 26–3). A speculum is placed into the vagina and the cervix cleansed with antiseptic soap solution. A 1.7-mm diameter polyethylene catheter with metal guide wire is then introduced through the cervix and guided to the chorion frondosum using real-time sector sonographic guidance (Fig. 26–4). The

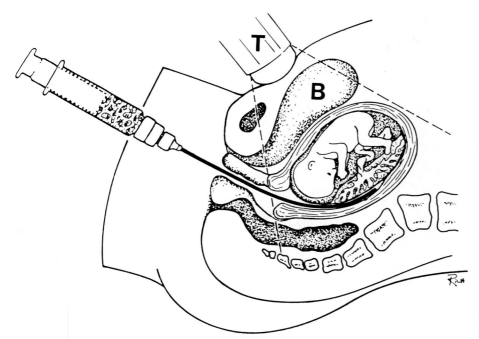

Fig. 26–3. Diagram illustrating technique of sonographically guided transcervical chorionic villus sampling.

catheter may be steered by shaping the curvature of the guide wire. Upward or downward pressure on the speculum will alter uterine position and is also useful in directing catheter placement.

The catheter should be directed in a plane between the inner uterine wall and gestational sac. While sonographic guidance is crucial, tactile sensation is also important. The catheter can be easily advanced if it is in the proper tissue plane, whereas resistance is encountered if it is directed against the uterine wall. Slight readjustment of the angle of direction can correct this problem. The catheter should be slowly advanced beneath the full length of the placenta. The guide wire is then removed and a 10-cc syringe attached. The sample is collected by aspiration using 2 to 8 cc of negative pressure as the catheter is slowly withdrawn. Slight distortion of the placental surface may be noted sonographically during this process, and larger villus fragments may be visualized as they pass through the catheter lumen.

The villus tissue is immediately analyzed under an inverted microscope (Fig. 26–5). Aspirated samples typically contain a mixture of villi and maternally-derived decidua. These tissues can be distinguished microscopically by virtue of their respective morphology. A minimum of 10 mg of tissue is required for most genetic analyses. If insufficient villi are present, a second aspiration may be performed.

Areas of retrochorionic hemorrhage may be observed immediately after CVS. These usually occur at the edge of the decidua basalis and have little if any clinical implication, except they may be associated with a transient elevation of maternal serum alpha fetopotein.[9]

Patients may resume normal physical activity immediately after CVS, although strenuous activity should be avoided. Sexual abstinence is recommended for a period of 5 days to minimize any risk of ascending infection. Approximately 14% of subjects experience light vaginal bleeding in conjunction with CVS. Delayed vaginal bleeding is even more common (44% incidence) and typically begins within 24 to 48 hours of the procedure. This is most commonly characterized as either "spotting" or light flow of 1 to 3 days' duration.

RISKS ASSOCIATED WITH CVS

Potential risks and reported complications of CVS include spontaneous abortion, maternal sepsis, perforation of the amniotic sac, and unexplained midtrimester oligohydramnios.[10–12] The impact of CVS on subsequent fetal growth and development is also of concern because the procedure is performed during a time frame when morphogenesis is in process.

Observed pregnancy loss rates among major centers performing CVS have varied from as low as 1.3% to as high as 5.0%.[8] First-trimester spontaneous abortion is, of course, a common event, occurring in one in every six clinically recognized pregnancies.[13] The observed rates of miscarriage in women undergoing CVS may therefore not be excessive.

Some data are available from first-trimester sonographic examinations performed for vaginal bleeding. These studies indicate that 5 to 11% of women will subsequently abort despite sonographic confirmation of fetal heart motion.[14,15] These patients, however, do not represent a suitable control group for determining the background risk of spontaneous abortion because vaginal bleeding carries an inherently greater risk of miscarriage.[15] Likewise, the risk of spontaneous abortion increases with advancing maternal age.[13] The majority of women undergoing CVS are 35 or older and therefore cannot be compared with younger women having first-trimester sonography. Finally, the risk of miscarriage is inversely related to gestational age at the time of the initial scan; ie, sonographic demonstration of fetal heart motion at 11 weeks' gestation carries a lower risk of later miscarriage than detection of cardiac activity at 7 weeks' gestation. An adequate CVS control population must therefore be similar with regard to each of these variables.

Table 26–3 provides data from a controlled prospective clinical trial of women undergoing either CVS or midtrimester genetic amniocentesis.[16] Both populations were comparable with regard to other variables that might influence the background risk of pregnancy loss

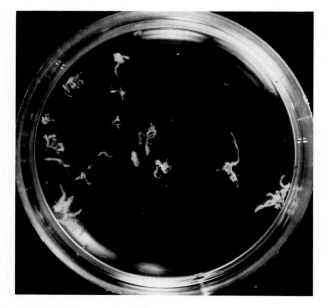

Fig. 26–5. Photograph of chorionic villus fragments under an inverted microscope following collection by CVS.

13. Warburton D, Fraser FC. Spontaneous abortion risks in man: Data from reproductive histories collected in a medical genetics unit. *Hum Genet*. 1964;16:1–25.

14. Mantoni M. Ultrasound signs in threatened abortion and their prognostic significance. *Obstet Gynecol*. 1985;65:471–475.

15. Wilson RD, Kendrick V, Wittman BK, McGillwray B. Spontaneous abortion and pregnancy outcome after normal first trimester ultrasound examination. *Obstet Gynecol*. 1986;67:352–355.

16. Crane JP, Beaver HA, Cheung SW. First trimester chorionic villus sampling versus mid-trimester genetic amniocentesis: Preliminary results of a controlled prospective trial. *Prenat Diagn*. 1988;8:355–366.

17. Martin AO, Simpson JL, Rosinksy BJ, Elias S. Chorionic villus sampling in continuing pregnancies. II: Cytogenetic reliability. *Am J Obstet Gynecol*. 1986;154:1353–1362.

18. Simoni G, Gimelli G, Cuoco C, et al. Discordance between prenatal cytogenetic diagnosis after chorionic villi sampling and chromosomal constitution of the fetus. In: Fraccaro M, et al, eds. *First Trimester Fetal Diagnosis*. Heidelberg: Springer-Verlag; 1985:137–143.

19. Cheung SW, Crane JP, Beaver HA, Burgess AC. Chromosome mosaicism and maternal cell contamination in chorionic villi. *Prenat Diagn*. 1987;7:535–542.

20. Hogge WA, Schonberg SA, Golbus MS. Prenatal diagnosis by chorionic villus sampling: Lessons of the first 600 cases. *Prenat Diagn*. 1985;5:393–400.

21. Karkut I, Zakrzewski S, Sperling K. Mixed karyotypes obtained by chorionic villi analysis: Mosaicism and maternal contamination. In: Fraccaro M, et al, eds. *First Trimester Fetal Diagnosis*. Heidelberg: Springer-Verlag; 1985:144–146.

22. Crane JP, Cheung SW. An embryogenic model to explain cytogenetic inconsistencies observed in chorionic villus versus fetal tissue. *Prenat Diagn*. 1988;8:119–129.

27 Amniocentesis

Roberto Romero • Marcos Pupkin • Enrique Oyarzun • Cecilia Avila • Michael Moretti

HISTORY

Amniocentesis is the oldest invasive procedure for prenatal diagnosis. It has been in use for over 100 years. Amniocentesis was first employed for the treatment of polyhydramnios in the 19th century[1-3]; subsequently, it has been used during amniography[4] and elective termination of pregnancy.[5-6] As a diagnostic procedure, amniocentesis gained popularity in the management of pregnancies complicated by isoimmunization.[7] Genetic amniocentesis has been in use since the early 1960s. In 1956, Fuchs and Riis[8] reported prenatal sex discrimination by analysis of the sex chromatin of cells obtained by amniocentesis. Human cytogenetics emerged as a field in 1966 when Steele and Breg reported the successful determination of a human karyotype from cultured amniotic fluid cells.[9] A year later, the first prenatal diagnosis of a chromosomal abnormality was reported, a balanced translocation.[10] Trisomy 21 was initially diagnosed in 1968 by Valenti.[11] The first congenital metabolic disorder diagnosed by amniotic fluid analysis was adrenogenital syndrome in 1965.[12]

INDICATIONS

Table 27–1 illustrates the most frequent indications for amniocentesis. The most common indication for amniocentesis is prenatal diagnosis. Evaluation of fetal lung maturity has been the leading use for the procedure in the third trimester.

TECHNICAL ASPECTS OF THE PROCEDURE

An ultrasound is performed before amniocentesis to establish fetal viability, gestational age, number of fetuses, placental location, adequacy of amniotic fluid volume, and the presence of any abnormality that might impact on the performance of the procedure (ie, uterine leimyoma, fetal anomaly, and so forth).

Gestational Age

Genetic amniocentesis is usually performed between 16 and 18 weeks. Early studies of amniocentesis indicated a lower success rate in retrieving amniotic fluid when the procedure was performed at gestational ages equal to or less than 15 weeks.[13,14] Amniocentesis performed between 16 and 18 weeks also provided adequate time for cytogenetic studies to be completed in time for pregnancy termination. Therefore, this gestational age has been considered the optimal time frame for genetic amniocentesis.

Improvements in amniotic fluid culture techniques and ultrasonography have led to a recent interest in performing "early amniocentesis" (at gestational ages of less than 15 weeks). This approach is attractive because it provides both early cytogenetic diagnosis and amniotic fluid for alpha fetoprotein (AFP) determinations for the assessment of neural tube defects. Therefore, early amniocentesis has been proposed as an alternative to chorionic villus sampling.[15-23] Similar findings have been noted by Elejalde and colleagues (unpublished data, 1987).

Amniocentesis can be performed at any gestational age for cytogenetic indications. The upper limit is a function of the time necessary to have cytogenetic results. In the past, most laboratories needed 3 to 4 weeks to report a karyotype. Improvements in tissue culture techniques have reduced this time to 1 or 2 weeks. Amniocentesis is often indicated at later gestational ages after the detection of structural abnormalities with ultrasound in view of the increased incidence of aneuploidy in these fetuses. However, if delivery is imminent when anatomic anomalies are first diagnosed, culturing amniotic fluid cells is not the most expeditious means of obtaining a karyotype. Cytogenetic studies of cord blood lymphocytes can provide results in 48 hours.

Needle Selection

Amniocentesis is performed with a regular spinal needle. It has been recommended that the needle bore should be between 20 and 22 gauge. Larger bore needles have been associated with an increased incidence of fetal loss.[13,24] Smaller bore needles prolong the period of time required to obtain amniotic fluid and are more difficult to guide if intraoperative manipulations are required. The standard length of a spinal needle is 8.89 cm, excluding the hub. Longer needles are required for procedures in obese patients. Recently, needles which optimize son-

TABLE 27–1. INDICATIONS FOR DIAGNOSTIC AMNIOCENTESIS

Reason for Amniocentesis	Specific Indications
Diagnostic use	Cytogenetic
	Metabolic disorders
	Neural tube defects (alpha fetoprotein and acetylcolinsterase)
	Isoimmunization
	Fetal maturity
	Intra-amniotic infection
	Confirmation of ruptured membranes
Therapeutic use	Drainage of hydramnios
	Medical treatment of fetal disorders

ographic visualization have been made commercially available (Cooke Catheter, Bloomington, Ind). Acoustic visualization is improved by "roughening" the needle, and Teflon coating is added to decrease needle friction.[25–28] Needles with side orifices are also commercially available. This design allows fluid to flow not only through the needle tip but also through the side orifices. This may have some advantages in cases of severe oligohydramnios. An adequate clinical trial of these new needle types has not been reported.

Ultrasound

Ultrasound has become an integral part of the amniocentesis procedure. The term "sonographically guided technique" refers to the use of ultrasound for selecting the site of needle insertion before amniocentesis; the needle is then inserted blindly into the amniotic cavity. On the other hand, the term "sonographically monitored technique" describes the continuous use of ultrasound throughout the procedure so that the movement of the needle and the fetus are under constant surveillance.[29]

The sonographically monitored technique has been shown to reduce the frequency of bloody and dry taps (and multiple needle insertions) when compared to amniocentesis performed with the sonographically guided technique.[29] The monitored technique also adds to the ease and expedience of the procedure, improves the patient's understanding of amniocentesis, and allows the inexperienced operator to acquire a satisfactory level of performance in a relatively short period of time. This technique also allows the operator to correct for potential difficulties during the procedure such as tenting of the membranes or uterine contractions.

Operative Technique

After the ultrasound examination, asepsis of the skin is performed with wide boundaries, and then the field is draped (Fig. 27–1). Needle insertion is performed under sonographic visualization. Several techniques have been described for this purpose. We have described a technique that continues to be employed in our institution.[29,30] A sterile coupling agent is then applied to the skin (Fig. 27–2). A non-sterile coupling agent is applied to the surface of a linear array real-time transducer, which is placed into a sterile glove or a sterile plastic bag (Fig. 27–3). A site for needle insertion is selected, trying to avoid the placenta, a localized contraction, a uterine lei-

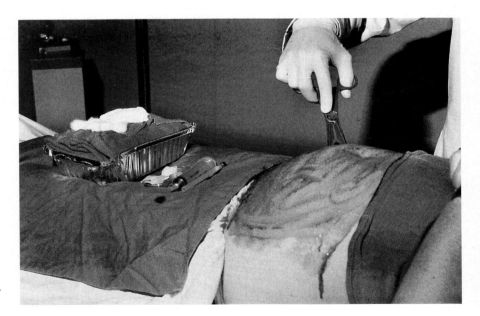

Fig. 27–1. Preparation of a sterile field using antiseptic and sterile drapes.

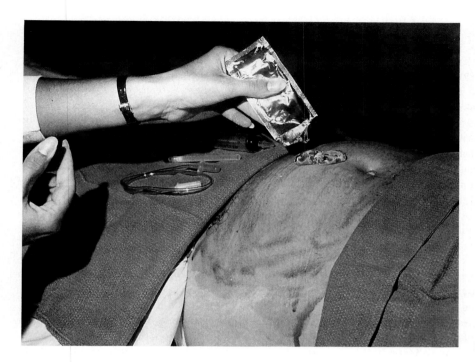

Fig. 27–2. Application of sterile gel.

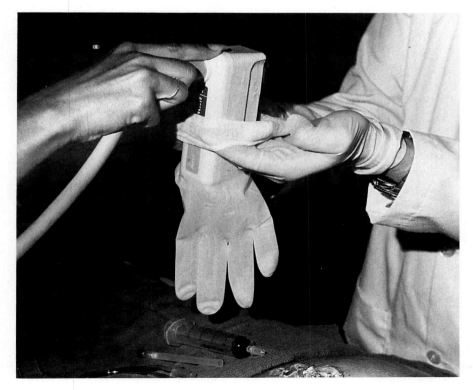

Fig. 27–3. Insertion of transducer into sterile glove.

myoma, or the umbilicus. An anterior placenta does not contraindicate the procedure, but if a transplacental puncture is necessary, preference is given to the thinnest portion of the organ. Once the insertion site has been selected, a finger is placed under the transducer. Decoupling of the transducer from the skin's surface produces a shadow that allows the identification of the needle path. Under direct sonographic visualization, the needle is inserted along the side of the transducer, and the tip, which appears as a bright echo, is continuously monitored throughout the procedure. The stylet is removed, and an extension tube is attached to the hub of the needle and connected to the syringe (Fig. 27–4). The purpose of the plastic tube is to allow the needle to float freely in the amniotic cavity, which decreases the likelihood of fetal injury. This method also prevents operator movements (ie, sneezing) from being transmitted to the needle. The first 0.5 mL of amniotic fluid is discarded to lower the likelihood of contamination of the fluid with maternal cells. After obtaining the fluid, the stylet is replaced and the needle removed. Fetal cardiac activity is documented with ultrasound after the procedure. An alternative method to performing a sonographically monitored procedure is to use a sector scanner to visualize the path of the needle. The advantage of this approach is that the needle can be visualized in its entirety and the transducer can be located away from the sterile field. This technique requires expertise with the needle–transducer spatial orientation. Besides these "free-hand" techniques, ultrasound manufacturers have developed special devices that

can be attached to the transducer and used as needle guides (Fig. 27–5). Although these devices are of potential value in percutaneous blood sampling, the free-hand approach seems sufficiently safe and accurate for the performance of routine amniocentesis.

At the conclusion of the procedure, either the syringe or the tubes in which the amniotic fluid will be transported to the laboratory are labeled with the name of the patient. The patient is asked to verify the identification of her own sample. An amniocentesis report should include the ultrasound findings, number of needle insertions, color and volume of amniotic fluid retrieved, whether or not the placenta was penetrated, and any other unusual finding or event occurring during the procedure. The patient is instructed to report any signs of infection or vaginal leakage of fluid. There is no evidence to support restriction of normal activity after an uneventful procedure. If the patient is Rh-negative nonsensitized, Rh immunoglobulin is administered.

Local anesthesia is not routinely employed at our institution. The administration of local anesthesia requires an additional needle puncture and will only provide subcutaneous and dermal anesthesia. However, some patients may benefit from its use. If used, administration of the anesthetic should be limited to the skin and subcutaneous tissue.

All patients undergoing genetic amniocentesis should have been fully informed about the objectives, procedure, and potential complications of amniocentesis. An informed consent is signed before the procedure.

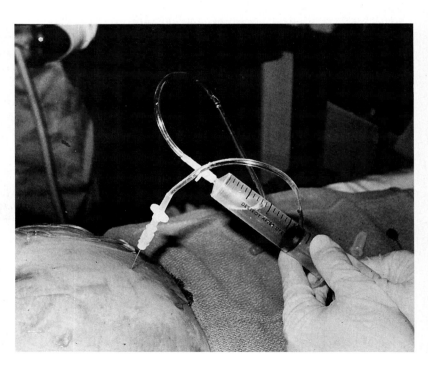

Fig. 27–4. Withdrawal of amniotic fluid using 22-gauge needle, extension tubing and 20 mL syringe.

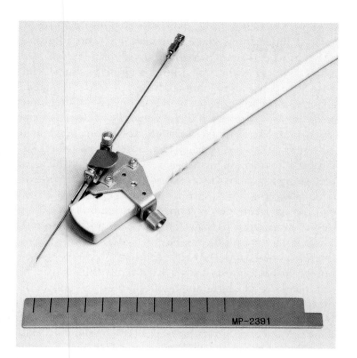

Fig. 27–5. Transducer with an attached needle guide device. (*Reproduced with permission from Corometrics Medical Systems, Inc.*)

Volume of Amniotic Fluid

The volume of amniotic fluid drawn at the time of genetic amniocentesis has varied from 8 mL to 45 mL. Most centers retrieve between 20 mL and 25 mL. This represents approximately 10% of the mean volume of amniotic fluid for 16 weeks of gestation. The effect of amniotic fluid volume on pregnancy loss has been the subject of contradictory reports. While the American Collaborative Study concluded that the volume removed was unrelated to fetal loss,[31] the Canadian report suggested an increased prevalence of neonatal complications when volumes removed are greater than 16 mL.[13] The volume of amniotic fluid retrieved in early amniocentesis programs (<15 weeks) has ranged between 8 and 25 mL. The standard recommendation is to draw 1 mL of fluid per week of gestation. The time required to replace the volume of fluid aspirated has not been established. Although a 3-hour period has been cited as an average replacement time for midtrimester amniocentesis (16 to 18 weeks), there are no adequate data to support this view.[32–34]

INTRAOPERATIVE COMPLICATIONS

Membrane Tenting

The term "membrane tenting" refers to the separation of the chorioamniotic membrane from the anterior uter-ine wall during needle insertion. It is a frequent cause of amniocentesis failure and of need for multiple needle insertions. The diagnosis is made when the tip of the needle is visualized within a clearly defined pocket and no fluid is obtained. The membranes can sometimes be visualized in contact with the tip of the needle. Tenting of the membranes can be overcome by twisting or re-directing the needle. If these maneuvers fail, another approach is to advance the needle into the posterior uterine wall, physically displacing the obstructing membrane down the shaft and away from the tip.[35–38] On occasion, patients will be referred to a different center when amniocentesis has failed and significant chorioamniotic separation has occurred. Amniocentesis can be deferred until reattachment is documented (1 or 2 weeks) or a transplacental needle insertion can be attempted, because membrane tenting is unlikely to occur at this site. Chorioamniotic membranes are more adherent on the surface of the chorionic plate.

Multiple Needle Insertions

The American Collaborative Study of midtrimester amniocentesis reported an increased frequency of spontaneous abortion and stillbirth after multiple needle insertions (>2).[31] Similarly, the Canadian trial found an association between multiple needle insertions (>2) and total fetal losses.[13] However, other studies examining this relationship have not confirmed these findings. Since the introduction of sonographic monitoring of amniocentesis, the frequency of dry taps and multiple needle insertions has decreased significantly.[29,39,40] For example, only 1.9% of all patients in the trial by Tabor and associates[39] required more than one needle insertion, and no patient required more than two needle insertions. These authors could not demonstrate an association between the number of taps and fetal loss.

Bloody Taps

Bloody amniotic fluid can result from contamination with maternal or fetal blood, or both. The prevalence of this complication has also decreased with the use of the sonographically monitored technique.[29,39–43] The American Collaborative Study did not demonstrate an increased risk of fetal loss with bloody taps,[31] whereas most other studies did not comment on this issue (ie, the Canadian and British Collaborative Studies).[42,44] Ron and colleagues[45] have specifically addressed the clinical significance of blood-contaminated amniotic fluid. They studied 706 women undergoing midtrimster amniocentesis. The first 2 mL of amniotic fluid were examined for the presence of blood after centrifugation. Electrophoresis was performed to determine whether the blood was of maternal or fetal origin. The prevalence of bloody taps was 25.5% (180/706). Maternal contamination occurred most frequently (84.4% [152/180]), and fetal contamination occurred in 15.5% (28/180). A mixture of fetal and maternal blood was present in eight cases. The incidence of spontaneous abortion was significantly greater in patients with bloody taps than in women with clear taps (maternal blood contamination = 6.6%; fetal blood contamination = 14.3%; and clear taps = 1.7%). The incidence of pregnancy loss when fetal blood contamination occurred was double that observed when maternal blood contamination was documented. However, this difference did not reach statistical significance. The authors did not provide separate risk figures for microscopic versus gross bloody taps.

Feto-maternal Transfusion

Feto-maternal transfusion (FMT) can be detected by performing a Kleihauer–Betke test after the procedure or by determinations of maternal serum AFP before and after the procedure.[46,47] The reported frequency of FMT depends on the test employed to diagnose this complication. The AFP method is more sensitive than the Kleihauer–Betke test. For example, Lele and coworkers[48] reported that the frequency of FMT was 1.8% and 7.02%, as detected with the Kleihauer–Betke test and the AFP method, respectively. However, it has been suggested that, in some cases, the rise of AFP concentration in maternal serum after the procedure is due to contamination with amniotic fluid and not FMT. Feto-maternal transfusion has importance because it can lead to isoimmunization (discussed later in this chapter) as well as an increased frequency of pregnancy loss. Mennutti and associates[47] reported that spontaneous abortion occurred more frequently in patients with an elevation of maternal serum AFP after amniocentesis than in women with no elevation (14.2% versus 0.98%).[4] Feto-maternal transfusion is more common with anterior placentae.

Discolored Amniotic Fluid

Brown- and green-stained amniotic fluid are occasionally obtained in midtrimester amniocenteses.[49–60] Brown amniotic fluid is considered an indicator of an intra-amniotic hemorrhage; green fluid had been attributed to meconium staining or an old hemorrhage. Recently, Hankins and colleagues[57] have presented compelling evidence to suggest that both green and brown amniotic fluid probably represent the occurrence of previous intra-amniotic bleeding.[5] Both green- and brown-stained amniotic fluids are positive for free hemoglobin. Furthermore, they have a similar spectrophotometric pattern that is consistent with the presence of oxyhemoglobin and free hemoglobin. It has been suggested that the color of the fluid correlates with the amount of hemoglobin present. In vitro experiments, in which amniotic fluid is contaminated with blood, indicate a sequential color change.

Green-colored fluid was seen after 3 days and brown-colored fluid after 7 days of incubation. This interpretation is consistent with the clinical observation that women with green or brown amniotic fluid have a positive history of vaginal bleeding. However, little is known about the etiology of the bleeding episode. Cassel and associates[61] have reported the recovery of *Mycoplasma hominis* and *Ureaplasma urealyticum* in four of 33 samples with discolored, second-trimester amniotic fluid.[6] It is possible that an intrauterine infection may lead to bleeding or that bleeding and clot formations provide an adequate nidus for microbial growth. Finally, the possibility that some green-stained amniotic fluid could be due to meconium passage cannot be entirely ruled out. The human fetus produces and can pass meconium before the 20th week of gestation.[62] Although the evidence is not consistent, most studies examining the prognostic significance of dark-stained amniotic fluid suggest an increased risk of pregnancy loss. The relative risk for spontaneous abortion after retrieval of discolored amniotic fluid has been reported to be 9.9 (1.0 = standard risk) by Tabor and coworkers.[39] King and colleagues[52] have suggested that the prognosis is worse if discolored fluid is associated with an elevated maternal serum AFP determined before the amniocentesis.[5] However, these findings are at variance with those of Hankis and associates[57] who did not find an increased frequency of poor pregnancy outcome after examining data from 83 patients with dark or green fluid (77 green and six brown) from a total of 1,227 women undergoing midtrimester amniocentesis.[5]

AMNIOCENTESIS RISKS

Maternal Risks

Maternal complications are extremely rare. They include perforation of an intra-abdominal viscera with subsequent intra-abdominal infection, bleeding, and blood group sensitization. One case of amniotic fluid embolism has been reported after a third-trimester amniocentesis.[63] The patient presented at 32 weeks of gestation with polyhydramnios. After draining of 200 mL, the mother developed respiratory distress and disseminated intravascular coagulation. The mother was treated with exchange transfusions and survived. The fetus died in utero. Severe hemorrhage due to laceration of the inferior epigastric vessels has also been reported after a third-trimester amniocentesis.[64]

Fetal Risks

Fetal complications can be grouped into fetal loss and needle injuries. Fetal loss can be idiopathic or due to direct fetal injury resulting in exsanguination or infection. The term "idiopathic" refers to unexplained fetal death that occurs during the procedure and in which post-mortem examination yields no demonstrable reason for the demise. In these cases, fetal heart activity is detected before but not after the amniocentesis. A neurogenic mechanism has been postulated; however, there is no evidence to support this hypothesis.

Amniocentesis may lead to intra-amniotic infection by introducing micro-organisms into the amniotic cavity (ie, contaminated instruments, passage of the needle through contaminated skin, or intra-abdominal viscera). Alternatively, if amniocentesis results in the rupture of membranes, ascending infection may occur. The mid-trimester period seems to be particularly vulnerable to microbial invasion, as the antibacterial activity of amniotic fluid is at its nadir.[65] Antibiotic prophylaxis is not a routine practice. Blood cultures obtained around the time of the procedure have been negative in a small study.[66]

The prevalence of intra-amniotic infection after mid-trimester amniocentesis is unknown. The nature of the evidence implicating infection as an etiologic factor for pregnancy loss after midtrimester amniocentesis is anecdotal. There have been case reports in which there was a temporal association between the procedure and clinical chorioamnionitis. Positive microbial cultures of amniotic fluid obtained at the time of midtrimester amniocentesis in asymptomatic patients suggest that, in some cases, intra-amniotic infection may precede the procedure rather than follow it.[61]

Ager and Oliver[65] have analyzed the results of 28 different reports of midtrimester amniocenteses published between 1977 and 1985.[6] The total fetal loss rate (total spontaneous abortions + stillbirths + neonatal deaths/effective total number of pregnancies) varies considerably among the studies (range: 2.4 to 5.2%). (Note: the effective total number of pregnancies = total number of pregnancies − [deaths prior to amniocentesis + total elective abortions + pregnancies lost to follow-up].) However, Ager and Oliver have concluded that these estimations of risk are questionable because of differences in amniocentesis procedures, patient populations, methods of risk estimation, and problems in the design and analysis of the different studies. Most studies do not have a control group, or the control group was the result of matching. Nonrandomized studies are susceptible to bias. Furthermore, most studies do not have the adequate sample size to detect a significant difference in the risk associated with the procedure (statistical power).

Tabor and coworkers[39] have recently reported a randomized, controlled trial of genetic amniocentesis in 4,606 low-risk women. This study provides the best risk estimation available in the literature.

Patients were invited to participate in a study in which they were randomly selected to have an amniocentesis or only an ultrasound in the midtrimester. The

patient population consisted of "low-risk" women. Patients at increased risk for chromosomal anomalies, neural tube defects, metabolic disorders, or spontaneous abortions were excluded. Amniocenteses were performed under sonographic guidance with a 20-gauge needle by a group of five physicians.[39] The rate of spontaneous abortion was higher in the study group (having amniocentesis) than in the control group (having ultrasound only) (1.7% versus 0.7%; $p < 0.01$). The increased spontaneous abortion rate of 1% (95% confidence limits = 0.3 to 1.5) corresponds to a relative risk of 2.3 (95% confidence limits = 1.3 to 4.0). There was a different distribution of the time elapsed between procedure and spontaneous abortion in the study and control groups. The median interval time in the study group was 21.5 days (range 5 to 67), and the median interval was 46.5 days (range 8 to 70) in the control group. An elevated maternal serum AFP (greater than 2 multiples of the median for gestational age), perforation of the placenta, and discolored amniotic fluid were identified as risk factors for spontaneous abortion. The relative risks for fetal loss were 8.3 (95% confidence limits = 2.4 to 19.8); 2.6 (1.3 to 5.4); and 9.9 (4.3 to 22.6), respectively. The authors pointed out that the 1% increased risk of spontaneous abortion after midtrimester amniocentesis may be an underestimation of the real risk. Termination of pregnancies with fetuses affected with chromosomal abnormalities (identified in the study group and not in the control group) may artificially reduce the rate of spontaneous abortion of the study group. Contrary to what has been reported in older studies, no correlation was found between the rate of spontaneous abortion and number of needle insertions, placental site, or experience of the operator.

While amniotic fluid leakage occurred more commonly in the study group than in the control group (1.7% versus 0.4%; $p < 0.001$), vaginal bleeding occurred with similar frequency in both groups (2.4% versus 2.6%). Other obstetric complications such as preterm delivery, spontaneous rupture of membranes, and abruptio placentae had similar prevalence in both groups.

The frequency of orthopedic congenital anomalies was not different in the amniocentesis and control groups. These results are compatible with the findings of a case-control study in which amniocentesis had not been performed more often in mothers of newborns with orthopedic abnormalities than in a control group.[67] In contrast, the British[44] and American[31] Collaborative Studies reported an increased incidence in orthopedic abnormalities (talipes equinovarus, congenital dislocation of the hip, and metatarsus abductus) in the newborns of mothers who underwent amniocentesis.

The prevalence of respiratory distress syndrome (RDS) was higher in neonates born to mothers in the study group than in those born to mothers in the control group (1.1% versus 0.5%; $p < 0.05$). A similar finding was reported for neonatal pneumonia (0.7% versus 0.3%; $p < 0.05$). These observations are of considerable interest because they are consistent with those of the British Collaborative Study,[44] in which there was an increased incidence of respiratory distress (defined as respiratory difficulties requiring oxygen and lasting more than 24 hours) in neonates born to mothers who had undergone amniocentesis compared with those in the control group (1.27% [30/2,370] versus 0.38% [9/2,402]).[39] In addition, the mean crying vital capacity, a measure of lung volume, has been found to be lower in ten neonates of mothers undergoing midtrimester amniocentesis when compared to that of a control group.[68] Experimental studies in monkeys (*Macaca fascicularis*), specifically designed to study the effect of amniocentesis on lung development, indicate that a reduction in the number of alveoli and in lung volume can occur after amniocentesis at a period equivalent to 14 to 17 weeks of gestation in humans.[69,70] Although other clinical studies have not demonstrated an increased incidence of pulmonary complications after amniocentesis, their design and sample size is not as adequate as that reported by Tabor and coworkers.[39]

Leakage of Amniotic Fluid. Transient vaginal leakage of small volumes of amniotic fluid is common after genetic amniocentesis, occurs in approximately 1 to 2% of all cases, and resolves spontaneously within 48 hours.[71] Chronic leakage of amniotic fluid is rare. Of the eight cases recently reviewed by Crane, preterm delivery (< 32 weeks) occurred in three, and club foot deformity in two, cases with chronic leakage. One death occurred in an infant delivered at 31 weeks of gestation with club deformity and Potter fascies.

Fetal Injuries Associated With Amniocentesis. Table 27–2 illustrates the fetal injuries that have been attributed to amniocentesis and whether or not ultrasound was employed during the procedure. The spectrum of lesions ranges from mild skin dimples to fetal death due to exsanguination.[72–98] Although fetal injuries are generally associated with bloody taps, they have also been reported after clear taps. If a fragment of tissue is retrieved with amniotic fluid, histologic examination is recommended to establish its origin. Fetal injuries have occurred even with the use of a sonographically monitored technique.

Several ocular injuries have been attributed to amniocentesis.[75,79,90,94,98] Typically, these are unilateral lesions detected shortly after birth. In one case, the newborn had a small and cloudy eye, a coloboma of the upper lid, and a hazy and edematous cornea. The combination of lesions in the eyelid and cornea suggests that the injury occurred before separation of the eyelids. The mother had an amniocentesis at 19 weeks; the first 2 mL of fluid

were bloody, but the subsequent 30 mL were clear.[90] In two cases, a red and photophobic eye in the newborn period was subsequently associated with the development of an enlarging cystic mass in the anterior chamber of the eye. The cystic lesions evolved over a period of several months and were lined by a stratified squamous epithelium.[75,79]

A porencephalic cyst in a newborn with two subcutaneous nodules in the right and left occipital region (suggesting a needle tract) have been reported. An amniocentesis had been performed at 18 weeks.[91] In utero injection of contrast in the ventricular system during the course of amniograms has also been reported.[73,74]

Thoracic lesions associated with amniocentesis include hemothorax,[76,95] pneumothoraces,[73,78] and fetal cardiac tamponade.[74] In the abdomen, injuries have ranged from laceration of the liver, kidney, and spleen to ileo-cutaneous fistula with ileal atresia.[77,83,84,89,92] In one case, a fragment of tissue retrieved during amniocentesis grew small bowel mucosa in culture, confirming intraoperative bowel injury.[92]

Limb lesions have included disruption of the patellar tendon[88] and gangrene of one arm (perforation of the subclavian artery).[80] Amniocentesis has been implicated by some authors in the etiology of amniotic band syndrome;[86,87,93,96] however, there is no agreement regarding a cause-effect relationship between this syndrome and amniocentesis.

Two cases of hematomas of the umbilical cord have been reported.[76,97] Fetal exsanguination due to vascular puncture has also been reported.[72,85]

The most frequent lesion associated with amniocentesis is skin puncture. Although a cause-effect relationship is difficult to establish, needle injuries should be suspected if the shape of the lesion resembles a needle tract or a depressed punctiform scar.[81,82,88]

ISOIMMUNIZATION

Fetal red blood cells contain the D antigen on their surface and are capable of immunizing the Rh-negative mother after a feto-maternal transfusion in the midtrimester. This event can occur spontaneously during pregnancy or after an amniocentesis. The World Health Organization (WHO) and the American College of Obstetrics and Gynecology (ACOG) have recommended the administration of the anti-D IgG to women after midtrimester amniocentesis. There is no agreement on the dose; the WHO recommends 50 μg, while the ACOG recommends 300 μg.[99]

The basis for this recommendation is that midtrimester amniocentesis has been associated with an in-

TABLE 27–2. FETAL INJURIES DUE TO AMNIOCENTESIS AND MONITORING TECHNIQUES USED

Author	Year	Lesion	Outcome	Bloody Amnio-centeses	US	GA	Indication for Amniocentesis
Misenhimer[72]	1966	Fetomaternal transfusion >100 mL	Newborn died—1 hour	Yes	N	35	Pre-eclampsia, PROM
		Fetomaternal transfusion >100 mL	Preterm labor—newborn died	-	N+	30	Placental localization
Creasman[73]	1968	Hematoma on thorax, skin dimple on arm	No limitation	No	N+	30	Placental localization
		Pneumothorax 40%	Thoracentesis	No	N	Term	?
		Subdural hemorrhage with brain damage: injection of contrast material into fetal brain and spinal cord	Stillborn	No	N+	28	Placental localization
Berner[74]	1972	Fetal cardiac tamponade	Stillborn	-	N	31	RH negative
Cross[75]	1973	Intermittent glaucoma, chronic irritation, coloboma, epithelial cyst (slow growth)	Enucleation, 2 years old	-	N	34	RH sensitive, diabetes
Grove[76]	1973	Pneumothorax	Thoracentesis, Neonatal death	Yes	N	42	Fetal assessment
Egley[77]	1973	Cord hematoma	Newborn healthy	No	N	Postterm	Gestational age
		Fetal spleen laceration	C/S fetal distress Discharged at 10 days	Yes	N	44(?)	Gestational age
Cook[78]	1974	Pneumothorax	Thoracostomy discharged at 32 days	Yes	N+	32	Placental localization, fetal assessment
Fortin[79]	1975	Corneal perforation	Enucleation at 4 months	-	N	39	Fetal lung maturity
Lamb[80]	1975	Fetal arm gangrene caused by supraclavicular puncture	Elective abortion at 16 weeks for anencephalia	-	Y	15	Genetic indication
Broome[81]	1976	Scar on arm	Normal newborn	No	-	17	Genetic indication
		Scars on arm and chest	Normal newborn	No	-	16	Genetic indication
		Scars on chest and thigh	Normal newborn	Yes	-	16	Genetic indication
		Scars on neck	Normal newborn	No	Y*	17	Genetic indication
		Scars on inferior limb and genital area	Normal newborn	No	Y*		Genetic indication
Karp[82]	1976	Punctate lesion on right arm	Normal newborn	No	-	15	Genetic indication
		Punctate lesion on abdomen	Normal newborn	No	-	14.5	Genetic indication
		Punctate lesion on back	Normal newborn	-	-	14.5	Genetic indication
		Punctate lesion on chest	Normal newborn	-	Y*	16	Genetic indication
Rickwood[83]	1977	Fistula and ileal atresia	After resection, normal	No	N	18	Genetic indication
Cromie[84]	1978	Renal trauma	Observation, normal evolution	Yes	N	35	Fetal assessment
Young[85]	1977	Fetal exsanguination	Stillbirth	Yes	Y*	22.5	Genetic indication
Rehder[86]	1978	Amniotic band syndrome: circular constriction and tibial necrosis on right leg	Spontaneous abortion (18.5 weeks)	No	-	14	Genetic indication
Rehder[87]	1978	Amniotic band syndrome	Premature malformed infant (born at 28 weeks; died within 4 minutes)	Yes	-	16	Genetic indication

TABLE 27–2. FETAL INJURIES DUE TO AMNIOCENTESIS AND MONITORING TECHNIQUES USED (Continued)

Author	Year	Lesion	Outcome	Bloody Amnio-centeses	US	GA	Indication for Amniocentesis
Epley[88]	1979	Patellar tendon disruption; multiple amniocenteses	Successful surgery	No	–	14–16	Genetic indication
Swift[89]	1979	Small bowel obstruction with a protruding, necrotic knuckle on abdominal wall	Resection and anastomosis Full recovery at 34 days	No	Y	16	Genetic indication
Merin[90]	1980	Coloboma of eyelid, corneal perforation	Unilateral undeveloped eye and blindness	Yes	Y*	19	Genetic indication
Youroukos[91]	1980	Porencephalic cyst (right occipital and temporal lobes)	Opsoclonus, slight left hemiparesia	Yes	Y	18	Genetic indication
Therkelsen[92]	1981	Ileal atresia	Pregnancy ended	No	Y**	16	Genetic indication
Moessinger[93]	1981	Amniotic band syndrome: constriction and amputation of fingers	Elective abortion (21 weeks)	No	Y*	17	Genetic indication
Isenberg[94]	1985	Scleral perforation with exposed uvea		No	Y*	20	Genetic indication
Achiron[95]	1986	Massive right hemothorax and laceration of pulmonary lobe	Neonatal death	Yes	Y**	32	Fetal lung maturity
Kohn[96]	1987	Amniotic band syndrome: shortened fingers with digital constriction and hypoplastic or absent nails	Delivery at term	–	N	16	Genetic indication
Morin[97]	1987	Cord hematoma	Spontaneous antenatal resorption	No	N	17	Genetic indication
Admoni[98]	1988	Leukocoria, globe perforation, retinal traction and detachment	No mention	Yes	Y**	17	–

US = ultrasound; GA = gestational age at amniocentesis; – = information not available; Y* = guided; Y** = monitored; N = none; N+ = amniography.

creased incidence of transplacental hemorrhage, a risk factor for isoimmunization. However, the precise risk of isoimmunization after midtrimester amniocentesis has not been well defined. The incidence of Rh isoimmunization in the randomized controlled clinical trial reported by Tabor and associates[39] was 0.3% (7/370) in the study group and 0.1% (3/347) in the control group (anti-D IgG was not administered to Rh-negative patients undergoing amniocentesis). Although this difference is not significant, the number of Rh-negative patients required to detect a difference of 1% between the amniocentesis and the control group would be 2,896 in each group.[39] The analysis of the previous reports suggests that midtrimester amniocentesis is associated with an increased risk of isoimmunization. The magnitude of the increased risk seems to be approximately 1%.[65]

Murray and colleagues[100] have provided a comprehensive analysis of the pros and cons of anti-D IgG administration. Among the objections that have been raised against the routine use of anti-D IgG is unproven efficacy. Isolated case reports indicate that sensitization can occur after anti-D IgG administration.[101,102] Another objection is that long-term safety has not been proved. Anti-D IgG crosses the placenta and coats Rh + fetal red cells. It is unclear if this could have adverse effects. The theoretic risk of augmentation has been suggested. This phenomenon consists of an enhancement of the immune response in the context of small amounts of antibody. Furthermore, the long-term effects of exposing the immunologically "naive" fetal immune system to human immunoglobulins are unknown.[103]

Although there is no incontrovertible evidence to support the routine administration of anti-D IgG after midtrimester amniocentesis, this has become the standard practice in the United States.

AMNIOCENTESIS IN MULTIPLE GESTATIONS

Multiple pregnancy was once considered a contraindication for midtrimester amniocentesis; however, this is no longer the case. The prevalence of a chromosomal abnormality is estimated to be higher in twins than in singleton pregnancies (for advanced maternal age indication).[104] Similarly, the incidence of neural tube defects in a patient with a previous history of a child with a neural tube defect is higher in a twin gestation (as high as doubled) than that in a singleton gestation.[65,104]

Before amniocentesis is carried out in a multiple gestation, the possible outcome, risks, and management alternatives need to be discussed with the patient. The major problem to be considered is the possibility of discrepant results regarding cytogenetic diagnosis. If only one fetus is affected, the options available to the patient

include abortion of both fetuses, continuation of the pregnancy, or selective termination of the affected fetus. Selective termination is associated with potential complications such as infection, disseminated intravascular coagulation, and spontaneous abortion.[105] Under these circumstances, pregnancy termination implies the abortion of an unaffected fetus.

The technique for amniocentesis in multiple gestations is different from that in singleton gestations. The number of fetuses, location within the uterine cavity, presence of an interamniotic membrane, placentation, sex, fetal biometry, and anatomy need to be documented. An important step is the topographic location of the fetus. This becomes critical in cases where discrepant results are reported and selective termination is considered. Identification of the fetuses should be based on their relationship to the maternal hemipelvis (left/right, anterior/posterior, and superior/inferior). We recommend that a diagram of the procedure be drawn and kept in the medical record for reference.

Amniotic fluid needs to be retrieved from each amniotic cavity. After amniotic fluid is obtained from the first sac, before removing the needle, an indicator dye is injected into the cavity. Indigo carmine is presently the dye of choice.[106–112] Other alternatives are Congo red[113,114] and Evan's blue.[115] The use of methylene blue is discouraged because of the risk of fetal hemolytic anemia due to metahemoglobinemia.[116,117] Comparative data regarding pregnancy outcome after the use of indicator dyes are limited. Of a total of nine reports, methylene blue was used in one ($n = 18$, fetal loss rate = 22.2%); Evan's blue in one ($n = 16$, fetal loss rate = 12.5%); Congo red in two ($n = 70$, fetal loss rate = 17.1%); and Indigo carmine in five ($n = 342$, fetal loss rate = 11.1%).[100,102,103,105–108,118] It is expected that clear amniotic fluid will be obtained when the second sac is punctured. The same procedure is applicable to amniocentesis for a multiple gestation with more than two fetuses. The technique consists of sequential injections of dye into different sacs before removal of the needle. The number of clear amniotic fluid aspirations should equal the number of fetuses.[106–119]

The overall success rate in obtaining amniotic fluid from both sacs is over 90%. A challenging situation occurs when one sac is behind the other. Under these circumstances, a lateral approach may not be possible. After obtaining amniotic fluid from the anterior sac, we have been able to sample the second sac by advancing the needle to penetrate the interamniotic membrane under direct visualization. The first 2 mL of amniotic fluid retrieved from the second sac are discarded to decrease the likelihood of contamination. Another difficult situation arises when an interamniotic membrane cannot be identified. This can occur in the setting of polyhydramnios and in monoamniotic twins. A practical approach consists of sampling two sites in close proximity to each fetus but distant from each other. We have found it helpful to place a linear array transducer along the transverse axis of the uterus and to monitor the turbulence created by the injection of the indicator dye. Before injection, the dye is diluted with 10 mL of amniotic fluid or sterile saline solution (at room temperature). The mixture is then injected into the amniotic cavity, producing a typical particulate image that identifies the boundaries of that sac. The operator must be ready to proceed with the second puncture because the image is short-lived.

Ager and Oliver[65] have conducted a detailed analysis of the risks of midtrimester amniocentesis in twin gestations.[6] The overall risk of total fetal loss rate is as follows: total spontaneous abortions + stillbirths + neonatal deaths = total number of losses. The mean total fetal loss is 10.8% (range 3.6 to 22.2%). At first impression, this figure seems to indicate that genetic amniocentesis in twin gestations is associated with a significant risk of fetal loss. However, Ager and Oliver have pointed out that this pregnancy loss rate is similar to that (spontaneous) observed in twin gestations after the 17th week of gestation. This assessment is based on the data from 12,392 twin pregnancies collected in Japan. The spontaneous fetal loss was 11.4%.[65,120]

REFERENCES

1. Prochownick L. Beitrage zur lehre vom fruchtwasser und seiner entstehung. Arch Gynaekol. 1877;11:304.
2. Lambl D. Ein seltener fall van hydramnios. Centralbl Gynaekol. 1881;5:329.
3. Von Schatz F. Eine besondere art von einseitiger polyhydramnie mit anderseitiger oligohydramnie bie eineiigen zwillingen. Archiv fur Gynaekol. 1882;19:329.
4. Menees TO, Miller JD, Holly LE. Amniography: Preliminary report. AJR. 1930;24:363.
5. Boero E. Intra-amniotiques. Semana Medica Buenos-Aires. 15 August 1935.
6. Aburel ME. Le declanchement du travail par injections intra-amniotques du serum sale hypertonique. Gynecologie Obstetrique. 1937;36:393.
7. Bevis DCA. Composition of liquor amnii in haemolytic disease of newborn. Lancet. 1950;2:443.
8. Fuchs F, Riis P. Antenatal sex determination. Nature. 1956;177:330.
9. Steele MW, Breg WR Jr. Chromosome analysis of human amniotic-fluid cells. Lancet. 1966;1:383.
10. Jacobson CB, Barter RH. Intrauterine diagnosis and management of genetic defects. Am J Obstet Gynecol. 1967;99:796.
11. Valenti C, Schutta EJ, Kehaty T. Prenatal diagnosis of Down's syndrome. Lancet. 1968;2:220. Letter to the Editor.
12. Jeffcoate TNA, Fliegner JRH, Russell SH, Davis JC, Wade AP. Diagnosis of the adrenogenital syndrome before birth. Lancet. 1965;2:553.
13. Simpson NE, Dallaire L, Miller JR, et al. Prenatal diagnosis of genetic disease in Canada: Report of a collaborative study. Canad Med Assoc J. 1976;115:739.
14. Golbus MS, Loughman WD, Epstein CJ, Halbasch G, Stephens JD, Hall BD. Prenatal genetic diagnosis in 3000 amniocenteses. N Engl J Med. 1979;300:157.
15. Henry G, Peakman DC, Winkler W, O'Connor K. Amniocentesis before 15 weeks instead of CVS for earlier prenatal cytogenetic diagnosis. Am J Hum Genet. 1985;37(suppl). Abstract 650.
16. Luthardt FW, Luthy DA, Karp LE, Hickok DE, Resta RG. Prospective evaluation of early amniocentesis for prenatal diagnosis. Am J Hum Genet. 1985;37(suppl). Abstract 659.
17. Luthy DA, Hickok DE, Luthardt FW, Resta RG. A prospective evaluation of early amniocentesis: An alternative to chorionic villus sampling for prenatal diagnosis. Presented at Sixth Annual Meeting of the Society of Perinatal Obstetricians; January 30–February 1, 1986; San Antonio, Tex. Abstract 268.
18. Hanson FW, Zorn EM, Tennant FR, Marianos S, Samuels S. Amniocentesis before 15 weeks' gestation: Outcome, risks, and technical problems. Am J Obstet Gynecol. 1987;156:1524.
19. Miller WA, Davies RM, Thayer BA, Peakman D. Success, safety and accuracy of early amniocentesis (EA). Am J Hum Genet. 1987;41(suppl). Abstract 835.
20. Weiner CP. Genetic amniocentesis at, or before, 14.0 weeks gestation. Presented at Seventh Annual Meeting of the Society of Perinatal Obstetricians; February 5–7, 1987; Lake Buena Vista, Fla. Abstract 63.
21. Godmilow L, Weiner S, Dunn LK. Genetic amniocentesis performed between 12 and 14 weeks gestation. Am J Hum Genet. 1987;41(suppl). Abstract 818.
22. Johnson A, Godmilow L. Genetic amniocentesis at 14 weeks or less. Clin Obstet Gynecol. 1988;31:345.
23. Benacerraf BR, Greene MF, Saltzman DH, et al. Early amniocentesis for prenatal cytogenetic evaluation. Radiology. 1988;169:709–710.
24. Lowe CU, Alexander D, Bryla D, Seigel D. The NICHD Amniocentesis Registry: The Safety and Accuracy of Midtrimester Amniocentesis. Washington, DC: 1978; US Department of Health, Education, and Welfare. DHEW publication NIH 78–190.
25. McGahan JP. Aspiration and drainage procedures in the intensive care unit: Percutaneous sonographic guidance. Radiology. 1985;154:531.
26. McGahan JP, Walter JP. Diagnostic percutaneous aspiration of the gallbladder. Radiology. 1985;155:619.
27. McGahan JP. Laboratory assessment of ultrasonic needle and catheter visualization. J Ultrasound Med. 1986;5:373.
28. McGahan JP, Tennant F, Hanson FW, Lindfors KK, Quilligan EJ. Ultrasound needle guidance for amniocentesis in pregnancies with low amniotic fluid. J Reprod Med. 1987;32:513.
29. Romero R, Jeanty P, Reece EA, et al. Sonographically

monitored amniocentesis to decrease intraoperative complications. *Obstet Gynecol.* 1985;65:426.

30. Jeanty P, Rodesch F, Romero R, Venus I, Hobbins JC. How to improve your amniocentesis technique. *Am J Obstet Gynecol.* 1983;146:593.

31. NICHD National Registry for Amniocentesis Study Group. Midtrimester amniocentesis for prenatal diagnosis, safety and accuracy. *JAMA.* 1976;236:1471.

32. Fuchs F. Volume of amniotic fluid at various stages of pregnancy. *Clin Obstet Gynecol.* 1966;9:449.

33. Abramovich DR. The volume of amniotic fluid in early pregnancy. *J Obstet Gynaecol Br Commonw.* 1968;75:728.

34. Finegan JK. Amniotic fluid and midtrimester amniocentesis: A review. *Br J Obstet Gynaecol.* 1984;91:745.

35. Platt LD, Manning FA, Lemay M. Real-time B-scan-directed amniocentesis. *Am J Obstet Gynecol.* 1978;130:700.

36. Benacerraf BR, Frigoletto FD. Amniocentesis under continuous ultrasound guidance: A series of 232 cases. *Obstet Gynecol.* 1983;62:760.

37. McArdle CR, Cohen W, Nickerson C, Hann LE. The use of ultrasound in evaluating problems and complications of genetic amniocentesis. *J Clin Ultrasound.* 1983;11:427.

38. Bowerman RA, Barclay ML. A new technique to overcome failed second-trimester amniocentesis due to membrane tenting. *Obstet Gynecol.* 1987;70:806.

39. Tabor A, Madsen M, Obel EB, Philip J, Bang J, Norgaard-Pedersen B. Randomized controlled trial of genetic amniocentesis in 4606 low-risk women. *Lancet.* 1986;1:1 287.

40. Williamson RA, Varner MW, Grant SS. Reduction in amniocentesis risks using a real-time needle guide procedure. *Obstet Gynecol.* 1985;65:751.

41. Dacus JV, Wilroy RS, Summitt RL, et al. Genetic amniocentesis: A twelve years' experience. *Am J Med Genet.* 1985;20:443.

42. Katayama KP, Roesler MR. Five hundred cases of amniocentesis without bloody tap. *Obstet Gynecol.* 1986; 68:70.

43. Crandon AJ, Peel KR. Amniocentesis with and without ultrasound guidance. *Br J Obstet Gynaecol.* 1979;86:1.

44. Chayen S, ed. An assessment of the hazards of amniocentesis: Report to the Medical Research Council by their working party on amniocentesis. *Br J Obstet Gynaecol.* 1978;85 (suppl 2):1.

45. Ron M, Cohen T, Yaffe H, Beyth Y. The clinical significance of blood-contaminated midtrimester amniocentesis. *Acta Obstet Gynecol Scand.* 1982;61:43.

46. Harwood LM. Detection of foetal cells in maternal circulation. *J Med Lab Technol.* 1961;19:19.

47. Mennuti MT, Brummond W, Crombleholme WR, Schwarz RH, Arvan DA. Fetal-maternal bleeding associated with genetic amniocentesis. *Obstet Gynecol.* 1980;55:48.

48. Lele AS, Carmody PJ, Hurd ME, O'Leary JA. Feto-maternal bleeding following diagnostic amniocentesis. *Obstet Gynecol.* 1982;60:60.

49. Robinson A, Bowes W, Droegemueller W, et al. Intrauterine diagnosis: Potential complications. *Am J Obstet Gynecol.* 1973;116:937.

50. Karp LE, Schiller HS. Meconium staining of amniotic fluid at midtrimester amniocentesis. *Obstet Gynecol.* 1977;50(suppl):47.

51. Seller M. Dark-brown amniotic fluid. *Lancet.* 1977;2:983.

52. King CR, Prescott G, Pernoll M. Significance of meconium in midtrimester diagnostic amniocentesis. *Am J Obstet Gynecol.* 1978;132:667.

53. Bartsch FK, Lundberg J, Wahlstrom J. One thousand consecutive midtrimester amniocenteses. *Obstet Gynecol.* 1980;55:305.

54. Crandall BF, Howard J, Lebherz TB, Rubinstein M, Sample WF, Sarti D. Follow-up of 2000 second-trimester amniocenteses. *Obstet Gynecol.* 1980;56:625.

55. Svigos JM, Stewart-Rattray SF, Pridmore BR. Meconium-stained liquor at second trimester amniocentesis—is it significant? *Aust NZ J Obstet Gynecol.* 1981;21:5.

56. Cruikshank DP, Varner MW, Cruikshank JE, Grant SS, Donnelly E. Midtrimester amniocentesis. *Am J Obstet Gynecol.* 1983;146:204.

57. Hankins GDV, Rowe J, Quirk JG, Trubey R, Strickland DM. Significance of brown and/or green amniotic fluid at the time of second trimester genetic amniocentesis. *Obstet Gynecol.* 1984;64:353.

58. Allen R. The significance of meconium in midtrimester genetic amniocentesis. *Am J Obstet Gynecol.* 1985; 152:413.

59. Hess LW, Anderson RL, Golbus MS. Significance of opaque discolored amniotic fluid at second-trimester amniocentesis. *Obstet Gynecol.* 1986;67:44.

60. Zorn EM, Hanson FW, Greve LC, Phelps-Sandall B, Tennant FR. Analysis of the significance of discolored amniotic fluid detected at midtrimester amniocentesis. *Am J Obstet Gynecol.* 1986;154:1234.

61. Cassell GH, Davis RO, Waites KB, et al. Isolation of Mycoplasma hominis and Ureaplasma urealyticum from amniotic fluid at 16–20 weeks of gestation: Potential effect on outcome of pregnancy. *Sex Transm Dis.* 1983;10:294.

62. Abramovich DR, Gray ES. Physiologic fetal defecation in midpregnancy. *Obstet Gynecol.* 1982;60:294.

63. Dodgson J, Martin J, Boswell J, Goodall HB, Smith R. Probable amniotic fluid embolism precipitated by amniocentesis and treated by exchange transfusion. *Br Med J.* 1987;294:1322.

64. Galle PC, Meis PJ. Complications of amniocentesis. *J Reprod Med.* 1982;27:149.

65. Ager RP, Oliver RWA. *The Risks of Midtrimester Amniocentesis.* Lancashire, UK: University of Salford; 1986. Monograph.

66. Klein SA, Gobbo PN, Ristuccia PA, Epstein H, Cunha BA. Diagnostic amniocentesis and bacteremia. *J Hosp Infect.* 1987;9:81.

67. Wald NJ, Terzian E, Vickers PA. Congenital talipes and hip malformation in relation to amniocentesis: A case-control study. *Lancet.* 1983;2:246.

68. Vyas H, Milner AD, Hopkin IE. Amniocentesis and fetal lung development. *Arch Dis Child.* 1982;57:627.

69. Hislop A, Fairweather DVI. Amniocentesis and lung growth: An animal experiment with clinical implications. *Lancet.* 1982;2:1271.

70. Hislop A, Fairweather DVI, Blackwell RJ, Howard S. The

effect of amniocentesis and drainage of amniotic fluid on lung development in *Macaca fascicularis*. *Br J Obstet Gynaecol*. 1984;91:835.

71. Crane JP, Rohland BM. Clinical significance of persistent amniotic fluid leakage after genetic amniocentesis. *Prenat Diagn*. 1986;6:25.

72. Misenhimer HR. Fetal hemorrhage associated with amniocentesis. *Am J Obstet Gynecol*. 1966;94:1133.

73. Creasman WT, Lawrence RA, Thiede HA. Fetal complications of amniocentesis. *JAMA*. 1968;204:91.

74. Berner HW, Seisler EP, Barlow J. Fetal cardiac tamponade: A complication of amniocentesis. *Obstet Gynecol*. 1972;40:599.

75. Cross HE, Maumenee AE. Ocular trauma during amniocentesis. *N Engl J Med*. 1972;287:993.

76. Grove CS, Trombetta GC, Amstey MS. Fetal complications of amniocentesis. *Am J Obstet Gynecol*. 1973;115:1154.

77. Egley CC. Laceration of fetal spleen during amniocentesis. *Am J Obstet Gynecol*. 1973;116:582.

78. Cook LN, Shott RJ, Andrews BF. Fetal complications of diagnostic amniocentesis: A review and report of a case with pneumothorax. *Pediatrics*. 1974;53:421.

79. Fortin JG, Lemire J. Une complication oculaire de l'amniocentese. *Can J Ophthal*. 1975;10:511.

80. Lamb MP. Gangrene of a fetal limb due to amniocentesis. *Br J Obstet Gynaecol*. 1975;82:829.

81. Broome DL, Wilson MG, Weiss B, Kellogg B. Needle puncture of fetus: A complication of second-trimester amniocentesis. *Am J Obstet Gynecol*. 1976;126:247.

82. Karp LE, Hayden PW. Fetal puncture during midtrimester amniocentesis. *Obstet Gynecol*. 1977;49:115.

83. Rickwood AMK. A case of ileal atresia and ileo-cutaneous fistula caused by amniocentesis. *J Pediatr*. 1977;91:312.

84. Cromie WJ, Bates RD, Duckett JW Jr. Penetrating renal trauma in the neonate. *J Urol*. 1978;119:259.

85. Young PE, Matson MR, Jones OW. Fetal exsanguination and other vascular injuries from midtrimester genetic amniocentesis. *Am J Obstet Gynecol*. 1977;129:21.

86. Rehder H. Fetal limb deformities due to amniotic constrictions (a possible consequence of preceding amniocentesis). *Path Res Pract*. 1978;162:316.

87. Rehder H, Weitzel H. Intrauterine amputations after amniocentesis. *Lancet*. 1978;1;382.

88. Epley SL, Hanson JW, Cruikshank DP. Fetal injury with midtrimester diagnostic amniocentesis. *Obstet Gynecol*. 1979;53:77.

89. Swift PGF, Driscoll IB, Vowles KDJ. Neonatal smallbowel obstruction associated with amniocentesis. *Br Med J*. 1979;1:720.

90. Merin S, Beyth Y. Uniocular congenital blindness as a complication of midtrimester amniocentesis. *Am J Ophthalmol*. 1980;89:299.

91. Youroukos S, Papedelis F, Matsaniotis N. Porencephalic cysts after amniocentesis. *Arch Dis Child*. 1980;55:814.

92. Therkelsen AJ, Rehder H. Intestinal atresia caused by second trimester amniocentesis. *Br J Obstet Gynaecol*. 1981;88:559.

93. Moessinger AC, Blanc WA, Byrne J, Andrews D, War-

burton D, Bloom A. Amniotic band syndrome associated with amniocentesis. *Am J Obstet Gynecol*. 1981;141:588.

94. Isenberg SJ, Heckenlively JR. Traumatized eye with retinal damage from amniocentesis. *J Pediatr Ophthalmol Strabismus*. 1985;22:65.

95. Achiron R, Zakut H. Fetal hemothorax complicating amniocentesis—antenatal sonographic diagnosis. *Acta Obstet Gynecol Scand*. 1986;65:869.

96. Kohn G. The amniotic band syndrome: A possible complication of amniocentesis. *Prenat Diagn*. 1987;7:303.

97. Morin LRM, Bonan J, Vendrolini G, Bourgeois C. Sonography of umbilical cord hematoma following genetic amniocentesis. *Acta Obstet Gynecol Scand*. 1987;66:669.

98. Admoni M, Ben Ezra D. Ocular trauma following amniocentesis as the cause of leukocoria. *J Pediatr Ophthalmol Strabismus*. 1988;25:196–197.

99. American College of Obstetricians and Gynecologists. Management of isoimmunization in pregnancy. Washington, DC: 1984. ACOG Technical Bulletin 80.

100. Murray JC, Karp LE, Williamson RA, Cheng EY, Luthy DA. Rh isoimmunization related to amniocentesis. *Am J Med Genet*. 1983;16:527.

101. Henry G, Wexler P, Robinson A. Rh-immune globulin after amniocentesis for genetic diagnosis. *Obstet Gynecol*. 1976;48:557.

102. Golbus MS, Stephens JD, Cann HM, Mann J, Hensleigh PA. Rh isoimmunization following genetic amniocentesis. *Prenat Diagn*. 1982;2:149.

103. Frigoletto FD, Jewett JF, Konugres AA, eds. *Rh Hemolytic Disease: New Strategy for Eradication*. Boston: GK Hall; 1982.

104. Hunter AGW, Cox DM. Counseling problems when twins are discovered at genetic amniocentesis. *Clin Genet*. 1979;16:34.

105. Rodeck CH, Mibashan RS, Campbell S. Selective feticide of the affected twin by fetoscopic air embolism. *Prenat Diagn*. 1982;2:189.

106. Elias S, Gerbie AB, Simpson JL, Nadler HL, Sabbagha RE, Shkolnik A. Genetic amniocentesis in twin gestations. *Am J Obstet Gynecol*. 1980;138:169.

107. Fribourg S. Safety of intra-amniotic injection of indigo carmine. *Am J Obstet Gynecol*. 1981;140:350.

108. Goldstein AI, Stills SM. Midtrimester amniocentesis in twin pregnancies. *Obstet Gynecol*. 1983;62:659.

109. Librach CL, Doran TA, Benzie RJ, Jones JM. Genetic amniocentesis in seventy twin pregnancies. *Am J Obstet Gynecol*. 1984;148:585.

110. Di-lin L, Zhi-long Z. Double sacs amniocentesis in twin pregnancy. *Chin Med J*. 1984;97:465.

111. Filkins K, Russo J, Brown T, Schmerler S, Searle B. Genetic amniocentesis in multiple gestations. *Prenat Diagn*. 1984;4:223.

112. Tabsh KMA, Crandall B, Lebherz TB, Howard J. Genetic amniocentesis in twin pregnancy. *Obstet Gynecol*. 1985;65:843.

113. Bovicelli L, Michelacci L, Rizzo N, et al. Genetic amniocentesis in twin pregnancy. *Prenat Diagn*. 1983;3:101.

114. Palle C, Andersen JW, Tabor A, Lauritsen JG, Bang J,

Philip J. Increased risk of abortion after genetic amniocentesis in twin pregnancies. *Prenat Diagn*. 1983;3:83.

115. Wolf DA, Scheible FW, Young PE, Matson MR. Genetic amniocentesis in multiple pregnancy. *J Clin Ultrasound*. 1979;7:208.

116. Cowett RM, Kakanson DO, Kocon RW, Oh W. Untoward neonatal effect of intraamniotic administration of methylene blue. *Obstet Gynecol*. 1976;48:74s.

117. Plunkett GD. Neonatal complications. *Obstet Gynecol*. 1973;41:476.

118. Field B, Picker R. Genetic amniocentesis in twin pregnancy. *Aust N Z J Obstet Gynecol*. 1982;22:71.

119. Gerbie AB, Elias S. Technique for midtrimester amniocentesis for prenatal diagnosis. *Semin Perinatol*. 1980; 4:159.

120. Imaizumi Y, Asaka A, Inouye E. Analysis of multiple birth rates in Japan. VII: Rates of spontaneous and induced terminations of pregnancy in twins. *Jpn J Human Genet*. 1982;27:235.

28 Fetal Blood Sampling

Roberto Romero • Apostolos P. Athanassiadis • Mona Inati

HISTORY

Valenti,[1] in 1972, was the first to obtain fetal blood under endoscopic visualization using a #18 F pediatric cystoscope. Further refinements were introduced in 1974 by Hobbins and Mahoney,[2] who developed a special cannula to obtain fetal blood in continuing pregnancies under endoscopic control (Fig. 28–1). This method was used in the prenatal diagnosis of hemoglobinopathies.[3] The standard procedure consisted of puncturing vessels on the surface of the placental chorionic plate (Fig. 28–2). This approach was fraught with difficulties because the chorionic vessels are small and, therefore, are a difficult target. In addition, contamination with maternal blood and amniotic fluid was a problem, as the tip of the needle was in close proximity to the amniotic cavity or the intervillous space (containing maternal blood). A major advance in fetoscopic blood sampling was introduced by Rodeck and Campbell in 1979.[4] They reported blood-drawing from the umbilical cord in its area of insertion into the placental mass (Fig. 28–3). This approach yielded fetal blood uncontaminated with maternal blood or amniotic fluid in the majority of cases. Advances in high resolution ultrasound allowed clear visualization of the umbilical cord and its vessels without endoscopic visualization (Fig. 28–4). Daffos and colleagues[5] in 1983 were the first to report percutaneous umbilical blood sampling (PUBS) under direct ultrasound guidance. More recently, other groups have developed techniques for fetal blood sampling under ultrasound guidance using minor modifications of the original procedure.[6-11] The terms PUBS, cordocentesis, or funiculocentesis are used interchangeably to refer to this technique.

TECHNIQUE OF FETAL BLOOD SAMPLING

Prior to fetal viability, PUBS can be performed in an outpatient facility. After viability, the procedure should be performed in proximity to an operating room as a cesarean section may be required if fetal distress develops during or after the procedure.[12] We perform cordocentesis in a clean suite used for sonographic examinations or in a labor room. A particle-size analyzer (Coulter Channelyzer) is available for determining the maternal or fetal origin of the blood sample.

An ultrasound examination is performed prior to the procedure to determine fetal viability, position, gestational age, biometry, location of the placenta, and the presence of associated anomalies. Clear identification of the insertion site of the umbilical cord in the placenta is a critical step. It is important not to confuse a loop of umbilical cord adjacent to the placental mass with the actual insertion site. Color Doppler can be helpful in difficult cases. Cordocentesis is easiest when the placenta is anterior. Access to an insertion site in a posterior placenta may be hampered by the fetus. A version or fetal displacement is occasionally required to gain access to the sampling site under these circumstances.[11]

The abdomen is cleaned with an antiseptic solution and draped. The use of local anesthesia for diagnostic procedures is a matter of choice.[7,13-15] We use maternal sedation (diazepam) and local anesthesia for prolonged therapeutic procedures. Diazepam is preferred to meperidine because the latter may induce nausea and vomiting.

Several different approaches can be used for cordocentesis. The general principle is to insert the needle under sonographic monitoring. The transducer is manipulated to maintain the tip of the needle under visualization. Two major considerations are the type of transducer and whether the operator employs a needle-guiding device or "a free-hand technique." We favor a sector over a lienar array transducer, as the latter is bulkier. However, tridimensional orientation with the linear array transducer is easier for those not thoroughly familiar with the sector transducer. Most experienced operators use "a free-hand technique" because of its flexibility in the adjustment of the needle path. A very acceptable approach is to employ a needle-guiding device attached to the transducer (Fig. 28–5). Modern real-time machines are equipped with an on-screen template of the needle tract that is used to target the sampling site. A disadvantage of the needle guiding device is that it restricts the lateral motion of the needle. However, in some cases it is possible to remove the guiding device as the needle approaches the target. In this manner, small corrections can be accomplished if necessary.

After the needle enters the umbilical cord, the stylet

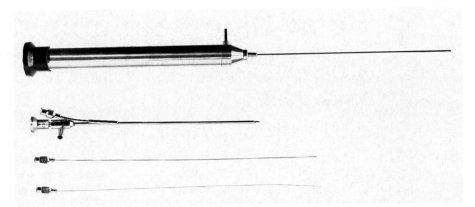

Fig. 28–1. Instruments used in fetoscopy: needlescope, blood sampling cannula, and 27-gauge needles.

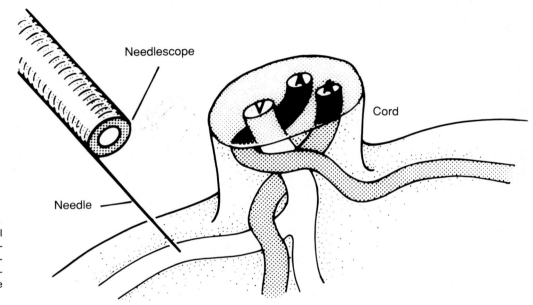

Fig. 28–2. Method for fetal blood sampling under fetoscopic visualization. The needle was inserted into the chorionic vessels on the surface of the chorionic plate.

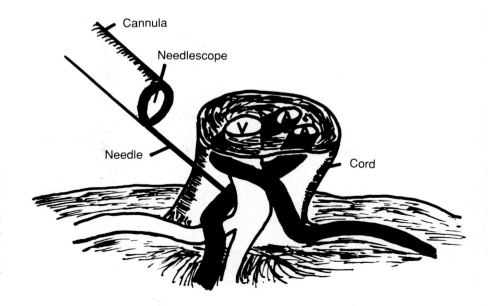

Fig. 28–3. Needle insertion into the umbilical cord. This method was introduced by Rodeck and constituted a major advance in fetal blood sampling technique. (*Reproduced with permission from Devore GR, Venus I, Hobbins JC, et al: Fetoscopy: General clinical approach. In: Rocker I, Laurence KM, eds. Fetoscopy. Amsterdam: Elsevier/North Holland Biomedical Press; 1981:59.*)

TABLE 28–2. COMPARATIVE FETAL (20–26TH WEEK) AND MATERNAL BIOCHEMISTRY (Mean and SD)

	Fetuses (n = 63)	Mothers (n = 63)
Glucose	2.8 ± 0.2 mmol/L (51 ± 3.8 mg/dL)	4.4 ± 0.1 mmol/L (79 ± 1.8 mg/dL)
Triglycerides	0.89 ± 0.03 mmol/L (78 ± 2 mg/dL)	1.4 ± 0.07 mmol/L (122 ± 6 mg/dL)
Cholesterol	1.5 ± 0.05 mmol/L (58 ± 2 mg/dL)	6.6 ± 0.2 mmol/L (255 ± 7 mg/dL)
Total protein	30.4 ± 0.6 g/L (3.04 ± 0.06 g/dL)	69.6 ± 0.9 g/L (6.96 ± 0.09 g/dL)
Albumin	21.4 ± 0.4 g/L (2.14 ± 0.04 g/dL)	34.9 ± 0.5 g/L (3.49 ± 0.05 g/dL)
Calcium	2.25 ± 0.2 mmol/L (9.02 ± 0.8 mg/dL)	2.27 ± 0.1 mmol/L (9.1 ± 0.4 mg/dL)
Phosphorus	2.65 ± 0.1 mmol/L (8.31 ± 0.29 mg/dL)	1.45 ± 0.1 mmol/L (4.55 ± 0.18 mg/dL)
Urea	2.6 ± 0.16 mmol/L (16 ± 0.1 mg/dL)	4.3 ± 0.2 mmol/L (26 ± 0.1 mg/dL)
Creatinine	64 ± 2 μmol/L (0.726 ± 0.021 mg/dL)	67 ± 1.5 μmol/L (0.765 ± 0.016 mg/dL)
Uric acid	167 ± 10 μmol/L (2.80 ± 0.17 mg/dL)	215 ± 9.5 μmol/L (3.62 ± 0.16 mg/dL)
Total bilirubin	26.8 ± 1 μmol/L (1.57 ± 0.06 mg/dL)	8.6 ± 0.4 μmol/L (0.504 ± 0.025 mg/dL)
Direct bilirubin	16.1 ± 0.6 μmol/L (0.943 ± 0.035 mg/dL)	0.9 ± 0.4 μmol/L (0.05 ± 0.02 mg/dL)

(Reproduced with permission from Forestier F, Daffos F, Rainaut M, et al. Blood chemistry of normal human fetuses at midtrimester of pregnancy. Ped Research. 1987;21:579.)

Complications

Table 28–3 summarizes the maternal and fetal complications of fetal blood sampling. The spontaneous abortion rate after diagnostic PUBS has been reported to be 0.8% and the in utero fetal death rate, 1.1%. Other complications associated with the procedure include bleeding from the puncture site, fetal bradycardia, infection, thrombosis of the umbilical vein, and formation of an umbilical cord hematoma.[19–21] The frequency with which bleeding occurs immediately after the procedure is variable. Daffos and associates[15] reported that bleeding for up to 60 seconds occurred in 32% of the cases, of 1 to 2 minutes in 6% of cases, and of more than 2 minutes in 2% of cases. No bleeding was reported in 59% of cases. Fetal exsanguination has been reported in two cases with Glatzmann's thromboasthenia.[15] It is interesting that in at least one of the cases the fetus did not bleed immediately after the procedure. The frequency of bradycardia in their series was 9%. Thrombosis and cord hematomas associated with intrauterine death have been noted after cordocentesis. In a pathologic study of 50 umbilical cords collected between 1 hour and 20 weeks after PUBS, one giant hematoma was noted.[21] In four additional cases,

TABLE 28–3. COMPLICATIONS OF FETAL BLOOD SAMPLING

Chorioamnionitis
Spontaneous rupture of membranes
Umbilical cord hematoma
Umbilical cord thrombosis
Fetal bradycardia
Fetal bleeding and hemorrhage
Fetal death
Feto-maternal transfusion

small hematomas encircling the vessels were documented. In this study, no relationship could be documented between transient fetal bradycardia or bleeding from the cord puncture site and the size of the hemorrhage in the umbilical cord at pathologic examination.[21] Preterm birth and intrauterine growth retardation has been reported in 5% and 8% of cases, respectively. Therefore, diagnostic PUBS does not seem to increase the incidence of these complications. Approximately 7% of patients have irregular uterine contractions after the procedure.[17] When reporting or reading the literature concerning complications of cordocentesis, it is important to separate diagnostic procedures from therapeutic cordocentesis. The prevalence and implications of complications are different.

Infection is a potentially serious complication of fetal blood sampling. It has been reported after both diagnostic and therapeutic procedures. This complication is the most common cause of pregnancy loss after the procedure. Chorioamnionitis may lead to the development of maternal sepsis and severe adult respiratory distress syndrome.[22] Despite the absence of scientific evidence, many centers have implemented a policy of antibiotic prophylaxis for the procedure.

Cordocentesis for diagnostic or therapeutic purposes has been associated with feto-maternal transfusion. In a study of 68 consecutive cordocenteses for Rh isoimmunization, feto-maternal hemorrhage was detected in 63% of cases with an anterior placenta and in 18% of cases with a posterior placenta.[23] The mean estimated hemorrhage was 2.4 mL (3.1% of the total feto-placental blood volume). A small series examining the prevalence of feto-maternal transfusions after diagnostic cordocentesis documented this complication in 57% of the cases.[24] These data indicate that there is a risk for isoimmunization with the procedure. Therefore, in any Rh negative patient, it is important to determine the fetal blood type and to administer Rh immunoglobulin to those patients carrying a Rh positive fetus.

Training

Who should perform PUBS? Fetal blood sampling is a surgical procedure. In the United States, PUBS is per-

TABLE 28–4. INDICATIONS FOR PERCUTANEOUS UMBILICAL BLOOD SAMPLING

Risk of fetal hemolytic disease
  Isoimmunization: anti-D, E, C, Kell
Rapid karyotype
  Mosaicism in amniocytes or CVS cultures
  Anatomic malformation
  IUGR
  Rapid sexing for X-linked disorders
Congenital infection
  Rubella, varicella, parvovirus, CMV, and toxoplasmosis
Hemoglobinopathies
  Alpha, Beta-thalassemia, sickle cell anemia
  Hemoglobin E, and so forth
Coagulopathies
  Hemophilia A and B, von Willebrand's disease
  Immune thrombocytopenia purpura, alloimmune thrombo-
    cytopenia, and Glantzmann's thrombasthenia
Immunodeficiency syndromes
  SCID
  Chronic granulamatous disease
  Wiskott–Aldrich
Fetal welfare (Blood gases—third trimester)
  IUGR
Other
  Fragile-X syndrome
  Single gene disorders
  Biochemical diagnoses, and so forth

formed by specialists in maternal–fetal medicine. Training is difficult to obtain because of the limited number of available cases in any given institution and the risks associated with the procedure. Ideally, the operator should have a strong background in obstetric ultrasonography and experience with invasive procdures of prenatal diagnosis. In our institution, training is first obtained with in vitro models. Once proficiency is acquired in vitro, the procedure is performed in patients having elective midtrimester terminations of pregnancy.[25,26]

INDICATIONS AND USES OF FETAL BLOOD SAMPLING

Table 28–4 summarizes the most common indications for fetal blood sampling. The role of the procedure in the evaluation and treatment of the fetus with isoimmunization has been discussed in Chapter 24.

Cytogenetic Diagnosis

Although amniocentesis is the method of choice for the prenatal diagnosis of chromosomal abnormalities in large populations, there has been growing interest in obtaining fetal karyotypes from cultured human lymphocytes obtained from fetal blood. This information is desirable under the following circumstances: (1) the presence of fetal structural anomalies, (2) the detection of mosaicism or pseudomosaicism in amniocyte culture or chorionic villus sampling, and (3) a diagnosis of fragile X or chromosomal instability syndromes when the feasibility of diagnosis using amniocytes or chorionic villi has not been established or has yielded equivocal results.

The work-up of a fetus with a structural anomaly is currently one of the most common indications for diagnostic cordocentesis. The objective of the procedure is to exclude the presence of chromosomal anomalies and congenital infection. Fetal karyotypes can be obtained through transabdominal chorionic villus biopsy in the second and third trimesters of pregnancy, but cordocentesis is the method of choice. The number of mitoses in tissue obtained by trophoblastic sampling at this gestational age is lower than that in cells obtained by blood sampling.[27] Recently, Eydoux and colleagues[28] reported a comprehensive study of the frequency of chromosomal anomalies in 936 fetuses with structural anomalies identified by ultrasound. The overall prevalence of chromosomal aberrations was 12.1% in cases of an isolated anomaly or 29.2% in cases of multiple anomalies. Table 28–5 illustrates the prevalence of chromosomal anomalies per structural defect. Trisomy 21, 18, 13 and monosomy X accounted for 80% of all anomalies. Triploidy (4.9%) and balanced (4.9%) and unbalanced (9.8%) non-Robertsonian translocations were also frequently found. These observations are consistent with other smaller reports.[29,30]

Another cytogenetic indication for cordocentesis is the finding of more than one cell line when performing karyotype studies of amniotic fluid cells. The key question is whether the fetus carries a true mosaicism or if there is another cause for this abnormal finding. Other causes could include in vitro changes in cultured amniotic fluid cells (pseudomosaicism), a postzygotic error that is restricted to the extraembryonic membranes (amnion or trophoblast), an unrecognized dizygotic twin pregnancy with early death of an abnormal twin, or contamination with maternal tissue. Similar problems could arise after chorionic villus sampling (CVS).

Recently, Gosden and coworkers[31] reported their experience with fetal blood sampling in the investigation of 41 patients with chromosomal mosaicism in amniotic fluid culture. After an abnormal finding, a second amniotic fluid sample and a fetal blood sample were karyotyped. Repeated studies were normal in 23 or 24 cases of autosomal and sex chromosomes trisomies. In one case, the second amniotic fluid sample confirmed the original finding of trisomy 20, but the karyotype

TABLE 28–5. CHROMOSOMAL ABNORMALITIES AND "ISOLATED" MALFORMATIONS

Assessment	No.	Chromosomal Abnormalities	%
Monomalformations	239	29	12.1
Central nervous system	51	4	7.8
Cardiovascular	21	3	14.3
Gastrointestinal	20	3	15.0
Genito-urinary	55	1	1.9
Facial	4	0	–
Extremities	7	0	–
Ventral wall defects	42	3	7.1
Hygromas	20	14	70.0
Fetal effusions	15	1	6.7
Placenta	2	0	–
Other	2	0	–
Polymalformations	65	19	29.2

(*Adapted from Eydoux, et al. 1989.*[28] *Prenat Diagn. 1989;9:255.*)

obtained from fetal blood was normal. On the other hand, 5 of 11 cases of structural rearrangement and four of six cases with de novo supernumerary marker mosaicism were confirmed by subsequent studies.[31] Our group has reported 21 blood sampling procedures that sought evidence of mosaicism in the fetus when mosaicism or pseudomosaicism has been demonstrated in amniotic fluid culture. Three of the 21 patients had mosaicism confirmed by blood sample analysis.[32] For more data on the subject of mosaicism, the reader is referred to specific reports.[33–36]

The identification of more than one cell line in amniotic fluid or CVS presents serious diagnostic dilemmas for which there are no perfect solutions. Patients should be informed that it is not possible to exclude that the mosaic cell line may be present in fetal tissues other than blood cells (ie, liver, brain, and so forth). For example, in trisomy 20, the chromosomal abnormality has not been detected in peripheral blood although it is present in other tissues.[37]

Fetal chromosomal analysis has also been valuable in the prenatal diagnosis of fragile X syndrome.[38] New advances in DNA technology have made it possible to prenatally diagnose fetuses at risk in most, but not all, families.[39,40] Currently, cytogenetic studies of cultured amniocytes coupled with DNA studies is the method for a definitive diagnosis. If results are equivocal, cordocentesis can be employed.[41]

Blood Sampling in the Assessment of Congenital Infection

Fetal blood sampling has been used in the prenatal diagnosis of several congenital infections including toxoplasmosis, rubella, cytomegalovirus, varicella, and parvovirus. The general approach to prenatal diagnosis consists of obtaining material to isolate the infectious agent and documenting a specific fetal immunoresponse. Materials for culture include fetal blood, ascites, and pleural and amniotic fluid. It is important to be aware that fetal immunoresponse to the infectious agent is an indirect method of diagnosis. As with any other biologic phenomenon, this response is variable, and it is influenced by the maturity of the fetal immune system. A consistent response may not be obtained before 20 to 22 weeks. The response could also be transient and, therefore, affected by the elapsed time between infection and blood sampling. Moreover, the response may be weak or nondetectable. Finally, the formation of antigen-antibody complexes under conditions of excess antigen may interfere with immunologic assays used to detect the immunoresponse. The documentation of a specific IgM response is diagnostic of infection. On the other hand, the absence of a response is nondiagnostic.

Toxoplasmosis. Of infants who have acquired toxoplasmosis during fetal life, 15% become infected in the first trimester, 25% in the second trimester, and 60% in the third trimester.[42] The incidence of fetal or congenital toxoplasmosis is 0.6% when the mother acquires the infection in the periconceptional period, 3.7% from 6 to 16 weeks and 20% from 16 to 25 weeks.[43] The clinical manifestations associated with transplacental infection vary, depending on the gestational age at which the infection occurs. Although more than 90% of fetal infections acquired in the third trimester are asymptomatic, those occurring in the first trimester often result in fetal death, abortion, or overt clinical disease.

Congenital transmission of *Toxoplasma gondii* only occurs when the acute infection is acquired during pregnancy.[44] Acute toxoplasmosis is diagnosed by demonstrating seroconversion from a negative to a positive test, the presence of IgM antibodies, or rising titers in the pregnant woman. Once the diagnosis of acute maternal toxoplasmosis is made, the challenge is to establish whether or not the fetus is infected. Daffos and associates[43] reported the largest world experience in the diagnosis and treatment of congenital toxoplasmosis. They studied fetuses at about 20 weeks of gestation. Studies included serology (specific IgM, total, and specific IgG), intraperitoneal inoculation into mice, and other fetal blood determinations (eosinophils, platelets, total IgM, glutamyl transpeptidase, and lactic dehydrogenase). Amniotic fluid was also studied by inoculation into mice and serologic examination (IgG and IgM).[43,45]

Table 28–6 illustrates the diagnostic indices of different parameters in the identification of congenital toxoplasmosis. With the above combination of tests, 92% (39/42) of the cases of congenital toxoplasmosis were prenatally identified.[43] As can be appreciated in this table,

TABLE 28–6. SPECIFICITY, SENSITIVITY, AND PREDICTIVE VALUE OF NONSPECIFIC DIAGNOSTIC TESTS FOR CONGENITAL TOXOPLASMOSIS

	Specificity (%)	Sensitivity (%)	Predictive Value	
			Positive Test (%)	Negative Test (%)
Ultrasound findings	99.8	45.0	95.0	96.8
Serologic tests				
Platelet count	98.4	28.0	52.0	95.8
Specific IgM	100.0	21.0	100.0	95.5
Total IgM	96.7	52.0	48.8	97.4
Gamma-glutamyltransferase	96.8	57.0	52.1	97.4
Lactic dehydrogenase	98.0	16.6	33.0	95.1
Eosinophil count	94.4	19.0	17.0	95.1
White-cell count	96.8	38.0	42.0	96.3
Gamma-glutamyltransferase plus total IgM	98.7	38.0	64.00	96.3
Gamma-glutamyltransferase plus white-cell count	99.8	26.0	91.0	95.7
Total IgM plus platelets	100.0	21.0	100.0	95.5
Total IgM plus white-cell count	99.8	21.0	90.0	95.5

Tests were done on a fetal blood sample after maternal acquisition of toxoplasmosis infection during pregnancy.
(*Reproduced with permission from Daffos, et al.* N Engl J Med. *1988;381:271.*)

IgM determinations had a sensitivity of only 21%. In three cases, the prenatal work-up was negative, but the infants were affected. One infant had subclinical infection with persitence of specific IgG at 8 months of age. The other two infants had symptomatic infection, one had intracranial calcifications, while the other had systemic infection with meningoencephalitis and chorioretinitis. There were three additional cases in which the infants had no clinical signs or specific IgG or IgM, but the parasite was recovered from the placenta. Prenatal work-ups were also negative in these cases. Treatment of the affected fetuses had been conducted with maternal administration of pyrimethmine and sulfadizine. In 11 of 15 infants treated in utero, there were no clinical signs of infection at birth.[43] However, assessment of the effectiveness of prenatal treatment requires more experience and long-term follow-up.

Rubella. It has been estimated that the risk of congenital rubella in infants born to seronegative pregnant patients is 0.5 per 1,000. The rate of transplacental infection varies with the gestational age at which the infection occurs. In the first 12 weeks of pregnancy, it is 80%; between 13 and 14 weeks it is 54%, and during the late second trimester it is 25%.[46–48]

Prenatal diagnosis of rubella infection has been attempted. Grangeot-Keros and coworkers[49] have evaluated 50 pregnant women with a confirmed rubella infection by measuring specific IgA and IgM by capture immunoassay. They found that control and non-infected fetuses had less than 6 mg/dL of specific IgM, while all infected fetuses had more than 10 mg/dL. Similar observations were noted with specific IgA. There was a good correlation between specific IgM and IgA levels. However, the concentration of IgA was consistently lower in both infected and noninfected fetuses. These results are at variance with those reported by Nigro and colleagues[50] who were unable to detect specific IgA in infected infants. Morgan-Capner and coworkers[51] have reported their experience with prenatal diagnosis at 19 to 25 weeks in four fetuses whose mothers had confirmed rubella infection in early pregnancy. No specific IgM was found in one fetus and the infant was unaffected at birth. Of the three fetuses with specific IgM, two pregnancies were terminated with IgM levels of 5.4 and 2.9 units. One fetus with a very low level (1 unit) went to term and was born with features of congenital rubella syndrome. They also reported four abortuses (from which the virus was recovered) whose postabortion sera were negative for specific IgM. These pregnancies were terminated before 20 weeks, and the lack of detectable antibodies emphasizes the need to wait until 22 weeks.

Cytomegalovirus. Congenital cytomegalovirus (CMV) infection is the most common intrauterine viral infection, with a prevalence ranging between 0.4 and 2.3 per 100 live births.[52] Although only 5 to 10% of infants are symptomatic at birth, 90% of these develop major sequelae.[53] The CMV virus can be transmitted to the fetus during the primary infection but also during a reactivation of a latent infection. The presence of maternal-specific immunoglobulin does not protect against reactivation of the viral disease or transmission to the fetus. It has been estimated that transmission to the fetus occurs in 42% of the cases of primary infection. The gestational age at which the infection occurs seems to have little effect on the rate of fetal transmission. The risk of a mother giving birth to an infant with severe congenital CMV disease has been estimated to be 5% after a primary infection.[54]

The feasibility of prenatal diagnosis of intrauterine infection has been reported by the detection of specific IgM antibodies in the blood of a 25-week fetus with nonimmune hydrops. The serum had been negative with a serologic test using an indirect fluorescent assay, but was clearly positive with a radioimmunoassay for CMV-specific IgM.[55] Amniotic fluid or any other body fluid (ascites or pleural effusion) has been used to make a prenatal diagnosis of this condition.[56] Failure to recover the virus from amniotic fluid does not rule out congenital infection.[57]

Congenital Varicella-Zoster Infection. After maternal chickenpox, the rate of intrauterine transmission of the infection has been estimated to be 24%.[54] No fetal infection has been documented after zoster. Infection in early pregnancy has been associated with a variety of congenital anomalies, including cicatricial skin lesions, microcephaly, brain calcifications, intrauterine growth retardation, limb hypoplasia, and club foot deformities. Recently, cordocentesis has been employed to diagnose congenital chickenpox by demonstrating the presence of specific antiviral IgM in fetal blood.[58] The mother had had chickenpox at 20 weeks of gestation. Ventriculomegaly and hydramnios were detected at 32 weeks of gestation. Specific IgM against three different components of the varicella-zoster virus was detected in fetal serum.

Parvovirus. Human parvovirus B19 is the etiologic agent of erythema infectiosum or "fifth disease." Transplacental transmission of the virus may lead to fetal infection. Nonimmune hydrops could be due to bone marrow hypoplasia or myocarditis. A prenatal diagnosis has been made by visualizing viral particles by electron microscopy in ascites fluid of a fetus affected with nonimmune hydrops.[59] Of interest is that the fetal serum was negative for anti-B18 IgM and IgG.[60]

Congenital Immunodeficiency

Four components of the immune system play a role in the defense of the host against infection. These involve phagocytosis, antibody-mediated immunity (B cells), cell-mediated immunity (T cells), and complement. Congenital disorders of any of these components can impair the ability of the host to deal with infection. These dis-

orders are serious and frequently result in early death due to opportunistic infections. Because all of these components of the effector limb of the immunoresponse are contained in blood, a logical extension of the development of fetal blood sampling techniques has been their application in the prenatal diagnosis of congenital immunodeficiency syndromes.

The severe combined immunodeficiency (SCID) syndrome includes a wide group of disorders (Table 28–7).[61] Prenatal diagnosis relies on counting specific fetal lymphocyte subpopulations. Functional assays, such as stimulation with PHA, are used adjunctively but must be interpreted with caution because of occasional high percentages of blast cells in peripheral blood.

A micromethod for cell counting was developed by Levinsky and associates[62] in 1982. A fetal blood sample of 200 to 500 μL is required. A leukocyte-rich fraction is prepared by sedimentation methods and then stained in microtiter plates with a panel of commercially available antibodies. In addition to cell counting, enzyme activity is helpful in the prenatal diagnosis of SCID due to adenosine deaminase deficiency, purine nucleoside phosphorylase, and orate phosphoribosyltransferase-orotidylate decarboxylase deficiencies. Two of these conditions have been diagnosed by assessing enzymatic activity in uncultured cells from CVS.[63]

Absence of both lymphocytes and granulocytes, known as a reticular dysgenesis, is the most severe form of SCID. The diagnosis could presumably be accom-

TABLE 28–7. SEVERE INHERITED IMMUNODEFICIENCY DISORDERS

Autosomal recessive inheritance
Severe combined immunodeficiency due to:
  Adenosine deaminase deficiency
  Purine nucleoside phosphorylase deficiency
  Absence of HLA class I or II or both (bare lymphocyte syndrome)
  Reticular dysgenesis
  SCID in association with short-limbed dwarfism
Leukocyte adhesion deficiency (leukocyte function antigen-1 deficiency)
Ataxia telangiectasia
Chronic granulomatous disease
Chediak–Higashi syndrome

X-linked inheritance
X-lined agammaglobulinaemia
Severe combined immunodeficiency
Wiskott-Aldrich syndrome
Chronic granulomatous disease
X-linked hyperimmunoglobulinaemia M
X-linked lymphoproliferative disease
X-linked properdin deficiency
X-linked agammaglobulinaemia with growth hormone deficiency

plished with fetal blood. Severe combined immunodeficiency due to "bare lymphocyte syndrome" has also been diagnosed prenatally. In this condition, there is deficient synthesis of the HLA class I or class II molecules. Diagnosis has been accomplished by membrane immunofluorescence using specific monoclonal antibodies for the HLA class I and class II molecules.[64]

Three forms of immunodeficiency are associated with short-limb dwarfism. Type I is associated with combined immunodeficiency syndrome, type II with cellular immunodeficiency, and type III with humoral immunodeficiency. The clinical course varies, depending on the immunologic defect. Short-limb dwarfism is present at birth, and this diagnosis would seem to be possible with ultrasound in a patient at risk. If ultrasound findings were equivocal, fetal blood studies could be used to support the diagnosis.

The diagnosis of Wiskott–Aldrich syndrome has been established by the detection of cellular dysfunction.[65–67] The diagnosis of congenital neutropenia should also be possible by enumerating granulocytes. We have excluded this diagnosis in two pregnancies in an at-risk family; both babies were born free of disease. Because neutrophil numbers in the peripheral circulation are very low before 18 weeks, diagnosis should probably not be undertaken before this time.

Chronic Granulomatous Disease. Chronic granulomatous disease (CGD) is a congenital immunodeficiency disorder due to abnormalities in the intracellular metabolism of phagocytic cells, which results in an increased susceptibility to pyrogenic infections. The disease is inherited either with an autosomal or X-linked recessive pattern.

Under normal circumstances, ingested bacteria are destroyed by the combined effect of the degranulation process and the oxidizing agents produced during "the respiratory burst" within the phagocytic cell. The term "respiratory burst" describes a metabolic pathway, dormant in resting cells, which is responsible for the synthesis of highly reactive microbicidal molecules by the partial reduction of oxygen. The basic problem of CGD is an impaired respiratory burst activity in phagocytic cells.

The most commonly used test for the diagnosis of CGD is the nitroblue tetrazolium dye reduction test. Nitroblue tetrazolium (NBT) is a yellow, water-soluble compound, which can be transformed into a deep blue dye (formazan) on reduction. Normal neutrophils can reduce the NBT, but neutrophils from patients with CGD cannot. The NBT reduction test is carried out using phagocytic cells from fetal blood that have adhered to a glass surface; the most effective stimulator of dye uptake is phorbol myristate acetate. Newburger and coworkers[68]

reported that NBT reduction was similar in adult (range 98–100%) and fetal cells (80 to 100%). Female carriers of X-linked CGD had fewer positive cells (18 to 64%), and almost no cells from patients with CGD reduced the dye (0–4%). This technique has successfully identified affected fetuses. Almost no fetal neutrophils showed dye reduction. The diagnoses were confirmed after midtrimester terminations of pregnancy, based on NBT reduction and superoxide production.[68,69] A possible alternative diagnostic method has been suggested using chemiluminescence to measure superoxide anions in fetal cells.[70] Fetal blood sampling should be conducted after the 18th week of gestation, when a significant number of phagocytic cells can be found in the peripheral circulation. Molecular biology techniques have been used recently for carrier detection of this condition. This will allow prenatal diagnosis using DNA methods.

Prenatal Diagnosis of Coagulopathies

Fetal blood has been used in the prenatal diagnosis of congenital hemostatic disorders involving both soluble clotting factors and platelets. This section will consider the relevant issues in the diagnosis of hemophilia A, hemophilia B, von Willebrand's disease, and thrombocytopenic disorders. Although the prenatal diagnoses of hemophilias A and B have heretofore required fetal blood, recent advances in the definition of the genes for factor VIII and factor IX now make is possible to diagnose both of these disorders in a large number of families through the use of DNA technology.

Factor VIII is a protein formed by two different fragments: a small molecule, known as VIII:Ag, coded by the X chromosome, and a large multimeric molecule, referred to as vWF:Ag, coded by an autosomal chromosome. Both hemophilia A and von Willebrand's disease result from a decrease in factor VIII activity. In hemophilia A, there is deficiency or absence of VIII:Ag, whereas in von Willebrand's disease there is deficiency of both vWF:Ag and VIII:Ag and also abnormalities of platelet function.

Factor VIII nomenclature uses the following abbreviations:

- VIII. Factor VIII coagulant activity as measured by clotting assay techniques
- VIII:Ag. Factor VIII coagulant antigen as measured by immunologic techniques using homologous antibodies
- vWF:Ag. Factor VIII-related antigen as measured by immunologic techniques using heterologous antibodies

Diagnosis of factor VIII disorders must consider the properties tested by the assay employed. Factor VIII is measured in a functional clotting assay, and its activity is defined by its ability to shorten the clotting time of hemophilic plasma. This assay was the method used for many years to assess factor VIII levels in the postnatal period. Shortcomings of this assay were that it required a relatively large amount of blood, and that it was affected by coagulation of the sample (VIII is not present in serum because it is consumed during normal clotting). A major advance was the development of an immunoradiometric assay for the antigenic portion of factor VIII. Antibodies against factor VIII develop in some hemophilic patients after transfusions. These antibodies can be used to detect an antigenic determinant of factor VIII. This antigen is present in both serum and plasma, and, therefore, the assay can be used in partially clotted blood. In addition, this assay is not significantly affected by contamination with amniotic fluid, whereas the functional clotting assay for VIII is. In normal individuals, the VIII activity and VIII:Ag level are highly correlated and inferences can be drawn from either assay. However, in some hemophilic patients, there is a discrepancy between VIII and VIII:Ag, with an excess of the latter. The substance responsible for this difference is a cross-reactive material (CRM), an antigenically recognizable protein without functional activity. A false-negative diagnosis of hemophilia A could occur if the clinician relies solely on the immunoradiometric assay of factor VIII:Ag. Therefore, for prenatal diagnostic purposes, it is important to know if the index case in the family has CRM. If the affected individual is CRM-positive, diagnosis will require a functional clotting assay. Ninety-five percent or more of families with severe hemophilia A (VIII activity < 1%) are CRM negative.

Prenatal Diagnosis of Hemophilia A. Hemophilia A is a congenital coagulopathy that is inherited through an X-linked recessive pattern. Its severity is related to the degree of reduction of VIII activity. The first step involved in the prenatal diagnosis of hemophilia A is an assessment of the carrier risk. This can be made by family history, laboratory techniques, or the demonstration of linkage between hemophilia A and other genetic markers.[71] Several laboratories have established normal values for factor VIII, VIII:Ag, and vWF:Ag for midtrimester fetuses that are disease free.[72–75] It is prudent that centers involved in the prenatal diagnosis of coagulopathies, however, derive their own control data prior to undertaking diagnostic efforts in patients at risk. Mibashan and Rodeck[76] have reported their results in the prenatal diagnosis of 153 consecutive male fetuses at risk for hemophilia A. Of these fetuses, 47 were found to be affected and all but two couples elected to terminate their pregnancies. Confirmation of the diagnosis by factor VIII assays in blood from abortuses was available in 38 cases. There were no false-positive or negative diagnoses in the abortuses or infants delivered at the time of the report. The incidence of CRM-positive families in their first 100

cases was 8%. In all cases, the correct diagnosis could be made by using a functional clotting assay for VIII. Recently, Daffos and associates[77] have reported their experience with the prenatal diagnosis of 79 cases of hemophilia A.

Prenatal Diagnosis of Hemophilia B. Hemophilia B, or Christmas disease, is inherited with an X-linked recessive pattern and is due to a deficiency in factor IX activity. Clinical presentation is quite similar to that of hemophilia A. The diagnosis of this condition is made by demonstrating reduced factor IX coagulant (IX:C) activity in a functional assay. An immunoradiometric assay is available for the detection of factor IX antigen (IX:Ag). It is important that a functional assay for factor IX be performed in all fetal blood samples because there is a high prevalence of CRM-positive families with severe hemophilia B, unlike the situation in hemophilia A.[78] Only when a proband had been clearly demonstrated to be CRM negative would it be sufficient to rely on IX:Ag measurement.

Mibashan and Rodeck[76] examined 19 male fetuses at risk for hemophilia B. Of these fetuses, 16 were normal and three were affected. The diagnoses were confirmed in blood specimens from the abortuses or from infants after birth. Daffos and associates[77] also reported their experience in the prenatal diagnosis of 12 fetuses at risk.

Prenatal Diagnosis of von Willebrand's Disease. The most common type of von Willebrand's disease is a coagulopathy inherited as an autosomal dominant trait and characterized by a prolonged bleeding time associated with qualitative or quantitative abnormalities of vWF:Ag. Although the levels of VIII are generally low, they may also be within normal range. The von Willebrand portion of the factor VIII complex is critical for normal platelet adhesion, and this explains the abnormalities in bleeding time. Von Willebrand's disease is the most common inherited bleeding disorder. Its precise incidence is difficult to establish because mild cases may not be noticed. The disease can be classified as homozygous or heterozygous. The type of interest for prenatal diagnosis is homozygous von Willebrand's disease because hemorrhagic manifestations are very severe. The disorder is characterized by low vWF:Ag and reduced VIII and VIII:Ag.

Mibashan and Rodeck[76] examined three couples at risk for an infant with homozygous disease. The diagnoses were excluded in two fetuses and made in one. The affected fetus had extremely low levels of all components of the factor VIII complex. Hoyer and colleagues[79] (1979) also reported the exclusion of the diagnosis of a couple at risk for homozygous disease. Daffos and associates[77] also examined two fetuses at risk for von Willebrand's disease.

Prenatal Diagnosis of Other Congenital Hemostatic Disorders. Several congenital hemostatic disorders are associated with a risk of intrauterine or early postnatal hemorrhage. Normal values for the activity of coagulation factors provide the framework for prenatal diagnosis (Table 28–8). Daffos and associates[77] have documented antenatal diagnoses of deficiency of factors V, VII, and XIII.

Prenatal Diagnosis of the Platelet Disorders. Fetal blood sampling can be very useful in the prenatal diagnosis and management of congenital thrombocytopenias, which include congenital amegakaryocytic thrombocytopenia, thrombocytopenia with absent radii (TAR) syndrome, Wiskott–Aldrich syndrome, alloimmune thrombocytopenia, and immune thrombocytopenic purpura.

Congenital amegakaryocytic thrombocytopenia is probably inherited as an autosomal recessive disorder. A prenatal diagnosis of an affected infant has been made by the detection of thrombocytopenia.[80] Fetal blood sampling is also indicated in fetuses in whom the radial ray deficiency has been detected on ultrasound. Thrombocytopenia would be diagnostic of TAR syndrome. However, other conditions, such as Fanconi's pancytopenia and Aase syndrome, also present with hematologic abnormalities.

Fetal blood sampling has been used for the diagnosis and prenatal management of alloimmune thrombocytopenia.[81] This condition has been estimated to occur in 5,000 births and involves the platelet-specific antigen PLA[1] in the majority of the cases (isoimmunization is also possible with other antigens). The disease can be considered as the counterpart of Rh isoimmunization in the platelet system. A PLA[1]-negative mother is immunized by fetal PLA[1]-positive platelets. An antiplatelet IgG crosses the placenta and produces thrombocytopenia in the PLA[1]-positive fetus. Severe intracranial hemorrhage at the time of vaginal delivery or during the perinatal period is a major cause of death.[80] The risk of fetal bleeding during pregnancy has been estimated to be 10%, whereas that in the early neonatal period is 20%. Cordocentesis can be employed for the prenatal diagnosis and management in the perinatal period. Blood sampling is performed at 20 weeks of gestation. Platelet typing can exclude the disease. If the fetus is PLA[1]-positive, then the pregnancy is followed with serial ultrasound examinations to monitor the occurrence of an intracranial hemorrhage and fetal platelet counts. Thrombocytopenia has been treated with serial platelet transfusions.[82] If platelet counts remain within normal limits, a cordocentesis is performed at term before delivery. If the platelet count is normal, vaginal delivery can be allowed. If thrombocytopenia is present, platelets are administered and delivery planned for the same day. Daffos and associates[77] have reported excellent results with this approach. The major problem with this, however, is the requirement of serial platelet counts and, possibly, platelet transfusions. Recently, a novel approach to this problem has been reported. Parenteral administration of immunoglobulin to the mother has resulted in improved pregnancy outcome of index pregnancies when compared to a previously affected pregnancy.[83] The role of steroids in the treatment of this disease is under current investigation.

Another condition for which blood sampling could be helpful is immune thrombocytopenic purpura.[84] The current approach to this condition is to wait for the mother to go into labor and perform a scalp platelet count as soon as the cervical dilatation permits it. A cesarean section is performed if the platelet count is less than 50,000.[84,85] Although this approach has been used quite successfully, it does not address the risk of intracranial hemorrhage before the onset or during early labor. Fetal blood sampling prior to the onset of labor could avoid the theoretical risks associated with early labor in a thrombocytopenic fetus or, more importantly, would permit a prenatal diagnosis of thrombocytopenia and pre-

TABLE 28–8. EVOLUTION OF COAGULATION FACTOR OF 103 NORMAL FETUSES DURING PREGNANCY RELATED TO THOSE OF THEIR MOTHERS (Mean ± SD)

Week of Gestation	VIII (%)	vWF:Ag (%)	IX:C (%)	V:C (%)	II:C (%)
Fetuses					
19–21 (n = 51)	40 ± 12	59 ± 12.5	9 ± 2.5	39 ± 11	13 ± 4
22–24 (n = 44)	39 ± 13.5	64 ± 13	9 ± 3	40.5 ± 5	14 ± 2
25–27 (n = 44)	42.5 ± 12	63 ± 13	12 ± 4	39 ± 9	14 ± 3.5
Mothers					
	160 ± 80	190 ± 110	90 ± 20	85 ± 10	95 ± 15

(Reproduced with permission from Forestier, et al. Pediatr Res. 1986;20:342.)

natal treatment with corticosteroids. Umbilical blood sampling could also be employed to monitor the effectiveness of the therapy. It must be stressed that all these advantages could be outweighed by the risk of fetal bleeding after the procedure. Therefore, this approach must be considered experimental at this time.

Glanzmann's thrombasthenia is a congenital platelet functional disorder for which a prenatal diagnosis has been made. The work-up consists of in vitro platelet aggregation and platelet membrane glycoprotein studies. Two cases of exsanguination after cordocentesis have been reported in fetuses affected with Glanzmann's thrombasthenia.[15,77,79]

Prenatal Diagnosis of Hemoglobinopathies

The hemoglobinopathies can be divided into two major groups. Those in the first group, the thalassemias, result from inherited defects in the rate of synthesis of one of the globin chains. The second group results from inherited structural alterations in one of the globin chains, as in sickle cell anemia.

Hemoglobin is a tetrameric molecule composed of four polypeptide chains in a stoichiometric fashion. Adult hemoglobin, or hemoglobin A, contains two alpha-globin chains and two beta-globin chains. The major fetal hemoglobin, hemoglobin F, has two gamma chains instead of beta chains. The fetal red blood cells are capable of synthesizing fetal and adult hemoglobin from early gestation.

Prenatal diagnosis of hemoglobinopathies is based on assessment of the rate of synthesis of different globin chains. Blood cells are incubated with radiolabeled leucine for two hours to label the nascent hemoglobin. Red cells are then lysed and the globin precipitated and separated into carboxymethylcellulose columns. The presence of both beta alpha- and betaS-globins would identify a fetus with sickle cell trait; the presence of betaS but no beta alpha would diagnose sickle cell anemia. Quantitation of the amount of beta-globin (or hemoglobin A) synthesized in relation to the amount of gamma-globin (or hemoglobin F) synthesized is necessary for the diagnosis of beta-thalassemia (Table 28–9). No beta chain will be synthesized in beta-thalassemia, and only a very small amount, if any, in beta-positive–thalassemia. Fetuses with beta-thalassemia trait will have intermediate beta/gamma ratios.[86]

Prenatal diagnosis techniques have been used in the diagnosis of over 11,000 fetuses at risk for hematologic disorders. The most common indications for evaluation have been thalassemia and sickle disorders. A major trend in prenatal diagnosis for these disorders has been a progressive shift toward the use of molecular biology techniques.[87]

Although prenatal diagnosis of alpha-thalassemia

with pure fetal blood is possible, this can be done simply with the use of DNA techniques in cultured amniotic fluid or chorionic villi cells.[88,89] The diagnosis of sickle cell disease can also be made with the use of restriction endonucleases in cultured amniotic cells.[90] However, it is anticipated that this technique will be useful in only 60 to 70% of families with infants at risk; the rest will require fetal blood analysis for prenatal diagnosis.

Evaluation of Discrepant Growth in Multiple Gestation

Differential growth may result from twin-to-twin transfusion syndrome, utero placental insufficiency, congenital infection, or a chromosomal anomaly. Fetal blood sampling is a rapid and informative method of assessing the etiology of the discrepancy.[91] Differences in the hematocrit are not a reliable means of identifying twin-to-twin transfusion syndrome. The injection of adult blood in one twin and the recovery of adult red blood cells in the circulation of the other has been recently employed in the diagnosis of this syndrome. (Rodeck CH, personal communication.)

Selective Termination. A serious clinical challenge results if only one of the members of a multiple gestation is affected. The options available to the patient include termination of the pregnancy, continuation, and selective termination. Techniques employed for selective termination include: (1) intracardiac injection of potassium chloride (5 to 15 mEq) to cause cardiac arrest, (2) cardiac puncture to achieve exsanguination, (3) intravascular air embolism (10 to 20 mL of air), and (4) intracardiac injection of calcium gluconate.[92–96] The most reliable method is intracardiac injection of potassium chloride.[93]

The first step consists of correctly identifying the affected fetus. This is easy in the presence of a gross structural anomaly or discordant gender. In the absence of an anatomic marker for the abnormal fetuses, fetal blood sampling for rapid karyotyping may be required before termination. After selective termination, a sample of blood should be obtained to confirm that the correct

TABLE 28–9. EVOLUTION OF HbA/HbFac RATIO BETWEEN 19 AND 36 WEEKS OF GESTATION (Mean ± SD)

Week of Gestation	No. of Cases	HbA HbFac
19–21	34	0.86 ± 0.13
22–24	44	0.92 ± 0.18
25–27	15	0.94 ± 0.21
28–30	7	1.00 ± 0.2
31–36	9	1.19 ± 0.18

(*Reproduced with permission from Forestier, et al. Pediatr Res. 1986; 20:342.*)

fetus was selected. Complications include intra-amniotic infection, disseminated intravascular coagulation, rupture of the membranes, and preterm labor. In the absence of vascular communications (dichorionic twinning), embolic phenomenon to the surviving co-twin should not occur. Patients should be followed with serial clotting studies because chronic disseminated intravascular coagulation may develop. Heparin treatment is an option for prolonging the pregnancy if such a complication occurs.

Intrauterine Growth Retardation

Severe and early intrauterine growth retardation (IUGR) is rapidly emerging as one of the main indications for diagnostic cordocentesis. The objectives are to exclude aneuploidy, to identify fetal infection, and to assess the hematologic and acid base status. Eydoux and colleagues[28] have reported that the prevalence of structural chromosomal abnormalities in 108 patients with isolated IUGR was 6.7%.[28] The most frequent anomalies are trisomies 21, 18, and 13, triploidy, and other structural anomalies. The prevalence was 27% (6/22) if IUGR was accompanied by polyhydramnios, 31.5% (18/57) when IUGR was associated with structural anomalies, and 50% (7/15) if associated with both polyhydramnios and congenital anomalies. In a study of 21 fetuses with early and severe IUGR (mean gestational age 29 weeks), Weiner and coworkers[97] reported a 23.8% (5/21) incidence of aneuploidy and two cases of congenital infection. In a study of 239 fetuses with IUGR, Bilardo and Nicolaides[98] reported a 17% prevalence of chromosomal anomalies. Triploidy was the most common anomaly found. Hematologic indices, acid-base parameters, and liver function tests can help assess the degree of stress and utero-placental insufficiency in the setting of IUGR. These studies hold great promise toward helping us understand the biology of IUGR.[99,100] More research is needed to define the role of these studies in daily clinical practice.[101,102]

REFERENCES

1. Valenti C. Endoamnioscopy and fetal biopsy: A new technique. *Am J Obstet Gynecol.* 1972;114:561.
2. Hobbins JC, Mahoney M, Goldstein LA. A new method of intrauterine visualization by the combined use of fetoscopy and ultrasound. *Am J Obstet Gynecol.* 1974;118:1069.
3. Hobbins JC, Mahoney MJ. In utero diagnosis of hemoglobinopathies: Techniques for obtaining fetal blood. *N Engl J Med.* 1974;290:1065.
4. Rodeck CH, Campbell S. Umbilical cord insertion as a source of pure fetal blood for prenatal diagnosis. *Lancet.* 1979;1:1244.
5. Daffos F, Capell-Pavlovsky M, Forestier F. A new procedure for fetal blood sampling in utero: Preliminary results of fifty-three cases. *Am J Obstet Gynecol.* 1983;146:985.
6. Ludomirsky A, Weiner S, Ashmead GG, Librizzi RJ, Bolognese RJ. Percutaneous fetal umbilical blood sampling: Procedure safety and normal fetal hematologic indices. *Am J Perinatol.* 1988;5:264.
7. Benacerraf BR, Barss VA, Saltzman DH, Greene MF, Penso CA, Frigoletto FD. Fetal abnormalities: Diagnosis or treatment with percutaneous umbilical blood sampling under continuous US guidance. *Radiology.* 1988;166:105.
8. Weiner CP. The role of cordocentesis in fetal diagnosis. *Clin Obstet Gynecol.* 1988;31:285.
9. Nicolaides KH. Cordocentesis. *Clin Obstet Gynecol.* 1988;31:123.
10. Nicolaides KH, Soothill PW, Rodeck CH, Campbell S. Ultrasound-guided sampling of umbilical cord and placental blood to assess fetal wellbeing. *Lancet.* 1986;1:1065.
11. Hobbins JC, Grannum PA, Romero R, Reece EA, Mahoney MJ. Percutaneous umbilical cord blood sampling. *Am J Obstet Gynecol.* 1985;152:47.
12. Benacerraf BR, Barss VA, Saltzman DH, Greene MF, Penso CA, Frigoletto FD. Acute fetal distress associated with percutaneous umbilical blood sampling. *Am J Obstet Gynecol.* 1987;156:1218.
13. Weiner CP. Cordocentesis. *Obstet Gynecol Clin North Am.* 1988;15:283.
14. Moise KJ, Carpenter RJ, Deter RL, Kirshon B, Diaz SF. The use of fetal neuromuscular blockade during intrauterine procedures. *Am J Obstet Gynecol.* 1987;157:874.
15. Daffos F, Capella-Pavlovsky M, Forestier F. Fetal blood sampling during pregnancy with use of a needle guided by ultrasound: A study of 606 consecutive cases. *Am J Obstet Gynecol.* 1985;153:655.
16. Forestier F, Cox WL, Daffos F, Rainaut M. The assessment of fetal blood samples. *Am J Obstet Gynecol.* 1988;158:1184.
17. Ludomirski A, Weiner S. Percutaneous fetal umbilical blood sampling. *Clin Obstet Gynecol.* 1988;31:19.
18. Nicolini U, Santolaya J, Ojo OE, et al. The fetal intrahepatic umbilical vein as an alternative to cord needling for prenatal diagnosis and therapy. *Prenat Diagn.* 1988;8:665.
19. Muller J, Giovangrandi Y, Parnet-Mathieu F, Cabrol D, Paniel BJ, Sureau C. Acute fetal distress after blood sampling. *Eur J Obstet Gynecol.* 1988;28:269. Case report.
20. Pielet BW, Socol ML, MacGregor SN, Ney JA, Dooley SL. Cordocentesis: An appraisal of risks. *Am J Obstet Gynecol.* 1988;159:1497.
21. Jauniaux E, Donner C, Simon P, Vanesse M, Hustin J, Rodesch F. Pathologic aspects of the umbilical cord after percutaneous umbilical blood sampling. *Obstet Gynecol.* 1989;73:215.
22. Wilkins I, Mezrow G, Lynch L, Bottone EJ, Berkowitz RL. Amnionitis and life-threatening respiratory distress after percutaneous umbilical blood sampling. *Am J Obstet Gynecol.* 1989;160:427.

23. Nicolini U, Kochenour NK, Greco P, et al. Consequences of fetomaternal haemorrhage after intrauterine transfusion. *Br Med J.* 1988;297:1379.

24. Bowell PJ, Selinger M, Ferguson J, Giles J, MacKenzie IZ. Antenatal fetal blood sampling for the management of alloimmunized pregnancies: Effect upon maternal anti-D potency levels. *Br J Obstet Gynaecol.* 1988;95:759.

25. Angel JL, O'Brien WF, Michelson JA, Knuppe. RA, Morales WJ. Instructional model for percutaneous fetal umbilical blood sampling. *Obstet Gynecol.* 1989; 73:669.

26. Timor-Trish IE, Yeh MN. In vitro training model for diagnostic and therapeutic fetal intravascular needle puncture. *Am J Obstet Gynecol.* 1987;157:858.

27. Pijpers L, Jahoda MGJ, Reuss A, Wladimiroff JW, Sachs ES. Transabdominal chorionic villus biopsy in second and third trimesters of pregnancy to determine fetal karyotype. *Br Med J.* 1988;297:822.

28. Eydoux P, Choiset A, Le Porrier N, et al. Chromosomal prenatal diagnosis: Study of 936 cases of intrauterine abnormalities after ultrasound assessment. *Prenat Diagn.* 1989;9:255.

29. Williamson RA, Weiner CP, Patil S, Benda J, Varner MW, Abu-Yousef MM. Abnormal pregnancy sonogram: Selective indication for fetal karyotype. *Obstet Gynecol.* 1987;69:15.

30. Nicolaides KH, Rodeck CH, Gosden CM. Rapid karyotyping in non-lethal fetal malformations. *Lancet.* 1986; 1:283.

31. Gosden C, Nicolaides KH, Rodeck CH. Fetal blood sampling in investigation of chromosome mosaicism in amniotic fluid cell culture. *Lancet.* 1988;1:613.

32. Watson MS, Breg WR, Hobbins JC, et al. Cytogenetic diagnosis using midtrimester fetal blood samples: Application to suspected mosaicism and other diagnostic problems. *Am J Med Genet.* 1984;19:805.

33. Kaffe S, Benn PA, Hsu LY. Fetal blood sampling in investigation of chromosome mosaicism in amniotic fluid cell culture. *Lancet.* 1988;1:284.

34. Bui TH, Iselius L, Lindsten J. European collaborative study on prenatal diagnosis: Mosaicism, pseudomosaicism and single abnormal cells in amniotic fluid cell cultures. *Prenat Diagn.* 1984;4:145.

35. Hsu LYF, Perlis TE. United States survey on chromosome mosaicism and pseudomosaicism in prenatal diagnosis. *Prenat Diagn.* 1984;4:97.

36. Worton RG, Stern RA. Canadian collaborative study of mosaicism in amniotic fluid cell cultures. *Prenat Diagn.* 1984;4:131.

37. Hsu LYF, Kaffe S, Perlis TE. Trisomy 20 mosaicism in prenatal diagnosis—a review and update. *Prenat Diagn.* 1987;7:581.

38. Chudley AE, Hagerman RJ. Fragile X syndrome. *J Pediatr.* 1987;110:821.

39. Barnes D. Fragile X syndrome and its puzzling genetics. *Science.* 1989;243:171.

40. Brown T, Gross A, Chan C, et al. Multilocus analysis of the fragile X syndrome. *Human Genet.* 1988;78:201.

41. Webb TP, Rodeck CH, Nicolaides KH, Gosden CM. Prenatal diagnosis of the fragile X syndrome using fetal blood and amniotic fluid. *Prenat Diag.* 1987;7:203.

42. Sever JL, Larsen JW, Grossman III JH. *Handbook of Perinatal Infections.* Boston: Little Brown; 1979.

43. Daffos F, Forestier F, Capella-Pavlovsky M, et al. Prenatal management of 746 pregnancies at risk for congenital toxoplasmosis. *N Engl J Med.* 1988;318:271.

44. Remington JS, Desmonts G. Toxoplasmosis. In: Remington JS, Klein JO, eds. *Infectious Diseases of the Fetus and Newborn Infant.* Philadelphia: Saunders; 1976:171.

45. Desmonts G, Daffos F, Forestier F, Capella-Pavlovsky M, Thulliez PH, Chartier M. Prenatal diagnosis of congenital toxoplasmosis. *Lancet.* 1985;1:500–3.

46. Miller E, Cradock-Watson JA, Pollock TM. Consequences of confirmed maternal rubella at successive stages of pregnancy. *Lancet.* 1982;2:781.

47. Freig BJ, South MA, Sever JL. Maternal rubella and the congenital rubella syndrome. *Clin Perinatol.* 1988; 15:247.

48. Cradock-Watson JE, Ridehalgh MKS, Anderson MJ, Pattison JR. Rubella reinfection and the fetus. *Lancet.* 1985;1:1039.

49. Grangeot-Keros L, Pillot J, Daffos F, Forestier F. Prenatal and postnatal production of IgM and IgA antibodies to rubella virus studied by antibody capture immunoassay. *J Infect Dis.* 1988;158:138.

50. Nigro G, Nanni F, Midulla M. Rubella reinfection and the fetus. *Lancet.* 1985;1:1040. Letter.

51. Morgan-Capner P, Rodeck CH, Nicolaides K, et al. Prenatal detection of rubella-specific IgM in fetal sera. *Prenat Diagn.* 1979;5:21.

52. Stagno S, Pass RF, Sworsky ME, et al. Maternal cytomegalovirus infection and perinatal transmission. *Clin Obstet Gynecol.* 1982;25:563.

53. Pass RF, Stagno S, Myers GJ, et al. Outcome of symptomatic congenital cytomegalovirus infection: Results of long-term follow up. *Pediatrics.* 1980;66:758.

54. Freij BJ, Sever JL. Herpes virus infections in pregnancy: Risks to embryo, fetus, and neonate. *Clin Perinat.* 1988; 15:203.

55. Lange I, Rodeck CH, Morgan-Capner P, et al. Prenatal serological diagnosis of intrauterine cytomegalovirus infection. *Br Med J.* 1982;284:1763.

56. Binder ND, Buckmaster JW, Benda GI. Outcome for fetus with ascites and cytomegalovirus infection. *Pediatr.* 1988;82:100.

57. Stagno S, Pass RF, Dworsky ME, et al. Congenital cytomegalovirus infection: The relative importance of primary and recurrent maternal infection. *N Engl J Med.* 1982;306:945.

58. Cuthbertson G, Weiner CP, Giller RH, Grose C. Prenatal diagnosis of second-trimester congenital varicella syndrome by virus-specific immunoglobulin M. *J Pediatr.* 1987;111:592.

59. Naides SJ, Weiner CP. Antenatal diagnosis and palliative treatment of non-immune hydrops fetalis secondary to fetal parvovirus B19 infection. *Prenat Diag.* 1989; 9:105.

60. Knisely AS, O'Shea PA, McMillan P, Singer DB. Electron

microscopic identification of parvovirus virions in erythroid-line cells in fatal hydrops fetalis. *Pediatr Path.* 1988;8:163.

61. Lau YL, Levinsky RJ. Prenatal diagnosis and carrier detection in primary immunodeficiency disorders. *Arch Dis Child.* 1988;63:758.

62. Levinsky RJ. Prenatal diagnosis of severe combined immunodeficiency. In: Rodeck CH, Nicolaides KH, eds. *Prenatal Diagnosis: Proceedings of the Eleventh Study Group of the Royal College of Obstetricians and Gynaecologists.* Chichester, England: Royal College of Obstetricians and Gynaecologists; 1984:137.

63. Perignon JL, Durandy A, Peter MO, Freycon F, Dumez Y, Griscelli C. Early prenatal diagnosis of inherited severe immunodeficiencies linked to enzyme deficiencies. *J Pediatr.* 1987;111:595.

64. Durandy A, Cerf-Bensussan N, Dumez Y, Grisell C. Prenatal diagnosis of severe combined immunodeficiency with defective synthesis of HLA molecules. *Prenat Diagn.* 1987;7:27.

65. Kenney D, Cairns L, Remold-O'Donnell E, Peterson J, Rosen FS, Parkman R. Morphological abnormalities in the lymphocytes of patients with the Wiskott–Aldrich syndrome. *Blood.* 1986;68:1329.

66. Pidard D, Didry D, Le Deist F, et al. Analysis of the membrane glycoproteins of platelets in the Wiskoff–Aldrich syndrome. *Br J Haematol.* 1988;69:529.

67. Fearon ER, Kohn DB, Winkelstein JA, Vogelstein B, Blaese RM. Carrier detection in the Wiskott–Aldrich syndrome. *Blood.* 1988;72:1735.

68. Newburger PE, Cohen HJ, Rothchild SB, et al. Prenatal diagnosis of granulomatous disease. *N Engl J Med.* 1979;300:178.

69. Borregaard N, Bang J, Berthelsen JG, et al. Prenatal diagnosis of chronic granulomatous disease. *Lancet.* 1982;1:114.

70. Matthay KK, Golbus MS, Wara DW, et al. Prenatal diagnosis of chronic granulomatous disease. *Am J Med Genet.* 1984;17:731.

71. Mibashan RS, Peake IR, Rodeck CH, et al. Carrier detection of hemophilia A in pregnancy by measurement of factor VIIIC/RAg and VIIICAg/RAg ratios. *Thromb Haemostasis.* 1981;46:187.

72. Firshein SI, Hoyer LW, Lazarchick J, et al. Prenatal diagnosis of classic hemophilia. *N Engl J Med.* 1979;300:937.

73. Mibashan RS, Rodeck CH, Thumpston JK, et al. Plasma assay of fetal factors VIIIC and IX for prenatal diagnosis of hemophilia. *Lancet.* 1979;2:1309.

74. Peake IR, Bloom AL, Giddings JC, et al. An immunoradiometric assay for procoagulant factor VIIIAg: Results in hemophilia, von Willebrand's disease and fetal plasma and serum. *Br J Haematol.* 1979;42:269.

75. Holmberg L, Gustavi B, Cordesius E, et al. Prenatal diagnosis of hemophilia B by an immunoradiometric assay of factor IX. *Blood.* 1980;56:397.

76. Mibashan RS, Rodeck CH. Haemophilia and other genetic defects haemostasis. In: Rodeck CH, Nicolaides KH, eds. *Prenatal Diagnosis. Proceedings of the Eleventh*

Study Group of the Royal College of Obstetricians and Gynaecologists. Chichester, England: Royal College of Obstetricians and Gynaecologists; 1984:179.

77. Daffos F, Forestier F, Kaplan C, Cox W. Prenatal diagnosis and management of bleeding disorders with fetal blood sampling. *J Obstet Gynecol.* 1988;158:939.

78. Kasper CK, Osterud B, Minami J, et al. Hemophilia B: Characterization of genetic variants and detection of carriers. *Blood.* 1977;50:351.

79. Hoyer LW, Lindsten J, Blomback RM, et al. Prenatal evaluation of a fetus at risk for von Willebrand's disease. *Lancet.* 1979;2:191.

80. De Vries LS, Connell J, Bydder GM, et al. Recurrent intracranial haemorrhages in utero in an infant with alloimmune thrombocytopenia. *Br J Obstet Gynaecol.* 1988;95:299.

81. Kaplan C, Daffos F, Forestier F, et al. Management of alloimmune thrombocytopenia: Antenatal diagnosis and in utero transfusion of maternal platelets. *Blood.* 1988;72:340.

82. Nicolini U, Rodeck CH, Kochenour NK, et al. In-utero platelet transfusion for alloimmune thrombocytopenia. *Lancet.* 1988;2:506.

83. Bussel JB, Berkowitz RL, Mc Farland JG, Lynch L, Chitkara U. Antenatal treatment of neonatal alloimmune thrombocytopenia. *N Engl J Med.* 1988;319:1374.

84. Scioscia AL, Grannum PA, Copel JA, Hobbins JC. The use of percutaneous umbilical blood sampling in immune thrombocytopenic purpura. *Am J Obstet Gynecol.* 1988;159:1066.

85. Moise KJ Jr, Carpenter RJ Jr, Cotton DB, Wasserstrum N, Kirshon B, Cano L. Percutaneous umbilical cord blood sampling in the evaluation of fetal platelet counts in pregnant patients with autoimmune thrombocytopenia purpura. *Obstet Gynecol.* 1988;72:346.

86. Alter BP. Prenatal diagnosis of hemoglobinopathies: Development of methods for study of fetal red cells and fibroblasts. *Am J Pediatr Hemat.* 1985;5:378.

87. Alter BP. Prenatal diagnosis of hematologic diseases: 1986 update. *Haemoglobin Proc Int Meeting.* London; 1986;78:137.

88. Cao A, Rosatelli C, Pirastu M. Prenatal diagnosis of inherited hemoglobinopathies. *J Genet Hum.* 34:413.

89. Cao A, Furbetta M, Angius A, Ximenes A, Angioni G, Caminiti F. Prenatal diagnosis of beta thalassemia: Experience with 133 cases and the effect of fetal blood sampling on child development. *Ann NY Acad Sci.* 1980;344:165.

90. Weatherall DJ, Old JM, Thein SL, Wainscoat JS, Clegg JB. Prenatal diagnosis of the common haemoglobin disorders. *J Med Genet.* 1985;22:422.

91. Cox WL, Forestier F, Capella-Pavlovsky M, Daffos F. Fetal blood sampling in twin pregnancies. *Fetal Therapy* 1987;2:101–108.

92. Aberg A, Mitelman F, Cantz M, et al. Cardiac puncture of fetus with Hurler's disease avoiding abortion of unaffected co-twin. *Lancet.* 1978;2:990.

93. Chitkara U, Berkowitz RL, Wilkins IA, Lynch L, Mehalek KE, Alvarez M. Selective second-trimester termination

of the anomalous fetus in twin pregnancies. *Obstet Gynecol.* 1989;73:690.

94. Kerenyi TD, Chitkara U. Selective birth in twin pregnancy with discordancy for Down syndrome. *N Engl J Med.* 1981;304:1525.

95. Rodeck CH. Fetoscopy in the management of twin pregnancies discordant for a severe abnormality. *Acta Genet Med Gemellol.* 1985;33:57.

96. Wittman BK, Farquharson DF, Thomas WDS, Baldwin VJ, Wadsworth LD. The role of feticide in the management of severe twin transfusion syndrome. *Am J Obstet Gynecol.* 1986;155:1023.

97. Weiner CP, Williamson RA. Evaluation of severe growth retardation using cordocentesis—hemotologic and metabolic alterations by etiology. *Obstet Gynecol.* 1989; 79:225.

98. Bilardo CM, Nicolaides KH. Cordocentesis in the assessment of the small-for-gestational-age fetus. *Fetal Therapy.* 1988;3:24–30.

99. Cetin I, Marconi AM, Bozzetti P, et al. Umbilical amino acid concentrations in appropriate and small for gestational age infants: A biochemical difference present in utero. *Am J Obstet Gynecol.* 1988;158:120.

100. Pardi G, Buscaglia M, Ferrazzi E, et al. Cord sampling for the evaluation of oxygenation and acid-base balance in growth-retarded human fetuses. *Am J Obstet Gynecol.* 1987;157:1221.

101. Soothill PW, Nicolaides KH, Rodeck CH, Gamsu H. Blood gases and acid-base status of the human second-trimester fetus. *Obstet Gynecol.* 1986;68:173.

102. Cox WL, Daffos F, Forestier F, et al. Physiology and management of intrauterine growth retardation: A biologic approach with fetal blood sampling. *Am J Obstet Gynecol.* 1988;159:36.

29 Ultrasound-Guided Fetal Invasive Therapy: Current Status

Frank A. Manning

The rapid development of very high quality dynamic fetal imaging methods now permits recognition of discrete developmental anomalies of fetal organ systems at an even earlier gestational age. It is now possible to monitor the progression of such anomalies in concert to determine their structural and functional sequelae. The observation of the "natural" history of anomalies has prompted the development of innovative, if largely unproven, invasive methods for averting the otherwise inevitable outcome.

Invasion of the fetal environment with therapeutic intent, although not a new concept in perinatal medicine (having been successfully practiced in alloimmunization syndromes since the landmark reports of Liley and Bowman[1,2]), has recently undergone a resurgence in interest and application. There are now many forms of invasive fetal therapy, yielding a range of proven and unproven benefits. The most well-established form of invasive fetal therapy involves creating a fetal intravascular communication by which fetal deficiencies may be corrected. Thus, direct intravascular transfusion of the alloimmunized anemic fetus has yielded amazing results in mortality and morbidity (see Chapter 24). An extension of this principle to replace missing or abnormal cell lines (stem cell therapy), gene products, or genes themselves is an area of active and promising research, but falls outside the scope of this summary.

Invasive intrauterine maneuvers designed to overcome intrinsic anomalous obstruction of fluid dynamics have been the object of recent intensive clinical study. In some conditions, such as simple obstructive uropathies, these therapies have yielded results that strongly suggest a true therapeutic benefit. In other instances, such as obstructive hydrocephalus, the benefits, if any, of in utero diversion therapies are much more obscured. The bulk of this chapter deals with these two sets of obstructive disorders, the data being derived from the International Fetal Medicine and Surgery Society Registry.[3] In other conditions, such as diaphragmatic hernia, aggressive in-utero surgical repair has been attempted; the number of cases to date is so few that comment on efficacy is currently unwarranted.

FETAL UROPATHY: FREQUENCY AND PATHOPHYSIOLOGY

Developmental anomalies of the fetal urinary tract are among the most commonly recognized congenital anomalies.[4,5] The incidence of lethal renal anomalies in the Manitoba study population is between 0.3 and 0.7 per 1,000 livebirths. Dynamic ultrasound imaging allows for assessment of both the structural and functional characteristics of the developing fetal urinary tract. Ultrasound assessment of the spectrum of congenital disease of the fetal urinary tract is neither simple nor direct, and diagnostic accuracy depends to a large degree on the experience of the ultrasonographer and the quality of equipment used. Serious diagnostic errors with this method have been reported.[6–8] Fortunately, the risk of diagnostic error is least with lower tract (outlet) obstructive uropathies,[6,7] the area of major concern to fetal surgeons.

In the normal fetus, the kidneys may be seen from as early as 12 weeks' gestation. As gestational age advances, renal mass and internal architecture become progressively well defined. With newer high-resolution ultrasound equipment, the renal arteries and arcuate arteries may be seen after 20 weeks' gestation, and renal blood flow patterns can be assessed. The fetal bladder is seen from as early as 14 weeks' gestation, and micturition pattern may be recorded as an indirect means of assessing fetal urine production rates.[9] In the male fetus, the external genitalia are usually recognized with certainty at about 16 to 20 weeks' gestation, and turbulence created by fetal voiding is often observed. Because fetal urine production is a major contributor to amniotic fluid volume in later pregnancy,[10] ultrasound assessment of amniotic fluid adequacy provides an important insight into the adequacy of renal function.

There is a very wide spectrum of congenital fetal uropathies ranging from complete absence of functioning renal tissue (renal agenesis) to minor and often transient dilatation of the renal pelvis. Although undetermined with certainty at present, it theoretically seems that few of these urinary tract diseases would benefit from in-utero therapeutic maneuvers. At the time of writing the diseases deemed amenable to fetal surgical diversion are restricted to those that produce bladder outlet obstruction, primarily urethral valve syndromes, urethral atresia, or possibly persistant cloacal syndromes.

It is evident from ovine fetal experiments that obstruction of the outflow tract produces pathologic renal changes, the extent and nature of which vary with the fetal age at obstruction. Ureteral ligation late in pregnancy in fetal sheep (22 weeks' human equivalent) produces simple hydronephrosis, whereas earlier obstruction (13 to 19 weeks' human equivalent) produces changes suggestive of renal dysplasia.[11,12] Ureteral occlusion in late gestation (29 weeks' human equivalent) causes simple hydronephrosis; in earlier gestation (16 weeks' human equivalent) it causes unequivocal renal dysgenesis, and lethal pulmonary hypoplasia occurs with obstruction at either age.[13–16] Of major importance is the observation that subsequent release of experimental obstruction halts the progression of both the renal and pulmonary effects.[14,15] These are landmark experiments because they provide insight into the pathogenesis of renal lesions and provide a rational basis for consideration of in-utero urinary diversion therapy in the affected human fetus.

The spectrum of outcomes in human fetuses with outlet obstruction fits reasonably well with these experimental models. When total obstruction occurs in very early human pregnancy, the most common result may be renal dysgenesis/agenesis and pulmonary hypoplasia, a uniformly lethal fetal condition. Lethal renal dysgenesis secondary to outlet obstruction in early human pregnancies has been reported.[8] The obstruction also can be either anatomically partial or anatomically complete but rendered functionally partial due to gross dilatation of the fetal bladder, ureters, and urachus, producing a less severe effect on the developing kidneys and lungs. Spontaneous cure of total obstructive uropathy can occur in utero by a pressure effect at the site of obstruction, by bladder rupture and urinary ascites,[17] or by urachal cyst formation and subsequent rupture into the amniotic space. We have observed spontaneous resolution of outlet obstruction uropathy due to persistant cloacal syndrome by the latter mechanism (Manning FA, Harman CR, Menticoglou S, unpublished data, 1986.) These experiments of nature appear to confirm that release of obstruction of the outflow tract can halt the natural progression of the renal and pulmonary effects of such obstruction.

The natural history of bladder outlet obstruction is, of course, the critical and key unanswered question. Assessment of whether or not benefits result from fetal surgery, and what they are, will depend on the answer.

However, at least part of the total picture may be seen. Persistent absence of renal function in utero as may occur with anatomical (renal agenesis) or functional (severe renal dysgenesis) defects frequently results in fetal death. The mechanism is assumed to be cord compression secondary to gross oligohydramnios. What proportion of all fetuses with outlet obstruction present in this manner is unknown, but is probably relatively high. The outcome of fetuses with outlet obstruction of either later onset or a less severe functional form appears to be highly variable. Many of these fetuses die in utero, again most likely as a consequence of oligohydramnios, but some will deliver as liveborns, often prematurely.

A second critical natural selection process becomes operative in the immediate postnatal period. The successful transition from fetal to neonatal life depends critically on the rapid establishment of adequate pulmonary function. Pulmonary hypoplasia, a common sequela of severe obstruction uropathy, prevents this successful transition. What proportion of liveborns with obstructive uropathy is lost at birth as a result of this lethal natural selection process is also unknown, but two separate observations suggest this proportion may be high. The International Fetal Surgery Registry report describes the outcome of 58 liveborn infants with obstructive uropathy treated in utero; 25 of these 58 liveborns (43%) died in the immediate newborn period from pulmonary hypoplasia.[3] Nakayama and colleagues[18] described the outcome in 11 liveborn infants with obstructive uropathy (posterior urethral valve syndrome) evident at birth; 5 of the 11 liveborns (40%) died in the immediate neonatal period from pulmonary hypoplasia.[18] The prognosis for those affected perinates who survive these two powerful selection periods, the fetal and immediate neonatal, improves dramatically. Survival rates of up to 95% are reported for infants with obstructive uropathy (posterior urethral valve syndrome) who survive the immediate neonatal period.[19]

It is this range of outcomes created by natural selection that accounts for much of the controversy surrounding indications for and efficacy of fetal surgical diversion therapy for obstructive uropathy. The experimental and serendipitous clinical evidence that release of fetal urinary tract obstruction can halt the progression of renal and pulmonary sequelae seems evident. The major challenge for fetal surgeons lies in case selection, specifically in the differentiation of those perinates who will die from disease in the fetal and immediate neonatal periods from those perinates who will survive to benefit from postnatal therapy. The secondary challenge is to devise effective therapeutic maneuvers to ensure maximal continued benefit to the selected at-risk fetus at minimal risk to the mother.

FETAL SURGERY: CASE SELECTION CRITERIA AND METHODS

Selection of those few fetuses who might benefit from in-utero surgical urinary tract diversion procedures may be best achieved by application of rigid exclusion criteria. Few of these have been subjected as yet to rigorous scientific scrutiny. Despite the optimistic enthusiasm of the fetal surgeon, there can be little doubt that neonatal repair of obstructive uropathies will almost always be a safer and more definitive procedure. Therefore, as the first principle, the fetus of sufficient age and maturity to sustain extrauterine survival should never be a candidate for in-utero surgery. A second principle is that the therapy should only be considered in the fetus with bladder outlet obstruction and bilateral progressive renal disease. The primary aim of therapy is to prevent both the renal and pulmonary sequelae. Penetrating the fetus with a needle, even when done by an experienced operator using the most sophisticated ultrasound guidance systems, is not without risk. Obstetricians have accumulated a great deal of experience with needle penetration of the fetal peritoneal cavity, and less experience with bladder puncture. For either method, the fetal death rate directly attributable to the procedure is about 5%.[3,20] Therefore, the issues must not be whether or not therapy is possible, for it nearly always is, but rather if such therapy will benefit the fetus and if the potential benefit outweighs any real fetal risk. Against this background, the justification for prenatal therapy for unilateral disease, as has been reported,[21,22] may be lacking, although in some cases an apparent amelioration of associated maternal disease has been described.[22]

The fetus with both obstructive uropathy and some other organ system(s) structural anomaly or karyotypic anomaly should not be considered a candidate for prenatal therapy. Such an association is not uncommon; of 72 treated cases reported to the International Fetal Surgery Registry, 5 (7%) had multiple organ system anomalies and 6 (8%) had karyotypic anomalies.[3] Thus, 11 of 72 fetuses (15%) had lethal anomalies, a rate that is 15 to 30 times higher than that of the general population. Although maternal morbidity has not been described as a complication of in-utero therapy for obstructive uropathy, severe maternal morbidity or death has been caused by other invasive intrauterine procedures such as amniocentesis[23] and intrauterine transfusion.[24] Serious and potentially life threatening maternal infection (chorioamnionitis) can occur as a consequence of diagnostic or therapeutic maternal percutaneous placement of a fetal bladder catheter.[25] It therefore follows that a detailed and complete ultrasound fetal organ system review should be a prerequisite to any therapeutic efforts. In theory,

such a review should detect all associated structural anomalies; in practice the detection rate is about 90%.[26] Confirmation that the affected fetus being considered for therapy has a normal karyotype has been a difficult problem because the traditional diagnostic method, amniocentesis for amniocyte culture, requires waiting up to 4 weeks for results. Further, in the presence of oligohydramnios, a frequent associated finding with obstructive uropathy, an amniotic fluid sample may not be obtainable. In such cases, fetal urine obtained by vesicocentesis may yield sufficient cells for culture,[27] but the reliability of this method is not uniform and considerable delay is again involved. The new technique of direct fetal umbilical vein blood sampling,[28,29] yielding karyotype results as early as in 2 days, can most certainly circumvent these problems.

The relationship between amniotic fluid volume, as estimated by ultrasound, and outcome in fetuses with obstructive uropathy is unclear. Hence the use of this variable for case selection remains controversial. Because fetal urine production is a major contributor to the dynamic amniotic fluid compartment in later pregnancy,[8] it follows that significant fetal obstructive disease should be associated with a reduction or absence of amniotic fluid (oligohydramnios). The data contained in the International Fetal Surgery Registry do not support this supposition. However, the majority of fetuses with obstructive uropathy do have oligohydramnios (78%). The survival rates are similar among treated fetuses with or without oligohydramnios (41% and 40% respectively).[3] Further, perinatal death due to pulmonary hypoplasia is observed among fetuses with obstructive uropathy and apparent normal amniotic fluid volume.

The discrepancy between the predicted and observed relationships of amniotic fluid volume to perinatal outcome in fetuses with obstructive uropathy may be due to a variety of factors. Amniotic fluid volume determination by ultrasound is often done by subjective assessment, and the use of objective criteria such as the largest fluid pocket measurement has not been uniform.[30] Under such subjective conditions, the true relationship remains uncertain. Alternately, in fetuses with partial or incomplete obstruction there may be sufficient outflow impedence to cause proximal dilatation and damage while urine efflux may be sufficient to maintain some amniotic fluid. Pulmonary hypoplasia is by far the most common cause of perinatal death in obstructive uropathies, accounting for 81% of deaths among treated pregnancies.[3] Chronic oligohydramnios, both in the experimental animal model and in the human, is associated with an increased incidence of lethal pulmonary hypoplasia.[31,32] It is tempting to suggest that the high incidence of pulmonary hypoplasia seen in fetuses with obstructive uropathy is therefore caused by this oligohydramnios. In the experimental animal model, reversal of experimental oligohydramnios restores lung growth and prevents pulmonary hypoplasia.[31] A similar recovery of lung growth is seen with corrected experimental obstructive uropathy.[12] The clinical human experience also clearly indicates that in-utero diversion therapy resulting in restoration of normal amniotic fluid volume may be associated with intact survival, even in the presence of pretreatment extreme oligohydramnios.[27,33] Thus, despite reported opinions to the contrary,[34] there is simply no evidence that oligohydramnios is a contraindication to therapy. However, the observation of lethal pulmonary hypoplasia with obstructive uropathy even in the presence of normal amniotic fluid volume indicates there must be more than one etiologic factor for pulmonary hypoplasia. Intrinsic pulmonary compression due to bladder and urinary tract dilatation may be another cause; diaphragmatic hernia, either experimental or clinical, is known to cause pulmonary hypoplasia by the same method.[35] Again, in such circumstances urinary tract decompression by in-utero diversion therapy may be expected to enhance lung growth and therefore improve survival.

An alternate explanation for the association of lung and urinary tract anomalies is that the primary insult, the nature of which remains entirely unknown, affects the endodermal lung primordia and the mesodermal genitourinary primordia simultaneously. Such a mechanism, while possible, is viewed as highly unlikely because most teratogens affect either all germ cell layers or a single layer, but rarely, if ever, affect only two of the three layers. Nonetheless, if such a mechanism is indeed operant, then the theoretical arguments for urinary tract diversion to prevent pulmonary hypoplasia are without foundation.

Fetal Renal Function

We have begun to learn at a very rapid rate how to evaluate fetal renal function. These data are becoming an integral part of individual case selection criteria. Initial attempts to assess renal function were based on noninvasive measurement of fetal urine production rates.[36] These methods are not easily applied to the fetus with obstruction to the urinary tract, and have not been of much benefit in case selection. Invasive evaluation of the fetal urinary tract, by ultrasound-guided percutaneous fetal bladder aspiration, is now the key step in individual case selection.

Temporary external drainage of the fetal bladder permits accurate measurement of fetal urine production rates, estimation of fetal glomerular filtration rate by a creatinine or iothalamate excretion test, and urine electrolyte composition.[25] These methods are being abandoned, however, because the risk of perinatal infection

is high (6%).[26] They have been replaced by a single procedure of needle aspiration and urine electrolyte composition determination.[37]

Fetal urine is produced from as early as 13 weeks' gestation and is an ultrafiltrate of fetal serum made hypotonic by selective tubular absorption of sodium and chloride. In the fetus with intact renal function, the urinary sodium is always less than 100 mEq/dL, the chloride less than 90 mEq/dL and the osmolality less than 200 mOsm/L. Fetal urine values above these levels are associated with poor renal function and perinatal loss.[37] Methods for prenatal detection of lethal pulmonary hypoplasia remain to be elucidated, although preliminary results by determination of lung density via ultrasound appear promising (according to Harman CR, personal communication, 1986).

The question remains: does the karyotypic and otherwise structurally normal immature fetus with sustained outflow tract obstruction and bilateral urinary tract dilatation, with known intact renal function and assumed healthy pulmonary tissue, benefit from in-utero urinary tract diversion (fetal surgery)? The development of the field of perinatal medicine is now advanced to the point where such highly selected fetuses can be identified with some certainty. The empirical answer to the question, based on experimental ovine fetal models and anecdotal clinical reports, would be affirmative. The specific human data base to irrefutably support this contention does not exist. The 73 treated cases of fetal obstructive uropathy recently reported offer incomplete evidence to support this premise because this group of fetuses has disease of diverse etiology and documentation.[3] Further, the potential for bias in any voluntary registry must be taken into account.

Within this larger group of fetuses, however, may be the subset that carries the critical information. Twenty-one of the 73 (28.8%) treated cases had an unequivocal diagnosis of posterior urethral valve syndrome. These cases may be the best model in which to evaluate the benefit, if any, of fetal therapy because the etiologic lesion in these cases was isolated and well described, was not associated with other karyotypic or structural anomalies, produced bilateral renal disease, and was usually associated with oligohydramnios. The survival rate for this subset of treated fetuses was 76.2% (16 of 21 cases). The survival rate of comparable, but nontreated fetuses, is unknown but cannot be 0% since the pediatric entity is well known. However, the survival rate in neonates born with posterior urethral valve syndrome is sharply different. Nakayama and associates[18] identified 11 neonates in whom the diagnosis of posterior urethral valves was made at birth. Because these neonates were subjected to aggressive resuscitative measures, it may be assumed that this population represents only a portion of those perinates born with the condition. Others may have been denied the resuscitative measures because of the observed anomalies at birth. Five of these anomalous fetuses died (45%), either within hours (three cases), or days (two cases), from respiratory insufficiency due to proven (four cases) or assumed (one case) pulmonary hypoplasia. All of the infants who perished exhibited extreme oligohydramnios in utero. These data, when compared to outcome data of similar fetuses treated in utero, reveal a nearly two-fold difference in mortality (45 to 22.8% mortality respectively).

The survival rates for post urethral valve syndrome in both treated fetuses and neonates are much lower than those reported among older children with this condition.[18,38] The powerful influence of natural selection in the prenatal period no doubt accounts for these differences. The long-term morbidity among survivors in the two groups also varies sharply. All untreated survivors with this condition exhibited serious morbidity. Four of six survivors had prolonged respiratory insufficiency suggestive of sublethal pulmonary hypoplasia, and five of six survivors had signs of chronic renal impairment, as evidenced by azotemia, defects in fixed acid excretion, and growth failure. In contrast, none of the 16 survivors of in-utero therapy exhibited clinical signs of respiratory insufficiency, and only one has developed chronic renal failure. The long-term outcome of these cases is, of course, unknown and must be determined because late-onset renal disease has been described with this condition.[39]

Comparison of outcome data between these somewhat similar groups presents a powerful argument for the benefits of in-utero surgery for this specific condition, posterior urethral valve syndrome. It may be argued that in view of the serious nature of the condition of the newborn, the disease in utero is unlikely to be less severe. Whether or not such comparisons establish the benefit of in-utero therapy beyond a reasonable doubt remains debatable. Definitive scientific evidence can only be garnered by a prospective trial in which diagnosed in-utero cases are randomly assigned to a treated or nontreated category. However, the rather clear experimental evidence in animals delineating the pathophysiology of the condition, the observed differences in perinatal outcome between treated fetuses and neonates born with the condition, and the anecdotal reports of successful outcome in treated fetuses, all suggest the therapy is beneficial among selected cases.

Treatment of Obstructive Uropathy

As indicated, only those fetuses with proven obstructive uropathy of a persistant and progressive nature and with known immaturity are considered candidates for in-utero diversion therapy. At our center, in addition to informed consent from both parents, case review and approval by a Fetal Therapy Committee, composed of a neonatologist, obstetrician, ultrasonographer, and members of the community at large, is required before the procedure is attempted.

Preoperative medications are based on a protocol tested extensively in patients requiring intrauterine fetal transfusion.[24] Prophylactic antibiotics (ampicillin 500 mg, cloxacillin 500 mg po tid) are begun the day prior to surgery and continued for a total duration of 48 hours. Morphine (10 to 15 mg IM) and scopolamine (0.67 mg IM) are given to the mother about 1 hour prior to the procedure to produce maternal and fetal sedation and analgesia. The procedure is done in an operating room with full aseptic technique.

Initially the fetal lie and bladder position is confirmed using a sterile ultrasound head. A fetal target site in the lower abdominal quadrant is identified and the maternal surface abdominal wall coordinates noted and marked. Two different methods for catheter placement are available: an overload system in which the catheter is loaded over a trocar and a hollow-needle system in which the catheter is threaded down the needle shaft. In our center, we have abandoned the overload system because offloading of the catheter may be very difficult and because the catheter may "accordian" along the trocar shaft with attempts to offload. Our system involves a thin-walled 17-gauge Toughy needle with a 15-degree angulation at the distal end. This needle is advanced under continuous ultrasound guidance to enter the fetal bladder; the position is confirmed by flow of urine, usually under some pressure. Confirmation that the needle tip is free in the bladder is confirmed by injection of $\frac{1}{4}$ mL to $\frac{1}{2}$ mL of air down the needle, and ultrasound observation of air bubbles within the bladder. A pre-cut no. 3 French single- or double-pigtail Teflon catheter with spiral side-holes is threaded on a wire guide and advanced through the needle. The catheter is cut so that at least 5 cm of catheter will protrude from the fetal abdomen into the amniotic sac. With the distal end of the catheter in the fetal bladder, the wire guide is withdrawn, allowing the pigtail to coil. The needle is then slowly withdrawn from the fetal abdomen while the catheter and guide wire are stabilized. As the needle tip leaves the fetus, the needle is tilted to maximize the angle within the fetal abdominal wall, and the guide wire is withdrawn. The needle is then slowly withdrawn as the catheter is advanced with the introducer. The pre-cut proximal end drops from the needle tip into the amniotic cavity, thereby creating a chronic vesico-amniotic shunt. The proximal end of the catheter is the most difficult to place; care must be taken not to place the entire catheter within the fetal bladder or the proximal end within the fetal abdomen, thereby creating vesico-peritoneal shunt and fetal urinary ascites.

Proximal catheter end placement is more difficult when oligohydramnios is present, but may be accomplished. In severe oligohydramnios, it may be reasonable to leave the proximal end of the catheter in the myometrium, allowing for fetal movement to draw the end into the amniotic space. We have observed one fetus in whom proper proximal end placement was achieved by this method.

Ultrasound is used to confirm successful catheter placement, and the changes observed are usually immediate and dramatic. Rapid bladder decompression and an increase in amniotic fluid volume, or in the case of preoperative oligohydramnios, the appearance of amniotic fluid, occurs within minutes of shunt placement. The proximal and distal ends of the catheter should be visible and the area of transabdominal passage noted. Failure to see those characteristics within the first 15 minutes after shunt procedure indicates improper placement and is an indication to repeat the procedure. Once a shunt is placed properly, it is essential to monitor shunt function frequently (once a week) because with fetal growth and movement, the proximal end may become dislodged or blocked. We have also observed one instance where the fetus apparently pulled the shunt from his abdomen. In the ideal case, vesico-amniotic shunt placement is a single short procedure. However, in our experience the procedure can be difficult, and in one case was impossible despite several attempts. The number of separate attempts at shunt placement before the procedure is abandoned varies among operators; at our center we agreed that no more than four attempts in an individual patient would occur.

Invasive Therapy for Obstructive Uropathy: Clinical Outcome

Seventy-three cases of obstructive uropathy treated by in-utero chronic placement of a vesico-amniotic shunt have been reported.[3,40] In total, 30 of 73 cases (41%) survived for at least the neonatal period (28 days) and up to 4 years after treatment. Survival was best among fetuses with proven posterior urethral valve syndrome

(76.2%) (Table 29–1). Forty-three perinates died, of which 14 were stillbirths and 29 were neonatal deaths (Table 29–2). Two of the stillbirths were the result of late second-trimester abortion (<22 weeks) for either associated chromosomal anomaly (trisomy 13) determined subsequent to shunt placement, or failure to detect renal function after shunt placement. Two stillbirths occurred more than six weeks after placement, the result of "cord entanglement" in one instance, and associated with major central nervous system anomaly in the other instance. Two stillbirths occurred within 1 week of shunt placement; in both, premature labor ensued and within 4 days of treatment, intrapartum fetal death occurred. In one instance, a diagnosis of acute chorioamnionitis was confirmed. Twenty-nine infants died in the neonatal period, all within the first 3 days of life and most (27 of 29) within the first few hours of life. Twenty-seven of 29 (93%) neonatal deaths were due to inability to establish ventilation due to suspect or proven pulmonary hypoplasia; only one neonatal death was due to absent renal function (Table 29–2).

No obvious relationship between the gestational age at the time of diagnosis and subsequent outcome was apparent. Survival ranged from 30% when the diagnosis was made between 20 and 24 weeks, and 100% when made between 26 and 28 weeks. Similarly, no relationship between gestational age and treatment and outcome was apparent. Survival ranged from 0% with treatment at 22 to 24 weeks, to 86% with treatment between 26 and 28 weeks. Therefore, earlier diagnosis and treatment did not appear to increase the probability of survival.

The presence of oligohydramnios determined by subjective assessment of amniotic fluid during ultrasound scanning was not related to survival.[40]

OBSTRUCTIVE HYDROCEPHALUS: CASE SELECTION CRITERIA AND METHODS

The case selection criteria for in-utero therapy of obstructive hydrocephalus, like the efficacy of the therapy,

TABLE 29–1. FETAL OBSTRUCTIVE UROPATHY: PRIMARY DIAGNOSIS[a] AND OUTCOME IN 73 TREATED CASES

Primary Diagnosis	No. of Cases	% of Total	No. of Survivors	% Survival by Diagnosis
Posterior urethral valve syndrome	21	28.8	16	76.2
Karyotype abnormality[a]	6	8.2	0	0
Renal dysplasia (by ultrasound[a])	5	6.8	0	0
Urethral atresia	5	6.8	1	20
"Prune belly" syndrome	3	4.1	3	100
Unknown Etiology	33	45.3	10	30.3
Total	73	100	30	

[a] Elective pregnancy termination.

tients who do not have a history of bleeding and who are not in their final weeks of pregnancy. Scans are performed after the transducer probe has been gently placed in the posterior vaginal fornix, with care taken to avoid direct pressure on the cervix. Transvaginal scanning is not advocated late in pregnancy because of the potential risk that the transducer may traumatize the cervix, placenta, or decidual veins, or potentiate infection. Furthermore, in all patients, if the transabdominal scan is technically satisfactory and the diagnosis of placenta previa is unequivocal, a transvaginal study is unnecessary and should not be performed.

A second reason for false-positive diagnosis of placenta previa is the presence of a myometrial contraction (Fig. 30–8). Contractions can distort the LUS in several ways. First, if the contraction is broad-based, it may involve a large portion of the uterus, including the lower uterine segment. A false-positive diagnosis of placenta previa may be made if such a contraction is mistaken for placental tissue.[18,23] This pitfall can be avoided if care is taken to identify the subplacental sonolucent region visible immediately beneath the placenta.[23] Second, a focal myometrial contraction beneath the placenta or between the placenta and internal os may also result in a false-positive diagnosis. Such a strategically located contraction can displace the placenta toward the cervical os and thereby mimic a previa. In the absence of a contraction,

myometrial tissue should be 1.5 cm or less in thickness. If the myometrium appears thicker than this, a delayed scan should be performed to confirm that the "previa" has disappeared.

In the final analysis, the phenomenon of placental "migration" is believed to relate the differing growth rates of the placenta and the LUS. The term "migration" is a misnomer because the placenta remains fixed; apparent movement is due to the relatively rapid growth rate of the lower portion of the uterus. This hypothesis is supported by the important observation that in two separate series, 100% of cases diagnosed as complete placenta previa during the second trimester persisted until term.[19,24] This suggests that if the placenta implants over the cervical os, it will remain fixed in this position for the duration of the pregnancy. In patients with a second trimester diagnosis of partial or marginal placenta previa, the majority of cases will appear normal at term and will not require cesarean section. In all likelihood, in these cases the implantation site was marginal, implying that at no point during the pregnancy did it actually encroach upon the internal cervical os. Preliminary experience with magnetic resonance imaging suggests that this new modality may play a role in selective cases for providing further definition of the relationship of the placenta to the internal cervical os.[25]

Although a false-positive diagnosis of placenta previa

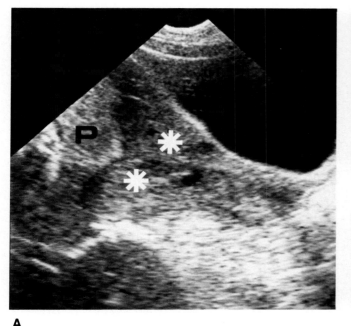

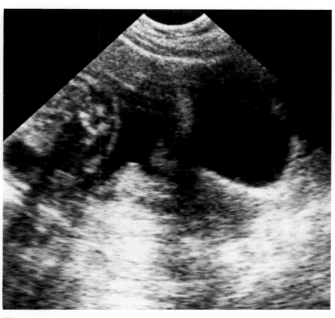

A   B

Fig. 30–8. A. In addition to an overly distended urinary bladder, a focal uterine contraction (∗) is present in the LUS. An apparent placenta previa (P) is seen. **B.** After the woman has partially voided and the contraction has subsided, the LUS has a normal appearance.

can cause emotional stress, it does not ultimately harm either the mother or fetus. By contrast, an undiagnosed placenta previa can result in fetal and maternal morbidity and mortality. Fortunately, false-negative diagnoses are uncommon, occurring in fewer than 2% of cases.[9,26,27] Several technical factors may contribute to these false-negative diagnoses. The most common problem is that the fetal head may prevent visualization of a posterior placenta previa.[10] In 98% of patients with cephalic presentations, posterior or low-lying placentas and their relationship to the internal os can be ascertained by scanning the mother in a Trendelenberg position and by applying gentle upward traction on the fetal head (Fig. 30–9).[21]

Two other situations exist that can cause confusion and potential failure to recognize and diagnose placenta previa.[28] Although most placentas are located on the anterior, posterior, or fundic portions of the uterus, occasionally attachment will be to the lateral wall in the vicinity of the lower uterine segment. Most sonographers diagnose placenta previa only when placental tissue is interposed between the presenting part and maternal bladder, or if the distance between the presenting part and sacral promontory is 1.5 cm or greater.[29] In women with lateral placenta previa, conventional anteroposterior scans may occasionally fail to disclose a placenta previa (Fig. 30–10). Before excluding a previa, it is necessary to carefully examine the LUS and cervical areas with multiple angled and oblique views.

A second potential problem in diagnosing placenta previa can occur in patients with blood in the region of the internal cervical os. If the blood is mistaken for amniotic fluid, it can result in a misdiagnosis of "normal" (Fig. 30–11). This problem can be overcome by careful scanning in an effort to reveal whether or not the fluid in question is interposed between placental tissue and the cervical os. This extremely important clue, which is commonly present in scans of women who have significant bleeding at the time of the ultrasound examination, should not be overlooked.

Placenta Accreta, Increta, and Percreta

Placenta accreta, increta, and percreta, represent a spectrum of abnormalities in which an abnormality or absence of the decidua basalis leads to direct attachment of the placenta to the myometrium. The least severe form, found in 60% of cases, is placenta accreta, with chorionic villi directly contacting the myometrium.[30] Placenta increta, present 20% of the time, implies that the chorionic villi invade the myometrium, while in placenta percreta (20% of cases) there is penetration of the chorionic villi through the myometrium and into adjacent contiguous tissues (Fig. 30–12). In an individual case, the degree of invasion into the myometrium is often variable. In addition, the amount of involved placental tissue also varies from case to case. The incidence of invasive placentation is usually reported as 1 in 7,000 deliveries,[31] although it

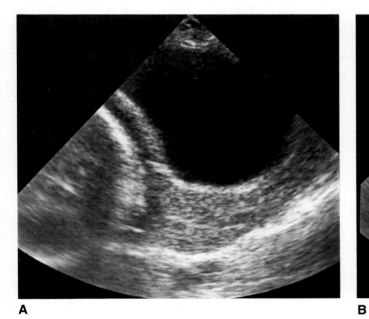

A

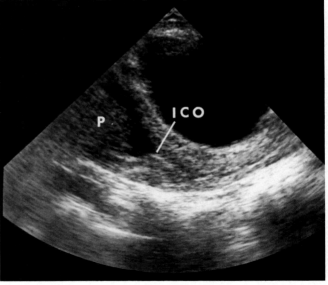

B

Fig. 30–9. A. This longitudinal scan shows the fetal head closely applied to the maternal urinary bladder. The placenta is not visible on this scan. **B.** Following a Trendelenberg traction maneuver, a marginal posterior placenta previa becomes visible (P). ICO = internal cervical os.

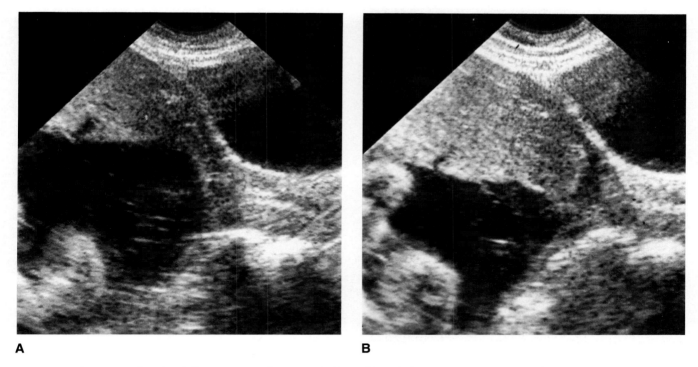

A   B

Fig. 30–10. A. This midline scan reveals an anteriorly positioned placenta without evidence for previa. **B.** An oblique scan toward the patient's left side reveals that the left lateral portion of the placenta is encroaching on the cervix. This patient required a cesarean section for a marginal placenta previa.

appears to be increasing and may be as high as 1 in 2,500 deliveries.[32]

Because the decidua basalis is defective or absent in these patients, it is not surprising that conditions that frequently lead to uterine scarring predispose to this entity. Placenta previa has been reported in association with invasive placentation in nearly two thirds of cases, and prior cesarean section is reported in approximately one quarter of cases.[32] Other conditions associated with uterine scarring and invasive placentation are increased maternal age, multiparity, prior dilatation and curettage, submucosal fibroids, and uterine synechiae (Asherman's syndrome).[30]

Several reports indicate that sonography may be able to diagnose this condition which, if not properly treated, can lead to maternal exsanguination.[30,33,34] A clue that suggests the diagnosis of placenta increta or percreta is absence of normally visible retroplacental sonolucent space (Fig. 30–12). This abnormality reflects a defect in vascularization of the decidua basalis. In women at high risk (placenta previa or prior cesarean section), these sonographic changes should be searched for in order to alert the obstetrician that the patient may experience severe postpartum hemorrhage. Because patients with placenta accreta do not have frank myometrial invasion, it is unlikely that this form of abnormal placentation can be di-

agnosed by ultrasound. Additionally, in patients with posteriorly implanted placentas, it may not be possible to adequately assess the placenta due to the interposed fetus.

CONDITIONS AFFECTING THE CERVIX

During pregnancy, the cervix undergoes appreciable widening. Its length remains similar to that measured in the nongravid state, namely 2.5 to 3 cm.[4] One ultrasonographic study that attempted to measure the cervix (with an empty maternal bladder) found that during pregnancy its length averaged 3.25 cm with a range of 2.3 to 4.5 cm.[20] Although ultrasonographic evaluation of the cervix should attempt to approximate length, from a diagnostic and clinical viewpoint, it is more important to evaluate the appearance of the endocervical canal. In a normal pregnancy, the mucous plug fills the nondilated endocervical canal and is readily visible as a highly echogenic line. At term and during labor, the cervix thins and dilates to accommodate fetal passage.

Three clinical situations have been described that result in cervical dilatation prior to term. These include premature labor, inevitable abortion, and incompetent cervix.[35] Because sonography is the most available im-

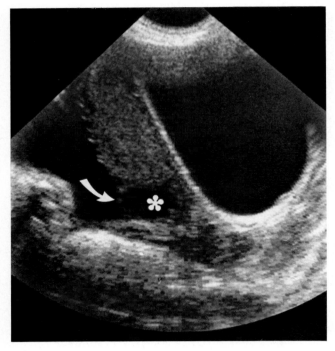

A

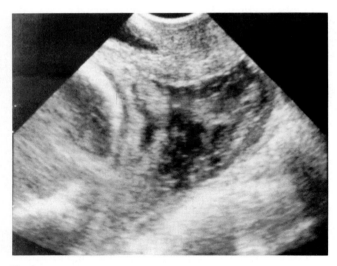

B

Fig. 30–11. A. This hypoechoic collection (∗) just above the cervix is due to blood. Note the insertion of the placenta (*arrow*) crossing over the internal os. This appearance is due to a marginal separation of a partial placental previa. **B.** Placental hemorrhage associated with placenta previa as depicted on TVS.

aging modality for visualizing the region of the internal os and endocervical canal, it can play a major role in aiding obstetric management for these conditions. The ultrasound findings for each of these conditions may be similar or identical. The clinical presentation and history are most useful for distinguishing one entity from another.

Premature labor consists of the spontaneous onset of palpable, regularly occurring uterine contractions between the 20th and 37th weeks of pregnancy.[36] The clinical diagnosis can be difficult. Waiting until labor is obvious is counterproductive, since therapeutic success is equated with the time at which it starts. Physical examination shows varying degrees of cervical effacement and/or dilatation, depending upon the course of labor. The decision of whether or not an attempt should be made to arrest premature labor must be an individual one. Sonographic demonstration of a closed endocervical canal is a favorable sign that may influence the obstetrician to attempt to delay labor in order to allow continued fetal growth and development. If, on the other hand, the sonographic examination reveals marked cervical dilatation with prolapse of the amniotic sac, therapy is of little value and spontaneous delivery soon occurs.[37]

Although women with an incompetent cervix may also have cervical dilatation, this group differs from women in premature labor or those experiencing inevitable abortion. In this condition, which typically occurs in the second trimester, cervical dilatation is painless, bloodless, and tends to recur with each successive pregnancy.[38] The causes of incompetent cervix are obscure and are probably multiple. A common theme appears to be cervical trauma; for example, women who have undergone dilatation and curettage, or cauterization, appear to be at increased risk.[3] Anatomic factors may also contribute to the development of cervical incompetence. There appears to be excessive smooth muscle with an altered collagen-to-muscle ratio within the cervices of these women.[39] An interesting but poorly understood association exists between incompetent cervix and women who have been exposed to diethylstilbestrol in utero. Five of nine patients with this history developed evidence of cervical incompetence and, in addition, had cervical hypoplasia. Finally, hormonal influences upon the sphincteric ring, which is thought to exist at the junction of the lower uterine segment and internal os, may also play a role in incompetent cervix.[4] This sphincter is normally tightly contracted during pregnancy, but is relatively relaxed under the influence of estrogen.

There are several indications for sonographic examination of women who carry the diagnosis of incompetent cervix. Because the best time to treat this condition is between the 14th and 18th weeks of pregnancy[40] (ie, before significant cervical dilatation occurs), it is important to assess the fetus for possible anomalies, or to ascertain that a molar pregnancy is not present. A second indication is for diagnosis or confirmation of this condition. The ultrasonographic hallmark of cervical incompetence is visualization of either fetal parts or amniotic fluid, or both, within a dilated endocervical canal (Fig.

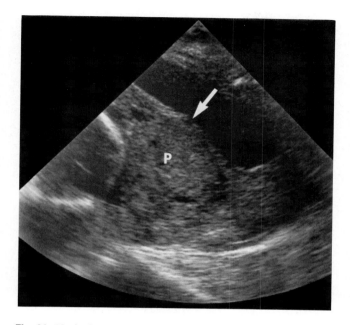

Fig. 30–12. An irregular contour at the bladder-uterine interface (*arrow*), as well as loss of the normally visible retroplacental clear space, allowed the correct diagnosis of placenta increta to be made. Note that a complete previa is also present. P = placenta.

30–13). Attention must be paid to technical aspects of the study because an overdistended maternal bladder compressing the anterior and posterior cervical walls can give the false impression of a closed cervix.[35,41] In suspicious cases, our clinic attempts to examine this area

using real-time equipment with the patient standing. In the erect position, gravitational pressure from uterine contents can force amniotic fluid into the proximal endocervical canal so that a mild, albeit significant, amount of cervical dilatation can be visualized at the earliest possible time. Unfortunately, this approach is not only technically difficult, but it is also frequently ineffective. Recently we have found that a better approach is to perform a transvaginal scan with the patient's bladder completely empty. This minimizes compression of the cervical walls against one another, allows the length of the cervical canal to be measured, and improves the sonographic diagnosis of incompetent cervix.[22]

The final indication for performing sonography in women with cervical incompetence is to evaluate the patient following placement of a cervical cerclage (Fig. 30–14). Both the 5-mm wide Mersiline tape suture used in the Shirodkar procedure and the No. 2 nylon suture used in the McDonald procedure can be visualized as hyperechoic linear structures with variable posterior acoustic shadowing.[42] Sonography can be used to locate the position of the suture material relative to the external os, and to evaluate for possible protrusion of membranes beyond the sutures before it is clinically evident.

CONCLUSION

Although the precise etiologies for placenta previa and premature cervical dilatation remain to be determined,

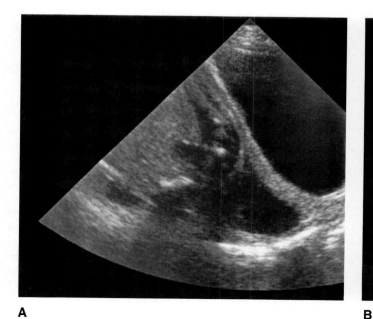

A

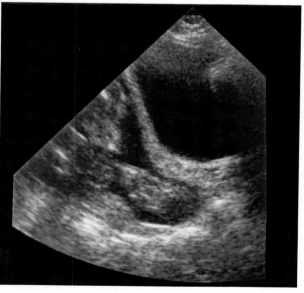

B

Fig. 30–13. A. Dilatation of the endocervical canal should be diagnosed when either amniotic fluid or **B.** a fetal part is present in the endocervical canal.

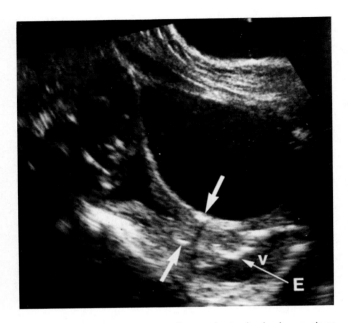

Fig. 30–14. A longitudinal scan in a patient who had a cerclage because of an incompetent cervix reveals high amplitude echoes with variable shadowing (*arrows*) due to suture material. The distance from the sutures to the external cervical os (E) can be readily measured after introducing water into the vagina (V). (*Reprinted with permission from Parulekar SG, Kiwi R.* J Ultrasound Med. *1982;1:223.*)

sonography has proven to be a major tool for diagnosing these important conditions. Prior to the advent of sonography, most patients with painless third trimester vaginal bleeding were treated expectantly (ie, they were put to bed and were given appropriate fluid replacement). They were all considered to have a placenta previa until a definitive double-setup vaginal examination was performed, usually at 36 to 37 weeks.[8] Ultimately, only one third of this group was diagnosed as placenta previa.[11] The economic and emotional strain on the patient, her family, as well as the obstetrician, was not inconsiderable. Fortunately, sonography can now be used to reassure the majority of these women that placenta previa is absent.

Evaluation of the endocervical canal by sonography can similarly reassure many patients and physicians by ascertaining that it appears normal. In patients in whom sonography diagnoses or confirms premature dilatation, an appropriate course of action can be undertaken at the earliest possible time.

REFERENCES

1. Taslitz N. Anatomy of the female reproductive system. In: Iffy, L, Kaminetzky HA, eds. *Principles and Practice of Obstetrics and Perinatology.* 1st ed. New York: Wiley; 1981:43–64.

2. Harrison RG. The urogenital system. In: Romanes GF, ed. *Cunningham's Textbook of Anatomy.* 10th ed. London: Oxford University Press; 1964:514.

3. Percival R. Normal pregnancy. In: *Holland and Brews' Manual of Obstetrics.* 14th ed. Edinburgh: Churchill Livingstone; 1980:66–67.

4. Greenhill JP, Friedman EA. Effects of pregnancy on the maternal organism. In: *Biological Principles and Modern Practice of Obstetrics.* 1st ed. Philadelphia: Saunders; 1974:105–109.

5. Percival R. Normal labour. In: *Holland and Brews' Manual of Obstetrics.* 14th ed. Edinburgh: Churchill Livingstone; 1980:317–319.

6. Zemlyn S. The length of the uterine cervix and its significance. *J Clin Ultrasound.* 1981;9:267.

7. Gillieson MS, Winer-Mural HT, Muram D. Low-lying placenta. *Radiology.* 1982;144:577.

8. Goplerud CP. Bleeding in late pregnancy. In: Danforth DN, Scott JR, eds. *Obstetrics and Gynecology.* 5th ed. Philadelphia: Lippincott; 1986:433–439.

9. Bowie JD, Rochester D, Cadkin AV, et al. Accuracy of placental localization by ultrasound. *Radiology.* 1978;128:177.

10. Scheer K. Ultrasonic diagnosis of placenta previa. *Obstet Gynecol.* 1973;42:707.

11. Greenhill JP, Friedman EA. Placenta previa. In: *Biological Principles and Modern Practice of Obstetrics.* 1st ed. Philadelphia: Saunders; 1974:415–425.

12. Kelly JV, Iffy L. Placenta previa. In: Iffy L, Kaminetzky HA, eds. *Principles and Practice of Obstetrics and Perinatology.* 1st ed. New York: Wiley; 1981:1105–1120.

13. Pritchard JA, MacDonald PC, Gant NF. Obstetric hemorrhage. In: Pritchard JA, MacDonald PC, Gant NF, eds. *Williams Obstetrics.* 17th ed. Norwalk, Conn: Appleton-Century-Crofts; 1985:395–412.

14. Gottesfeld KR, Thompson HE, Holmes JH, et al. Ultrasonic placentography: A new method for placental localization. *Am J Obstet Gynecol.* 1966;96:538.

15. Wexler P, Gottesfeld KR. Second trimester placenta previa. *Obstet Gynecol.* 1977;50:709.

16. Mittelstaedt CA, Partain CL, Boyce IL Jr, et al. Placenta praevia: Significance in the second trimester. *Radiology.* 1979;131:465.

17. King DL. Placental migration demonstrated by ultrasonography. *Radiology.* 1973;109:167.

18. Artis AA III, Bowie JD, Rosenberg ER, et al. The fallacy of placental migration: Effect of sonographic techniques. *AJR.* 1985;144:79.

19. Townsend RR, Laing FC, Nyberg DA, et al. Technical factors responsible for "placental migration": Sonographic assessment. *Radiology.* 1986;160:105.

20. Bowie JD, Andreotti RF, Rosenberg ER. Sonographic appearance of the uterine cervix in pregnancy: The vertical cervix. *AJR.* 1983;140:737.

21. Jeffrey RB, Laing FC. Sonography of the low-lying placenta: Value of Trendelenburg and traction scans. *AJR.* 1981;137:547.

22. Brown J, Shah D, Thieme G, Fleischer A, Boehm F. Evaluation of the cervix with transabdominal and transvaginal US. *Am J Obstet Gynecol.* 1986;155:721–726.

MOLAR PREGNANCIES

Pathogenesis and Clinical Aspects

The pathogenesis of hydatidiform mole has remained a subject of considerable speculation for many years. Recently, however, the work of Kajii and Ohama[9] demonstrated that hydatidiform mole results from the fertilization of an "empty egg," that is, an ovum without any active chromosomal material. The chromosomes of the sperm, finding no chromosomal complement from the ovum, reduplicate themselves, resulting in a 46XX molar pregnancy. This has also been called a "complete mole" or "classic mole." In complete mole, there is complete lack of fetal development, so there are no identifiable fetal parts or fetal membranes that can be seen in this situation. Complete moles are associated with varying degrees of trophoblastic proliferation, and may follow either a benign or malignant clinical course. Only about 20% of cases will eventually pursue a malignant course.[4]

Some cases of hydatidiform mole are found to contain a small complement of fetal structure, such as a placenta with membranes, or even a developed fetus. This is referred to as a "partial mole." These cases usually involve some edema of the villi, but relatively little trophoblastic proliferation. Hydropic degeneration is present, but with some elements associated with fetal structures, the designation partial mole has been made.[10] Although subsequent malignancy has been reported, "partial moles" are almost always benign.[11] In partial mole, the fetus usually has significant congenital anomalies as well as a triploid karyotype.[12] Two sets of chromosomes are of paternal origin and the third set is of maternal origin.

A fetus with a coexisting molar pregnancy can occur. This is much less common than a partial molar pregnancy; however, it can grossly appear similar to the partial mole. This disorder is thought to result from a dizygotic pregnancy, with one fetus resulting from a normal fertilization and the other being a complete molar pregnancy.[13] In these patients, a fetus and normal placenta can usually be identified, in contrast to a partial molar pregnancy where a normal placenta is not present.

Hydropic degeneration of the placenta may give a similar sonographic appearance to complete and partial mole but, histologically, it is not associated with trophoblastic proliferation. The villi and hydropic degeneration of the placenta are swollen and edematous and may thus resemble abnormal trophoblastic tissue. Microscopic examination will usually reveal the absence of cisternal formation; only hydropic swelling is seen. Hydropic degeneration may be seen in 20% to 40% of placentae from abortuses.[4]

The most common presenting clinical sign of molar pregnancy is vaginal bleeding, which may be seen in 89% to 97% of cases; in approximately half of the cases, the bleeding may be severe enough to produce anemia.[14]

A uterus that is enlarged beyond what is expected based on gestational age is considered "classic" for molar pregnancy. However, this is only seen in from 33% to 51% of cases.[14] In approximately 50% of cases, patients will present with what is easily recognized as a molar pregnancy based on the passage of vesicular tissue via the vagina.[15] If there has been significant expulsion of molar tissue prior to presentation, the uterus may appear normal for size or even small for dates, both clinically and sonographically.

Molar pregnancies should always be considered in the differential diagnosis of a patient presenting with severe preeclampsia prior to 24 weeks' gestation without underlying renal disease. While this presentation is considered classic for hydatidiform mole, it is only seen in 6% to 12% of cases of molar pregnancy.[14]

Theca lutein cysts are often encountered in patients with molar pregnancies. The actual incidence of these cysts in association with molar pregnancy has been reported in various series to range from 18% to 37%.[16,17] Compared to clinical examination, sonography can more accurately assess the presence or absence of theca lutein cysts (Figs. 31–4 and 31–5).[18] In one large series, theca lutein cysts were detected clinically in 10% of patients with molar pregnancy, compared to 37% of patients when examined by sonography.[17] The presence or absence of theca lutein cysts does not seem to be an accurate predictor of later development of an invasive mole or choriocarcinoma.[17] However, review of a recent series at the University of Southern California has suggested that patients with theca lutein cysts have a two-fold increase of malignant sequalae.[19] In most patients who undergo spontaneous resolution of hCG levels, the cysts also regress spontaneously. However, they may occasionally un-

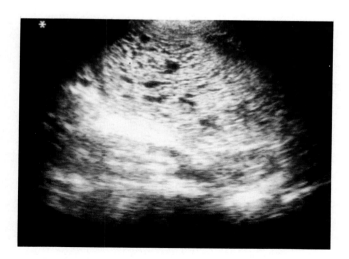

Fig. 31–4. Typical sonographic appearance of hydatidiform mole with small vesicular cystic spaces.

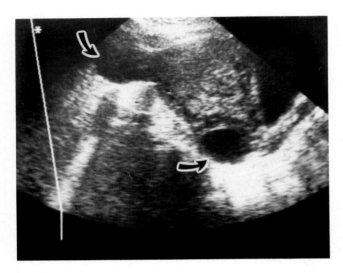

Fig. 31–5. Complete hydatidiform mole, demonstrating two theca lutein cysts, one superior to the fundus (*curved arrow*), one in the cul-de-sac (*curved arrow*).

dergo torsion and, therefore, require surgical intervention.

The laboratory findings for molar gestation are usually diagnostic. Measurement of human chorionic gonadotropin, specifically the beta subunit, is almost always abnormally elevated in molar gestations. The assay is not foolproof, since it can be spuriously elevated in twin gestations or may occasionally fail to show significant elevation in a molar pregnancy.[20]

As soon as the diagnosis of molar pregnancy is confirmed, the uterus should be evacuated. This typically involves suction curettage (dilation and evacuation, or D & E). Prior to evacuation, a chest x-ray should be obtained to exclude metastatic disease that might already be present. The patient should also be evaluated as to her pulmonary status, cardiac status, thyroid status and to be sure that adequate coagulation factors are present.[14] After D & E, serial beta-hCGs are obtained weekly to assess the status of any remaining trophoblastic tissue. The level of this glycoprotein hormone should return to normal approximately 10 to 12 weeks after evacuation; however, it may occasionally take longer.[21] As previously mentioned, theca lutein cysts will usually regress after successful treatment of molar pregnancy. Their presence or absence should not be taken as absolute indication of the presence or activity of residual trophoblastic disease.[22]

Sonography has an important role in evaluating those patients in whom the beta-hCG subsequently rises. It can detect the presence or absence of intrauterine pregnancies that may occur after the initial evacuation. It can also detect the small number of patients with molar ges-

tation that have a coexisting normal pregnancy.[23] It may also detect the presence of residual trophoblastic disease and can detect invasion of the myometrium by this residual trophoblastic tissue.[2]

Sonographic Features

The sonographic appearance of a hydatidiform mole is quite distinctive.[1] In most cases, a sonographic pattern arising from molar tissue consists of echogenic intrauterine tissue that is interspersed with numerous punctuate sonolucencies (Fig. 31–4). Irregular sonolucent areas may occur secondary to internal hemorrhage or an area of unoccupied uterine lumen.

The sonographic appearance of a hydatidiform mole varies according to its gestational duration and the size of the hydropic villi.[24] For instance, hydatidiform moles that occur from 8 to 12 weeks typically appear as homogeneously echogenic intraluminal tissue, since the villi at this stage have a maximum diameter of 2 mm (Fig. 31–5). As the hydatidiform mole matures to 18 to 20 weeks, the vesicles have a maximum diameter of 10 mm, which is readily delineated as cystic spaces on sonography (Fig. 31–6).

In contrast to the complete mole, partial molar pregnancy, hydatidiform mole coexistent with fetus, and hydropic degeneration of the placenta are associated with the presence of a fetus or fetal parts. Although it may be difficult to differentiate between a partial molar pregnancy and a complete mole with a coexistent fetus on the basis of sonography, these two entities can be differentiated from a complete mole when an identifiable fetus is present.[13,15] In addition, the complete mole with a coexistent fetus typically has a fetus with a separate normal placenta as well as the molar mass. This contrasts with a partial mole in which only a portion of the placenta is normal and most of it has a vesicular pattern.

Sonography can also delineate the theca lutein cyst that enlarges under the influence of high levels of beta-hCG elaborated by trophoblasts. These cysts appear as multiloculated cystic masses that are usually located superior to the uterine fundus or, less commonly, in the cul-de-sac (Fig. 31–5).

Rarely, there can be massive enlargement of the ovaries with luteinization of several follicles in apparently normal pregnancies. This condition, which is termed hypereactio luteinalis, may be a result of hypersensitivity of the woman's ovary to high circulating levels of hCG (Fig. 31–7).

Sonographic Differential Diagnosis

Hydropic degeneration of the placenta associated with incomplete or missed abortions is the most common condition that can simulate the appearance of a molar pregnancy (Fig. 31–8). The hydropic areas may be focal or

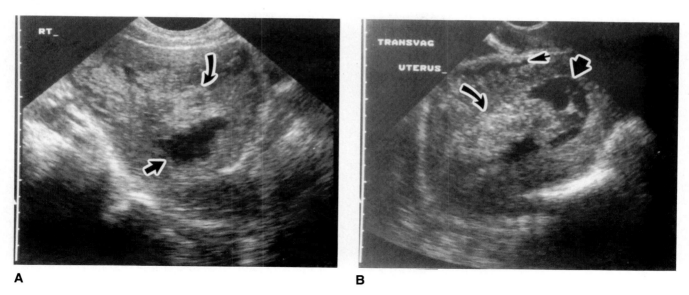

Fig. 31–6. Hydatidiform mole with cystic spaces. **A.** Transabdominal longitudinal scan demonstrating echogenic material (*curved arrow*) within enlarged uterus, as well as irregular cystic region along lower uterine lumen (*straight arrow*). **B.** Semicoronal transvaginal sonogram demonstrating echogenic material (*curved arrow*) within the uterine lumen, representing trophoblastic tissue and irregular cystic space inferiorly. A myometrial vein is distended (*arrowhead*).

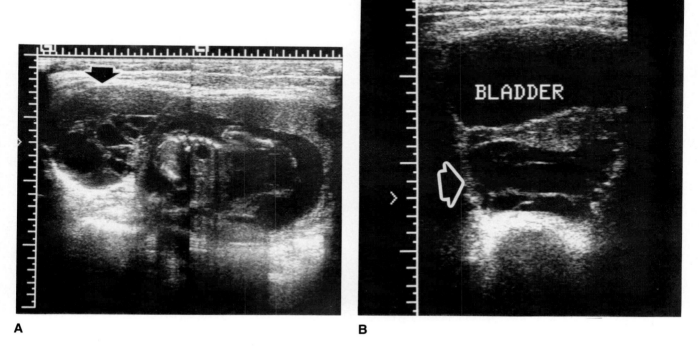

Fig. 31–7. Hypereactio luteinalis. **A.** Composite obstetric sonogram demonstrating multi-loculated cystic mass (*arrow*) superior to the uterine fundus. **B.** Same patient demonstrating a second multi-loculated cystic mass (*arrow*) in the cul-de-sac. At surgery, massively enlarged ovaries that contained multiple luteinized cysts were found. (*Courtesy of Bill Wilson, MD.*)

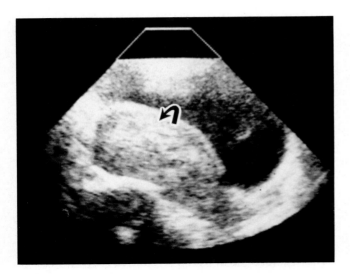

Fig. 31–8. Choriocarcinoma appearing as an echogenic area (*arrow*) within myometrium of the anterior corpus.

diffuse, and appear as anechoic space within the placenta (Fig. 31–8). This is due to the sonographic similarity of a hydropic placenta with marked swelling of the villi to molar tissue. A fetus may or may not be present with hydropic degeneration of the placenta. Serum beta-hCG levels are generally lower in hydropic degeneration than in partial or complete moles, probably due to the reduced number of functioning trophoblasts. Hydropic changes in the placenta can be associated with triploidy.[25]

Technical factors that may be used to improve the ability to distinguish partial from complete moles or hyropic degeneration have been described.[3] Specifically, detailed examination of the entire intrauterine contents with transducers that are optimally focused to a particular region within the uterus has been stressed. Transvaginal scanning may be helpful in some cases in which the molar tissue cannot be adequately delineated transabdominally. Using this technique, the typical vesicular texture arising from molar tissue can be correctly distinguished from tissue texture emanating from retained products of conception or leiomyomata.[3]

Recently, pulsed Doppler sonography has been used to assess the presence of invasive trophoblastic disease.[26] This technique is discussed in greater detail in the section devoted to invasive trophoblastic diseases.

Occasionally, the sonographic appearance of a uterine leiomyoma may mimic that of a hydatidiform mole. However, as illustrated in Chapter 37, uterine leiomyoma typically have a whorled internal consistency which is distinctly different from the vesicular pattern encountered in the hydatidiform mole. They may also contain areas of hyaline and myxomatous degeneration that can simulate the sonographic appearance of hemorrhage

within a hydatidiform mole. We have also encountered some partially solid ovarian tumors that simulate the appearance of a hydatidiform mole. Patients with this type of mass can usually be distinguished from those with molar pregnancies by clinical and laboratory methods because the beta-hCG is not elevated in nonpregnant conditions.

Finally, patients with retained products of conception with hemorrhage can simulate the sonographic appearance of molar pregnancies. However, one is usually not able to demonstrate a vesicular pattern of tissue associated with retained products.

Although absolute distinction between the various trophoblastic disorders may not always be possible on the basis of sonography, the sonographic evaluation of these disorders can have clinical importance. Specifically, it is known that the malignant potential of a complete mole is greater than that of a partial mole or hydropic degeneration. Thus, the sonographic findings can have a significant clinical impact on the treatment and management of these disorders.

INVASIVE MOLE AND CHORIOCARCINOMA

Pathogenesis and Clinical Aspects

The majority of patients who develop malignant trophoblastic disease will have a history of an antecedent molar pregnancy. In a series of patients reported from Duke University, 86% of patients who developed malignant trophoblastic disease did so after a hydatidiform molar pregnancy.[24] Approximately 10% of patients had a history of a previous full-term pregnancy, and another 5% had an abortion or some other form of pregnancy event. In patients who presented with high-risk disease, there was a larger proportion of patients presenting after full-term pregnancy, abortions, and other types of pregnancy events.

Histologically, invasive moles differ from choriocarcinoma. A villous structure is maintained in invasive mole, and is always absent in choriocarcinoma. Both disorders are associated with excessive trophoblastic proliferation and invasion of the myometrium. In general, choriocarcinoma is associated with a great deal of hemorrhage and necrosis.

Generally, an invasive mole is first suspected in a patient with a history of evacuation of a hydatidiform mole who subsequently presents with continued uterine bleeding, or a persistently elevated hCG level, and/or persistenty enlarged theca lutein cysts. This clinical picture, however, can also be seen in patients who histologically are found to have choriocarcinoma. However, since hysterectomy is rarely performed in the current management of trophoblastic diseases, these entities are not recognized separately in the clinical staging system. Patients with choriocarcinoma that extends outside the uterus can present for the first time with manifestations of metastatic spread to the lungs, liver, or brain. In the lungs, metastatic chroriocarcinoma has a rather specific radiographic appearance of radiodense masses with hazy borders, due to the hemorrhage around the metastases. The metastases may undergo rapid regression after therapy has been instituted. Since these diseases are responsive to chemotherapeutic agents, their early clinical and sonographic recognition is imperative for institution of appropriate therapy.

The sonographic appearance of invasive trophoblastic tissue is that of a focal irregular echogenic region within the uterine myometrium (Figs. 31–8 and 31–9). Irregular hypoechoic areas may surround the more echogenic trophoblastic tissue that corresponds to areas of myometrial hemorrhage.

Due to its proximity to the uterus, myometrial implants may be best delineated with transvaginal scanning (Fig. 31–9). Pulsed Doppler sonography has been used to assess the presence and relative aggressiveness of myometrial implants by depicting increased and typically turbulent flow to these tumors through the uterine arteries.[26]

In addition to the echogenic intrauterine areas, sonography is helpful in the detection of theca lutein cysts associated with trophoblastic disease. These cysts are typically bilateral multiloculated cystic masses that characteristically measure between 4 cm and 8 cm in diameter. Sonography has been shown to be more sensitive than physical examination in the detection of these cysts because it may be difficult to palpate a cyst that is displaced high in the pelvis by an enlarged uterus. The presence of theca lutein cysts may be an indication of persistent trophoblastic activity because it has been shown that malignant trophoblastic disease develops more commonly in patients with persistent theca lutein cysts.[19] However, because it can take up to 4 months for these cysts to regress after evacuation of a molar pregnancy, their presence or absence during the period of follow-up cannot be taken as an accurate indication of the presence or activity of remaining trophoblastic tissue.

Sonography and pulsed Doppler analysis of the uterus can be useful, when used in combination with serial beta-hCG assays, in the evaluation of tumor response to chemotherapy.[24] Serial evaluation of tumor volume can be accomplished using sonography; reduced volume follows closely the diminution in beta-hCG values in successfully treated patients. Preliminary reports also describe the sensitivity of pulsed Doppler techniques for detection of tumor growth or regression.[26] The presence of tumor is implied when the Doppler waveforms obtained from the uterine arteries show increased systolic and diastolic flow with low resistance similar to that typically seen in third-trimester pregnancy.

Sonography also is helpful in evaluation of the liver for metastatic disease in patients with malignant, metastatic trophoblastic disease.[13] Typically, the metastases associated with choriocarcinoma appear as echogenic foci within the liver. The kidneys can also be evaluated for

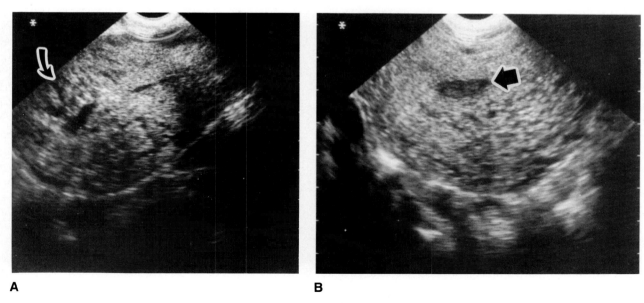

A   **B**

Fig. 31–9. Locally invasive trophoblastic disease. **A.** Long axis transvaginal sonogram, demonstrating irregular area in right side of uterine fundus (*curved arrow*). **B.** Transvaginal semiaxial sonogram showing hypoechoic tumor focus (*arrow*), measuring approximately 3 × 7 mm.

the presence of obstructive uropathy, which is important not only to rule out metastatic involvement, but also because effective chemotherapy often requires adequate renal function.

SUMMARY

As discussed and illustrated in this chapter, sonography has an important role in the evaluation of patients with benign and malignant gestational trophoblastic disease. The sonographic features of hydatidiform mole and its variants are usually diagnostic. If malignant trophoblastic disease is suspected clinically, sonography can be used to establish the presence and extent of disease, as well as in the serial evaluation of patients undergoing treatment.

REFERENCES

1. Fleischer A, James A, Krause D, et al. Sonographic patterns in trophoblastic disease. *Radiology.* 1978;126:215.
2. Berkowitz RS, Birnholz J, Goldstein DP, et al. Pelvic ultrasonography and the management of gestational trophoblastic disease. *Gynecol Oncol.* 1983;15:403.
3. Requard C, Mettler F. Use of ultrasound in the evaluation of trophoblastic disease and its response to therapy. *Radiology.* 1980;135:419.
4. Reid M, McGohan JO. Sonographic evaluation of hydatidiform mole and its look-alike. *AJR.* 1983;140:307.
5. Jones H III. Gestational trophoblastic disease. In: Jones H Jr, Jones S, eds. *Novak's Textbook of Gynecology.* 10th ed. Baltimore: Williams & Wilkins; 1981:659–689.
6. Hertz R, Lewis JL Jr, Lipsett MB. Five years experience with the chemotherapy of metastatic choriocarcinoma and related trophoblastic tumors in women. *Am J Obstet Gynecol.* 1961;82:631.
7. Hammond CB, Borchert LG, Tyrey L, et al. Treatment of metastatic trophoblastic disease: Good and poor prognosis. *Am J Obstet Gynecol.* 1973;115:451.
8. Surwit EA, Hammond CB. Treatment of metastatic trophoblastic disease with poor prognosis. *Obstet Gynecol.* 1980;55:565.
9. Kajii T, Ohama K. Androgenetic origin of hydatidiform mole. *Nature.* 1977;168:633.
10. Vassilakos P, Riotton G, Kajii T. Hydatidiform mole: Two entities: A morphologic and cytogenetic study with some clinical considerations. *Am J Obstet Gynecol.* 1977;127:167.
11. Szulman A, Surti J, Berman M. Patient with partial mole requiring chemotherapy. *Lancet.* 1978;1:1099.
12. Szulman A, Surti N. The syndromes of hydatidiform mole. I: Cytogenic and morphologic correlations. *Am J Obstet Gynecol.* 1978;131:665.
13. Munyer T, Callen P, Filly R, et al. Further observations on the sonographic spectrum of gestational trophoblastic disease. *J Clin Ultrasound.* 1981;9:349.
14. Gordon AN. Gestational trophoblastic disease. In: Kase NG, Weingold AB, eds. *Principles and Practice of Clinical Gynecology.* 2nd ed. New York: John Wiley & Sons; 1988.
15. Szulman AE, Surti V. The clinicopathologic profile of the partial hydatidiform mole. *Obstet Gynecol.* 1982;59:597.
16. Kobayashi M. Use of diagnostic ultrasound in trophoblastic neoplasms and ovarian tumors. *Cancer.* 1978;38:441.
17. Santos-Rasmos A, Forney J, Schwartz B. Sonographic findings and clinical correlations in molar pregnancies. *Obstet Gynecol.* 1980;56:186.
18. Pritchard J, Hellman L, eds. *Williams' Obstetrics.* New York: Appleton-Century-Crofts; 1971:578.
19. Montz FJ, Schlaerth JB, Morrow CP. Natural history of theca lutein cysts. *Gynecol Oncol.* 1987;26:414.
20. Callen P. Ultrasonography in evaluation of gestational trophoblastic disease. In: Callen P, ed. *Ultrasonography in Obstetrics and Gynecology.* Philadelphia: Saunders; 1983:259–270.
21. Goldstein D, Berkowitz R, Cohen S. The current management of molar pregnancies. *Curr Prob Obstet Gyn.* 1979;3:1.
22. MacVicar J, Donald I. Sonar in the diagnosis of early pregnancy and its complications. *J Obstet Gynaecol Br Commonw.* 1968;70:387.
23. Jones W, Lauerson N. Hydatidiform mole with coexistent fetus. *Am J Obstet Gynecol.* 1975;122:267.
24. Hammond CB, Weed JC, Currie JL. The role of operation in the current therapy of gestational trophoblastic disease. *Am J Obstet Gynecol.* 1980;136:844.
25. Crane J, Beaver H, Cheung S. Antenatal ultrasound findings in fetal triploidy syndrome. *J Ultra Med.* 1985;4:519–522.
26. Taylor KJW, Schwartz PE, Kohorn EI. Gestational trophoblastic neoplasia: Diagnosis with Doppler US. *Radiology.* 1987;165:445–448.

32 Postpartum Ultrasonography

J. Patrick Lavery • Kathleen A. Gadwood

The puerperium refers to the 6-week period following delivery. During this time, physical recovery and regression takes place from the dramatic physiologic changes that developed throughout the course of pregnancy. In other words, it is during the puerperium that the female organs are attempting to regain their prepregnancy function and size.

Robinson[1] used diagnostic ultrasound to investigate puerperal changes as early as 1972. Malvern and Campbell[2] availed themselves of this diagnostic modality to evaluate postpartum bleeding in 1973. Thus, almost from its introduction into clinical medicine, sonography has been a valuable adjunct to the clinician in assessing puerperal pathology as well as affording an understanding of normal anatomic changes. With the vastly improved resolution and sensitivity of current equipment, it can be anticipated that diagnostic ultrasound will play an increasingly prominent role in the assessment of puerperal changes, both normal and abnormal.

Although the postpartum period is a time of physiologic resolution, complications will occur in a significant number of patients. These are primarily due to hemorrhage or infection.[3] Conditions such as endomyometritis, postpartum hemorrhage, wound abscess, and urinary tract infection are but some of the diagnoses accounting for the 5 to 10% morbidity seen after delivery.[4]

The purpose of this chapter is to discuss the normal and pathologic findings that may be appreciated sonographically during the puerperium. Major emphasis will be placed on changes within the genital tract. However, other systems that are occasionally the site of clinically significant complications during the puerperium will also be described and discussed. Normal variations and common pathologic findings will be highlighted in order to acquaint the reader with the spectrum of uses that sonography offers for the understanding and management of conditions occurring in the puerperal period.

NORMAL ANATOMY

The Uterus

In the nonpregnant state, the uterus occupies a midline position and measures approximately 8 cm in length.[5] Uterine size may be influenced by gravidity as well as pathologic conditions such as leiomyomata or adenom-

yosis.[6] Physiologically, the pregravid uterus grows from a weight of approximately 140 g to a final term weight of 1 kg.[7] Blood flow to the uterus increases during pregnancy from 50 cc/minute to 500 cc/minute at term. During the puerperium, the uterus regresses to nearly its pregravid weight. Factors such as parity, breast or bottle feeding, and route of delivery have not been demonstrated to influence the rate of uterine involution[8,9] (Fig. 32–1).

The process of uterine involution is perhaps the most dramatic aspect of the anatomic changes in the puerperium. It is a dynamic physiologic reversal of the growth changes that occurred during pregnancy. In this regression process, there is no cell destruction. Cell size is reduced with concomitant loss and reabsorption of tissue fluid and contractile protein. Animal experiments show an orderly process of cellular restitution where cytoplasmic and collagen disintegration take place without tissue necrosis.[10]

The most rapid phase of uterine involution occurs during the first week postpartum when a near 50% reduction in size is seen.[8,9,11] By this time, the term size gravid uterus will have come from its subxyphoid position to a point approximately halfway between the umbilicus and the pubic symphysis. The mean measurements of uterine size obtained sonographically in a group of 37 normal parturients are shown in Table 32–1.[8] Uterine involution appears to occur more rapidly after preterm deliveries, both clinically and sonographically, than after term deliveries.

The myometrium has a heterogeneous echo appearance on the sonogram, which is related to the anatomic changes in the vascular structure, changes in uterine blood flow, as well as the degree of resolution of tissue edema and fluid content taking place in this organ during the postpartum period. Variations will be seen among normal patients at different times after delivery, depending on the respective stage of resolution when viewed. Significantly enlarged vascular channels mediating intramural blood flow during pregnancy may be seen early in the puerperium, only to disappear in subsequent evaluation as the vessels constrict and involute (Fig. 32–2).

The endometrial cavity appears to maintain a consistent size of less than 2 cm in antero-posterior diameter during the early puerperium. This cavity wall, however,

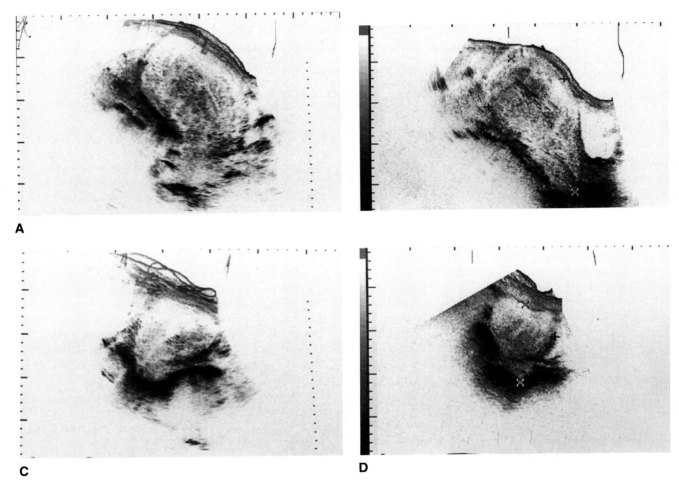

Fig. 32–1. Series of sonograms showing a normal uterus in involution during the first 2 weeks after delivery. Longitudinal views are shown at **A.** 24 hours, **B.** 48 hours, **C.** 1 week, and **D.** 2 weeks postpartum.

has a remarkable variation in appearance among clinically normal and uncomplicated cases. Sonographic studies show patterns ranging from smooth, well-defined mural linings to those with irregular, nonhomogeneous borders[8] (Fig. 32–3). The length and width of the endometrial echo will decrease in proportion to overall uterine in-

TABLE 32–1. THE UTERUS DURING INVOLUTION: MEAN MEASUREMENTS (IN CM) TAKEN DURING THE FIRST TWO WEEKS IN 37 NORMAL SINGLETON GESTATIONS

Time After Delivery	Length	Width	A-P Diameter	Endometrial Cavity (A-P)
24 Hours	17.5	12.3	9.0	1.2
48 Hours	16.3	11.3	8.7	1.3
1 Week	12.9	9.4	7.8	1.3
2 Weeks	11.0	7.7	6.6	1.0

Used with permission from Lavery JP, Shaw L. Sonography of the puerperal pelvis. *J Ultrasound Med.* 1989;8:481.

volution.[9] On occasion, small echogenic areas may be seen within the uterus, which may represent residual small clots or pieces of membranes not expelled at time of delivery (Fig. 32–4). It is sometimes difficult to distinguish normal variations from pathologically retained products of conception. A significantly enlarged endometrial cavity (>2.5-cm diameter) may also be associated with a hypotonic uterus in the early postpartum period. Clinical correlation is mandatory to distinguish between the normal variant and the abnormal thickening seen with retained material or uterine hypotonia.

The Broad Ligament

The broad ligament (Fig. 32–5) is a reflection of the parietal peritoneum extending medially from the bony pelvic sidewall beneath the infundibulo-pelvic ligament, to the lateral margin of the uterus bilaterally, and extending inferiorly to the pelvic floor. It contains the vascular supply to the uterus as well as to the fallopian tubes. Although

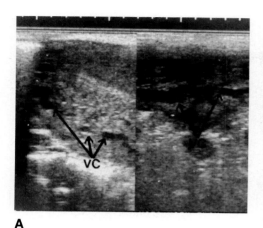

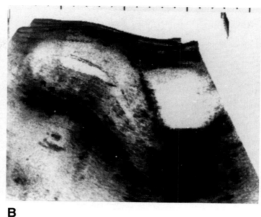

Fig. 32–2. A. Longitudinal and transverse sonograms of an early involuting uterus showing large vascular channels (VS with *arrows*). **B.** Subsequent longitudinal sonogram of the same uterus showing where these channels have been obliterated (*arrows*).

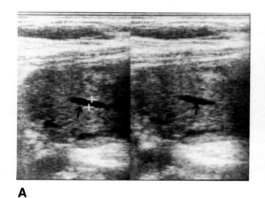

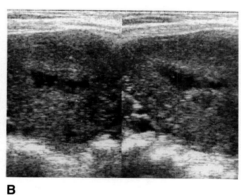

Fig. 32–3. A. Endometrial cavity appearing as a well-defined echogenic smooth-walled space. **B.** Another clinically uncomplicated patient with irregular and ill-defined endometrial lining in transverse view containing residual fluid. Both sonograms were made 1 week following normal delivery.

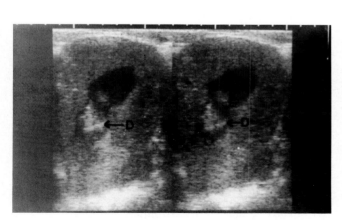

Fig. 32–4. Echogenic debris (D) found in normal postpartum patient. This may represent small clots or membranes not expelled at delivery.

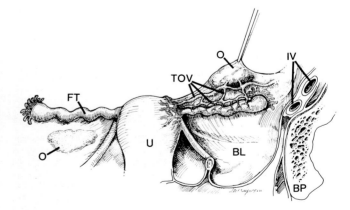

Fig. 32–5. Schematic illustration of the broad ligament, the peritoneal sheet containing loose areolar tissue supporting the uterus and containing the vascular supply to the uterus and fallopian tubes. U = uterus; BL = broad ligament; FT = fallopian tube; TOV = tuboovarian vessels; O = ovary; IV = iliac vessels; BP = bony pelvis.

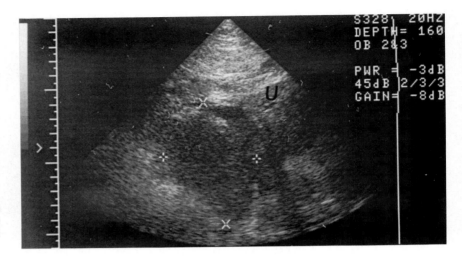

Fig. 32–6. Hematoma (defined by ∗s) of the broad ligament following cesarean section appearing as a heterogeneous mass lateral to the uterus (U).

difficult to visualize sonographically in the normal patient because of the homogeneous nature of the areolar tissue that acts as its supporting structure and the frequent shadowing of bowel gas above it, the broad ligament may be a location of significant pathologic findings. Because the minimally resistant loose areolar tissue encompasses the uterine vessels medially, and the vascular supply to the fallopian tubes and ovaries superiorly, the broad ligament is potentially the site of hematoma, abscess or phlegmon formation in the puerperal period (Fig. 32–6).

The Ovaries

The ovaries, normally found within the true pelvis in the nonpregnant state, are extrapelvic in location during much of the puerperium. They can be demonstrated sonographically approximately 50% of the time[8] (Fig. 32–7). After the first trimester, when cysts are commonly present, the ovary does not undergo any significant change in size or contour related to pregnancy. However, the condition of a luteoma of pregnancy has been described.[12]

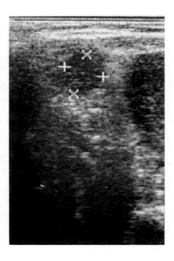

Fig. 32–7. Ovary (*caliper marks*) appears as an extra pelvic mass adjacent to the uterus (U).

This represents a solid enlargement of the ovary because of stromal hypertrophy, which is an exaggerated luteinizing reaction secondary to the hormonal stimulus of pregnancy. In this unusual condition, the ovary regresses in size during the puerperium in contrast to the case of a true neoplasm, which persists even after the elevated levels of pregnancy-associated hormones regress.

The Cul-De-Sac

The cul-de-sac is a potential space posterior to the uterus created by the peritoneal reflection between the uterus and the rectum. Free fluid in the abdomen may settle in this dependent recess. Ascites from any cause, including hypoalbuminemia or severe preeclampsia, will be visualized in this area (Fig. 32–8). In the absence of free fluid, however, this area is not easily defined sonographically, either during pregnancy or in the normal puerperium.

PATHOLOGY

Postpartum Hemorrhage

Hemorrhage represents one of the most significant factors of maternal morbidity following childbirth. Postpartum hemorrhage (PPH) is divided into two diagnostic entities according to the time of its clinical presentation: primary and secondary.

Primary PPH occurs during the first 24 hours after delivery and is associated with acute clinical problems such as coagulopathies, dysfunctional and prolonged labors, chorioamnionitis, placental implantation abnormalities (eg, previa and accreta), the use of uterine relaxing agents such as halothane or magnesium sulfate, and incomplete manual removal of the placenta. Clinical circumstances at the time of delivery usually point to the diagnosis and guide the therapeutic endeavors.

Secondary PPH occurs more than 24 hours after

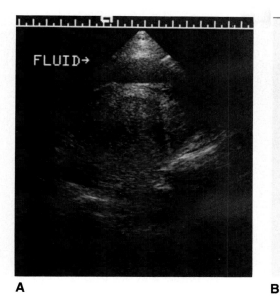

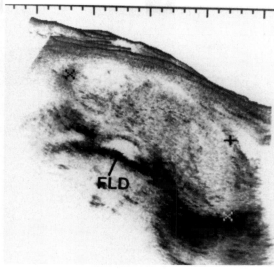

Fig. 32–8. Examples of free fluid (FLUID) **A.** around the uterus and **B.** behind the uterus (FLD) above the cul-de-sac in two patients with severe preeclampsia.

delivery and is seen in 1% of patients. It is caused by either retained placental tissue or subinvolution of the placental site (Fig. 32–9). Surgical intervention by dilatation and curettage (D & C) during the puerperal period increases the probability of uterine scar formation (senechiae) with the consequence of Asherman's syndrome and susequent infertility.[13] Dewhurst[14] has shown that only 32% of a series of 89 patients, all subjected to a D & C for secondary PPH, had pathologically confirmed tissue obtained. Lee and colleagues[15] confirmed this statistic in a study in which 56 patients underwent ultrasound evaluation for PPH, and only 14 (25%) required a D & C because of sonographic evidence of retained products of conception.[15] In the remaining 42 patients, where there was no ultrasound evidence of retained secundines, all patients responded satisfactorily to medical therapy. Hence, the use of ultrasound and judicious surgical intervention can minimize the need for operative intervention and subsequent reproductive complications in some patients suffering from PPH.

Other aspects of PPH specifically related to operative delivery are discussed later in this chapter.

Postpartum Infection

Puerperal infectious morbidity develops in 3 to 4% of vaginal births and in 10 to 15% of cesarean deliveries, although significantly higher rates have been noted in certain populations at risk.[16,17] Factors that predispose to puerperal infectious morbidity are listed in Table 32–2. The most common source of puerperal sepsis is from organisms normally present in the vagina, including both aerobic and anaerobic species. *Escherichia coli*, bacteroides species, aerobic and anaerobic streptococci, and

enterococci are the most common organisms isolated in these infections.

Endomyometritis is difficult to diagnose sonographically, but certain findings are associated with the condition when clinical suspicion is present. These include a dilated or irregular endometrial cavity occasionally containing fluid, shadowing echoes because of gas, and often the presence of fluid in the cul-de-sac (Fig. 32–10). Retained products of conception predispose infection and serve as a nidus for bacterial growth. Endomyometritis usually presents within the first 3 to 4 days after delivery. Later febrile illness is more likely related to abscess formation, to wound infection, or to the development of a

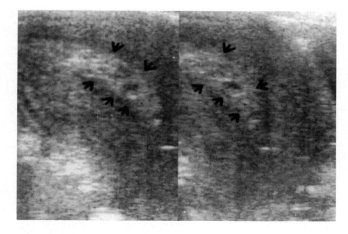

Fig. 32–9. Retained placental fragment (*arrows*) associated with postpartum bleeding appears as a heterogeneous mass enlarging the endometrial cavity. Blood clots (anechoic areas) are also present.

TABLE 32–2. FACTORS ASSOCIATED WITH INCREASED RISK OF PUERPERAL INFECTION

Medical	Surgical
Premature membrane rupture	General anesthesia
Internal fetal monitoring	Operator expertise
Obesity	Intraoperative delay and complications
Anemia	Classical uterine incision
Multiple pelvic exams	
Chorioamnionitis	**Social**
Prolonged labor	Low socio-economic status
Retained secundies	Poor hygiene
	Smoking, ethanol, and drug abuse

phlegmon, an indurated inflammatory mass often confluent with the uterus and the broad ligament[18] (Fig. 32–11). A phlegmon is a nonfluctuant inflammatory mass that on ultrasound appears to be of lower density and less well-circumscribed or encapsulated than an abscess. It requires prolonged and intense antibiotic medical therapy, as opposed to the surgical or percutaneous catheter drainage warranted with an abscess. In one series, phlegmons represented 19% of infectious complications following cesarean delivery.[19]

Abscesses appear as complex masses that are primarily cystic with internal echoes. They have a wall or margin around them, the thickness of which depends on their stage of development. Rarely, acoustic shadowing from gas formation may be seen (Fig. 32–12). The presence of a wall or capsule distinguishes an abscess from a phlegmon. Reliable sonographic diagnosis of abscesses

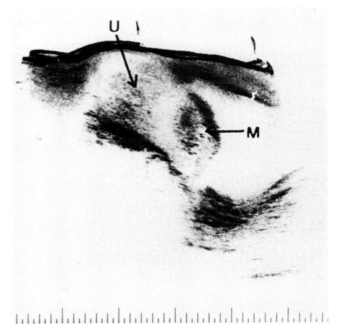

Fig. 32–11. A phlegmon developing from the anterior wall of the uterus (U) following cesarean section. At laparotomy this nonfluctuant mass (M) was found to extend into the broad ligament.

has been reported by Taylor and associates[20] in a series of 67 nonpuerperal patients.

Abscess formation can occur deep in the pelvis, in the broad ligament, in the uterus, or at any point along the line of the surgical incision. An abscess or an infected hematoma can be indistinguishable from a sterile hematoma when viewed ultrasonographically. Needle aspiration may be necessary for diagnosis and, in some cases, therapy. Sonography can aid in the localization of

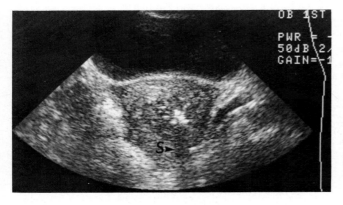

Fig. 32–10. Case of endomyometritis typified by poorly defined and thickened appearance of the endometrial wall and showing inferior shadowing (S) related to possible gas or retained material.

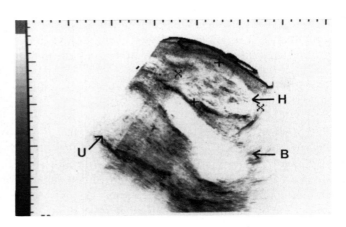

Fig. 32–12. Infected hematoma (H) creating abscess cavity seen as a mass with defined borders and heterogeneous echoes. Inflammatory process was suprafascial. U = uterus; B = bladder.

33 Sonographic Evaluation of Maternal Disorders During Pregnancy

Arthur C. Fleischer • Dinesh M. Shah • Stephen S. Entman

Because of its ability to evaluate the uterus, placenta, and fetus, and because it does not use ionizing radiation, sonography is the diagnostic modality of choice for several maternal disorders that occur during pregnancy. Those disorders that will be discussed in this overview include pelvic masses, cholecystitis, and renal disorders.

PELVIC MASSES DURING PREGNANCY

The pregnant patient who has a pelvic mass palpated or delineated sonographically presents a special management problem for the obstetrician. Factors that affect obstetric management include the size of the mass, its internal consistency, its most-likely histologic composition, the possibility of it becoming torsed or incarcerated, and whether or not it could hinder vaginal delivery. Sonography has an important role in documenting enlargement or regression of a mass. Sonographic delineation of the internal contents of a pelvic mass assists in narrowing its differential diagnosis. Masses that contain irregular septae, papillary excrescences, or large solid areas are more suspicious for malignancy than simple cysts.

This section will discuss and illustrate the role of sonography in evaluation of pelvic masses that can be encountered in a pregnant patient. An attempt will be made to differentiate those masses that may require immediate surgical intervention from those that usually do not.

Clinical Aspects

Sonography provides important clinical information in the evaluation of a patient with a pelvic mass. In fact, some pelvic masses may first be discovered by the initial sonographic exam. A pelvic mass may become clinically manifest during pregnancy if it is palpated during physical examination or produces abdominal pain, or in later stages of pregnancy if it impedes labor. Detection of pelvic masses by palpation can be limited during pregnancy because of the difficulty of distinguishing a pelvic mass from an enlarged uterus. This problem is particularly encountered in large or obese patients. Because it is often

difficult to establish the size, extent, and nature of a pelvic mass during pregnancy by physical examination alone, sonography is particularly helpful.

In general, conservative management is followed in a gravid patient who has a pelvic mass that is less than 5 cm in size, is not painful, and does not enlarge on serial examinations.[1] However, if the mass is greater than 5 cm in size and appears to be enlarging or causing significant pain, surgical intervention may be indicated. Surgical intervention is also indicated if there is a possibility of torsion or rupture of the mass itself, or both. Torsion is much more likely to occur if the mass is located on a pedicle. The probability of rupture of a pelvic mass during pregnancy may also be increased if it is incarcerated in the cul-de-sac region.

Along with establishing the parameters of a pelvic mass, sonography has an important role in establishing the exact gestational age of the pregnancy. This is helpful because most operative procedures requiring manipulation of the gravid uterus are preferably performed during the second trimester. Such timing lessens the possibility of spontaneous abortion in the first trimester and avoids the potential problem in the third trimester of limited surgical access to the abdomen because of the large uterus. Sonographic demonstration of the internal structure of a pelvic mass may also enter into deciding whether or not to perform surgery. Sonographic demonstration of a simple cyst, for example, might preclude immediate surgery. If a mass contains solid irregular areas, the chance of malignancy is increased and surgery prior to delivery may be indicated. Thus, sonography plays an important role in determining if and when to do surgery.

SONOGRAPHIC EVALUATION OF PELVIC MASSES

This discussion covers pelvic masses that are cystic, complex, and solid. Although some types of pelvic masses can demonstrate a variety of sonographic appearances, one can usually narrow the differential diagnosis down to one or two of the most probable diagnoses based on sonographic features of a pelvic mass.

Cystic Masses

The most common cystic mass that occurs during pregnancy is a corpus luteum cyst. During the first few weeks of pregnancy, the corpus luteum produces progesterone that sustains the decidualized endometrium. Typically, corpora lutea appear as 2- to 3-cm anechoic masses located within the ovary (Fig. 33–1). They can enlarge up to 5 to 10 cm. Most corpus luteum cysts are asymptomatic, nonpalpable, and primarily detected by sonography rather than palpation (Fig. 33–2). They usually do not require intervention because they regress prior to 16 to 18 weeks.[2] Occasionally, they can contain internal echoes and septae secondary to internal hemorrhage or separation of the luteinized lining from the wall of the cyst. Uncomplicated paraovarian or peritoneal inclusion cysts may have a similar sonographic appearance to corpus luteum cysts.

Theca lutein cysts represent an exaggerated corpus luteum response in patients with high levels of human chorionic gonadotropin (hCG). Occasionally, theca lutein cysts can undergo marked enlargement, resulting in multiloculated pelvo-abdominal cystic masses associated with pregnancy. These masses typically contain uniformly sized 2- to 3-cm anechoic spaces representing the cystic portions of the mass (Fig. 33–3). Theca lutein cysts are frequently present with hydatidiform moles and other forms of gestational trophoblastic diseases, as well as in some isoimmunized pregnancies.

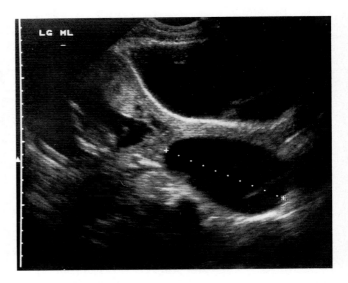

Fig. 33–2. Transabdominal sonogram demonstrating cystic mass (between + s) posterior to lower uterine segment. On a follow-up exam 4 weeks later, the mass had completely regressed. Most likely this represented a corpus luteum cyst.

In addition to corpus luteum cysts, there are several other types of pelvic masses that may appear as anechoic adnexal structures on sonography. These include a hydrosalpinx, peritoneal inclusion cyst, and developmental or remnant cyst (paraovarian) cyst. Peritoneal inclusion cysts typically are irregularly shaped because they form between the peritoneal surfaces of organs and may not have a true wall. Usually, there is a history of pelvic surgery in patients with peritoneal inclusion cysts. Hydrosalpinges typically occur as sequela to pelvic inflammatory disease. When small, their fusiform configuration and origin from the cornual areas of the uterus can usually be depicted on transvaginal sonography. When enlarge, however, they can assume a rounded configuration similar to other ovarian cysts. Paraovarian cysts arise from the mesoovarium in remnants of the Gartner's duct.[3] They can remain adnexal in location or, when enlarged, can project superior to the uterine fundus. Rarely, these masses may have thin internal septations similar to ovarian epithelial tumors. Most of these masses are asymptomatic and do not require surgical intervention during pregnancy.

There are several types of ovarian neoplasms that appear as predominantly cystic pelvic masses (Figs. 33–4 through 33–6). In general, ovarian epithelial neoplasms are the most common cystic tumor to demonstrate significant enlargement during pregnancy.[4] As in the nongravid patient, mucinous or serous cystadenomas can contain various amounts of internal septation (Fig. 33–5). Multiple thick septations are typically found in mucinous cystadenomas, whereas serous tumors tend to be uni-

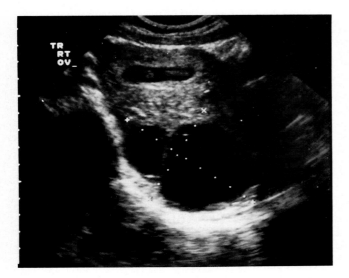

Fig. 33–1. Transvaginal sonogram of 5-week pregnancy with two corpora luteum cysts (between + s) associated with ovulation induction.

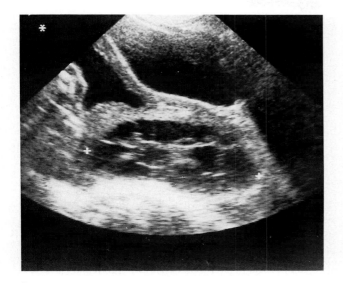

A

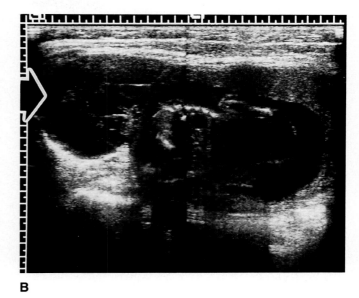

B

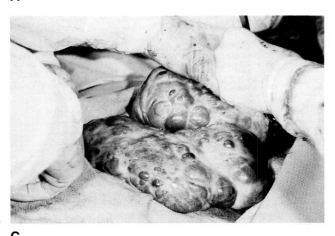

C

Fig. 33–3. Enlarged ovaries containing theca luteum cysts. A. Enlarged ovary (between + s) within the cul-de-sac containing several cystic spaces. B. Composite scan demonstrating enlarged ovary (*arrow*) superior to the fundus, containing several cystic spaces. C. At surgery, massively enlarged ovaries that contained multiple theca lutein cysts were found. (*Courtesy of Bill Wilson, MD, and Lonnie Burnett, MD.*)

locular (Fig. 33–6). Cystic masses that contain irregular solid components, papillary excrescences, or both should be distinguished from those that are unilocular. In general, masses that contain internal septations or papillary excrescences are more likely to have borderline or malignant histology (Fig. 33–7). The presence of maternal ascites with a cystic pelvic mass increases the likelihood of a malignant lesion.

Torsion of a cystic mass may be suggested if there is unusual thickening of the wall of the mass. Usually, torsion of a pelvic mass is associated with severe pelvo-abdominal pain. Torsion of an ovarian mass is typically associated with intraperitoneal fluid related to obstruction of venous and lymphatic drainage.[5] Over the course of a pregnancy, a torsed ovary can be observed to enlarge significantly, probably due to vascular engorgement within the affected ovary. Often, the affected ovary is lodged within the cul-de-sac.

Complex Masses

The term "complex" implies that the mass contains both cystic and solid components. Complex masses can be further categorized into those that are predominantly cystic and those that are predominantly solid. Complex masses can be cystic and contain echogenic components or solid masses that contain areas of cystic degeneration.

The most common complex mass encountered during pregnancy is a dermoid cyst. This is because dermoids are the most common tumor in the reproductive age group. These masses are thought to arise parthenogenetically from germ cells within the ovary. As a consequence of this method of development, dermoid cysts usually contain heterologous tissue elements including teeth, hair, skin, and fat in various proportions. Tooth elements can usually be recognized by their dense echogenicity with distal shadowing. Fat, hair, and skin elements usually produce a moderately echogenic ap-

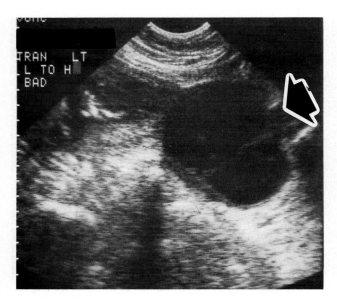

Fig. 33–4. Ovarian abscess (*arrow*) adjacent to the gravid uterus.

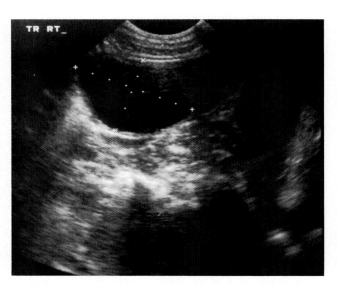

Fig. 33–6. Completely cystic mass (between + s) superior to uterine fundus representing a serous cystadenoma.

pearance (Fig. 33–8). Some dermoid cysts that contain sebaceous material can demonstrate layering of this material above that of serous fluid.

Because most benign teratomas arise within the ovary, they are prone to undergoing torsion. They typically present as masses superior to the uterine fundus. Slow leakage from a dermoid cyst can result in granulomatous peritonitis, whereas sudden rupture can lead to an acute abdominal crisis.

Other complex masses include those that contain internal solid components or hemorrhage. Occasionally, an endometrioma can appear as a complex mass with internal echoes arising from clot.

Solid Masses

The most common solid masses encountered during pregnancy are those that arise from the smooth muscle and connective tissue within the myometrium. Uterine

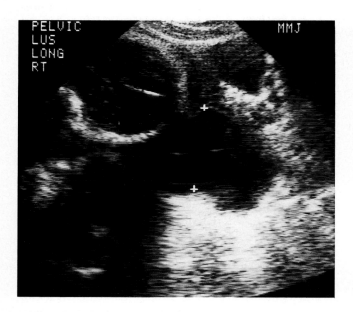

Fig. 33–5. Cystic mass (between + s) containing an irregular septation and solid components near lower uterine segment. A mucinous cystadenoma was surgically removed at time of cesarean section.

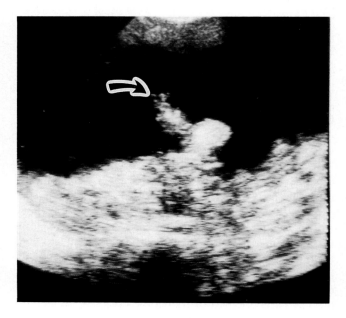

Fig. 33–7. Large cystic mass containing solid areas with papillary projections (*arrow*). This represented an immature teratoma containing papillary excrescences of tumor.

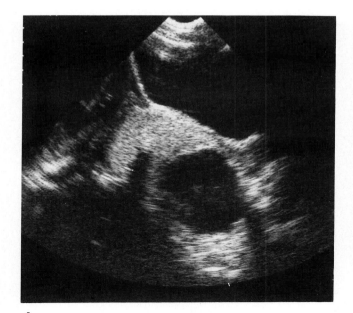

A

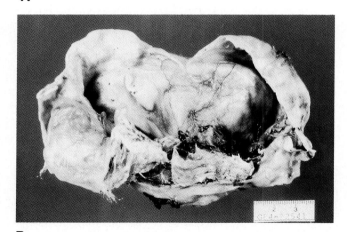

B

Fig. 33–8. Dermoid cyst. **A.** Complex mass in cul-de-sac consisting of echogenic material with central echogenic focus corresponding to calcified area. **B.** Opened specimen showing hair and solid elements within this dermoid cyst.

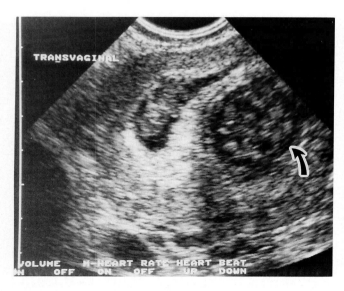

Fig. 33–9. Transvaginal sonogram of 8-week intrauterine pregnancy, showing a fibroid (*curved arrow*) in the lower uterine segment. The fibroid is a stationary well-defined area of hypoechogenicity, as opposed to a uterine contraction which blends into surrounding myometrium.

leiomyomas demonstrate a spectrum of sonographic appearances, the most common of which is a relatively hypoechoic mass traceable within the uterine wall (Fig. 33–9). Because leiomyomas may appear similar to a contracted portion of the uterus, a repeat examination in 20 to 45 minutes may help delineate if a mass arising from the myometrium is indeed a well-circumscribed myoma or a focal contraction of the uterus. One can also assess the relative position of the uterine fibroids to the placenta.

Sonograhic appearance of a uterine fibroid is related to the relative amount of smooth muscle to collagen as well as the presence and amount of hyaline or hemor-rhagic degeneration. Fibroids that are made up of mostly connective tissue tend to be more echogenic than those that are mostly made up of smooth muscle.

It has been the predominant view in obstetrics that uterine fibroids enlarge during pregnancy and involute during the puerperium. A change in estrogen and progesterone levels in pregnancy may be related to fibroid tumor growth.[6] It has been shown that myoma cells have a greater number of estrogen receptors than surrounding normal myometrial cells. It is possible that these cells may be more responsive to increased concentrations of estrogen during pregnancy and exceed the growth of surrounding myometrium. Progesterone may inhibit the growth of fibroids and even induce degenerative changes and involution. This may become most evident in late pregnancy when there are increased progesterone levels. Another theory implicates the arterial supplies of fibroids as causes of degenerative and size changes. Fibroids are typically supplied by one or two nutrient arteries entering the periphery and encircling the tumor mass. As a result of passive stretching of the uterine wall and active muscle contraction, these arteries may become twisted. This may result in carneous degeneration of fibroids related to venous obstruction or accelerated arterial infarction of these tumors.

In a recently completed study that sonographically monitored changes in fibroid size during the three trimesters of pregnancy, the enlargement or involution of a fibroid was found to be related to its size in early pregnancy.[6] Small fibroids (average dimension, 2 to 6 cm) tended to increase in size during the first or second trimester and decrease in the third trimester. Larger fibroids (between 6 and 12 cm) tended to increase in size only in the first trimester, but decreased in size during the second and third trimesters.

Fibroids may demonstrate a change in their texture during pregnancy. It is not uncommon for hypoechoic fibroids to develop cystic spaces, which may be the result of hyaline degeneration. Fibroids can demonstrate an echogenic rim corresponding to areas of calcification around the periphery of the tumor.

There is a relationship between the presence of multiple fibroids and a higher frequency of retained placental tissue, bleeding during pregnancy, malpresentation, and premature uterine contractions. Large fibroids located in the lower uterine segment may obstruct labor and necessitate cesarean section. Most fibroids detected in the lower part of the uterus during the first trimester are likely to migrate cephalically with growth of the uterus and may not pose any difficulty by the time of delivery. Thus, the location of a fibroid is an important parameter to be determined by sonographic examination.

Other Masses

Sonography can detect other masses that arise from the pelvis during pregnancy, such as those related to the bowel (Fig. 33–10). In some masses, there can be concomitant obstruction, ileus of bowel, or both. Fluid-filled, distended loops of small bowel appear as numerous tubular structures that have periodic projections from the wall corresponding to valvulae conniventes (Fig. 33–10.B). Large bowel can be distinguished from the small bowel by the thicker and more regular haustral indentations.

Sonographic detection of appendicitis during pregnancy is difficult due to the inability to completely delineate the right lower quadrant adjacent to an enlarged uterus. Most appendiceal abscesses, however, can be detected as a tubular complex mass in the right lower quadrant or higher in the abdomen because the appendix migrates cephalically during pregnancy.[7]

Occasionally, solid masses secondary to uterine fusion abnormalities may simulate the appearance of a solid mass or fibroid. It may be difficult to delineate the nongravid uterine horn in the later stages of pregnancy. In the first trimester, the nongravid bicornuate horn typically has a rounded solid structure with an echogenic central interface related to the decidual reaction that occurs in the nonpregnant horn. However, as the uterus enlarges, it may be more difficult to delineate this nongravid horn due to compression and axial rotation by the gravid uterus.

Pelvic kidneys may appear as a fusiform or rounded solid structure near the bladder with a central echogenic interface arising from the renal pelvis.

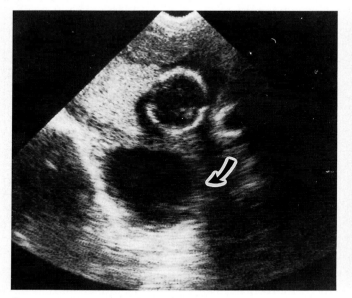

A

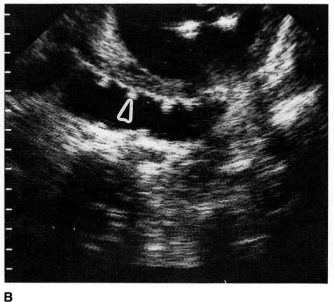

B

Fig. 33–10. Cystadenoma with associated bowel obstruction. **A.** Hypoechoic well-defined cystic mass (*curved arrow*) in cul-de-sac representing a cystadenoma. **B.** Multiple loops of dilated small and large bowel superior to the uterine fundus. The valvulae conniventes (*arrowhead*) could be identified projecting into the lumen of the small bowel loops.

MATERNAL DISORDERS

Sonography has an important role in the evaluation of the pregnant patient who presents with pain in the upper abdomen, flank, leg, or pelvic areas.

In a patient who presents with upper abdominal pain, sonography can delineate conditions such as cholelithiasis/cholecystitis, subcapsular liver hemorrhage associated with toxemia, and renal stones and/or infection (Fig. 33–11). These conditions should be considered in the pregnant patient presenting with pain. The hypervolemic state of pregnancy can also contribute to rupture of vascular aneurysms. Sonography can also detect conditions such as retroplacental hemorrhage or abruption that may result in pelvo-abdominal pain.

The incidence of gallstones in women is twice that of men. Pregnancy is thought to be one possible cause of the increased incidence of gallbladder disease in women. The exact mechanism of formation and deposition of biliary calculi is not fully understood. However,

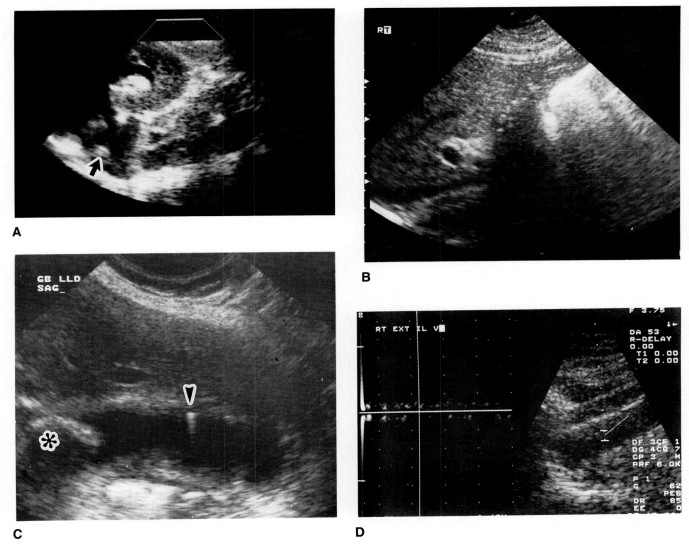

Fig. 33–11. Miscellaneous maternal disorders. **A.** Coronal image of maternal left kidney showing echogenic focus (*arrow*) within renal pelvis corresponding to renal calculi. **B.** Contracted gallbladder containing several calculi. **C.** Gangrenous gallbladder wall with a large obstructing calculus (∗) in gallbladder neck, and an echogenic focus within gallbladder secondary to air (*arrowhead*). This condition would require immediate surgery because of the possibility of rupture. **D.** Duplex Doppler examination of right external iliac vein of a woman who was 12 weeks pregnant demonstrating no Doppler flow and thrombus filling the lumen.

it is thought that, as a result of pregnancy with its increase in circulating steroid levels, there is an increased concentration of cholesterol in the bile. This combined with biliary stasis and changes in the physiochemical nature of bile salts may contribute to the increased incidence of cholelithiasis in women.[8,9] Gallbladder calculi appear as echogenic foci with distal shadowing. It is not uncommon to detect this viscid bile or sludge even in the asymptomatic pregnant patient. If there is focal gallbladder wall thickening or pericholecystic fluid collection, acute cholecystitis should be highly suspected (Fig. 33–11.C). Fluid surrounding a gallbladder with an impacted stone may be an indication that rupture has occurred.

It may be difficult to evaluate the pregnant patient with physiologic hydronephrosis for the presence of an obstructing renal calculus because the renal pelvis and ureter distend as early as 15 to 20 weeks and remain distended throughout pregnancy. However, if one delineates a markedly distended (over 1-cm) ureter, calculus obstruction should be considered. The right kidney usually demonstrates more pelvicalyceal distension than the left. Distension of the collecting systems is thought to result from mechanical pressure from the enlarging uterus compressing the ureter between the maternal pelvis and the gravid uterus and smooth muscle relaxation induced by progesterone and prostaglandins.[10] This distension of the collecting system and ureter begins as early as 10 weeks and returns to a nondistended configuration approximately 6 weeks after delivery.

Calculi that remain in the renal collecting system appear as echogenic foci. If associated with pus, low level echogenic material can be seen within the collecting system (Fig. 33–11.A). In order to delineate a renal calculus within the ureter, coned down radiographs of the maternal abdomen after contrast injection may be necessary. In these cases, shielding of the fetus should be attempted.

Acute painful swelling of the lower extremity of a pregnant patient usually deserves immediate work-up because of the possibility of deep venous thrombosis with subsequent pulmonary embolism. Duplex Doppler, with or without color flow mapping, is accurate in determining the presence and extent of venous thrombosis involving the femoral, popliteal, and tibioperoneal veins (Fig. 33–11.D).[11] Color flow Doppler facilitates the detection of both partially and totally occluded vessels. Ovarian vein thrombosis can also be detected using this method.

SUMMARY

This overview has discussed and illustrated the sonographic features of the most common pelvic masses that can be encountered in pregnant patients. Sonographic evaluation allows delineation of the size, consistency, and location of pelvic masses that occur during pregnancy. It has an important role in establishing the enlargement or regression of pelvic masses that occur during pregnancy. Sonography also has an important role in the diagnosis of cholecystitis and upper urinary tract obstruction or infections in the pregnant patient.

REFERENCES

1. Bezjian A. Pelvic masses in pregnancy. In: Sabbagha RE, ed. *Diagnostic US Applied to Obstetrics and Gynecology*. Philadelphia: Lippincott; 1987.
2. Nelson MJ, Cavalieri R, Graham D, Sanders RC. Cysts in pregnancy discovered by sonography. *J Clin Ultrasound*. 1986;14:509–512.
3. Alperin M, Sandler M, Madrazo B. Sonographic features of paraovarian cysts and their complication. *AJR*. 1984; 143:157.
4. Beischer N, Buttery B, Fortune D, Macafee C. Growth and malignancy of ovarian tumors in pregnancy. *Aust NZ J Obstet Gynecol*. 1971;11:208.
5. Warner M, Fleischer A, Bundy A, Edell S. Adnexal torsion: Sonographic findings and clinical implications. *Radiology*. 1985;154:773.
6. Lev-Toaff AS, Coleman BG, Arger PH, Mintz MC, Arenson RL, Toaff M. Leiomyomas in pregnancy: Sonographic study. *Radiology*. 1987;164:375–380.
7. Jeffrey RB, Laing FC, Townsend RR. Acute appendicitis: Sonographic criteria based on 250 cases. *Radiology*. 1988;167:327.
8. Williamson SL, Williamson MR. Cholecystosonography in pregnancy. *J Ultrasound Med*. 1984;3:329–331.
9. Stauffer RA, Adams A, Wygal J, Lavery JP. Gallbladder disease in pregnancy. *Am J Gynecol*. 1982;144:661.
10. Fried AM, Woodring JH, Thompson DJ. Hydronephrosis of pregnancy: A prospective sequential study of the course of dilatation. *J Ultrasound Med*. 1983;2:255–259.
11. Foley WD, Middleton WD, Lawson TL, Erickson S, Quiroz FA, Macrander S. Color Doppler ultrasound imaging of lower-extremity venous disease. *AJR*. 1989;152:371–376.

34 Normal Pelvic Anatomy as Depicted by Transvaginal Sonography

Arthur C. Fleischer • Donna M. Kepple

Transvaginal sonography (TV US) affords improved resolution of the uterus and ovaries over that which can be obtained with the conventional transabdominal approach (TA US). While the proximity of the transducer/probe to the pelvic organs allows their more detailed depiction, it may be more rather than less difficult for the sonographer to become oriented to the images obtained on a TV US when compared to conventional, TA US. This is because of the limited field-of-view and unusual scanning planes depicted with TV US. However, as one develops a systematic approach to the examination of the uterus and adnexal structures with TV US, the examination becomes much easier to perform. In this chapter, the sonographic appearances of the uterus, ovary, and other adnexal and pelvic structures will be described with particular emphasis on how they are best depicted on a real-time, TV US examination.

SCANNING TECHNIQUE AND INSTRUMENTATION

The three scanning maneuvers that are used in TV US include:

1. Vaginal insertion of the probe with side-to-side movement within the upper vagina for sagittal imaging.
2. Transverse orientation of the probe for imaging in various degrees of semi-axial to semi-coronal planes.
3. Variation in depth of probe insertion for optimal imaging of the fundus-to-cervix by gradual withdrawal of the probe into the lower vagina for imaging of the cervix.

In contrast to conventional TA US, bladder distension is not necessary for TV US. In fact, overdistension can hinder TV US by placing the desired field-of-view outside the optimal focal range of the transducer. Minimal distension is useful in a patient with a severely anteflexed uterus to straighten the uterus relative to the imaging plane.

As is true for conventional sonographic equipment,

one should select the highest-frequency transducer possible that allows adequate penetration and depiction of a particular region of interest. Thus, 5.0-MHz and 7.5-MHz transducers are preferred, but these higher frequency transducers limit the field-of-view to within only 6 cm of the probe.

The major types of transducer/probes that are used for transvaginal scanning include those that contain a single-element oscillating transducer, multiple small transducer elements that are arranged in a curved linear array, and those that consist of multiple small elements steered by an electronic phased array (see Chapter 3). All of these depict the anatomy in a sector format that usually encompasses 100°. In our experience, the greatest resolution is achieved with a curved linear array that contains multiple (up to 124) separate transmit–receive elements. Mechanical sector transducers may be subject to minor image distortions at the edges of the field due to the hysteresis (lag in effect when stopping and starting) that occurs with an oscillating transducer. Reverberation artifacts can be created by suboptimal coupling of the condom/probe/vagina surfaces. Although degradation of image quality by side lobe artifacts can occur in the far field in a phased-array transducer, they do not significantly degrade the image in the near field. Therefore, phased-array transducers have similar resolution capabilities to sector as curved linear-array transducers for use in transvaginal examinations.

After completely covering the transducer/probe with a condom and securing the condom to the shaft of the probe with rubber bands, the probe is inserted into the vagina and manipulated around the cervical lips and into the fornix so as to depict the structures of interest in best detail. When the transducer is oriented in the longitudinal or sagittal plane, the long axis of the uterus can usually be depicted by slight angulation off midline. The uterus is used as a landmark for depiction of other adnexal structures. Once the uterus is identified, the probe can be angled to the right or left of midline in the sagittal plane to depict the ovaries. The internal iliac artery and vein appear as tubular structures along the pelvic sidewall. Low-level blood echoes can occasionally be seen streaming within these pulsating vessels. The ovaries typically lie medial to these vessels. After appropriate images are obtained in the sagittal plane, the transducer can be turned 90° to depict these structures in their axial or semicoronal planes.

Particularly in larger patients, it is helpful for the sonographer to use one hand to scan while the other is used for gentle abdominal palpation to move structures such as the ovaries as close as possible to the transducer/probe.

UTERUS

Examination of the uterus (Fig. 34–1) begins with its depiction in long axis. The endometrial interface, which is typically echogenic, is a useful landmark to depict this in long axis. Once the endometrium is identified in long axis, images of the uterus can be obtained in the sagittal and semi-axial/coronal plane.[1]

It may be difficult to determine the flexion of the uterus on the hard copy images obtained solely from transvaginal scanning, except in extreme cases of anteflexion or retroflexion. However, one can obtain an impression of uterine flexion during the examination by the relative orientation of the transducer/probe needed to obtain the most optimal images of the uterus. For example, retroflexed uteri are best depicted when the probe is in the anterior fornix and angulated in a posterior direction.

The endometrium has a variety of appearances, depending on its stage of development. In the proliferative phase, the endometrium measures 3 to 5 mm in anterior–posterior (AP) dimension (width). This measurement includes two layers of endometrium. A hypoechoic interface can be seen within the luminal aspects of echogenic layers of endometrium in the periovulatory phase and probably represents edema in the inner layers of endometrium. In the few days after ovulation, a small amount of secretion into the endometrial lumen can be seen. During the secretory phase, the endometrium typically measures between 5 and 8 mm in width and is surrounded by a hypoechoic band representing the inner layer of the myometrium.

Endometrial volume may be calculated by measuring its long axis, and multiplying by the AP and transverse dimension. One can use the axial-plane landmark where the endometrium invaginates into the area of ostia in the region of the uterine cornu.

Because of the proximity of the transducer/probe to the cervix, the cervix is not as readily depicted as the remainder of the uterus. However, if one withdraws the probe into the vagina, images of the cervix can be obtained. The mucus within the endocervical canal usually appears as an echogenic interface. This may become hypoechoic during the periovulatory period as the cervical mucus has a higher fluid content.

OVARIES

Ovaries (Fig. 34–2) are typically depicted as oblong structures measuring approximately 3 cm in long axis, 2 cm in AP and transverse dimension. On angled long-axis scans, they are immediately medial to the pelvic vessels. They are particularly well-depicted when they contain a mature follicle that is typically in the 1.5- to 2.0-centimeter range. It is not unusual to depict multiple immature or atretic follicles in the 3-mm range.

The size of an ovary is related to the patient's age and phase of follicular development. When the ovary contains a mature follicle, it can become twice as large in volume as one that does not contain mature follicles. However, the greatest dimension of a normal ovary typically is less than 3 cm.[2] The ovaries of postmenopausal women may be difficult to recognize because they are relatively small and usually do not contain follicles that enhance their sonographic recognition.

OTHER PELVIC STRUCTURES

Transvaginal sonography can depict several other pelvic structures (Fig. 34–3) besides the uterus and ovaries. These include bowel loops within the pelvis, iliac vessels, and occasionally distended fallopian tubes. Even small amounts (1 to 3 cc) of intraperitoneal fluid can be detected in the cul-de-sac or surrounding the uterus.

The pelvic vessels appear as straight tubular structures on either pelvic sidewall. The internal iliac arteries have a typical width of between 5 mm and 7 mm and tend to pulsate with expansion of both walls. The iliac vein is larger (approximately 1 cm) but does not demonstrate this pulsation. Occasionally, low-level "blood echoes" will be seen streaming within the vein. The transducer can be manipulated or pivoted to demonstrate these vessels in their long axis. Occasionally, a distended distal ureter may have this appearance but does not demonstrate pulsations. In most patients, the larger branches of the uterine vessels will be demonstrable by TV US as tubular structures coursing in the paracervical area.

The nondistended fallopian tube is difficult to depict on TV US, which is probably related to its small intraluminal size and serpiginous course. Occasionally, one can identify the origin of the tubes by finding the invagination of endometrium depicting the area of the tubal ostia and following these structures laterally in the axial or coronal plane. The ovarian and infundibulopelvic ligaments usually cannot be depicted.

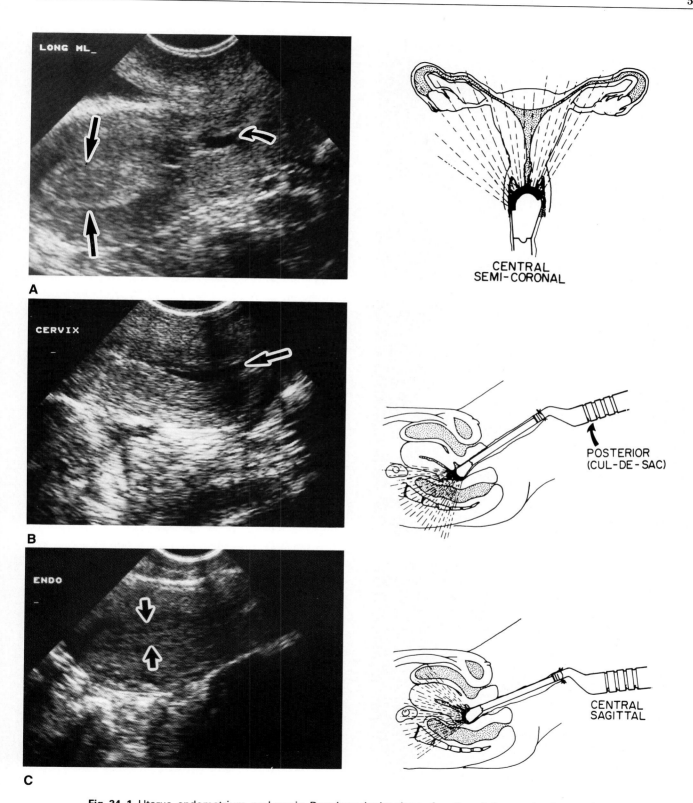

Fig. 34–1. Uterus, endometrium, and cervix. Drawings depict plane of section. **A.** Long axis of uterus in semi-coronal plane showing endometrium (*arrows*) and cervix. There is a small amount of fluid (*curved arrow*) within the endocervical canal. **B.** Same patient after withdrawing the probe into the mid-vagina. The endocervical canal with its fluid mucus (*arrow*) is clearly seen. **C.** Long axis of endometrium (*arrowheads*) during the proliferative phase. It is hypoechoic at this stage. (*Figure continued.*)

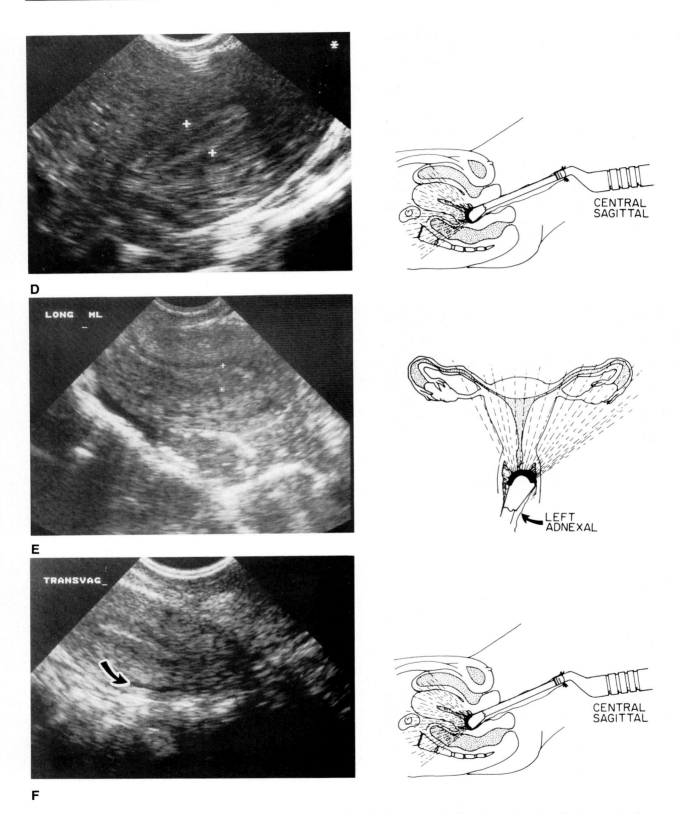

Fig. 34–1. (continued). Uterus, endometrium, and cervix. Drawings depict plane of section. **D.** Long axis of endometrium (*arrowheads*) during the periovulatory phase showing hypoechoic inner layer. The multilayered endometrium is clearly seen between the +s. **E.** Long axis of endometrium (between +s) in secretory phase, appearing as echogenic tissue (reversed orientation with uterine fundus to right of image). **F.** Oblique image showing veins (*arrow*) within outer myometrium.

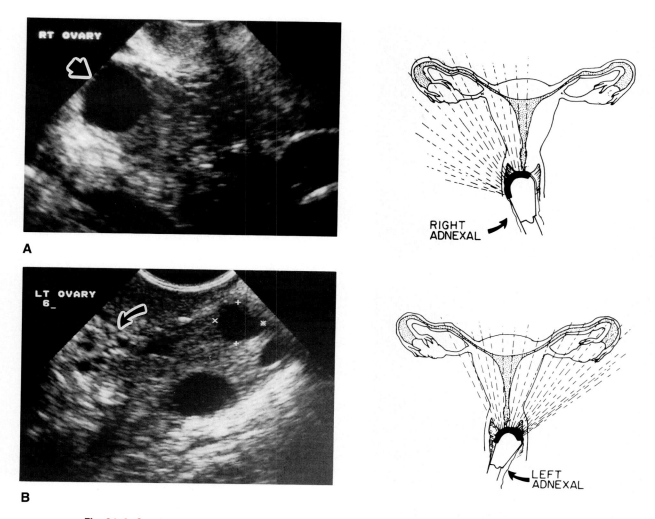

Fig. 34–2. Ovaries. Drawings depict plane of section. **A.** Right ovary containing a mature follicle (*arrow*) in a spontaneous cycle. **B.** Left ovary containing a fresh corpus luteum (+s). The wall is thick and irregular secondary to luteinization. Some pericervical vessels (*curved arrow*) are also seen.

Sonographic delineation of the tubes is facilitated by intraperitoneal fluid that may be present in the cul-de-sac.[3] By placing the patient in a reverse-Trendelenburg position, the fluid can be collected around the tube. When surrounded by fluid, the normal tube appears as a 0.5- to 1-cm in width tubular echogenic structure that usually comes from the lateral aspect of the uterine cornu posterolaterally into the adnexal regions and cul-de-sac. The flairing of the fimbriated end of the tube can be appreciated in some patients as it approximates its nearby ovary. Endosonographic depiction of the tubes is also facilitated when they contain intraluminal fluid.

The endosonographic appearances of the round ligaments are somewhat similar to that arising from a nondistended tube, except that its course is straighter and more parallel to the uterine cornu.

Bowel typically can be recognized as a fusiform structure that frequently contains intraluminal fluid and changes in configuration due to active peristalsis. If there is fluid within the lumen, periotic intraluminal projections—resulting from the valvulae conniventes—can be recognized from small bowel or the haustral indentations that are characteristic of large bowel.

SUMMARY

Transvaginal sonography affords detailed depiction of the uterus and ovaries. However, it requires a systematic evaluation of these pelvic structures for their complete delineation because of the limited field-of-view of transvaginal transducer/probes. This can be achieved by understanding the anatomic relationship of these structures from previous experience with TA US combined with anticipated findings from prior palpation of these structures during pelvic examination.

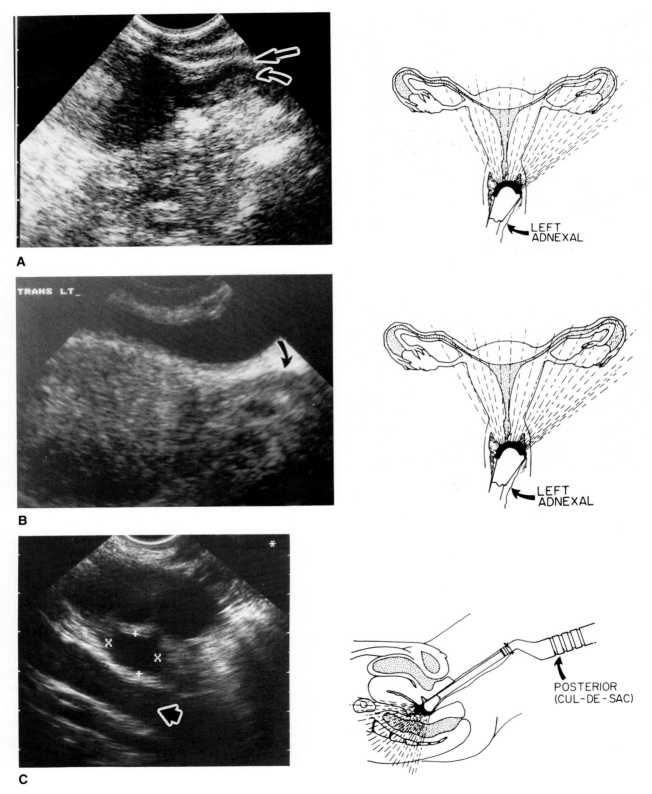

Fig. 34–3. Other pelvic structures. Drawings depict plane of section. **A.** Normal left tube (*curved arrow*) arising from cornual area adjacent to the uterine attachment of the round ligament (*straight arrow*). **B.** Normal left uterine tube (*curved arrow*) extending from left uterine corpus. **C.** Internal iliac vein (*arrow*) and artery in long axis adjacent to a follicle-containing ovary. (*Figure continued.*)

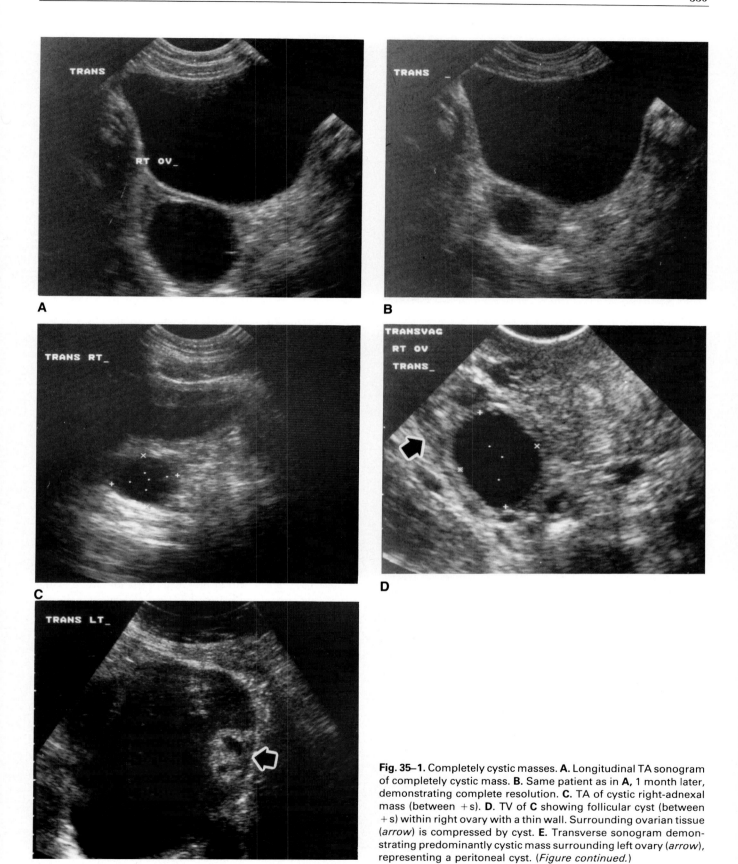

Fig. 35–1. Completely cystic masses. **A.** Longitudinal TA sonogram of completely cystic mass. **B.** Same patient as in **A,** 1 month later, demonstrating complete resolution. **C.** TA of cystic right-adnexal mass (between +s). **D.** TV of **C** showing follicular cyst (between +s) within right ovary with a thin wall. Surrounding ovarian tissue (*arrow*) is compressed by cyst. **E.** Transverse sonogram demonstrating predominantly cystic mass surrounding left ovary (*arrow*), representing a peritoneal cyst. (*Figure continued.*)

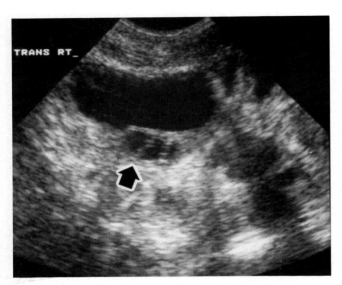

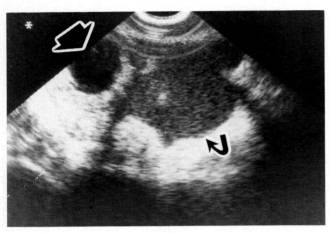

Fig. 35–1. (continued). Completely cystic masses. **F.** TV US of luteal cyst demonstrating thicker wall than follicular cyst, and rim of ovarian tissue containing several immature follicles (*arrow*) surrounding cyst. **G.** TV US of ruptured hemorrhagic corpus luteum cyst (*arrow*), surrounded by echogenic clotted blood in cul-de-sac (*curved arrow*).

due to its limited field of view and unusual image orientation, it is best used as an adjunct to a standard transabdominal scan. In particular, TV US is indicated for:

1. Determination of the presence or absence, and evaluation of, relatively small (less than 5- to 10-cm) adnexal masses.
2. Determination of the origin of a mass (uterine, ovarian, or tubal).
3. Detailed evaluation of its internal consistency with particular emphasis on the presence or ab-

sence of polypoid excrescences, septations, or internal consistencies (blood, pus, serous fluid).
4. Guiding transvaginal aspiration of certain masses.
5. Evaluation of endometrial or myometrial disorders related to pelvic masses.

For masses less than 10 cm in size, TV US can afford detailed delineation of the mass and determine its origin.[11–14] Specifically, masses that arise or are contained within the ovary can be differentiated from those of uterine origin. In addition, anatomic distortion of the tube by dilatation or inflammatory thickening can be identified with this technique. This is particularly helpful in differentiating inflammatory disease that may involve the tube or ovary—such as a tubo-ovarian abscess—from simple hydrosalpinx. The relative mobility of the pelvic organs can also be assessed when the probe comes into contact with the uterus or ovary.

Transvaginal sonography is particularly helpful in patients with fibroids because the ovaries can be identified as separate from the uterine abnormality. Conversely, some masses that are associated with uterine disorders (such as tubo-ovarian abscess with associated endometritis) can be identified.

Transvaginal sonography has been used as a means to guide abscess drainage.[15] It is conceivable that simple cysts with serous fluid could be safely aspirated using TV US. However, intraperitoneal spillage of the contents of "complicated" cysts such as endometriomas, dermoid cysts, or neoplastic cysts, might produce peritonitis or peritoneal spread from rupture and such cysts probably should not be aspirated.

Similarly, TV US affords a means to consider transvaginal aspiration of those pelvic masses thought to be benign serous cysts. These masses should demonstrate smooth and well-defined borders with no internal echoes. The sonographer should be aware that low-level artifactual echoes can be observed most with higher-frequency transducer/probes—even with completely serous cysts. But US findings of calcification, gravity-dependent layering material, or papillary excrescences should dissuade consideration of TV aspiration because these may indicate "complicated" cysts. (See previous discussion.) Accepting these limitations, however, there may be a role for TV aspiration with or without instillation of sclerosing agents for simple serous cysts. More extensive experience with follow-up after aspiration is needed before the clinical utility and indications for this procedure will be known.

Although it is tempting to speculate about the use of sonography as a means to screen for ovarian carcinoma in postmenopausal women, the incidence of this disorder would require that hundreds of patients be scanned for a single positive examination. In addition, most masses that are less than 5 cm in size are benign, according to one study demonstrating a 3% incidence of malignancy

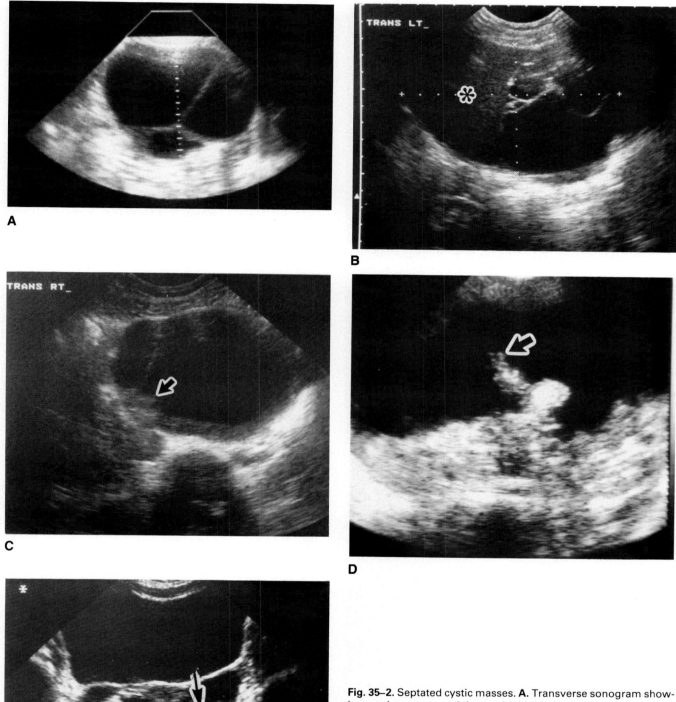

Fig. 35–2. Septated cystic masses. **A.** Transverse sonogram showing cystic mass containing multiple thin internal septations, representing mucinous cystadenoma. **B.** Transverse TA US showing septated mass with echogenic material (*) in upper loculated area. The echogenic material was mucin within this mucinous cystadenoma. **C.** Malignancy was suspected due to thickened septation (*arrow*) within this mucinous cystadenocarcinoma. **D.** Papillary projections (*arrow*) were found within this malignant teratoma. **E.** Transverse sonogram of complex predominantly cystic right-adnexal mass with calcific focus (*arrow*), arising from tooth within this dermoid cyst.

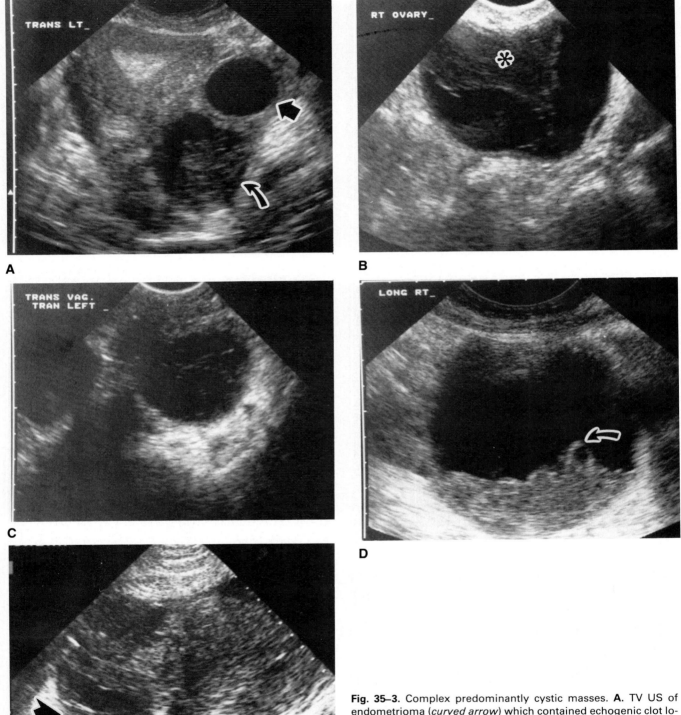

Fig. 35–3. Complex predominantly cystic masses. **A.** TV US of endometrioma (*curved arrow*) which contained echogenic clot located adjacent to mature follicle (*straight arrow*). **B.** TV US of tubo-ovarian abscess. Abscess cavity was surrounded by ovarian tissue (*). **C.** TV US of hemorrhagic corpus luteum cyst, with torsed right ovary (*arrow*). **D.** TV US of complex predominantly cystic masses with irregular solid area and some papillary excrescences (*curved arrow*). **E.** Transverse TA US showing cystic right-adnexal mass (*arrow*) within, representing appendiceal abscess in postpartum patient.

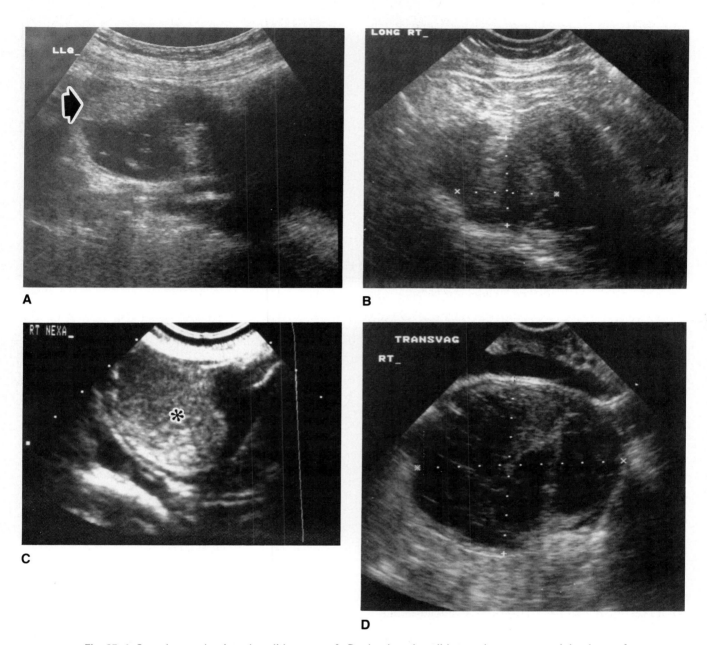

Fig. 35–4. Complex predominantly solid masses. **A.** Predominantly solid, complex mass containing layer of echogenic material (*arrow*) arising from sebum within this dermoid cyst. **B.** TA US of granulosa cell tumor. **C.** TV US of dermoid cyst with layer of echogenic sebum. (*Courtesy of Dr. Rebecca Pennell.*) **D.** TV US of hemorrhagic ovarian cyst containing irregular solid area corresponding to displaced hemorrhagic ovarian tissue surrounding area of hemorrhage. (*Figure continued.*)

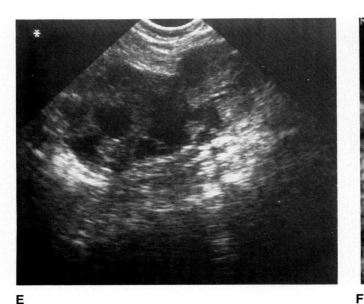
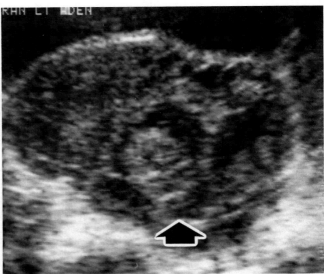

E   F

Fig. 35–4. (continued). Complex predominantly solid masses. **E.** Longitudinal TA US of ovarian cystadeno-carcinoma containing irregular solid areas. **F.** Magnified transverse TA US of cul-de-sac hemorrhage (*arrow*) resulting from ruptured ectopic pregnancy.

in masses of less than 5 cm.[16] Clearly, however, TV US has a role in delineation of the ovaries in obese, post-menopausal women in whom the incidence of carcinoma is high and pelvic examination is less than optimal.[34]

Additional investigation is necessary to determine whether or not the improved resolution afforded by TV US of the internal content of a mass would aid in its diagnostic specificity. Our initial impressions based on three years of experience is that TV US adds diagnostically specific information in over three fourths of women studied.[17] TV US is particularly helpful in determining the origin of a pelvic mass (intra- or extraovarian), and documentation of tubal, endometrial, and myometrial disorders. TV US also adds sensitivity over transabdominal sonography (TA US), particularly in obese patients.

On TV US, masses that appear hypoechoic on transabdominal sonography may demonstrate echogenic material suspended within the mass. The echogenic material most frequently represents blood in various degrees of coagulation. However, pus, mucous, or sebaceous material can be echogenic. Thus, it can be difficult to distinguish hemorrhagic from neoplastic cysts with TV US, and TV aspiration may be warranted.

In summary, the major roles of TV US for evaluation of adnexal masses include demonstration of the origin and internal consistency, as well as a means for guided aspiration. Transvaginal aspiration may have a role in guidance for aspiration of those masses that by clinical and sonographic criteria appear to be benign. But, because of the remote possibility of peritoneal spillage after an aspiration procedure, one should limit the application of transvaginal aspiration to only those masses that appear to be completely cystic with well-defined borders within adnexal structures that are freely mobile.

SONOGRAPHIC DIFFERENTIAL DIAGNOSIS OF PELVIC MASSES

This discussion of the sonographic differential diagnosis of pelvic masses is organized according to the most frequently seen sonographic appearance of particular types of pelvic masses. If a particular pelvic mass has a spectrum of sonographic appearances, it is mentioned in more than one category. Masses that are difficult to localize relative to a particular organ or category are considered "indeterminant." These may represent lesions related to the bowel, for example.[18,19]

This scheme for differential diagnosis should be used only as a general approach to the sonographic characterization of a pelvic mass (Table 35–1). Exceptions will undoubtedly occur, and the importance of correlating clinical and laboratory findings with the sonographic features of a pelvic mass is stressed.

Cystic Masses

Several types of pelvic masses can appear as cystic adnexal masses on sonography (see Figs. 35–1 and 35–2).

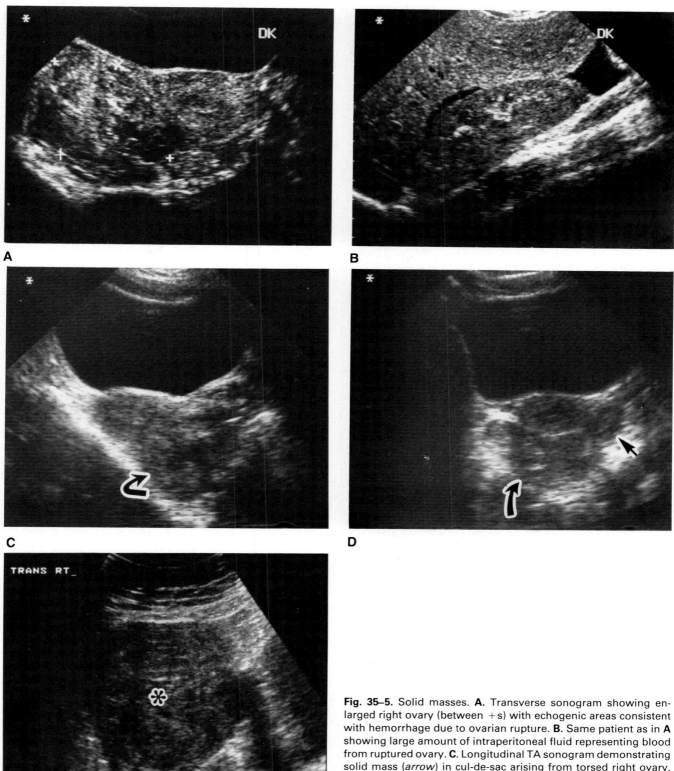

Fig. 35–5. Solid masses. **A.** Transverse sonogram showing enlarged right ovary (between + s) with echogenic areas consistent with hemorrhage due to ovarian rupture. **B.** Same patient as in **A** showing large amount of intraperitoneal fluid representing blood from ruptured ovary. **C.** Longitudinal TA sonogram demonstrating solid mass (*arrow*) in cul-de-sac arising from torsed right ovary. **D.** Transverse TA US of same patient as **C** showing left ovary (*arrow*) is normal in size and adjacent to torsed right ovary (*curved arrow*). **E.** Interligamentous fibroid appearing as solid pelvic mass. (*Figure continued.*)

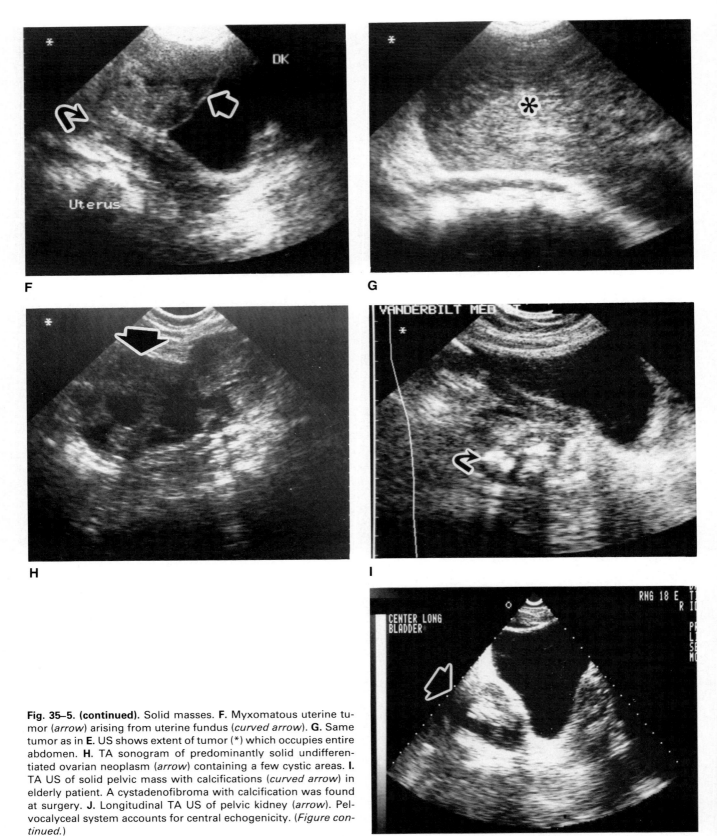

Fig. 35–5. (continued). Solid masses. **F.** Myxomatous uterine tumor (*arrow*) arising from uterine fundus (*curved arrow*). **G.** Same tumor as in **E.** US shows extent of tumor (*) which occupies entire abdomen. **H.** TA sonogram of predominantly solid undifferentiated ovarian neoplasm (*arrow*) containing a few cystic areas. **I.** TA US of solid pelvic mass with calcifications (*curved arrow*) in elderly patient. A cystadenofibroma with calcification was found at surgery. **J.** Longitudinal TA US of pelvic kidney (*arrow*). Pelvocalyceal system accounts for central echogenicity. (*Figure continued.*)

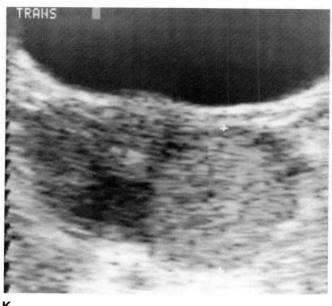

K

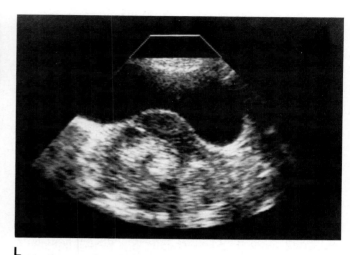

L

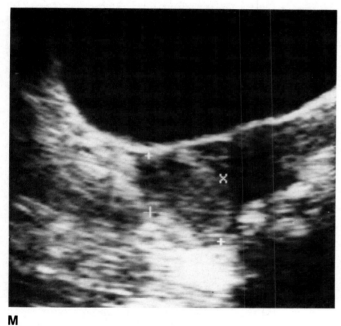

M

Fig. 35–5. (continued). Solid masses. K. Magnified transverse TA US showing solid left-adnexal mass (between +s) which represented hemorrhagic corpus luteum cyst. L. Longitudinal TA US of solid teratoma with calcified areas. M. Magnified TA US of solid mass (between +s) representing hemorrhagic corpus luteum cyst.

They include physiologic (follicular or luteal) ovarian cysts, hydrosalpinges, cystadenomas, parovarian cysts, and endometriomas. In general, physiologic cysts are the most common mass to appear as a well-defined anechoic, adnexal mass. Luteal cysts may have a slightly thicker wall than follicular cysts. Rarely, cysts that do not arise from the ovary—such as parovarian cysts or cysts of Morgagni—can mimic the sonographic features of an ovarian cyst.[20,21] These cysts will not demonstrate a rim of ovarian tissue, however. It may be helpful to use transvaginal scanning to determine whether or not a mass is surrounded by a rim of ovarian tissue in order to confirm its intraovarian location.

Even with the similar sonographic appearance of several types of cystic adnexal masses, the diagnostic possibilities can usually be narrowed to one or two entities based on clinical presentation and evaluation. In general, most cystic masses that arise within the pelvis

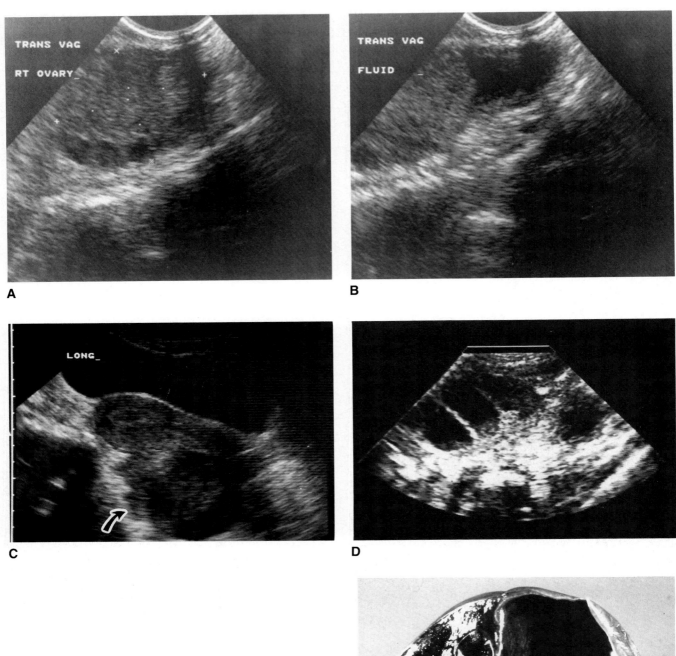

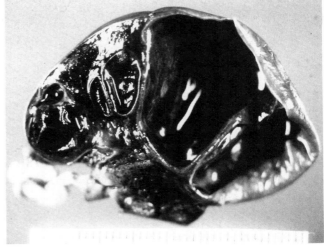

Fig. 35–6. Adnexal (ovarian) torsion. **A.** TV US showing enlarged right ovary (between +s) with mildly echogenic area resulting from internal hemorrhage. **B.** Cul-de-sac fluid adjacent to left side of uterus in same patient. **C.** 2 days later, ovary has enlarged secondary to re-torsion. On TA US, enlarged size of ovary relative to uterus can be better appreciated. **D.** Magnified TA US of enlarged ovary with two cystic spaces in 2-month-old girl. **E.** Bi-valved specimen shows torsed vascular pedicle. (*Figure continued.*)

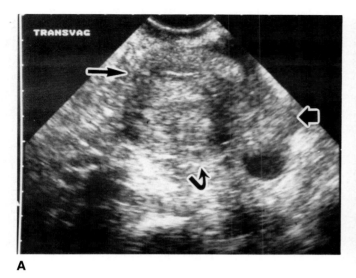

A

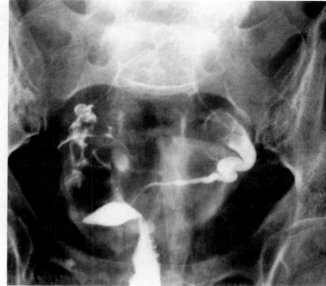

B

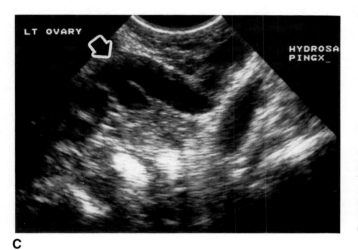

C

Fig. 35–8. Tubal disorders depicted by TV US. **A.** Transvaginal sonogram demonstrating mass (*arrow*) arising from left Fallopian tube, representing Fallopian tube carcinoma. Adjacent to uterus (*long arrow*) is a pedunculated subserous fibroid (*curved arrow*). **B.** Hysterosalpingogram in postmenopausal woman with vaginal bleeding, showing intrinsic filling defect in distal left uterine tube. **C.** Long axis of hydrosalpinx (*arrow*).

SUMMARY

This chapter has discussed and illustrated pertinent points in the differential diagnosis of pelvic masses by transabdominal and transvaginal sonography. Although the sonographic features of a pelvic mass may not allow a specific diagnosis, clinically useful information can usually be obtained. In general, transvaginal sonography is a useful adjunct to transabdominal sonography because it adds specificity in determining intra- versus extra-ovarian masses and endometrial and myometrial disorders. Transvaginal sonography affords an accurate means for evaluation of the ovaries and is particularly useful in obese, postmenopausal women in whom the incidence of ovarian carcinoma is especially high.[34,35]

REFERENCES

1. Fleischer A, James AE Jr, Millis J, et al. Differential diagnosis of pelvic masses by gray-scale sonography. *AJR.* 1978; 131:469–474.

2. Moyle J, Rochester D, Sider L, et al. Sonography of ovarian tumors: Predictability of tumor type. *AJR.* 1983; 141:985–991.

3. Warner M, Fleischer A, Edell S, et al. Uterine adnexal torsion: Sonographic findings. *Radiology.* 1985; 154:773–775.

4. Khan O, Cosgrove DO, Fried AM, Savage PE. Ovarian carcinoma follow-up: US versus laparotomy. *Radiology.* 1986; 159:111–113.

5. Mitchell DG, Mintz MC, Spritzer CE, et al. Adnexal

masses: MR imaging observations at 1.5T, with US and CT correlation. *Radiology.* 1987; 162:319–324.

6. Bluth E, Ferrarri B, Sullivan M. Real-time ultrasonography of the pelvis as an adjunct to the digital examination. *Radiology.* 1984; 153:789–791.

7. Callen P, DeMartins W, Filly R. The central uterine cavity echo: A useful anatomic sign in ultrasonographic evaluation of the female pelvis. *Radiology.* 1979; 131:187–190.

8. Meire J, Ferant P, Guha T. Distinction of benign from malignant ovarian cysts by ultrasound. *Br J Obstet Gynaecol.* 1978; 85:893–899.

9. Graif M, Shalev J, Strauss S, et al. Torsion of the ovary: Sonographic features. *AJR.* 1984; 143:1331–1334.

10. Worthen NJ, Gunning JE. Percutaneous drainage of pelvic abscesses: Management of the tubo-ovarian abscess. *J Ultrasound Med.* October 1986; 5:551–556.

11. Mendelson EB, Bohm-Velez M, Joseph N, Neiman HL. Gynecologic imaging: Comparison of transabdominal and transvaginal sonography. *Radiology.* 1988; 166:321–324.

12. Lande IM, Hill MC, Cosco FE, Kator NN. Adnexal and cul-de-sac abnormalities: Transvaginal sonography. *Radiology.* 1988; 166:325–332.

13. Vilaro MM, Rifkin MD, Pennell RG, et al. Endovaginal ultrasound: A technique for evaluation of nonfollicular pelvic masses. *J Ultrasound Med.* 1987; 6:697–701.

14. Timor-Tritsch I, Rottem S, eds. *Transvaginal Sonography.* New York: Elsevier; 1988; 125–141.

15. Nosher JL, Winchman HK, Needell GS. Transvaginal pelvic abscess drainage with US guidance. *Radiology.* 1987; 165:872–873.

16. Rulin M, Preston A. Adnexal masses in postmenopausal women. *Obstet Gynecol.* 1987; 70:578–581.

17. Fleischer A, Entman S, Gordon A. TV and TA US of pelvic masses: *J Ultra Med Biol.* 1989; 15:529–533.

18. Schnur P, Symmonds R, Williams T. Intestinal disorders masquerading as gynecologic problems. *Surg Gynecol Obstet.* 1969; 128:1016–1022.

19. Rifkin MD, Needleman L, Kurtz AB, et al. Sonography of nongynecologic cystic masses of the pelvis. *AJR.* 1984; 142:1169–1174

20. Alpern M, Sandler M, Madrazo B. Sonographic features of paraovarian cysts and their complications. *AJR.* 1984; 143:157–160.

21. Athey P, Cooper N. Sonographic features of paraovarian cysts. *AJR.* 1985; 144:83–86.

22. Guttman P. In search of the elusive benign cyst in teratoma "tip of the iceberg sign." *J Clin Ultrasound.* 1977; 5:403–406.

23. White E, Filly R. Cholesterol crystals as the source of both diffuse and layered echoes in a cystic ovarian tumor. Case report. *J Clin Ultrasound.* 1980; 8:241–243.

24. Baltarowich OH, Kurtz AB, Pasto ME, Rifkin MD, Needleman L, Goldberg BB. The spectrum of sonographic findings in hemorrhagic ovarian cysts. *AJR.* 1987; 148:901–905.

25. Reynolds T, Hill MC, Glassman IM. Sonography of hemorrhagic ovarian cysts. *J Clin Ultrasound.* 1986; 14:449–453.

26. Friedman H, Vogelzang R, Mendelson E, et al. Endometriosis detection by ultrasound with laparoscopic correlation. *Radiology.* 1985; 157:217–220.

27. Swenson M, Sauerbrei E, Cooperberg P. Medical implications of ultrasonographically detected polycystic ovaries. *J Clin Ultrasound.* 1981; 9:219–222.

28. Fleischer A, Daniell J, Rodier J, et al. Sonographic monitoring of ovarian follicular development. *J Clin Ultrasound.* 1981; 9:275–280.

29. Hall D, Hann L, Ferrucci J, et al. Sonographic morphology of the normal menstrual cycle. *Radiology.* 1979; 133:185–188.

30. Bass I, Haller J, Freidman A, et al. The sonographic appearance of hemorrhagic ovarian cysts in adolescents. *J Ultrasound Med.* 1984; 3:509–513.

31. Towne B, Maholar H, Wooley M, et al. Ovarian cysts and tumors in infancy and childhood. *J Pediatr Surg.* 1975; 10:311–320.

32. Gross B, Silver T, Jaffe M. Sonographic features of uterine leiomyomas: Analysis of 41 proven cases. *J Ultrasound Med.* 1983; 2:401–406.

33. Stephenson WM, Laing FC. Sonography of ovarian fibromas. *AJR.* 1985; 144:1239–1240.

34. Campbell S, Gosamy R. Screening for ovarian carcinoma with ultrasound. *Clin Ob/Gyn.* 1984; 10:621–643.

35. Granberg S, Wikland M. A comparison between ultrasound and gynecologic examination for detection of enlarged ovaries in a group of women at risk for ovarian carcinoma. *J Ultrasound Med.* 1988; 7:59–64.

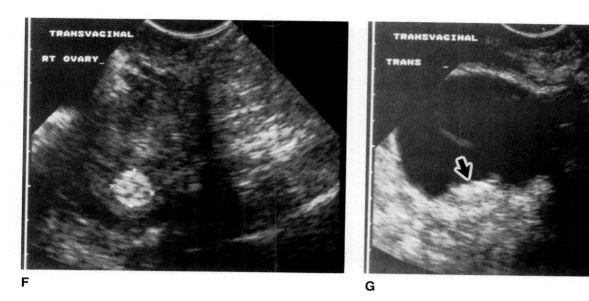

Fig. 36–3. (continued). TV US of benign ovarian masses. **F.** Dermoid cyst in right ovary with sebum in dermoid plug. **G.** Same patient with dermoid cyst in left ovary with layering sebum (*arrow*).

face of the hemi-diaphragms. At present, there is no established imaging procedure that accurately detects these small miliary-like metastases.[8]

Clearly, the prognosis of CaO is related to the stage of disease at initial presentation. Differences in the behavior of the various histologic grades of CaO may also influence long-term survival. It has been stated that the histologic grade of the tumor and the size of the largest individual mass after primary operation are the only statistically significant factors relative to survivorship.[3]

THE ROLE OF SONOGRAPHY (BOTH TRANSVESICULAR AND TRANSVAGINAL)

There have been a few large scale studies that evaluated the role of sonography in early detection of CaO. In one ongoing study reported in 1983, which utilized transabdominal real-time sonography for the study of 1,083 women, approximately 3% of the screened population were found to have an adnexal mass, and a third of these were ovarian carcinoma.[9] A recent update to this study reported the results of screening over 5,000 women. Nine CaOs were detected with transabdominal US, five were primary tumors, and four were metastasis. Interestingly enough, all of the primary tumors detected were confined to the ovary (stage I). This shows that transvesicular (scans performed through a fully distended bladder) and TV US are capable of detection of even those ovarian neoplasms that are contained in normal to minimally-enlarged ovaries.[19]

A similar study by Andolf[10] indicated that sonography could detect CaO in a screened population of asymptomatic women. In this study of over 800 patients who were at risk for CaO due to age, 39 masses (5% of the screened population) were found and 35 of these were abnormal. In 24, ovarian epithelial tumors were found, 8 of which were not palpated prior to the sonographic study.[10]

In a study that utilized transvaginal scanning, Higgins has shown that TV US is an accurate means for early detection of CaO, even though several benign tumors will be detected for every carcinoma found.[20] It has been postulated, however, that up to 15% of benign tumors have the potential for malignant transformation, therefore, their detection and treatment is clinically efficacious.[21]

It should be clearly stated that the small size and location of the typical postmenopausal ovary may make it difficult to image sonographically (Fig. 36–2). The ovary in the postmenopausal woman averages less than 1.5 cm in size (>3 mL volume) and very frequently is located deep to bowel.[11] Factors that may increase the volume of the ovary in postmenopausal women include multiparity, obesity, or hormonal replacement treatment. Transvesical scans may be helpful by identifying the ovary by its surrounding vessels (ie, internal iliac vein and artery). Transvaginal sonography may be limited in some postmenopausal women due to the small size of the vagina, hindering sonographic accessibility to the ovary.

It has been suggested by one respected authority that it is important to image the ovaries in postmenopausal

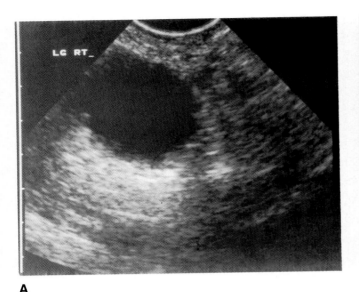

A

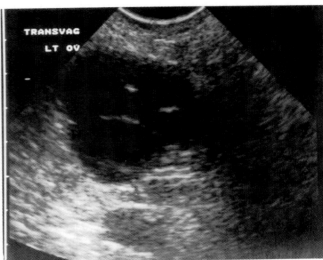

B

Fig. 36–4. TV US of ovarian tumors. **A.** 3 cm serous cystadenoma
in right ovary. **B.** Same patient with septated-cyst ovarian tumor
in left ovary. This was another serous cystadenoma. **C.** Metastasis
to ovary from gastrointestinal primary tumor showing papillary
excrescences.

C

women with both transvesicular and transvaginal approaches (S. Campbell, MD, personal communication). In our experience with 33 older postmenopausal (60 to 80 years of age) patients scanned prior to transabdominal hysterectomy and bilateral salpingo-oophorectomy for endometrial carcinoma, only about 60% of "normal" postmenopausal ovaries can be identified.[21] Some studies have considered the lack of identification of an adnexal mass in proximity to normal pelvic vessels around the expected position of ovaries as evidence of normalcy. We do not consider this "diagnosis of exclusion" an acceptable concept for early detection of CaO because tumors in their earliest stages may only minimally enlarge the ovary. In our study that evaluated the ability to delineate normal postmenopausal ovaries in women undergoing hysterectomy and bilateral salpingo-oophorectomy for

endometrial carcinoma, we found that only about 60% of normal postmenopausal ovaries could be delineated preoperatively. This factor may limit the accuracy of identifying early tumors as textural abnormalities within normal-sized ovaries. In addition, some small solid tumors (0.5 to 2.5 cm) were missed. All of these were benign.

In a study that evaluated 150 masses in postmenopausal women without regard to their sonographic features, of masses less than 5 cm in size, only 3% were malignant.[12] Several studies have shown that the incidence of malignancy in completely cystic masses in this age group is exceedingly low (less than 1 to 2%).[22,23,24] Sonographic findings that are highly suggestive of malignancy include demonstration of omental or peritoneal masses, liver metastases, ruptured capsules, pseudomyxoma peritonei, and intraperitoneal fluid (Fig. 36–4).[13]

The goal of any attempts to detect CaO should emphasize its early detection prior to the development of metastatic disease. This may entail the use of transvaginally-guided biopsy/aspiration. However, there remains a healthy reluctance to perform aspiration on a potentially malignant lesion due to the possibility of its later intraperitoneal spread.

A recently presented study from England in 41 asymptomatic women reported detection of 3 CaOs as well as a number of patients with an unsuspected endometrial disorder.[14] Depending on the inclusion criteria, most studies will find between 1 and 10% of the screened population to be abnormal.

It seems clear that the goal of TV US should be identification of ovarian tumors in ovaries that are not significantly enlarged (Figs. 36–3 and 4). It is also clear that for every malignancy detected, several benign masses will be found. Initial results with color Doppler sonography indicate that ovarian masses can be distinguished by their flow characteristics.[25,26] More extensive experience with this technique is required before it can be used clinically for this purpose.

COMBINED SCREENING/TESTING PROTOCOLS

Transvaginal sonography might be one of several screening tests used for early detection of CaO. In practical terms, an imperfect screening test should be more sensitive than it is specific. Transvaginal sonography could be used effectively as a secondary means to differentiate patients with true serum screening tests versus those with false-positive tests.

Today, carcinoma of the cervix is screened effectively by evaluation of exfoliated cells of the cervix taken in a Pap smear. Not only can noninvasive cervical cancer be detected with this test but the precursors to this neoplasm can also be found. Because the incidence of CaO is higher than carcinoma of the cervix, it seems logical that screening for CaO could be medically indicated. Some practical problems with this include patient reluctance to submit

TABLE 36–2. DETECTION OF CaO WITH CA 125, CLINICAL EXAM, AND TRANSABDOMINAL SONOGRAPHY

	Sensitivity	Specificity
Clinical exam	68%	85%
Transabdominal sonography	78%	92%
CA 125	84%	92%

Finkler N, et al. *Obstet Gyn.* 1988;72:659.

to a transvaginal study and primary physicians who may not be insistent in recommending the study to their patients. However, the transvaginal study is clearly less anxiety-provoking than sigmoidoscopy, which is currently a recommended screening procedure for detection of cancer of the rectum.[15]

There is a variety of tagable antibodies used in both serum and imaging that are under investigation for early detection of CaO. One of these, called CA 125, has been shown to be an accurate means for detection of recurrent tumors in women with known CaO.[10] It seems to be most sensitive in nonmucinous tumors.[16] For example, one case report does describe its use in detection of CaO when an ultrasound exam showed a 2- × 3-cm ovary that was nonpalpable.[14] However, its poor sensitivity of only 46% in one series substantially limits its use as the only screening test for early detection of CaO (Table 36–1).

In a recently completed study involving 102 patients, the relative sensitivity and specificity of pelvic examination, CA 125, and routine transabdominal sonography, were compared. The relative accuracy of transabdominal sonography and CA 125 were comparable, indicating that when results are abnormal, these tests can be additive and complementary (Table 36–2).[17] It is clear that an elevated CA 125 level in association with an abnormal sonographic finding is highly indicative of ovarian malignancy.

In a recently published study of 1,010 postmenopausal women in England, the combination of CA 125, pelvic exam, and transabdominal sonography was found to be nearly 99% specific (Table 36–3).[7] These findings indicated that, although no single screening test had an acceptable specificity for CaO, the combination of tests

TABLE 36–1. SUMMARY OF CLINICAL STUDIES WITH CA 125[a]

	(n = 141)
	mean; range
Sensitivity	33/72 (46%; 34–58%)
Specificity	68/69 (99%; 91–99%)
Positive predictive value	33/34 (97%; 84–99%)
Negative predictive value	31/49 (64%; 54–73%)

[a] 95% Confidence interval.
(*Courtesy of Centocor, December 7, 1987.*)

TABLE 36–3. MULTIMODALITY SCREENING FOR CaO WITH CA 125 AND SONOGRAPHY[a]

	With CA 125	Without CA 125
With Pelvic Exam	True + US+ (1) US− (0)	False + US+ (10) US− (17)
Without Pelvic Exam	False + US+ (2) US− (28)	True − US not done

[a] Study of 1,010 postmenopausal women.
(*Jacobs I, et al. Lancet. 1988;6:268–271.*)

achieved acceptable specificity and is the best hope for a specific and sensitive method for early detection of CaO.[7]

Tagged monoclonal antibody imaging may be useful in identifying metastatic disease.[20] Similar findings have been noted by M. Sandler, MD, and H. Jones, MD (personal communication). However, it cannot be used as a screening test, and seems to be best suited to document the extent of disease once it is diagnosed. With tagging of the antibodies to ^{125}I after ^{111}In, it has the potential for detection and treatment of tumor foci.

SUMMARY

Perhaps the best scheme for early detection of CaO would be an initial pelvic sonogram (transabdominal and transvaginal) combined with serum CA 125 and monoclonal antibody imaging if the sonogram and CA 125 are positive. At Vanderbilt University Medical Center, we are currently evaluating the clinical efficacy of such a scheme. It will take many subjects (an estimated 5,000 to 30,000) and multiple clinical sites for complete assessment of the efficacy of this approach, but conceptually it does seem promising.[18]

Acknowledgments

I would like to dedicate my work in this area to the late Conrad Julian, MD, who provided guidance and encouragement to me during my clinical training. I also thank Stephen S. Entman, MD, and Martin P. Sandler, MD, for their cooperation and encouragement. The thoughtful comments of Stuart Campbell, MBChB, Peter Callen, MD, Roy Filly, MD, and Ellen Mendelson, MD, Debra Hall, MD, and Gerald Holzman, MD, are also appreciated.

REFERENCES

1. Silverberg E, Lubera A. Cancer statistics. *CA.* 1988;38:9.
2. Mendelson EB, Böhm-Velez M, Neiman HL, Russo J. Transvaginal sonography in gynecologic imaging. *Semin Ultrasound, CT, MRI.* 1988;9:102–121.
3. Julian C. General concepts and characteristics of ovarian Ca. H. Jones, G. Jones, eds. *Novak's Textbook of Gynecology.* 10th ed. Baltimore: Williams & Wilkins, 1981:543.
4. Heintz AP, Hacker NF, Lagasse LD. Epidemiology and etiology of ovarian cancer: A review. *Obstet Gynecol.* 1985;66:127–135.
5. Woodruff JD. History of ovarian neoplasia: Facts and fancy. In: Winn RM, ed. *Obstet and Gynecol Annual.* New York: Appleton-Century-Crofts; 1976;5:331–344.
6. Bennington JL, Ferguson BR, Haber SL. Incidence and relative frequency of benign and malignant neoplasms. *Obstet Gynecol.* 1968;32:627–632.
7. Jacobs I, Bridges J, Reynolds C, et al. Multimodal approach to screening for ovarian cancer. *Lancet.* 1988;6:268–271.
8. Megibow AJ, Bosniak MA, Ho AG, Beller U, Hulnick DH, Beckman EM. Accuracy of CT in detection of persistent or recurrent ovarian carcinoma: Correlation with second-look laparotomy. *Radiology.* 1988;166:341–345.
9. Goswamy RK, Campbell S, Whitehead MI. Screening for ovarian cancer. *Clinics Obstet Gynecol.* 1983;10:621–643.
10. Andolf E, Svalenius E, Astedt B. Ultrasonography for early detection of ovarian carcinoma. *Br J Obstet Gynaecol.* 1986;93:1286–1289.
11. Granberg S, Wikland M. Comparison between endovaginal and transabdominal transducers for measuring ovarian volume. *J Ultrasound Med.* 1987;6:649–653.
12. Rulin MC, Preston AL. Adnexal masses in postmenopausal women. *Obstet Gynecol.* 1987;70:578–581.
13. Moyle JW, Rochester D, Sider L, Shrock K, Krause P. Sonography of ovarian tumors: Predictability of tumor type. *AJR.* 1983;141:985–991.
14. Smith B. The use of vaginal sonography as the basis of a perimenopausal ovarian and uterine screening program. Presented at the First World Congress on Vaginosonography in Gynecology; June 1988; Washington, DC.
15. Eddy D. Guidelines for cancer related checkup: Recommendations and rationale. *CA.* 1980;30:321.
16. Zurawski VR, Knapp RC, Einhorn N, et al. An initial analysis of preoperative serum CA 125 levels in patients with early stage ovarian carcinoma. *Gynecol Oncol.* 1988;30:7–14.
17. Finkler NJ, Benacerraf B, Wojciechowski C, Lavin PT, Knapp RC. Comparison of serum CA 125, clinical impression, and ultrasound in the preoperative evaluation of ovarian masses. *Obstet Gynecol.* 1988;72:659.
18. Berkowitz R. *Gynecologic Oncology.* New York: Macmillan; 1988:208.
19. Campbell S, Bham V, Royston P, et al. Transabdominal screening of early ovarian cancer. *Br Med J.* 1989; 299:1363–1367.
20. Higgins R, VanNagell J, Donaldson E. Transvaginal sonography as a screening method for ovarian cancer. *Gynecol Oncol.* 1989; 34:402–406.
21. Fleischer A, McKee M, Gordon A, et al. Transvaginal sonography of postmenopausal ovaries with pathologic correlation. *J Ultra Med.* In press, 1990.
22. Hall D, McCarthy K. The significance of the postmenopausal single adnexal cyst. *J Ultrasound Med.* 1986;5:503.
23. Goldstein S. Subvamanyam B, Synder J, et al. The postmenopausal cystic adnexal mass: The potential role of ultrasound in consecutive management. *Obstet Gynecol.* 1989;8:743.
24. Andolf E, Jorgenson C. Cystic lesions in elderly women diagnosed by ultrasound. *Br J Obstet Gynaecol.* 1989; 96:1076.
25. Fleischer A, Rao B, Keppler D. Transvaginal color Doppler sonography: Preliminary experience. *Gyn Cardiovasc Imaging.* In Press, 1990.
26. Boorne T, Campbell S, Steer C. Transvaginal color flow imaging: A possible new screening technique for ovarian cancer. *Br J Med.* 1989;299:1367–1370.

37 Sonographic Evaluation of the Uterus and Related Disorders

Arthur C. Fleischer • Stephen S. Entman

The ability of sonography, particularly transvaginal sonography (TV US), to depict subtle changes in the myometrium and endometrium makes it the diagnostic modality of choice for the evaluation of many uterine disorders. With sonography, the uterus can be imaged in several scan planes. Because the images are obtained in real time, the sonographer can empirically alter the scanning plane and gain settings for optimal depiction of the endometrium and myometrium. Because of its proximity to the uterus, a transvaginal transducer/probe can enhance the sonographic depiction of the uterus and endometrium.

Once a uterine lesion is suspected clinically, sonography can be used to establish the presence, size, extent, and internal consistency of the lesion, as well as to detect associated pathology such as liver metastases. Sonography has a major role in differentiating palpable uterine masses from those that arise from adnexal structures. The specific diagnosis can be confirmed by endometrial biopsy, through dilatation and curettage, by other imaging techniques such as hysterosalpingography, and, in some cases, even by direct hysteroscopic visualization. Magnetic resonance imaging (MRI) and computed tomography (CT) can also demonstrate uterine and para-uterine anatomy and are particularly useful in staging known uterine neoplasms.

This chapter discusses and illustrates the sonographic features of the most common uterine malformations and disorders. For the sonographer and sonologist to distinguish normal from pathologic findings, a short discussion of the sonographic features of the normal uterus follows comments about scanning technique.

SCANNING TECHNIQUE

Both transvaginal and transabdominal sonography (TA US) have a role in the evaluation of the uterus. Whereas transvaginal sonography affords detailed images of the uterus, larger uteri or those with masses greater than 5 cm may be better depicted by transabdominal sonography.

For transabdominal sonography, sonographic evaluation of the uterus should be performed when the patient has a fully distended bladder. A fully distended bladder displaces gas-filled bowel loops from the pelvis and places the uterus in a more horizontal plane. This orientation of the uterus relative to the transducer is advantageous because the uterus can be imaged using the better characteristics of axial, as opposed to lateral, resolution. Occasionally, the urinary bladder can be overly distended, placing the uterus out of the focal range of a focused transducer. In such cases, partial voiding will place the uterus in a more optimal focal range. In some patients with very large uterine masses, full distension of the bladder may be impossible, and adequate sonographic visualization of the uterus must be attempted without having the bladder fully distended.

When examining a pelvic mass thought to be of uterine origin, it is important to establish the continuity of that mass with the uterus. Establishing that a mass is uterine involves showing that the vagina leads into the mass and that a linear echogenic interface in the uterus—the endometrium—is present. Transvaginal sonography can be used to optimize depiction of these features.

A water enema can be used to further delineate possible masses arising from the posterior aspect of the uterus. In this technique, lukewarm water is slowly introduced into the rectum and followed using real-time sonography. After about 50 to 100 mL of water is introduced, the rectosigmoid colon distends, thereby improving delineation of structures in the posterior pelvic compartment.[1]

For transvaginal sonography, the urinary bladder should not be overly distended. The uterus should be imaged in its long axis first, sweeping from right to left by angulating the probe. Short axis images are then obtained. The relative position of the uterus can be inferred by the orientation of the probe that best images the uterus. For example, if the uterus is best imaged with a posterior inclination, the uterus is probably retroflexed.

The endometrium can be demonstrated in most patients as an echogenic interface or a group of interfaces in the center of the uterus. The sloughed pieces of the endometrium during menstruation usually produce a thin, broken echogenic interface. The endometrium thickens and becomes echogenic as it develops in the secretory phase. The thickness of the endometrium can usually be estimated by the distance from the proximal to distal interfaces between the hypoechoic halo that surrounds the endometrium (corresponding to the compact and relatively hypovascular inner layer of myometrium) and the more echogenic endometrium. The "natural contrast" provided by the endometrium can be used to definitively localize the uterus in relation to other masses that may surround or distort it.[2]

SONOGRAPHIC FEATURES OF THE NORMAL UTERUS

Sonography can accurately depict the position, size, shape, and texture of the uterus. Each of these features should be carefully assessed and documented sonographically (Figs. 37–1 to 37–4).

The position of the normal uterus is immediately

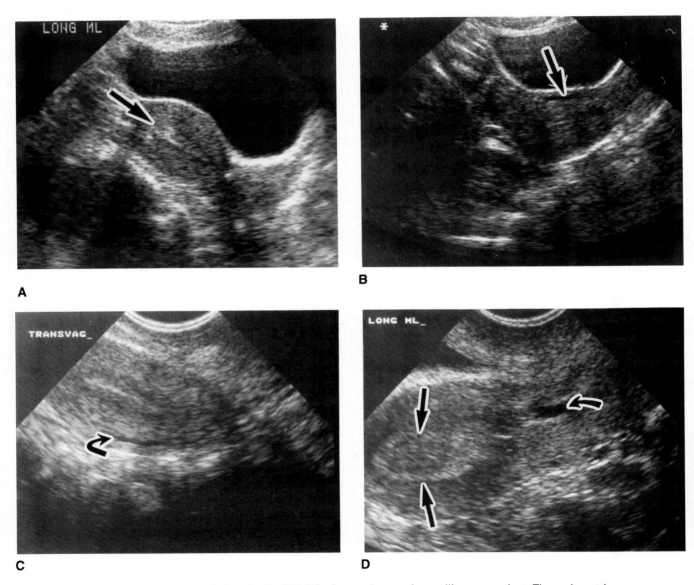

Fig. 37–1. Normal uterus. **A.** Longitudinal TA US of normal uterus in a nulliparous patient. The endometrium (*arrow*) appears as a group of linear, echogenic interfaces in center of uterus. **B.** Transverse TA US through uterus demonstrating arcuate vessel (*arrow*) coursing in outer myometrium. **C.** TV US demonstrating arcuate vein (*arrow*) in outer myometrium. **D.** TV US semicoronal plane demonstrating entire uterus. The endometrium (*between arrows*) is thick and echogenic, consistent with early secretory-phase endometrium. Within the endocervical canal is fluid-like mucus (*curved arrow*) seen in periovulatory period.

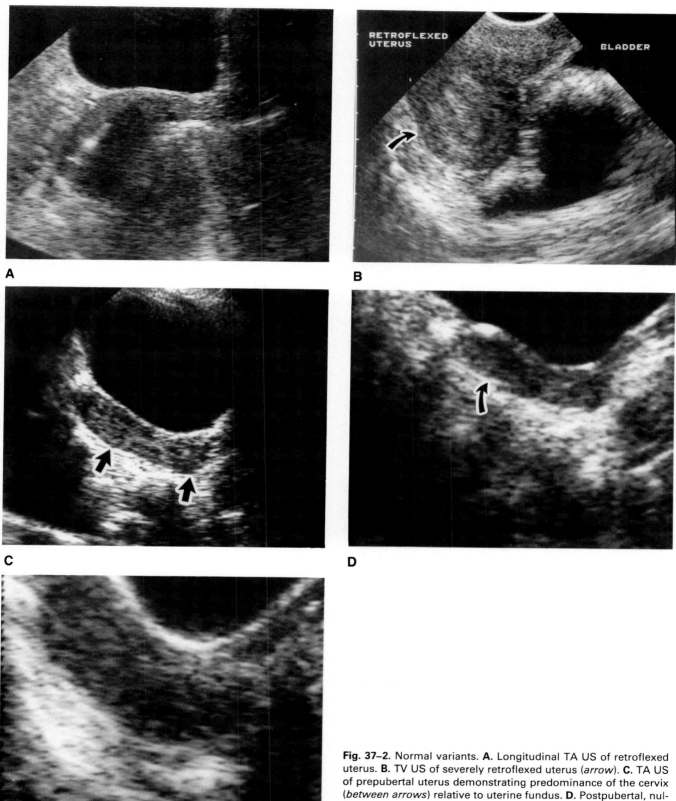

Fig. 37–2. Normal variants. **A.** Longitudinal TA US of retroflexed uterus. **B.** TV US of severely retroflexed uterus (*arrow*). **C.** TA US of prepubertal uterus demonstrating predominance of the cervix (*between arrows*) relative to uterine fundus. **D.** Postpubertal, nulliparous uterus as shown in long axis. The fundus (*curved arrow*) is now larger than the cervix. **E.** Magnified longitudinal TA US of a postmenopausal uterus demonstrating size comparable to a prepubertal uterus.

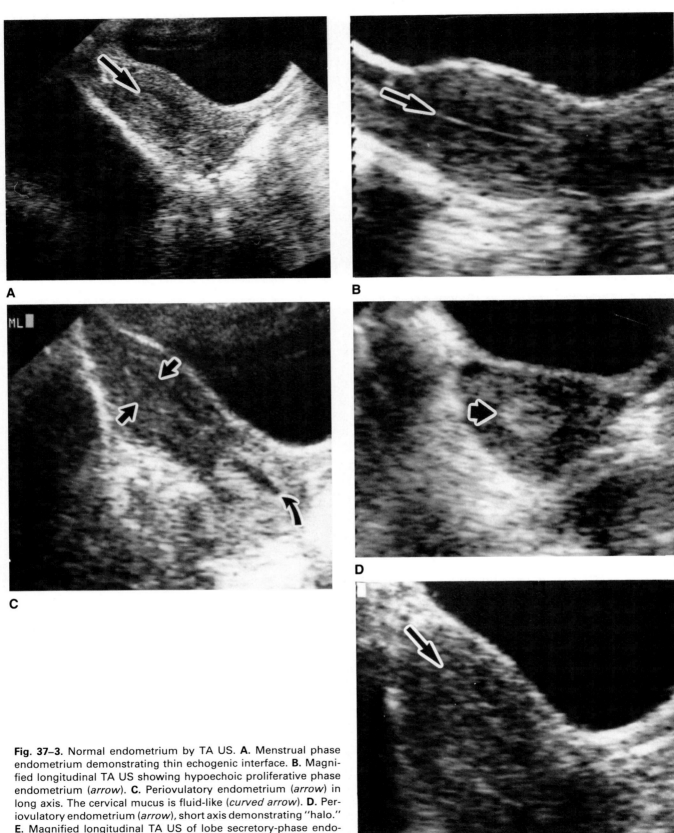

Fig. 37–3. Normal endometrium by TA US. **A.** Menstrual phase endometrium demonstrating thin echogenic interface. **B.** Magnified longitudinal TA US showing hypoechoic proliferative phase endometrium (*arrow*). **C.** Periovulatory endometrium (*arrow*) in long axis. The cervical mucus is fluid-like (*curved arrow*). **D.** Periovulatory endometrium (*arrow*), short axis demonstrating "halo." **E.** Magnified longitudinal TA US of lobe secretory-phase endometrium (*arrow*).

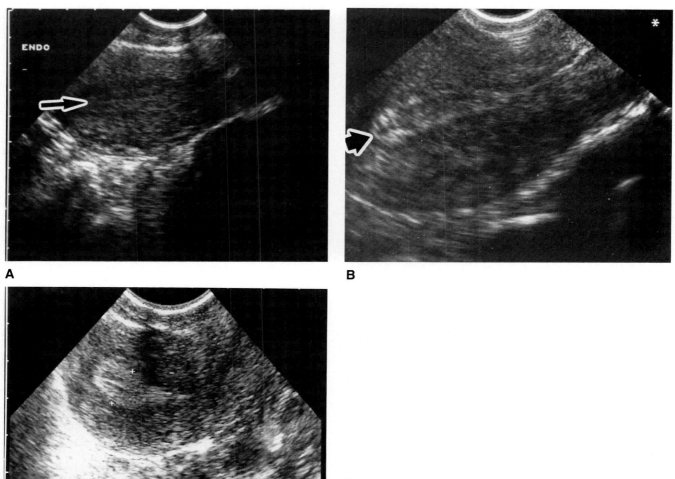

Fig. 37–4. Normal endometrium by TV US. **A.** Proliferative phase endometrium (*arrow*) in long axis as depicted by TV US. **B.** Periovulatory endometrium (*arrow*) demonstrating multiple layers. The inner hypoechoic layer probably results from edema. **C.** Secretory phase endometrium (between +s) on long axis, as seen with TV US.

posterior to the floor and dome of the urinary bladder. The fundus is usually anteriorly flexed when compared to the cervix (anteflexed). Although a retroflexed uterus can be a normal variant, this uterine configuration should raise suspicion of posterior pelvic compartment pathology. Retroflexed uteri appear more lobular in contour than anteflexed uteri, partly because there tends to be altered venous drainage with consequent myometrial suffusion. Transvaginal scanning can improve depiction in most of these cases. However, because of the posterior position and curved surface of the fundus, it may be difficult to obtain detailed images of the fundal portion of a retroflexed uterus. Furthermore, the endometrial layer may not be seen with transabdominal sonography. In some severely retroflexed uteri, an interface perpen-

dicular to the endometrial lumen can be seen; this probably results from an indentation and compression of the myometrium and uterine serosa.

On transverse sonograms, a significant range of variation in the right-to-left or anterior-posterior position of the uterus can be observed in normal individuals. These positional variants are in part dependent on the degree of bladder and rectal distension present when the patient is examined.

The flexion and position of the uterus is not as readily depicted by transvaginal scanning as by transabdominal scan. In general, if the uterus is best depicted on transvaginal scanning when there is a posterior orientation of the probe, the uterus is most likely retroflexed. Conversely, if the uterus is best depicted when the probe is placed in the posterior vaginal fornix and aimed anteriorly, the uterus is most likely anteflexed.

Before discussing the size and shape of the uterus, the various anatomic segments of the uterus are noted here. There are three main divisions of the uterus: the fundus, the corpus or body, and the cervix. The segment of the uterus that lies superior to the entrance of the uterine tubes is designated the fundus. Inferior to the fundus and superior to the internal cervix is the corpus. The lower portion of the corpus is sometimes termed the isthmus. Although the isthmus has been designated as a separate segment of the uterus, this designation is debatable because it is not distinct—on the basis of function or anatomy—from the corpus. There is a transition from the smooth muscle wall of the fundus and corpus to the cervix, which consists of mostly fibrous tissue.

The size and shape of the uterus varies according to the patient's pubertal status, age, and parity.[3] Before puberty occurs, the uterus measures 1.0 to 3.3 cm in length and 0.5 to 1.0 cm in width. The cervix and isthmus comprise a greater proportion of the uterus (up to two thirds of the total length), and are thicker than the fundus. In contrast, the nulligravidous, normal postpubertal uterus measures 7 cm in length, 4 cm in width, 4 cm in height, and has a relatively thicker fundus and shortened cervix. The multiparous woman typically has a uterus that measures an average of 1.2 cm greater in all directions, compared to the nulligravida.[4] A postmenopausal woman has a uterus that is smaller than the normal postpubertal woman. The average dimension of the postmenopausal uterus ranges from 3.5 to 6.5 cm in length, and is 1.2 to 1.8 cm thick.[5]

The texture of the normal myometrium is consistent throughout all age groups, and is of a homogenous low to medium echogenicity. Small vessels (between 1 and 2 mm in diameter) can sometimes be seen within the outer myometrium. It is not unusual to have calcification of these arcuate arteries in the outer layers of myometrium in older women. The endometrium in postmenopausal women should be relatively thin (less than 6 to 8 mm) because it is typically atrophic.

Sonography, particularly transvaginal sonography, can depict a variety of images of the endometrium that correspond to the major developmental stages (menstrual, proliferative, or secretory). The innermost layers of the endometrium appear as a central linear echogenicity—most prominent during menses. Surrounding this echogenic interface is a hypoechoic band that probably corresponds to the compact and relatively hypovascular inner layer of the myometrium. The endometrium thickens from 3 to 5 mm (in the proliferative phase) to 6 to 12 mm (in the secretory phase) in total anterior-posterior width.[6] The hypoechoic texture of the endometrium most frequently seen in the proliferative phase is related to

the particular arrangement of the enlarging glands and stroma. A small amount of intraluminal fluid can be observed during the periovulatory and secretory phase of the cycle.[7] In addition, the innermost layer of endometrium may be edematous, giving rise to a multilayered pattern (as seen in long axis) or a "halo" configuration (as depicted on transverse scans).[8] The endometrium appears thickened and echogenic during the secretory phase. The echogenic texture of the secretory endometrium is probably related to the hypertrophied and tortuous glands which contain a mucinous secretion. The masses contained within the endocervical canal are observed to become more hypoechoic as the canal becomes more fluid-filled near the time of ovulation.

CONGENITAL MALFORMATIONS AND RELATED DISORDERS

On pelvic examination, a malformed uterus may be confused with an adnexal mass (Fig. 37–5). Similarly, the sonographic appearance of malformations is sometimes mistaken for uterine fibroids. The most common congenital uterine malformations arise from anomalies of fusion. A T-shaped uterus is associated with a history of diethylstilbestrol (DES) ingestion by the mother of the patient. Hematometra can be secondary to congenital malformation, but also can be acquired secondary to cervical stenosis. Each of these entities is discussed here as it relates to sonographic findings.

Fusion Anomalies
Early in embryonic development of the female fetus, the wolffian and müllerian duct systems interact to form the

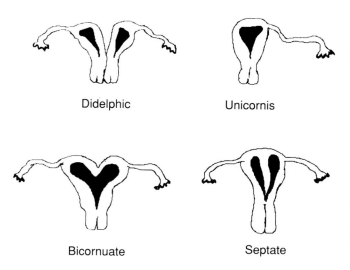

Fig. 37–5. Diagram of common uterine malformations. (*Courtesy of C. R. Odwin, RT, RDMS.*)

internal genitalia. The wolffian system regresses, and the uterus, oviduct, ovary, and vagina are formed from paired müllerian structures that eventually fuse in the midline.

The most common anomalies of the internal genitalia result from defects in fusion of the paired structures that form the uterus, cervix, and vagina. The degree of failure can range from partial to complete.[3] If there is total failure of fusion, a uterus didelphys will result. In patients with uterus didelphys, two vaginas, two cervices, and two uteri are present. Partial fusion of the müllerian duct derivatives range from uterus bicornis bicollis (two uterine horns, two cervices) or uterus bicornis unicollis (two uterine horns, one cervix) to uterus arcuatus (mildest fusion anomaly, with saddle-shaped lumen). In all of these fusion anomalies, a common central wall between the two uteri is present. Incomplete resorption of the sagittal septum within the uterus results in a uterus septus or subseptus, depending on the size of the septum.

Uterine malformations can be suspected from findings on pelvic examination, and are diagnosed definitively by hysterosalpingography. The lesions become important to the sonologist because they can be encountered on pelvic sonography as an incidental finding and confused with an adnexal mass.

Arrested development of the müllerian ducts results in uterine aplasia; if this occurs unilaterally, a uterus unicornis unicollis is formed. The suffix "cornis" refers to the uterine horns; "collis" refers to the cervix.

Although it is usually not possible to distinguish with any confidence between the more subtle types of uterine anomalies (septated versus bicornuate uterus) on the basis of sonography, it is important to remember that other congenital defects may be associated with these uterine malformations. Specifically, renal anomalies, such as renal agenesis, may be encountered on the same side as the uterine malformation.[14] Thus, if a uterine anomaly is suspected, one should scan the region of the kidneys.

Duplication of the uterus can be associated with an obstructed horn, resulting in hematometra. A bicornuate uterus can mimic the sonographic appearance of a parauterine solid mass. However, the typical pear shape of the uterus can be recognized on multiple sagittal scans. Sonographic recognition of a uterine septum in a gravid patient is important because of predisposition to premature labor, fetal malpresentation, and third-trimester bleeding.

One of the most common uterine anomalies detected on sonography is the gravid bicornuate uterus (Fig. 37–6). There are usually no symptoms to bring the patient to the attention of the physician, and the anomaly is often first discovered when a nodular mass is palpated. The empty horn of the uterus can be mistaken for a parauterine mass on pelvic examination.

The nongravid bicornuate uterus usually appears sonographically as a binodular structure that is best delineated on transverse scans. It can appear quite similar to leiomyomata, except that the myometrium has a homogeneous texture as opposed to the whorled appearance of a leiomyoma. During menstruation, two uterine lumina may be identifiable.

Hydrometrocolpos and Hematometrocolpos

These conditions can be associated with either congenital or acquired malformation of the uterus or vagina.[10–12] They result from accumulation of secretions or blood within the uterus or vagina, which occur because of congenital or acquired obstruction of a uterine horn, cervix, or vaginal tract.

Obstruction of menstrual flow can be congenital and symptomatic, as in delayed menarche with imperforate hymen or vaginal atresia, or it can be asymptomatic, as in a blind horn. Previously healthy women may have neoplastic obstruction of the uterine outflow tract. In either of these cases, retrograde menstruation can occur.[13]

Premenarchal girls may accumulate clear secretions in the vagina. Patients with this condition may be asymptomatic or can present with vague pelvic discomfort or pain during defecation or urination due to compression of the rectum or bladder by the pelvic mass. Similar to delayed menarche in the otherwise healthy girl, hematometrocolpos can be encountered in patients with an imperforate hymen or vaginal atresia.

Sonographically, the distended uterus or vagina appears as a pear-shaped structure with either anechoic or echogenic internal contents. If clotted blood is contained within the uterus, echoes emanating from the clotted blood can be seen. These are usually mobile when the patient is scanned in various positions.

A small amount of fluid or blood can be present within the endometrial cavity during menstruation or in pelvic inflammatory disease. Intraluminal fluid may be associated with endometritis from pelvic inflammatory disease. In postmenopausal women, intraluminal fluid can be associated with endometrial carcinoma.[9]

T-Shaped Uterus

A specific uterine anomaly has been encountered in women whose mothers received DES as a part of a therapeutic regimen. DES was widely prescribed to pregnant women between 1940 and 1960 as an anti-abortifacient. A great many women who were exposed to DES in utero have multiple benign abnormalities of the genital tract.[16] Additionally, over 300 cases of clear-cell adenocarcinoma of the vagina have been reported to date.[4]

Sonography can be useful in detecting the so-called T-shaped uterus associated with DES exposure. The volume of the T-shaped uterus, calculated from length,

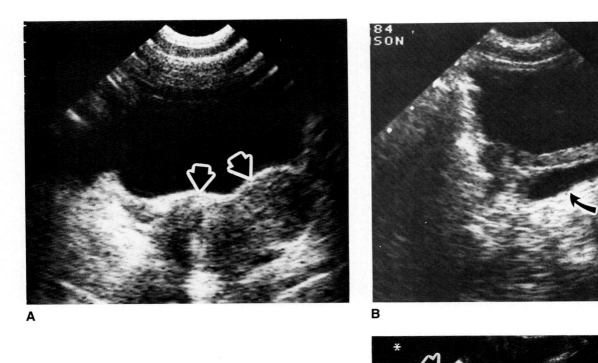

A

B

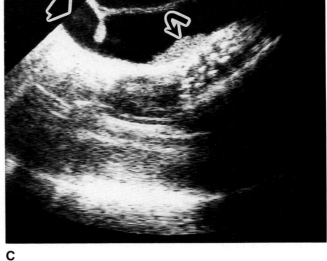

Fig. 37–6. Uterine malformations. **A.** TA US of bicornuate uterus as imaged in transverse plane. The two uterine cornua (*arrows*) are seen. **B.** Hematocolpos (*arrow*) secondary to an imperforate hymen. **C.** TA US of severe hydrometrocolpos (*arrow*). A collection of clotted blood is within the lower vagina (*curved arrow*).

C

width, and anterior-posterior dimension, has been reported to be significantly less than a control group of women at similar ages.[10] The T-shaped uterus derived its name from the hysterographic appearance of the uterine lumen. The abnormal shape and decreased size of the uterus can be detected sonographically by a greater-than-usual transverse dimension, as well as decreased thickness of the fundus.[3]

INFLAMMATORY DISORDERS

Pyometrium or suppurative endometritis may occur as a sequela to postpartum infection, or after an attempted

abortion with septic complications (Fig. 37–7). Pyometrium may also result from cervical stenosis secondary to radiation treatment of the uterine cervix for cervical carcinoma.[12] Endometritis is occasionally seen with salpingitis. Endometritis can also cause thickening of the endometrial interfaces, particularly as depicted by transvaginal sonography.

The sonographic appearance of the postpartum uterus is discussed in Chapter 32. Normally, the linear intraluminal interface is centrally located and the endometrial layers are closely opposed.

Puerperal infection is usually due to retrograde contamination of the uterine cavity by normal or pathogenic

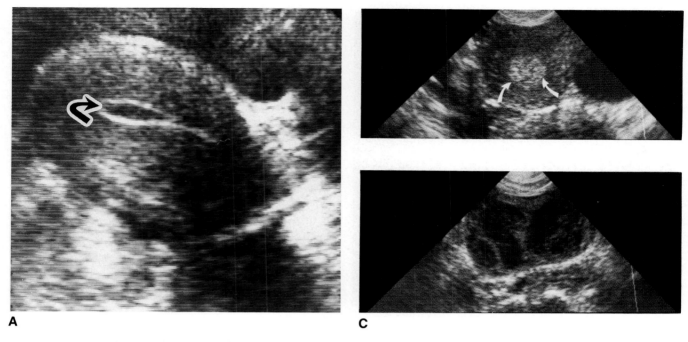

Fig. 37–7. Miscellaneous uterine conditions. **A.** TA US of patient with pelvic inflammatory disease with a small amount of intraluminal fluid (*curved arrow*) probably related to endometritis. **B.** TV US of patient with pelvic inflammatory disease demonstrating echogenic and thick endometrium (*arrows*) that may have been the result of endometritis. **C.** Same patient as in **B,** TV US of tubo-ovarian abscess. (*Courtesy of E. Mendelson, MD and M. Bohm-Velez, MD.*)

vaginal flora introduced during labor. Prolonged labor, premature rupture of membranes, retention of placental tissue, and cervical and vaginal lacerations are known risk factors. Clinically, this condition is suspected when a yellowish green-to-black discharge is found in the lochia. The endometritis can progress to myometritis, parametritis (pelvic lymphangitis), pelvic abscess, and septic pelvic thrombophlebitis.

It is clinically helpful to have a sonographic evaluation of the extent of the disease or involvement of the adnexa. The sonographic appearance of pelvic and adnexal inflammatory disease is discussed in Chapter 35. Endometrial inflammatory suppuration can be depicted as irregular hypoechoic areas in an enlarged uterus.

ACQUIRED ABNORMALITIES

Adenomyosis of the uterus is a condition in which clusters of endometrial tissue implant deep within the myometrium. During menstruation, significant pain can be caused by bleeding of the endometrial tissue within the muscle of the uterus. The uterus may be slightly enlarged. Occasionally, this condition can be diagnosed sonographically because of a thickened and "Swiss cheese" appearance of the myometrium caused by areas of hemorrhage and clot within the muscle. In addition, the endometrial implants that burrow into the myome-

trium may contribute to increased echogenicity of the myometrium.[27]

Endometrial hyperplasia typically follows prolonged endogenous or exogenous estrogenic stimulation. Adenomatous hyperplasia is thought to be a precursor of endometrial carcinoma. Endometrial hyperplasia may be suspected sonographically with abnormal thickening (greater than 6 mm) of the endometrium. Polyps of endometrial tissue may appear as thickening of the central endometrial interfaces. Because of the risk of endometrial hyperplasia and carcinoma, the sonographic finding of an abnormally thickened (over 10 mm) and echogenic endometrium should prompt further clinical evaluation. Endometrial hyperplasia and carcinoma lead the differential diagnosis for this sonographic finding.

UTERINE LEIOMYOMATA

Clinical Aspects

Uterine leiomyomata are benign tumors that consist of smooth muscle and connective tissue. They are the most common tumors encountered in gynecologic practice, and are commonly referred to as fibroids (Fig. 37–8). It is estimated that leiomyomata are present in 20% of women over 35 years of age. Such tumors are estrogen-dependent and usually regress after menopause. Leiomyomata are most prevalent in black women and other

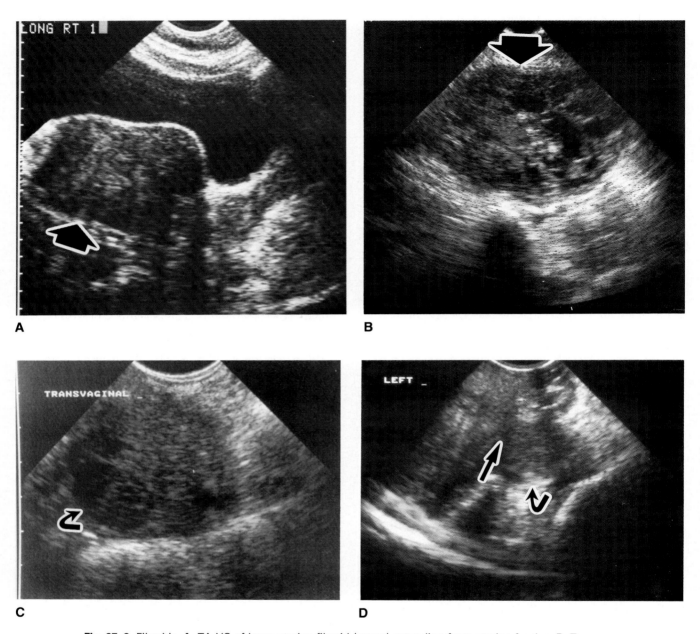

Fig. 37–8. Fibroids. **A.** TA US of large uterine fibroid (*arrow*) extending from uterine fundus. **B.** Transverse TA US of degenerated fibroid (*arrow*) with cystic regions. **C.** TV US of intramural fibroid appearing as hypoechoic area of the uterine corpus. **D.** TV US of pedunculated subserosal fibroid (*curved arrow*) extending from the left uterine corpus by a broad peduncle (*straight arrow*).

dark-skinned groups. The usual clinical picture is a palpable mass in a middle-aged woman, but leiomyomata may be associated with excessive menstrual bleedings and pelvic pain. They may cause infertility due to distortion of the isthmic portion of the tube. In addition, fibroids can contribute to uterine dystocia and endometrial interfaces, or to pelvic obstruction in the laboring patient.

The fibroid is important to the sonologist for two reasons. First, as a neoplasm, fibroids do have a small malignant potential. More commonly, however, the clinician needs to differentiate a palpable mass of uterine origin from an adnexal mass. For these reasons, detailed sonographic examination of fibroid tumors is warranted.

Leiomyomata usually develop in the myometrium of the upper contractile fundal and corporeal portions of the uterus. Only 3% of the leiomyomata are of cervical origin. Microscopically, these tumors arise from the smooth muscle and connective tissue that surround the smaller vessels coursing within the outer layers of the myometrium. Intramural leiomyomata cause the uterus to contract, and the resultant compression of these tumors is believed to displace them either toward the peritoneal surface to form subserous nodules or toward the endometrial cavity to produce submucous nodules. Intraligamentary nodules can arise by extrusion of the intramural nodule retroperitoneally into the areolar tissue between the leaves of the broad ligament. Also, rarely, leiomyomata can develop from fibro-muscular structures in the round ligament or from those surrounding the vessels.

Leiomyomata of the uterus are usually multiple and of various sizes. A solitary nodule is found in only 2% of patients; the number of tumors in a uterus may reach hundreds. The size ranges from microscopic to massive, with 100 pounds being the largest single fibroid reported.[14] Microscopically, each nodule is delineated by a pseudocapsule through which vascular channels enter and arborize within the tumor. As the tumor increases in size, it may eventually outgrow the blood supply and central ischemia is followed by various stages of degeneration.

Degenerative processes may be benign or malignant, asymptomatic or symptomatic. Asymptomatic benign degenerative processes include atrophic, hyaline, cystic, myxomatous, lipomatous, and carneous degeneration.

The symptomatic group includes carneous degeneration, infarction, and infection. Under the effect of strong uterine contractions, rotation of nodules within the pseudocapsule may shear supplying vessels and result in necrobiosis of the tumor. This process is most frequently seen during pregnancy.

Both subserous and submucous nodules may become pedunculated and undergo torsion of the pedicle, with subsequent infarction, degeneration, necrosis, and potential infection. For some pedunculated nodules whose circulation is occluded, attachment to the omentum or intestine allows the entry of new vessels and a revitalized blood supply. Under such circumstances, the pedicle may atrophy and the nodule become completely detached from the uterus—giving rise to a so-called parasitic fibroid.

Submucous fibroids are prone to necrosis because their blood supply is frequently insufficient to support the tumor mass. More importantly, their exposed position subjacent to the uterine lumen predisposes them to ascending infection. Pelvic inflammatory diseases may involve adjacent fibroids by direct extension or through the lymphatics; curettage can injure submucous nodules

and introduce bacteria. Occasionally, when the fibroid is infected, the central core may be filled with purulent material.

Malignant change in the tumor is a generative, not a degenerative process. Although the occurrence of leiomyosarcoma in pre-existing leiomyomata is 0.2% or less, the prevalence of leiomyomata results in this form of sarcoma being the most common malignant stromal uterine tumor (25%). Malignancy in a fibroid is seldom diagnosed preoperatively because there are no characteristic symptoms to distinguish this entity from pre-existing fibroid nodules. Sudden accelerated growth in a previously static tumor and postmenopausal enlargement should suggest the possibility of a superimposed malignant process.

The clinical manifestations of fibroids are variable and depend on the size and number of the tumors, age of the patient, proximity of the tumor to the endometrial cavity, mobility of the fibroid (sessile or pedunculated), and presence or absence of degenerative processes. Submucous tumors typically encroach on the endometrium and distort the endometrial cavity. Due to pressure necrosis, alteration in the vascular architecture of the endometrium may occur and cause excessive menstrual bleeding to be the presenting symptom. When submucous fibroids outgrow their blood supply, surface necrosis, slough, and bloody discharge may result. Pain is not a common symptom except in the presence of degenerative changes or torsion of the pedicle of a subserous nodule. Pelvic discomfort due to pressure on the surrounding organs may be present with large tumors, but often the only symptoms are abdominal enlargement and a palpable mass. Pedunculated submucous leiomyomas ("fibroid polyps") can be partially or completely extruded through the cervical canal and can cause infection, necrosis, and ascending endometritis. This event may also be associated with invasion of the uterus. Larger fibroids, particularly of the intraligamentous type, may compress the ureter with resultant hydroureter and hydronephrosis.

Sonographic Features

The typical sonographic appearance of leiomyomata consists of mildly-to-moderately echogenic intrauterine mass(es) that cause nodular distortion of the uterine outline. Small intramural or submucous leiomyomata may be recognized by their distortion of the normally linear central endometrial echoes. The solid nature of a fibroid often may cause an indentation on the bladder or rectum.

The echogenicity of a fibroid depends upon the relative ratio of fibrous tissue to smooth muscle. With a more fibrous component, there is increased echogenicity of the nodule. The sonographic texture of fibroids also depends on the type and presence of degeneration and on the vascular supply. Interfaces beween the normal myometrium and the pseudocapsule of the mass can sometimes be demonstrated. With transvaginal sonography, the distortion of the endometrial lumen associated with the fibroid can be demonstrated. In some fibroids, the whorled internal architecture can be appreciated. The whorled appearance corresponds to bundles of smooth muscle and connective tissue that are arranged in a concentric pattern. In some cases, leiomyomas are only minimally echogenic and appear as cystic masses, except that their posterior wall is not as prominent as expected. Irregular anechoic areas may be seen within leiomyomata if cystic degeneration has occurred. Calcific degeneration within a leiomyoma is quite common and can be recognized as clusters of high-level echoes that are associated with distal acoustical shadowing.

The most common cause of calcification within the uterus is calcific degeneration within a fibroid. Twenty-five percent of one series of 75 cases of fibroids had calcifications.[17] The pattern of calcification varied from a few small foci to a large rim of globular calcification. If the calcification is extensive and located along the anterior portion of the fibroid, it may prohibit complete sonographic delineation of the mass. Intrauterine calcifications can also be encountered in uterine sarcomas, but this condition is much less common than in leiomyomata.

Other types of degeneration within leiomyomas that produce sonographically recognizable changes in uterine texture include cystic, myxomatous, and hyaline degeneration. Among these, hyaline degeneration is the most common and appears as anechoic areas within a fibroid. Areas of hyaline degeneration can be distinguished from areas of cystic degeneration in that areas of cystic degeneration will usually demonstrate distal wall enhancement.

Leiomyomas that are pedunculated can be confused with other adnexal masses if their pedicle is not visualized. The most common location of pedunculated leiomyomas is superior to the uterine fundus. In most cases, an echogenic interface corresponding to the tissue plane connecting the fibroid and fundus can be delineated. Pedunculated subserosal fibroids can also extend into the broad ligament, and thus appear as an extra-uterine mass. However, the typical whorled configuration of the fibroid usually can be recognized. In order to ascertain whether or not a mass is connected to the uterus by a pedicle, applying slight pressure to the mass while scanning has been suggested.[17,18] The mass will move with the uterus if the two are connected. This procedure should be performed by an experienced gynecologist and monitored with real-time sonography.

Submucous leiomyomata can be difficult to differentiate from intramural leiomyomata. Both may produce distortion of the endometrial interfaces. Submucosal fibroids are best documented by hysterosalpingography.

Fibroids can be particularly difficult to detect in the retro-flexed uterus. Because the uterine fundus curves posteriorly in the retro-flexed uterus, this area may be relatively hypoechoic. Appropriate gain settings and TCG curves should be used; a hypoechoic area within the fundus of a retro-flexed uterus could be technical in origin rather than a fibroid.

Serial sonographic evaluation of leiomyomata can be of significant clinical value. Follow-up scans of the fibroid uterus of a pregnant woman can help assess the growth and accelerated degeneration of this mass. A recent study of fibroids during pregnancy revealed that the size of most fibroids remains stable during pregnancy.[17] (See Chapter 33.) Because fibroids should regress after menopause, serial sonograms can objectively document enlargement or regression of leiomyomata in the older woman. Due to its ability to portray larger areas of interest, transabdominal sonography is needed in fibroids that enlarge the uterus to over 8 to 10 weeks in size. When the uterus is smaller than this, transvaginal sonography is recommended. Depiction of the endometrial interfaces by transvaginal sonography is particularly helpful in identifying myometrial masses by their displacement of this interface.

Sonographic Mimics of Fibroids

Occasionally, solid masses that are adjacent to the uterus appear as masses within the uterine contour (Fig. 37–9). This finding has been referred to as "the indefinite uterus sign."[20] In such a setting, a retro-uterine mass may be misdiagnosed as an enlarged uterus. The most common solid masses to simulate the sonographic appearance of a fibroid are the solid ovarian tumors. In particular, cystadenofibromas can calcify, simulating the appearance of a fibroid. Metastases that settle and enlarge in the cul-de-sac, such as those associated with breast tumors, can also produce apparent enlargement of the uterine contour.

Transvaginal sonography can be helpful in distinguishing fibroids from other adnexal or ovarian masses. In particular, transvaginal sonography is helpful in identifying the ovaries in patients with fibroids because it usually is difficult to distinguish a fibroid from the ovary by palpation. We have also been able to distinguish a mass, representing a tubal carcinoma, from a fibroid by using transvaginal sonography.

Lesions of the Cervix

Transvaginal sonography also affords a means to evaluate several types of cervical masses and disorders. For this application, the transvaginal transducer/probe is usually

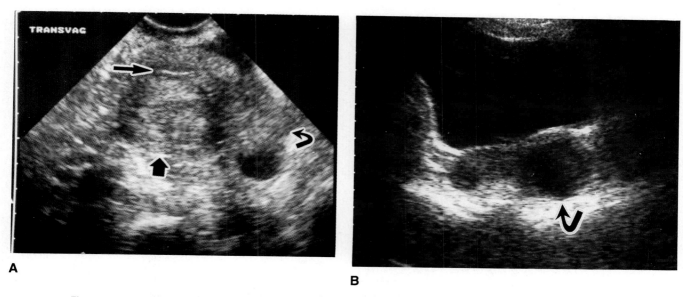

Fig. 37–9. Pelvic masses which mimic fibroids. **A.** TV US of tubal carcinoma (*curved arrow*) adjacent to an uterine fibroid large (*arrow*). Endometrium (*straight arrow*) is thin and atrophic. **B.** Transverse TA US of a hematoma adjacent to the uterus status postlaparoscopy.

placed a few centimeters into the vagina so that the cervix itself can be delineated.

Cervical inclusion cysts (nabothian) can be clearly identified by transvaginal sonography as cystic structures within the cervix.[21] The presence of cervical carcinoma, however, may be difficult to delineate in its early stages by transvaginal sonography. When more advanced, it usually appears as a hypoechoic irregular enlargement of the cervix.

Because most cervical carcinomas can be identified by visual inspection and histologic studies, sonography does not have a major role in their detection or staging. Cervical carcinoma may be present in enlarged cervices; on the other hand, enlarged patulous cervices can be normal. Detection of invasion into surrounding tissues is most important in assessing patients with cervical carcinoma. For this application, CT and MRI have better capability than sonography in detecting parametrial extension. In addition, these modalities have a higher accuracy in detecting lymphadenopathy associated with cervical carcinoma.

In the pregnant patient, sonographic delineation of the cervix by transvaginal sonography may have important implications in the detection of clinically suspected or unsuspected cervical incompetence. This topic is addressed at length in Chapter 30.

Both carcinoma of the cervix and of the endometrium may be associated with intraluminal fluid. In cervical carcinoma, this is usually related to cervical stenosis which can occur after radiation therapy.

CARCINOMA OF THE OVIDUCT

Carcinoma of the oviduct is a rare gynecologic neoplasm. It is mentioned here because its sonographic appearance can mimic intraligamentary or pedunculated uterine fibroids. Most patients with this malignancy remain undiagnosed both sonographically and clinically until time of surgery. Sonographically, one patient presented with an ill-defined, complex, fusiform mass concomitant with a large intramural leiomyoma. In another, a reniform, complex mass with central echogenic core surrounded by sonolucent halo was encountered. At surgery the mass depicted by pelvic sonography corresponded to a loop of jejunum infiltrated by surrounding tumor. Figure 37–9 shows a transvaginal sonogram of a patient with a known mass that filled the lumen of the left tube on hysterosalpingography. On transvaginal sonography, an unsuspected pedunculated fibroid was found rising from the uterine fundus, as well as a fusiform solid left-adnexal mass that corresponded to the fallopian tube carcinoma.

ENDOMETRIAL DISORDERS

Sonography has an increasingly important role in evaluating certain disorders of the endometrium (Figs. 37–9 to 37–11).[20] Although not a primary means for diagnosis of endometrial hyperplasia, a sonographic examination performed to evaluate a pelvic mass, for

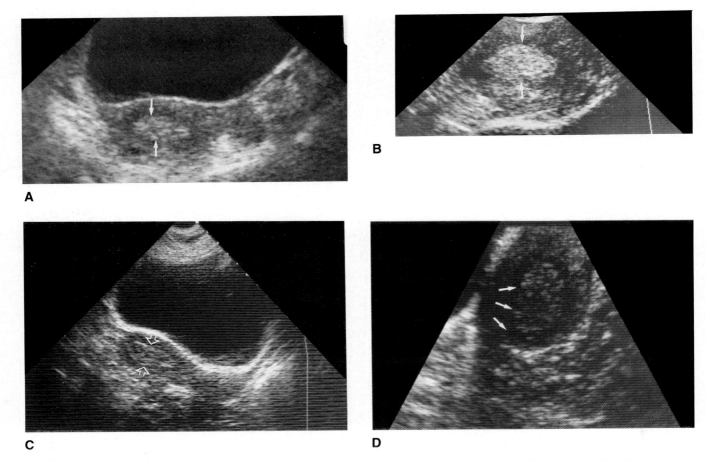

Fig. 37–10. Endometrial hyperplasia. **A.** TA US of patient with endometrial hyperplasia. The endometrium is thickened (*between arrows*). **B.** TV US of patient in **A,** better delineating the thickened hyperplastic endometrium (*between arrows*). (*Courtesy of E. Mendelson, MD.*) **C.** TA US of thickened irregular endometrium. **D.** TV US of patient in **C,** showing hyperplastic polyps (*arrows*). (*Courtesy of E. Mendelson, MD and M. Bohm-Velez, MD.*)

example, can detect this disorder.[5] It can also be helpful when dilatation and curettage is difficult (as in cervical stenosis).

The endometrium in a postmenopausal woman should be thin (no more than 6 to 8 mm anterior-posterior dimension) and regular. This size may be altered by certain medications (such as estrogen prescribed for osteoporosis).

When the endometrium is over 10 mm thick in a postmenopausal woman, one should consider performing dilatation and curettage, particularly if there is postmenopausal bleeding. Occasionally, blood or mucus retained within the lumen can give the false impression of endometrial thickening. Endometrial hyperplasia should be suspected when the endometrial mass is over 10 mm in thickness. Endometrial polyps can also distend the lumen with irregular punctuate echogenic tissue.

Myometrial invasion by endometrial carcinoma usu-

ally produces a disruption in a subendometrial halo, along with thickening and irregularity of the central endometrial interfaces. The actual tumor may be hypoechoic or echogenic, depending on its grade.[23] In general, the more highly differentiated tumors that produce mucin and have glandular elements tend to be echogenic, as opposed to lower grade tumors that do not form glandular elements. In addition, the echogenicity of the tumor is probably also related to the number of interfaces created by the infiltrating tumor. Exophytic tumors associated with myometrial thinning may be most difficult to distinguish from truly invasive tumors. It is also conceivable that adenomyosis might simulate myometrial invasion.[27,28] In some cases, intraluminal scanning may be indicated.[24] This procedure requires anesthesia, and is usually performed immediately prior to intracavitary tandum placement. We encourage the use of polyps forceps for removal of polyps during the initial dilatation and

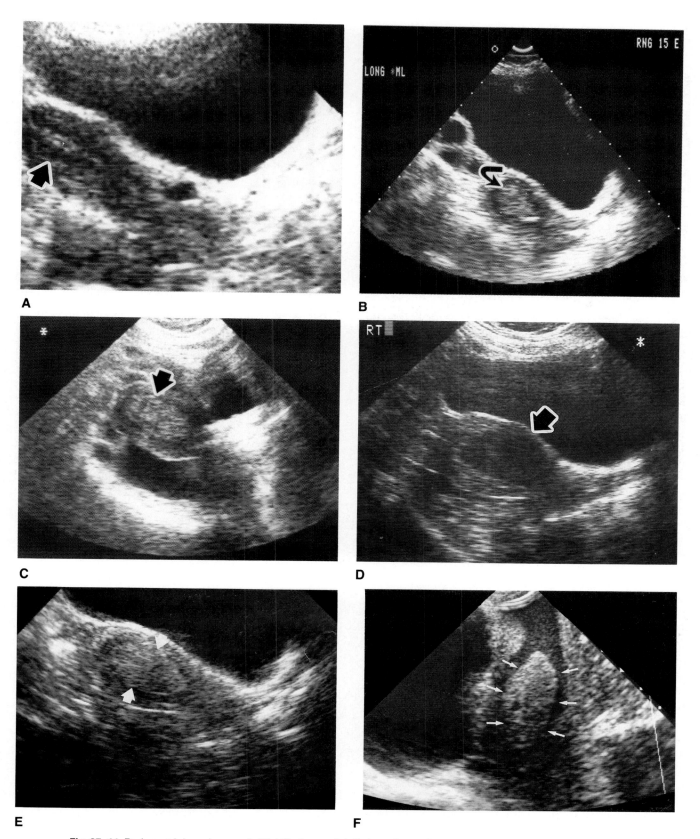

Fig. 37–11. Endometrial carcinoma. **A.** TA US of superficially invasive endometrial carcinoma. The hypoechoic "halo" is focally thickened in the area of the tumor (*arrow*). **B.** Large endometrial polyp (*arrow*) containing carcinoma. The hypoechoic "halo" is intact, indicating a noninvasive tumor. **C.** Invasive endometrial carcinoma (*arrow*) associated with ascites resulting from peritoneal spread of tumor. **D.** Hypoechoic low-grade endometrial carcinoma invasive to the uterine serosa (*arrow*). **E.** TA US showing a thickened endometrial interface in patient with uterine bleeding (*between arrows*). **F.** TV US of patient in **E,** showing moderately invasive endometrial carcinoma. (*Courtesy of E. Mendelson, MD and M. Bohm-Velez, MD.*)

curettage in order to decrease the likelihood of misdiagnosing an exophytic tumor for a deeply invasive one.

In some institutions, preoperative determination of amount of myometrial invasion has a role in determining whether or not intracavitary radiation should be used. With deeply invasive tumors (over 50% of myometrial width), some oncologists use preoperative intracavitary radiation to decrease the likelihood of lymphatic spread.

POSTHYSTERECTOMY EVALUATION

Patients who have undergone hysterectomy have altered anatomic relations in the pelvis, and may be difficult to evaluate adequately by manual pelvic examination.[25] Detection of pelvic mass in these patients may require additional clinical and diagnostic imaging evaluation.

Pelvic masses not related to the uterus can be encountered in the patient who has undergone hysterectomy or salpingo-oophorectomy. For instance, a small ovarian remnant may enlarge and produce a pelvic mass even though most of the ovary has been removed. The potential for resumption of ovulatory function remains, however, and the patient may resume production of ovarian sex steroids. The enlarged ovarian remnant is often adherent to the pelvic side wall and may also produce partial obstruction of the ureter due to compression.[26]

Hematomas and nondistended loops of bowel may appear as masses within the pelvis of a posthysterectomy patient, depending on the organization of the hematoma. They appear as anechoic to hypoechoic masses. In the postmenopausal patient, the ovary should be small and difficult to delineate.

A portion of omentum may be rounded and appear as a soft tissue mass. This may be adherent to the vaginal cuff or cul-de-sac and mimic the appearance of an ovary. It is indeed difficult to distinguish these two entities by sonography. Postoperative peritoneal adhesions may enclose fluid, causing a peritoneal retention cyst.

Transvaginal sonography can be helpful in evaluation of masses adjacent to the vaginal cuff, or adnexa in patients who have undergone hysterectomy. Due to the relatively close proximity of the transvaginal probe to the ovary, these structures can be identified and masses arising from them detected. Sometimes, however, the ability to use transvaginal sonography is limited in patients who have atrophic or short vaginas due to hysterectomy.

The use of the water enema technique, with simultaneous monitoring by real-time scanning, is advocated for further evaluation of the posthysterectomy patient when initial sonography suggests the presence of a pelvic mass. Water distension of the rectum affords a detailed evaluation of the posterior compartment of the pelvis in a posthysterectomy patient. Only small remnants of supravaginal tissue should be present between the urinary bladder and rectum of these patients.[25]

Radiation therapy, given to a patient with cancer, can cause areas of fibrosis, making pelvic examination more difficult. With radiation therapy, the vaginal vault becomes foreshortened, stenotic, and rigid. It is difficult to examine the adnexa or the suprapubic area. Sonography and CT can be, therefore, an important diagnostic adjunct in the follow-up of such patients. Ideally, the initial examination should serve as a baseline for comparison with future studies.

Occasionally, a patient is encountered who has had a supracervical hysterectomy. This operation consists of removal of the uterus, leaving the cervix in place, creating the potential for clinical confusion of the cervix with a pelvic mass as well as for development of cervical carcinoma. This type of hysterectomy is not commonly performed anymore. Because edematous changes in the cuff persist for about six weeks, a delay in performing a baseline sonogram for two to three months after surgery is suggested. The size of the vagina and "cuff" will vary from patient to patient, depending on her age, amount of atrophic changes, type of surgery, and amount of irradiation received—if any. In general, the older the patient, the more extensive the surgery, or the greater the amount of irradiation, the smaller the residual vagina. Cuff size is also dependent on surgical technique. The degree of tissue incorporated and the type of suture used in closure will affect the cuff size. Usually, the cuff appears as a 1- to 1.5-cm structure along the upper pole of the vagina. Once the size and configuration of the vaginal cuff are established on baseline examination, the cuff should not enlarge on later studies. As the patient ages, the cuff size usually decreases. If an increase is noted on follow-up examination, the possibility of tumor recurrence should be considered. Adherent bowel, or an ovary adjacent to the upper vagina, can mimic recurrent tumor around the cuff. Whenever the appearances are unusual, a water enema might be helpful in identifying structures relating to small and large bowel.

Seromas and inclusion cysts may form in the incision site. Inclusion cysts form from fluid collecting between free leaves of the peritoneum or around adhesions. They are typically irregularly shaped and do not conform to any particular anatomic compartment.

INTRAUTERINE CONTRACEPTIVE DEVICE LOCALIZATION

Sonography is useful in determining the exact location of an intrauterine contraceptive device (IUCD) relative to the endometrial lumen (Fig. 37–12). In most cases, the actual shaft of the intrauterine device (IUD) can be

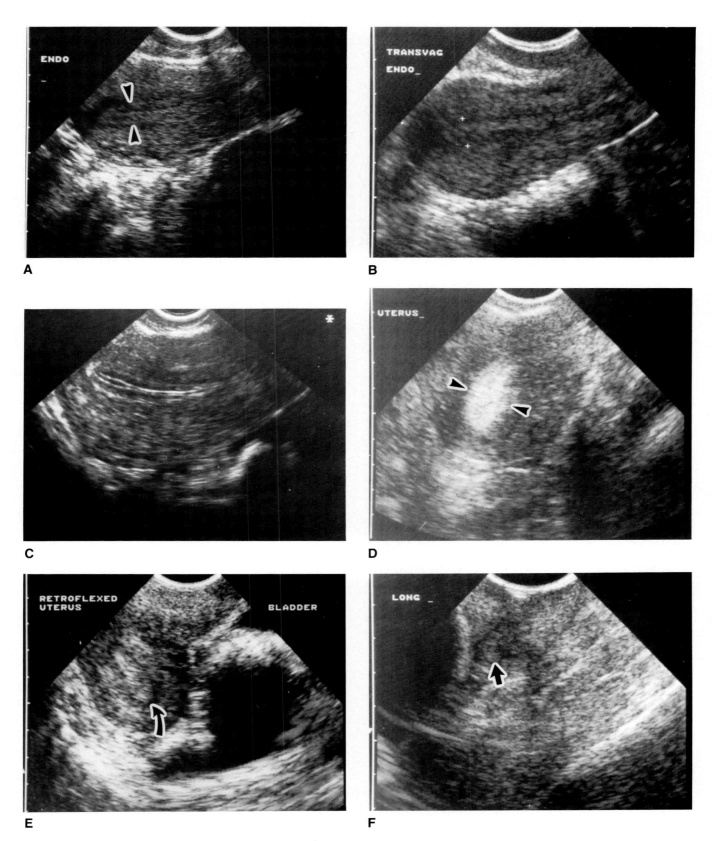

Fig. 38–4. Normal cyclical changes of the endometrium. **A.** Proliferative-phase endometrium (between +s), appearing as isoechoic to the myometrium. **B.** Late proliferative endometrium (between +s). Fluid-filled bowel is adjacent to the uterus. **C.** Late proliferative/early secretory phase endometrium showing multilayered endometrium. **D.** Secretory-phase endometrium (*between arrowheads*) appearing as echogenic tissue compared to surrounding myometrium. **E.** Midsecretory phase endometrium (*curved arrow*) in a severely retroflexed uterus. **F.** Normal atrophic endometrium (*arrow*) in a postmenopausal woman.

thickens between 4 and 8 mm and has a isoechoic or slightly hyperechoic texture relative to the outer myometrium (Fig. 38–4.B). In the late proliferative or periovulatory phase of endometrial development, a multilayered endometrium can be depicted (Figs. 38–4.B and C).[3] The inner hypoechoic area probably represents edema in the compact layer of the endometrium. As imaged in a semi-axial or semi-coronal plane, the endometrium has the configuration of a theta (θ) with respect to the hypoechoic areas (Fig. 38–4.D). In the secretor phase, the endometrium achieves a width of between 8 and 16 mm and is echogenic, most likely related to the increased mucus and glycogen within the glands as well as the increased number of interfaces created by tortuous glands in this phase (Fig. 38–4.E). The endometrium typically achieves its greatest thickness in the midsecretory phase of a spontaneous cycle, measuring up to 14 mm in width.

Endometrial volumes can be estimated by measurement of the long-axis AP and transverse widths of the endometrium and of the height in the semi-axial plane (Fig. 38–2). The location at which the endometrium invaginates into the region of the tubal ostia can be used as a landmark for measurement of the endometrium in its transverse plane. The endometrial volumes in our study of 10 normal women between 19 and 39 years of age with spontaneous cycles demonstrate a statistically significant difference ($P > 0.02$) between proliferative (1.6 $\pm$ 0.4 mL) and secretory phase endometrium (3.6 $\pm$ 0.8 mL).

The endometrium in postmenopausal women should be thin and is histologically atrophic (Fig. 38–4.F). Mucus trapped within the lumen may give the sonographic impression of a thickened endometrium. Postmenopausal women taking estrogen replacement may have relatively thick endometria (over 8 mm in width) in response to the medication.[4] However, the actual range of normal thickness and texture for this group of patients has not been reported to date, and one has to rely on subjective assessments.[5]

DECIDUAL CHANGES IN EARLY INTRAUTERINE PREGNANCY

Transvaginal sonography has had a major impact on the evaluation of patients with complicated early pregnancy. In particular, transvaginal sonography facilitates early detection of intrauterine pregnancy, thereby virtually excluding the possibility of an ectopic gestation. The possibility of a heterotopic (ectopic and intrauterine) pregnancy should be suspected, however, in women taking ovulation-induction medication because multiple implantations of the viable concepti can occur.

If pregnancy is achieved, the endometrium continues to be thick after the secretory phase of the conception cycle. The endometrium also becomes more transonic due to its increased fluid content (Fig. 38–5.A). At 3½ to 4 weeks' menstrual age, the endometrium appears as a thickened interface similar to that seen in endometrial disorders such as endometritis and endometrial hyperplasia.

After approximately 4 weeks, the chorionic sac can be delineated as an echogenic region within the decidualized endometrium (Fig. 38–5.B). The decidua appears as an echogenic area surrounding the hypoechoic sac. Early in embryonic development, the hypoechoic "gestational" sac is seen within the echogenic chorionic mass[6] (Fig. 38–5.C). With further differentiation of the choriodecidua, two layers of choriodecidua can be seen representing the chorion frondosum/decidua capsularis surrounded by the decidua parietalis or vera and chorionic laeve.

DECIDUAL CHANGES IN ECTOPIC PREGNANCY

Comprehension of the decidual changes that occur within the endometrium in intrauterine pregnancies is helpful in distinguishing them from the decidual reaction occurring in ectopic pregnancy. In ectopic pregnancy, the endometrium undergoes decidual changes without formation of chorionic villi. The pseudogestational sac of an ectopic pregnancy in the 6- to 8-week menstrual age period is frequently confused with an early intrauterine pregnancy decidual reaction. Here, there has been decidualization of the endometrium but, due to poor luteal support, areas of hemorrhage and necrosis occur within the decidua (Fig. 38–6). On transvaginal sonography, these appear as anechoic areas within the decidua as well as internally, where there can be fluid collection within the lumen, simulating a gestational sac. However, the pseudogestational sac associated with an ectopic pregnancy is rarely the size expected for a sac of comparable gestational age in an intrauterine pregnancy. The sac itself is also irregular.[7]

BENIGN ENDOMETRIAL DISORDERS

Although it is not possible to definitively differentiate benign from malignant endometrial disorders based on sonographic appearance with transvaginal sonography, many patients with endometrial disorders will present after histologic evaluation of material obtained at D & C. Most of these patients present with dysfunctional uterine bleeding or a history of pelvic inflammatory disease.

Hyperplasia of the endometrium is thought to occur

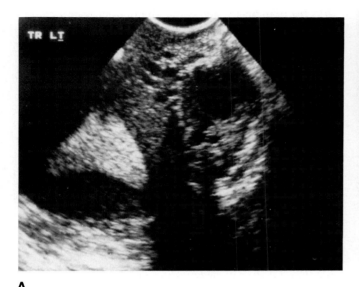

A

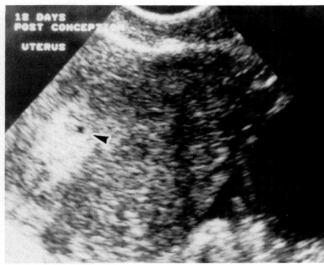

B

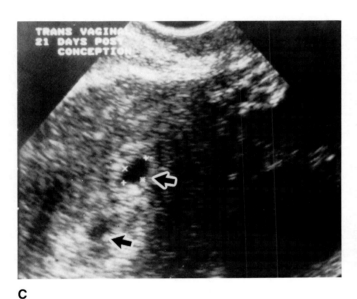

C

Fig. 38–5. Decidual changes. **A.** Thickening of the endometrium secondary to decidualization at 2 weeks 5 days since last menstrual period. **B.** Chorionic sac (*arrowhead*) identified at 18 days postconception in successful in vitro fertilization cycle. **C.** Same as **A**, 21 days postconception showing two gestational sacs (*arrowheads*).

secondary to the trophic influence of unopposed estrogen. The endometrium thickens and the endometrium itself becomes pseudopolypoid in configuration. In mild cases, the polyps are microscopic, but in more severe cases the polyps can measure up to 5 cm in size. In these patients, thickening of the endometrium beyond what is expected for women of comparable age is usually detected on transvaginal sonography. (Fig. 38–7). In perimenopausal women, endometria of greater than 14 mm in thickness should be considered for further evaluation, whereas in the postmenopausal patient, endometria over 10 mm should be considered abnormal. The sonographic findings must be interpreted in light of the patient's clinical presentation and laboratory findings.

Endometritis with or without intraluminal fluid can produce increased echogenicity and thickening of the endometrium (Fig. 38–8.A). In some cases, the hydropyosalpinx/tubo-ovarian abscess associated with pelvic inflammatory disease can be identified by transvaginal sonography as well.[1]

Occasionally, unclotted blood within the lumen is hypoechoic. Fluid can also be present within the endometrial lumen in a variety of disorders related to fluid overload or as a reflection of retained secretions related

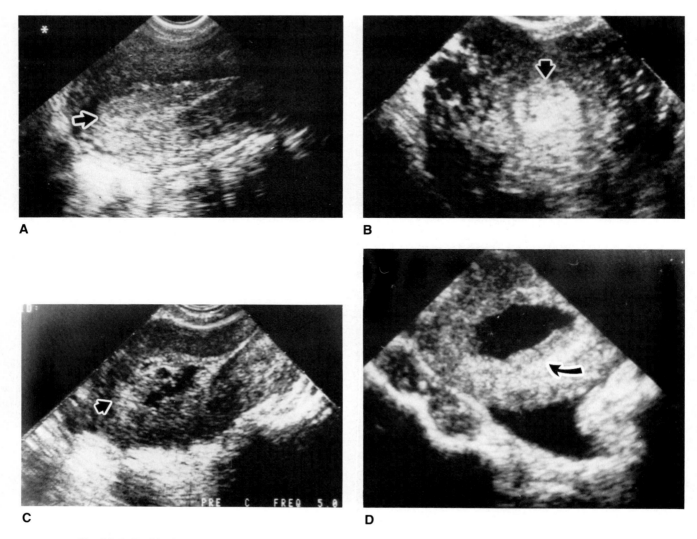

Fig. 38–6. Decidual changes in ectopic pregnancy. **A.** Decidualized endometrium (*arrow*) in an unruptured ectopic pregnancy in long axis. **B.** Decidualized endometrium (*arrow*) in short axis in an ectopic pregnancy. (*Courtesy of R. Pennell, MD.*) **C.** Necrotic decidualized endometrium (*arrow*) in an advanced ectopic pregnancy. (*Courtesy of R. Pennell, MD.*) **D.** Decidual cast (*curved arrow*) with intraluminal fluid in an advanced ectopic pregnancy. (*Courtesy of R. Pennell, MD.*)

to cervical stenosis from cervical carcinoma or radiation-induced fibrosis with hematometrocolpos.

MALIGNANT ENDOMETRIAL DISORDERS

Sonography has an important role in management decisions concerning preoperative radiation therapy in patients with stage I adenocarcinoma of the endometrium.[8] In patients that demonstrate deep invasion (over 50% of myometrium), preoperative radiation therapy may be administered with ovoids and tandem to reduce the likelihood of pelvic recurrence.[9] Transvaginal sonography

seems to be accurate in determining whether invasion is deep or superficial (defined as less than 50% of myometrial width) (Fig. 38–9). Preliminary results in 21 patients have shown that transvaginal sonography accurately depicted the extent of invasion in 17, with two overestimates and two underestimates. (A.N.G., A.C.F., unpublished data, 1989.)

Polypoid tumors (over 3 cm) may cause an apparent distension of the endometrial lumen and extrinsic thinning of the myometrium (Figs. 38–9.A and B). However, in noninvasive tumors the hypoechoic layer of the inner myometrium surrounding the endometrium is usually intact, indicating that the tumor is, at most, superficially

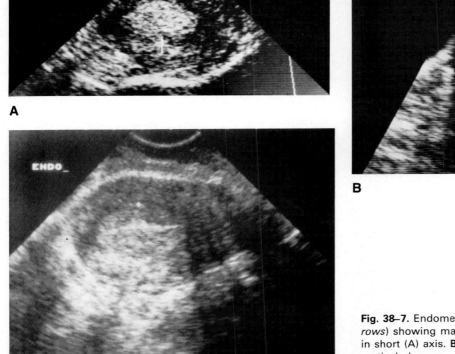

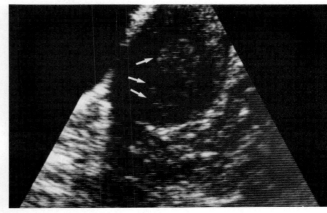

Fig. 38–7. Endometrial hyperplasia. **A.** Polypoid hyperplasia (*arrows*) showing marked thickening (*arrows*) of the endometrium in short (A) axis. **B.** The polypoid nature of the endometrium is particularly apparent when imaged in a semi-coronal plane. (*Courtesy of M. Bohm-Velez, MD.*) **C.** Hyperplastic endometrium (between +s) with polyps.

invasive. In some cases, it is difficult to delineate the endometrial/myometrial interface. However, the likelihood of invasion clearly is related to the bulk or volume of the endometrial tissue (Table 38–2). Problems in estimation of the extent of invasion may also occur if this subendometrial hypoechoic layer, which corresponds to the "junctional zone" on magnetic resonance imaging (MRI), is not detectable or if the myometrium is extremely attenuated due to muscular atrophy. One should therefore be most cautious in estimating the extent of myometrial invasion when the tumor is bulky or if the myometrium is quite thin (less than 1 cm).

The accuracy of MRI compared to transvaginal sonography for assessment of myometrial invasion will require a study that uses both modalities on the same patients with similar state-of-the-art equipment. Our feeling, based on preliminary studies, is that transvaginal sonography and MRI have comparable accuracies for de-

termining tumor invasion confined within the uterus, but that extrauterine extension and involvement of lymph nodes are better detected by MRI.[10] Certainly, transvaginal sonography is much more operator-dependent than MRI, but transvaginal sonography is less expensive and more extensively available.

MISCELLANEOUS CONDITIONS

Transvaginal sonography of the endometrium has an important role in delineating the exact location of masses such as uterine fibroids within the myometrium. By depicting the displacement or distortion of the endometrium by myometrial masses, the relative size of the myometrial mass can be inferred (Figs. 38–9.B and C).

Sonographic depiction of the endometrium has an important role in identifying the endometrial lumen in

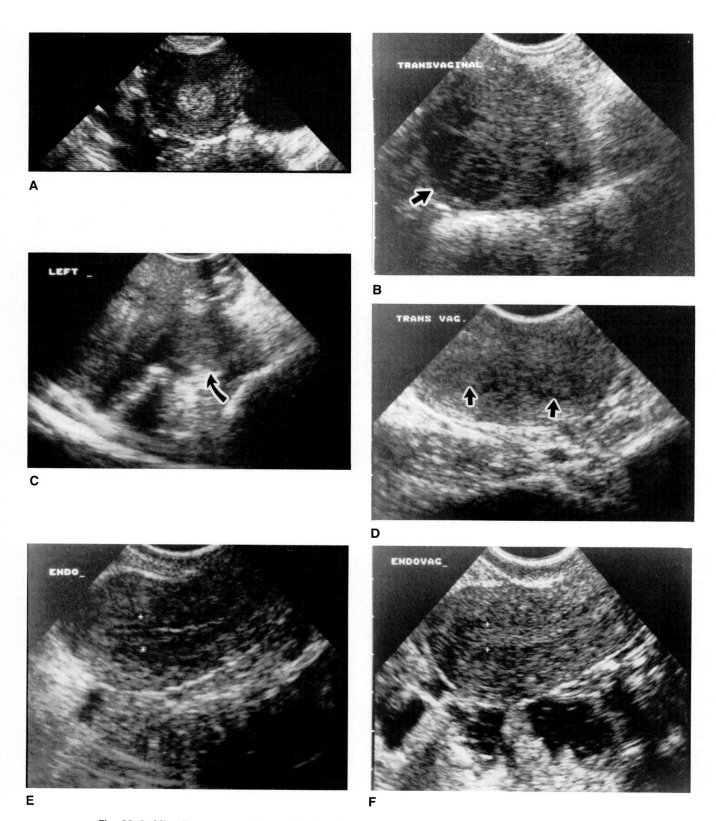

Fig. 38–8. Miscellaneous conditions affecting the endometrium. **A.** Endometritis appearing as thickened endometrium, depicted in short axis. (*Courtesy of E. Mendelson, MD.*) **B.** Intramural myoma (*arrow*) appearing as a hypoechoic area within the middle and external layers of the myometrium. **C.** Pedunculated subserosal fibroid (*arrow*) extending from the left uterine corpus by a peduncle (*curved arrow*). **D.** Bicornuate uterus with two separate endometria (*arrowheads*). **E.** Multilayered midcycle endometrium (between +s) in a successful in vitro fertilization conception cycle. **F.** Thin midcycle endometrium (between +s) in a nonconception in vitro fertilization cycle.

40 Guided Aspiration/Biopsy with Transvaginal Sonography

Arthur C. Fleischer • Carl Morse Herbert III • Robert L. Bree

Sonography, due to its real-time capability of delineating location of needles placed within the body, has multiple applications involving precise guidance for interventional procedures. These applications are particularly useful in the pelvis where pelvic structures can be sonographically accessed from the vagina, through a distended urinary bladder, or transrectally. For each of these approaches, sonography can provide a means for real-time delineation of the location of a biopsy or aspiration needle.

This chapter describes the techniques and advantages of sonographically guided interventional procedures in the pelvis, as well as some potential complications. The use of transvaginal probes that have attachable needle guides is emphasized.

INSTRUMENTATION AND TECHNIQUE

There are currently a variety of transvaginal probes that can be used for aspiration/biopsy guidance. The three major types of transvaginal transducer/probes include multielement curved linear array, single-element mechanically sectored, and multiple-element phased array. The field-of-view of these probes typically covers an 80° to 100° sector, and up to 10 cm in depth. Of these, the multielement large aperture arrays that afford the greatest line density and field-of-view are preferred (Fig. 40–1).

Each type of transducer/probe has its own set of advantages and limitations. First, for transvaginal guidance and aspiration, one wants a relatively small probe so that there is ample maneuverability. For deeper structures, one would prefer probes that offer deeper penetration. This may necessitate a relatively lower-frequency transducer and an adjustable focus or magnified view in order to achieve the greatest line density.

Probably the most important aspect of the instrumentation used for transvaginal aspiration guidance is the attachable needle guide. On most probes, the needle guide is flush to the end of the probe shaft. Basically, the needle guide insures a needle path that is within the incidental beam. In mechanically sectored transducers, the needle guide must be angled relative to the shaft of the probe. This creates some inconvenience in that the

needle guide may touch the urethral area, causing some discomfort to the patient. This would occur when the probe and its needle guide are placed in an anterior position for posteriorly directed aspiration. This situation is relatively rare, because in most aspirations the probe/needle guide is directed laterally within the vagina. The scanner should have a display that clearly shows the needle path and also should be equipped with a video cassette recorder for recording the study in real time (Fig. 40–2).

As in other biopsy needles, it is helpful to have a needle with a scored tip for transvaginal aspiration. This affords greater echogenicity, and therefore enhances the ability to locate the tip of the needle as it is passed into the structure of interest (Fig. 40–3). The needle should fit snugly into the needle guide, because if there is a significant space to move within the needle hole, it may contribute to inaccurate needle placement.

For transvaginal aspirations, the probe should be covered by a condom and local anesthesia should be used in the anticipated area for needle entrance. The probe itself can be used to manipulate the structure so that the shortest distance between the probe and the structure to be aspirated is obtained. This is particularly helpful in follicular aspiration where the ovary can be "trapped" in the ovarian fossa by manipulating the probe (Fig. 40–4).

FOLLICULAR ASPIRATION

There are several routes that can be used for sonographic guidance for follicular aspirations (Fig. 40–5). They vary according to the approach used for aspiration and the type of scanning used for guidance. The most commonly used include:

1. Transvaginal aspiration and guidance.
2. Transurethral–transvesical aspiration with transabdominal guidance.
3. Percutaneous transvesical aspiration with transabdominal guidance.

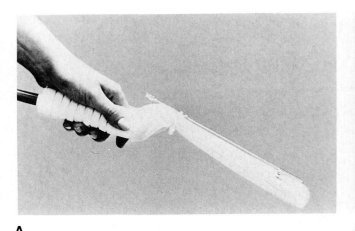

A

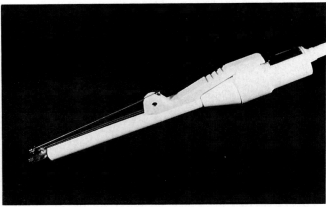

B

Fig. 40–1. Transvaginal probes and needle guides. **A.** Multielement curved linear array with transvaginal probe, with a needle guide attached over a condom. The needle guide is flush with shaft of the probe. **B.** Single-element mechanical sector transvaginal probe with an attached needle guide.

There have been only a few randomized studies to determine which approach results in the highest pregnancy rate in in vitro fertilization and embryo transfer (IVF-ET).[1] Although there is controversy as to whether or not the pregnancy rate is affected by the approach used, it is clear that the approach should be tailored to each patient's anatomy. For example, a transvesicular approach may be needed for patients with ovaries that are anteriorly located, whereas transvaginal approaches are preferred in women whose ovaries are located in the cul-de-sac. In general, if the ovary is greater than 3 cm from the probe, it may be better accessed by an alternative approach rather than transvaginally.

One should realize the difficulty in controlling the variables that are factors in determining whether or not pregnancy is achieved. These include the etiology of infertility, the type of medications used for ovulation induction, the number and quality of the retrieved oocyte, the fertilization and cleavage rate, and the state of endometrial development at implantation.

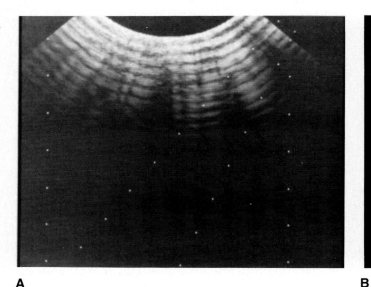

A

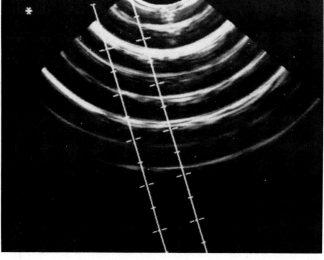

B

Fig. 40–2. Needle path display. **A.** The two lines of cm dots show projected needle path. **B.** Projected needle path is between the two graduated lines.

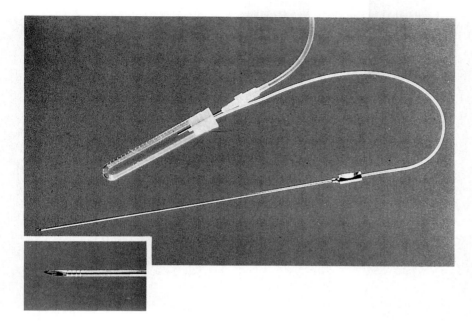

Fig. 40–3. Needle used for follicular aspiration. Magnified image shows the scored tip that facilitates its sonographic delineation.

Most IVF centers use the transvaginal approach, although some use the periurethral–transvesical approach. The advantages of the transvaginal approach include the use of only mild sedation and local anesthesia, high patient acceptance, and low complication rate. Some studies have reported a high fertilization rate and pregnancy rate for the periurethral–transvesical approach.[2] Similar findings have been noted by Parsons, Pampiglione, Sadler, and Booker (unpublished data). Except for transient hematuria, no significant complications were reported.[2]

For transvaginal follicular aspiration there is some data that suggest that preoperative antibiotic administration decreases the possibility of infection from the transvaginal aspiration procedure.[3] Because the vagina contains various bacterial flora, one theoretic concern is the possibility of contamination. However, the actual incidence of this seems to be very low.

Immediately prior to transvaginal aspiration, the vagina should be cleansed with a sterile saline solution. Once the desired area is lined up with the beam path, the needle can be passed through the vagina under constant sonographic visualization. One should avoid passing through the areas where the larger uterine vessels lie to either side of the cervix and laterally toward the pelvic sidewalls where the iliac vessels course (Fig. 40–6). If multiple follicles are present, the needle does not have to be withdrawn totally from the vagina between needle advances. It is best placed first within the ovary where the follicle is aspirated in the proximal portion of the ovary and then re-directed while located within the ovary.

Once the proper advancement of the needle is achieved, mild negative pressure (100 mm Hg) is applied for aspiration with transfer of the follicular fluid into a test tube (Fig. 40–3). Although most use a manual technique for achieving the proper amount of needle advancement, some advocate the use of a spring-loaded device.[4] The contents of the test tube are then examined under a microscope for the presence of an ovum (Fig. 40–5). Most follicular aspirations involve flushing the follicle with a buffered solution several times in order to obtain any ovum that may be floating within the follicle.

One should be careful not to confuse the short-axis view of a pelvic vessel for a mature follicle (Fig. 40–7). If a vessel is entered, the needle should be withdrawn as soon as possible. External pressure on the area can be applied by using the probe as a form of ballottement. Similarly, some hydrosalpinges may mimic the sonographic appearance of a mature follicle (Fig. 40–7.B).[4]

Transabdominal sonography can be used to guide follicular aspiration using the transurethral approach. For this procedure, the needle is placed within the tip of a Foley catheter, which is passed through the urethra. Once the Foley and needle are within the urinary bladder, the needle is popped out from the end of the Foley catheter and directed through the posterior bladder wall and into the follicle. Using this procedure, follicles can be aspirated successfully. However, this procedure causes more patient discomfort when the needle passes through the bladder wall into the follicle than in the transvaginal route.

The success rates for transvaginal, transvesicular,

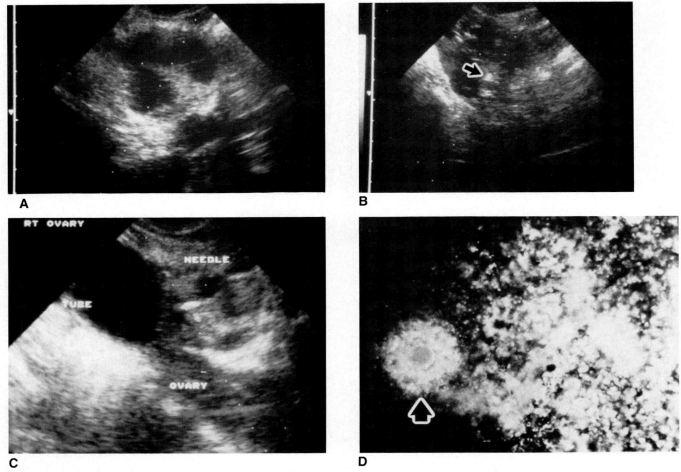

Fig. 40–4. Follicular aspiration. **A.** Preaspiration, a mature follicle is lined up in the beam path as depicted by the cm dots. **B.** During aspiration, the multiple interfaces arising from the scored needle tip (*arrow*) are seen within the follicle. **C.** Guided aspiration of a follicle adjacent to a hydrosalpinx. **D.** Picture of a retrieved ovum with surrounding cluster of granulosa cells (*arrow*).

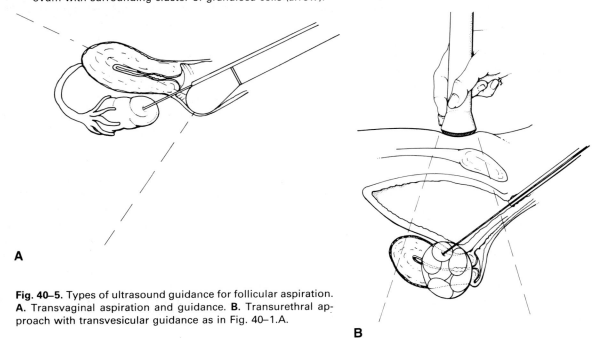

Fig. 40–5. Types of ultrasound guidance for follicular aspiration. **A.** Transvaginal aspiration and guidance. **B.** Transurethral approach with transvesicular guidance as in Fig. 40–1.A.

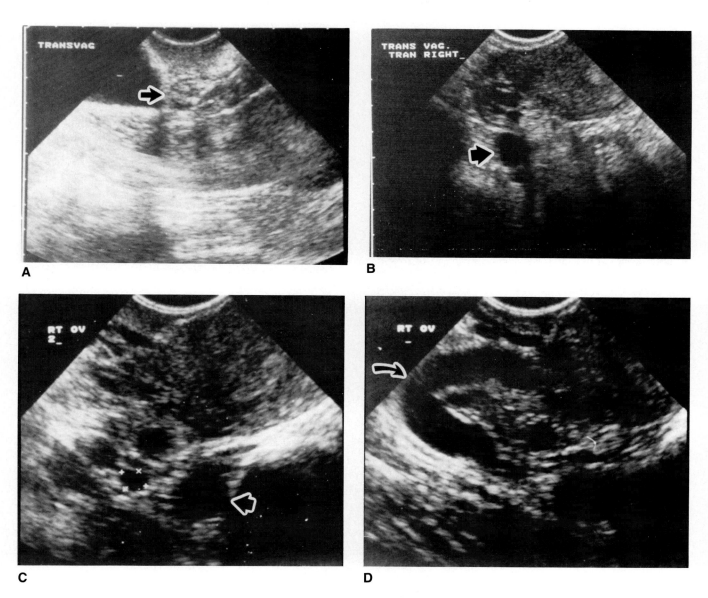

Fig. 40–6. Sonographic mimics. **A.** Uterine vessels (*arrow*) adjacent to the cervix. These vessels should be avoided during aspiration. **B.** Iliac vein (*arrow*) immediately posterior to the right ovary. **C.** A hydrosalpinx appearing initially as a rounded structure resembling a mature follicle (*arrow*). **D.** Same patient showing a fusiform structure of a typical simple hydrosalpinx (*curved arrow*). Doppler showed venous flow, though.

and laparoscopic ovum retrieval seem to be comparable (Table 40–1).[1] However, major advantages of the transvaginal route include no need of general anesthesia and high patient acceptance. These factors substantiate this method as the method-of-choice for follicular aspiration.

In a recently reported large series of patients undergoing transvaginal ultrasound-directed oocyte collection for IVF, a 98.7% rate of success was documented. In addition, the high (80%) fertilization rate associated with this technique was greater than from laparoscopic ovum pick-up reported in a previous series. This study

also described the incidence of complications that could be attributed to transvaginal aspiration.[5]

The complications that were reported included three pelvic abscesses and three pelvic hematomas. The abscesses were successfully treated after transvaginal needle aspiration of their contents, followed by instillation of antibiotics combined with a course of intravenous antibiotics. This group advocates the use of intraoperative antibiotics, particularly in patients with known endometriosis.[5] The three patients with pelvic hematomas were managed conservatively, and there was no signif-

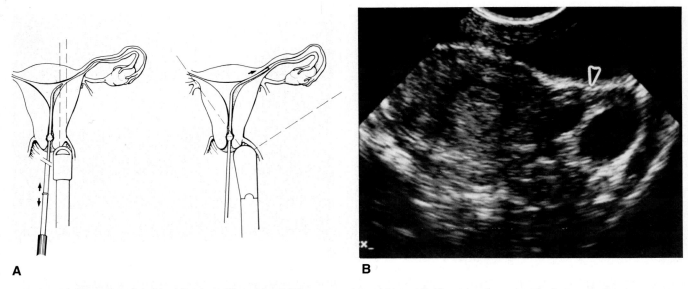

Fig. 40–7. Other applications of transvaginal sonography guidance. **A.** Diagram of transvaginal sonography guidance of transcervical catheterization of the left tube for GIFT procedure. **B.** Normal proximal left tube (*arrowhead*) on transvaginal sonography.

icant fall in hemoglobin level in any case. Five patients experienced vaginal bleeding immediately postprocedure, requiring insertion of a vaginal pack. One patient suffered a 200 mL blood loss immediately after withdrawal of the aspirating needle, requiring suturing.

GUIDED ASPIRATION/BIOPSY OF PELVIC MASSES

A transvaginal approach can be used for aspiration of completely cystic pelvic masses and aspiration/biopsy of those pelvic masses throught to be benign or seen in elderly or high-risk patients. In the patient undergoing IVF-ET, a cystic mass such as a follicular cyst may be present in the follicular phase of the cycle and may in-

terfere with eventual oocyte retrieval, particularly if a transvaginal route is used. These masses can be aspirated transvaginally in the early part of the cycle so that follicle stimulation and subsequent follicular aspiration can be optimized (Fig. 40–8).

Transvaginally guided aspiration can also be used for aspiration of completely cystic adnexal masses and aspiration biopsy of some selected pelvic masses that are thought to be benign. In patients who are elderly, or at high risk for surgery because of pelvic adhesions, a transvaginal approach for aspiration of cystic pelvic masses can be used. The sonographic findings that favor benign findings are a smooth wall, no internal echoes, and no papillary excrescences or tumor nodules. One can therefore aspirate most, if not all, completely cystic masses using the transvaginal route (Fig. 40–9). Some cystic masses,

TABLE 40–1. RESULTS OF OVUM PICKUP BY THREE METHODS

	Laparoscopic	Transvesicular	Transvaginal
Oocytes recovered/patient	6.4 ± 0.9	6.2 ± 0.3	5.7 ± 0.6
Oocytes recovered/follicle (%)	93.0	86.0	82.0
Fertilization rate (%)	73.6	72.3	70.9
Cleavage rate (%)	82.6	79.4	81.6
Number embryos transferred	3.9 ± 0.6	3.2 ± 6.4	3.6 ± 0.3
Pregnancy rate/per pickup (%)	23.7	22.3	21.6
Pregnancy rate/transfer (%)	26.6	26.7	25.9
Pregnancy rate/cycle (%)	20.2	22.6	21.1

From Feldberg, Goldman, et al,[1] with permission.

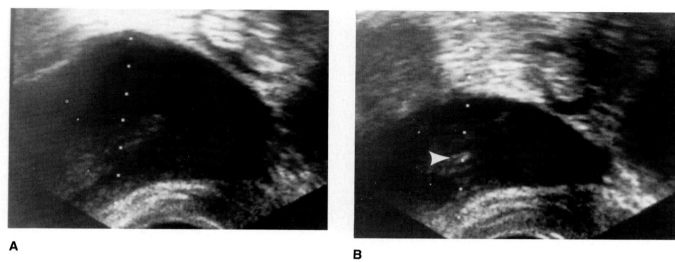

A   **B**

Fig. 40–8. A. Transvaginal scan (image oriented with vagina at bottom) on an IVF patient early in the cycle demonstrates a large cystic mass in the pelvis. The patient had a history of endometriosis and an endometrioma is suspected. Because this mass could interfere with the aspiration procedure, it was elected to aspirate the mass prior to beginning the cycle. **B.** Scan performed during aspiration demonstrates needle within the partially collapsed mass (*arrowhead*). The row of dots indicates the path of the needle. The mass was completely aspirated and the follicle aspiration procedure was easily performed during that cycle.

particularly in younger women, will reoccur following aspiration if there is inflammatory or hormonal stimulation (Fig. 40–10). Other masses with higher risks of malignancy should only be aspirated if no surgical approach is possible.[6] Other data (R.L.B., unpublished data) report performance of diagnostic procedures on five ovarian masses in high-risk patients. All masses had be-

nign characteristics on ultrasound image and benign cytologic features. Patients with prior history of gynecologic neoplasms and suspected recurrence can be biopsied via a transvaginal approach with ease and safety.[7,8] Patients with suspected pelvic abscesses are also good candidates for transvaginal aspiration, either for diagnosis or definitive treatment (Fig. 40–11). The cystic contents of a

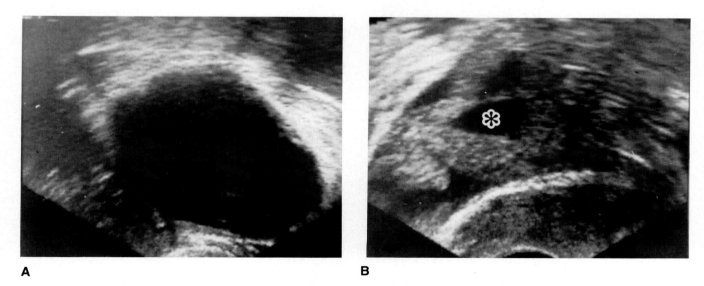

A   **B**

Fig. 40–9. An elderly woman was found to have a cystic pelvic mass on routine transabdominal ultrasound. Her surgical risk factors were high and transvaginal aspiration was recommended. **A.** Transvaginal scan shows large cystic pelvic mass that contains no internal echoes. The chance of this being a benign cyst is very high. **B.** Scan obtained following aspiration demonstrates small residual fluid within the cyst (∗). The surrounding echogenic tissue indicates that the mass is ovarian in origin. Cytologic evaluation of the fluid yielded benign cells.

uterus in a patient with a recurrent endometrial carcinoma with cervical stenosis have also been aspirated using the transvaginal approach.

Theoretic complications of transvaginal aspiration include inadvertent aspiration of an ovarian tumor with subsequent peritoneal spread, aspiration of an abscess with spread of septic fluid intraperitoneally, and aspiration of dermoid cysts or endometriomas with intraperitoneal spread of their contents, which may cause peritonitis. The actual incidence of these complications has not been documented and awaits further experience with a large series of patients. Availability of an operating room suite for surgical management of these complications must be maintained when aspiration procedures are performed.

OTHER APPLICATIONS

Transvaginal sonography can also be used for guided aspiration of cul-de-sac fluid in patients with suspected ruptured ectopic pregnancies. For this indication, an appropriate pocket of fluid is identified and entered under real-time sonography. Culdocentesis is indicated in patients with emergent clinical findings and suspicion of ectopic pregnancy. The aspiration of free nonclotted blood indicates a high probability of ruptured ectopic pregnancy and can shorten the time between the patient's initial presentation and surgery.

Transvaginal sonography may be employed for the transvaginal placement of drainage catheters for nonsurgical treatment of tubo-ovarian abscesses (TOA). Most

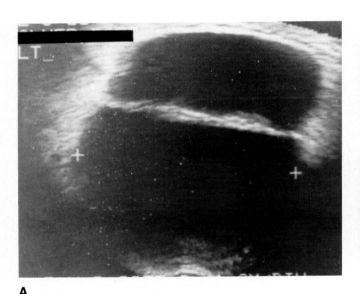

A

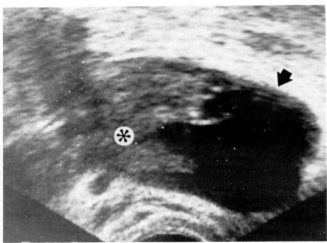

B

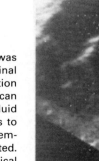

C

Fig. 40–10. A young woman with recurrent ovarian cysts was scanned during an episode of acute pelvic pain. **A.** Transvaginal scan demonstrates a large cystic pelvic mass with a septation within. **B.** Transvaginal aspiration was performed and the scan following the aspiration shows a small amount of residual fluid within the mass (*arrow*). When collapsed, the mass appears to arise from the ovary (∗). **C.** The scan obtained 5 days later demonstrates recurrence of the mass, which is now multiloculated. The pain in the pelvis recurred and the mass required surgical removal.

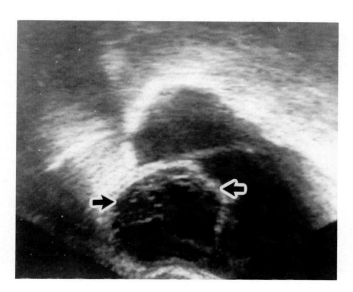

Fig. 40–11. Pelvic abscess. A multiloculated cystic mass was found in a patient with fever and pelvic pain. A pelvic abscess was suspected and a transvaginal scan demonstrates a multiloculated cystic mass with a portion of the mass containing internal echoes and septations (*arrows*). This mass was aspirated and thin purulent material was removed. The abscess was able to be completely collapsed following aspiration, without immediate recurrence.

importantly, a TOA must be clearly distinguished from a simple hydrosalpinx by demonstration of the abscess cavity within the ovary. Then transvaginal aspiration of the intra-ovarian mass can be performed.[9]

Transvaginal sonography can also be used for guidance of catheters into the area of the proximal tubal ostia for gamete intrafallopian tube transfer (GIFT) techniques. Prior to this procedure, one should evaluate carefully where the endometrium invaginates into the area of the proximal tubal ostia. The catheter is then manipulated to allow passage out into the tubal isthmus. The proximal portion of the uterine tube can be delineated in some patients, particularly if it is surrounded by intraperitoneal fluid (Fig. 40–7).

Sonography has been used for catheter placement in embryo transfer.[5] For this, transabdominal placement of the probe is used to monitor the location of the embryo-loaded catheter relative to the fundal portion of the uterine lumen as it is placed transvaginally. Theoretically, this ensures transfer of the embryo to the proper intrauterine location.

SUMMARY

In conclusion, sonography, particularly with transvaginal scanning, is a useful means to guide aspiration/biopsy of pelvic structures. It is extensively used for follicular aspiration, but can be used for aspiration/biopsy of selected pelvic masses.

REFERENCES

1. Feldberg D, Goldman JA, Ashkenazi J, Shelef M, Dicker D, Samuel N. Transvaginal oocyte retrieval controlled by vaginal probe for in vitro fertilization: A comparative study. *J Ultrasound Med.* 1988;7:339–343.
2. Wisanto A, Braeckmans P, Camus M, et al. Periurethral ultrasound-guided ovum pickup. *J In Vitro Fertilization Embryo Transfer.* 1988;5:107–111.
3. Dellenbach P, Nisand I, Moreau L, Feger B, Plumere C, Gerlinger P. Transvaginal sonographically controlled follicle puncture for oocyte retrieval. *Fertil Steril.* 1985;44:656–662.
4. Kemeter P, Feichtinger W. Transvaginal oocyte retrieval using a transvaginal sector scan probe combined with an automated puncture device. *Hum Reproduction.* 1986; 1:21–24.
5. Strickler RC, Christianson C, Crane JP, Curato A, Knight AB, Yang V. Ultrasound guidance for human embryo transfer. *Fertil Steril.* 1985;43:54–61.
6. deCrespigny LCH, Robinson HP, Davaren RAM, Fortune DW. Ultrasound guided puncture for gynecologic and pelvic lesions. *Aust NZ J Obstet Gynecol.* 1985;25:227–229.
7. Nash JD, Burke TW, Woodward JE, et al. Diagnosis of recurrent gynecologic malignancy with fine needle aspiration cytology. *Obstet Gynecol.* 1988;71:333–337.
8. Ganjei P, Nadji M. Aspiration cytology of ovarian neoplasms. *Acta Cytologica.* 1984;28:329–332.
9. Nosher JL, Winchman HK, Needell GS. Transvaginal pelvic abscess drainage with US guidance. *Radiology.* 1987; 165:872–873.

41 Sonography of the Breast

Arthur C. Fleischer • Valerie P. Jackson •
Peter J. Dempsey • Alan C. Winfield

Sonography has become an established diagnostic modality for the evaluation of patients with breast disorders. Years of comparative studies with x-ray mammography and breast sonography have documented their specific roles in breast diagnosis. Their complementary use in the clinical setting has resulted in an increase in the overall accuracy of breast imaging in diagnosing breast cancer.

DEVELOPMENTAL PERSPECTIVES

The first reference to the application of sonography for the diagnosis of breast disease was in 1951 when Wild and Neal described the acoustic characteristics of two breast tumors, one benign and one malignant, in the intact, in vivo breast.[1] They demonstrated three different acoustic tissue textures or tissue "signatures" based on acoustical impedance for normal breast tissue and for benign and malignant breast tumors.

The following year, 1952, Wild and Reid published the results of ultrasound examination in 21 breast tumors, 9 benign and 12 malignant, and in two of these cases also included the first two-dimensional echograms or B-mode sonograms of breast tissue ever published.[2]

In 1953, Howry, Stott and Bliss published two-dimensional images of in vitro breast tumors using a scanner that employed a lower-frequency pulse-echo system combined with focusing elements to reduce beam width.[3] These modifications improved resolution and produced images of better diagnostic quality.

During the 1960s, continuing research work on breast ultrasound was centered in Japan, Australia, and the United States. In Japan, work begun in the 1950s continued into the 1960s with emphasis on focused, single-transducer systems designed to examine the patient in the supine position, using a water bag as the coupling medium.[4]

In Australia, work began by Jellins and associates at the Commonwealth Acoustic Laboratories on a scanner, initially employing a "double breasted coupling" technique with the patient in the supine position. This was found unsatisfactory, and a supine, single-breast uncompressed technique was substituted. This research group also incorporated gray-scale technique along with a fo-cused transducer format and described the principles of gray-scale echography relating to all soft tissues.[5–8]

In the United States, Kelly-Fry began research with an on-line, computer-controlled system in the late 1960s.[9,10] Her efforts signaled a shift in the clinical emphasis from tissue characterization of known masses to an effort at early detection of small, subclinical breast abnormalities. Her efforts are also noteworthy in that an extraordinarily meticulous protocol was pursued in an effort to define and document the most ideally suited transducer system for examination of the breast. She recognized that a failure of previous systems resulted from very poor lateral resolution.

The mid-1970s saw the initiation of the development of the Octoson scanner under the auspices of the Department of Health of the Australian Government.[7,10] Multipurpose in design, the Octoson was also well-suited to examination of the breast. It used eight single-focus transducers that could be used either alone or in combination to produce either sector or compound scans.

Following the success of the Octoson scanner in Australia, and encouraged by Baum, who recognized the need for dedicated breast ultrasound equipment,[11] automated breast scanners were introduced in the United States in the middle to late 1970s. The most recently introduced dedicated scanner uses a high-resolution, 7.5-MHz PVDF transducer developed by Kelly-Fry laboratory[12] and examines the patient in a supine position through a water bag with the breast "autocompressed."

However, at present, the most commonly used technique for sonographic evaluation of the breast continues to employ the hand-held real-time high-frequency transducer. This technique provides sufficiently accurate information concerning the location, size, and consistency of most palpable breast masses, but lacks the systematic and global depiction of the breast afforded by dedicated breast scanners.[13–16]

Clinical and engineering research continues concerning improvement of the resolution and application of breast sonography. This research involves optimizing transducer design and other sonographic parameters that might enhance the diagnostic specificity of breast sonography.

In this chapter, the clinical applications of both hand-held and dedicated breast scanners are discussed and illustrated. Pertinent aspects concerning instrumentation used for breast sonography are presented as they relate to optimizing image quality and diagnostic capability.

CLINICAL ASPECTS

Carcinoma of the breast is one of the two leading causes of cancer deaths among women. It is estimated that one in every eleven women in the United States will develop breast cancer in her lifetime.[17] Currently, there is no known way to prevent breast cancer. Effort, therefore, has been directed toward early detection of breast cancers before they become palpable. The purpose of early detection by screening is to reduce the mortality rate for breast cancer in the screened population. Data that substantiate this theorem have been published by Tabar,[18] documenting a reduction in mortality for breast cancer by 31% in a population screened with x-ray mammography. A recently published summary of the results from the Breast Cancer Demonstration Project has indicated a 5-year survival rate of 95% in those cancers found at a minimal stage.[17] Thus, early detection clearly can reduce the morbidity and increase the 5- and 10-year survival rates for breast cancer.

It is crucial, however, to recognize that sonography presently has *no* role as a screening modality for breast cancer. With present automated or hand-held equipment, sonography cannot reliably detect small solid tumors or microcalcifications. However, ultrasound does have an important role as an adjunctive technique to high quality x-ray mammography in selected patients. It must be emphasized that for most symptomatic patients, except those that are very young, a preliminary x-ray mammogram (XRM) is indicated.

Sonography has a role in the following breast situations:

1. Evaluation of a palpable or nonpalpable mass that is of indeterminate etiology or not seen on x-ray mammography.
2. Evaluation of palpable masses in very young patients (often with limited, if any, XRM findings).
3. Evaluation of palpable breast masses in the pregnant or lactating patient.
4. Evaluation of the augmented breast.
5. Further evaluation of radiographically nondiagnostic "dense" areas on mammography or asymmetrical patterns.
6. Guided biopsy or fine-needle aspiration of cystic and solid breast lesions.

SCREENING VERSUS DIAGNOSIS

To understand the current role of breast sonography, it must be clear that there is an absolute distinction between screening and diagnosis.[19,20] The purpose of screening is to detect breast cancer at the earliest stage possible in asymptomatic women, which, as stated before, results in reduced mortality in the screened population. Although on occasion screening may be diagnostic, it need not be so. The role of screening is to identify those women who need a definitive diagnosis established. X-ray mammography is currently the *only* method used to screen asymptomatic women for occult breast cancer, as it is fast, repeatable, low in cost, and proven effective as a reliable detector of minimal cancers.[21,22]

Breast imaging as applied to the diagnosis of symptomatic breast disease is a totally different category of problem from pure screening. Although one may progress from screening to diagnosis in the same visit, the approaches must be considered separately. From the diagnostic standpoint, the only two meaningful symptoms or signs of breast cancer are the presence of a lump or the presence of a bloody or serous nipple discharge. Skin thickening and axillary adenopathy may also raise suspicion of breast carcinoma. If these symptoms or signs are present, then it should be the goal of the breast imaging specialist to define them as precisely as the imaging techniques allow.

Other than errors of interpretation, the false-negatives in x-ray mammography usually result from the superimposition of data, generally caused by the presence of dense fibroglandular tissue.[23,24] An XRM is a summation image in which three dimensions of tissue are portrayed in one plane. If anything other than complete fatty replacement exists, the possibility for superimposition of data, and for error, exists. It is in this context of superimposition of data that an additional (not alternative) form of breast imaging, ultrasound, can increase the overall clinical accuracy.[25-28] Furthermore, ultrasound does not simply provide the same parenchymal information as x-ray mammography. The most basic example of this is the ability of ultrasound to distinguish a pure cyst from a solid mass. X-ray mammography is incapable of this distinction. In addition, ultrasound provides this data in a slice-type or tomographic format, thus obviating concerns about possible superimposition of data.

When a local abnormality is suspected, either from physical examination or from asymmetry, on the XRM, ultrasound can be extremely helpful in establishing whether a definite lesion really does exist. It is particularly helpful in the situation of finding a palpable mass on physical examination that cannot be imaged on an XRM. In one of the author's (P.J.D.) experience, this situation occurs in approximately 6% of cancers. This is a potentially dangerous situation because in some instances a "negative" mammogram report may delay a biopsy of a significant lesion, with grave consequences. If a palpable lesion exists, it is incumbent on the breast imaging specialist to define that lesion and dictate a parenchymally accurate report.

INSTRUMENTATION AND SCANNING TECHNIQUES

There are a variety of sonographic scanners and probes that are commercially available for examination of the breast. While B-mode static scanning of the breast can be done, today the preferred method of hand-held breast ultrasound is with high-resolution real-time equipment.

Real-time hand-held probes can be classified into two major types: linear array and the sector scanners. Linear-array probes are ideally suited to the linear configuration of the breast (Fig. 41–1). These probes use either 5- or 7.5-MHz transducer elements and are oriented along a linear scan plane. The footprint is the area of the breast that is covered by the transducer and should be between 2 and 5 cm in length. Longer probes are difficult to couple to the breast, while smaller probes have a limited field-of-view. These transducers are typically focused to the near-field range, optimally between 1 and 3 cm from the transducer face. A standoff pad can be used to image superficial or skin lesions that are outside the focal zone of the transducer. Sector-scanning probes operate in one of two ways: with single-element me-

chanically driven crystals, or with electronic or phased steering. Both of these require a significant offset, because the apex of the sector would limit the field-of-view image. Thus, for most single-element mechanical sectors, a water path is needed for the probe.

The configuration of the hand-held probe allows the examiner to palpate while examining the breast. It is often helpful to place the palpable mass between the examiner's fingers during sonographic scanning. With hand-held devices, significant limitations include inability to systematically evaluate the entire breast and to reproduce examination on a follow-up study. For real-time evaluation of the breast, one relies on the examiner's ability to instantaneously evaluate the image while performing the study and to record pertinent images. For this reason, real-time sonography of the breast is often performed by a physician, rather than technologist.

Hand-held transducers allow for preoperative guided needle placement for fine-needle aspiration biopsy. The use of a needle-guide attachment is advocated because this keeps the needle in the beam path of the transducer, thus improving the accuracy of needle placement. Such needle guides currently are under development and will be available commercially in the near future. Ultrasound-guided aspiration is particularly useful in masses that are difficult or impossible to palpate. Sonographically guided fine-needle aspiration biopsy can

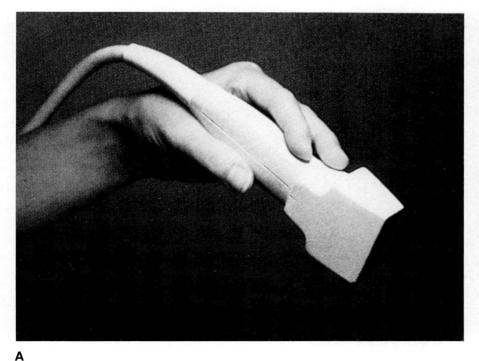
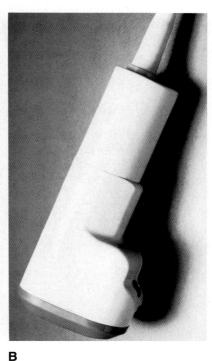

A

B

Fig. 41–1. Hand-held transducers. **A.** High frequency linear array transducer. (*Courtesy of Toshiba, Inc.*) **B.** Water-path offset high frequency sector transducer. (*Courtesy of Diasonics, Inc.*)

improve the confidence level of a negative aspirate by allowing visual confirmation that the needle is within the area of abnormality.

Two types of needle guides are currently available. The most commonly used is an attachment to the real-time probe that allows insertion of the needle at a predetermined angle into the area of abnormality. The second type of guide is an actual real-time transducer with a central needle-path hole. In the needle-path area, there are no transducer elements and therefore no image is visualized. However, by slight angulation of the needle, the tip of the needle may be visualized with these slotted transducers. Another technique that is helpful for needle-tip visualization is rotating the needle so that the bevel is parallel to the beam path. This exposes the largest echogenic interface to the beam.

Dedicated Systems

There are two major types of dedicated automated systems available for breast sonography, supine and prone. In the former, the patient is examined in the supine position by a transducer that is mounted on an articulated arm and surrounded by a small water path (Fig. 41–2.A). Prone scanners use one to four transducers mounted on a scanning gantry, using the long water path to examine the breasts with or without compression (Fig. 41–2.B). The patient is examined in the prone position with her breasts suspended in a large water bath.

The advantage of these systems include the ability to systematically delineate the entire breast in a tomographic fashion. The major disadvantage is the high cost of the systems ($80,000–$100,000) relative to their clinical efficacy. Certainly, they become more cost effective in clinics that do a high volume of mammography, as opposed to clinics that use breast ultrasound only on an infrequent basis.

SONOMAMMOGRAPHY AND X-RAY MAMMOGRAPHY

Although x-ray mammography clearly remains the primary diagnostic modality for the breast, the use of ultrasound can improve the diagnostic accuracy and confidence level in a variety of breast disorders. Because x-ray mammography depicts the entire breast in two planes, the superimposition of densities may obscure lesions or make their characterization difficult. However, ultrasound is a tomographic image that allows one to see within

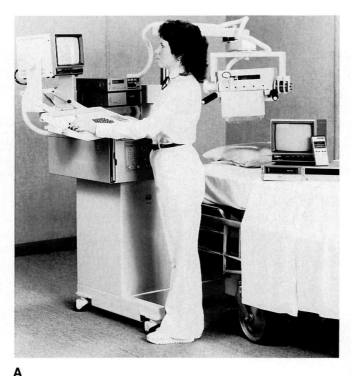

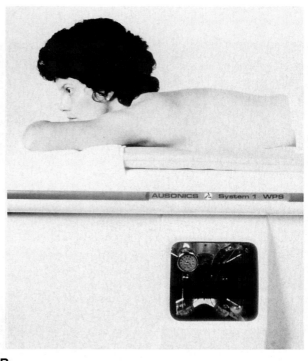

A   **B**

Fig. 41–2. Dedicated breast scanners. **A.** Dedicated breast scanning system (Labsonics) consisting of single 7.5 MHz transducer, which is attached to a scanning arm and moves in a water path. The scanning gantry and water path is placed on the breast with the patient in the supine position. **B.** Ausonics scanner.

the breast tissue in order to improve lesion detection and determination of the matrix of a mass.

Each of these imaging modalities has advantages and limitations. X-ray mammography is accurate in evaluation of the patient with fatty breasts. With increasing radiographic density, the detection of soft tissue masses becomes more difficult. Ultrasound can determine the internal matrix of a mass in any type of breast, but it is often most useful in the evaluation of masses in radiographically dense breasts. Ultrasound cannot reliably detect microcalcifications and is often poor for visualizing small solid masses in predominantly fatty breasts, and therefore it has no role as a screening modality for breast cancer.

There have been several studies comparing the relative accuracy of sonography and XRM in detection of breast tumors.[22,25,29–31] Cole-Beuglet and colleagues[29] found the sensitivity of ultrasound to be 79% in the detection of breast carcinoma when the findings of the x-ray mammogram and clinical examination were known. Sickles and coworkers[22] found only 58% accuracy of sonography in detection of early breast carcinoma when compared to the 97% accuracy of x-ray mammography, which included magnification views.[22] Egan and Egan[30] studied 176 solid lesions, including 107 proven carcinomas. Sonography was found to be positive in 6 cases of carcinoma where mammograms were interpreted as negative. Thus, it can be estimated that approximately 7% of all carcinomas might be detected by breast sonography that are not found on x-ray mammography. One large study that evaluated the diagnostic virtues and limitations of single modality and multimodality breast imaging concluded that 95% of cancers can be detected with the multimodality approach. When all tests (primarily XRM, ultrasound) were negative, 7% of cancer would be missed.[31]

SONOGRAPHIC FEATURES OF THE NORMAL BREAST

Sonographically, the normal breast is composed of three types of tissue. These are the echogenic fibroglandular tissue, the echogenic stromal or supportive structures, and relatively hypoechoic fat. The amount and arrangement of each of these tissue elements varies according to the age and functional state of the breast (Fig. 41–3). The pectoralis muscles, retromammary fat layer, ribs, and the costochondral junctions can also be seen (Fig. 41–3).

SONOGRAPHIC FEATURES OF BREAST MASSES

Certain parameters should be evaluated in the sonographic diagnosis of breast masses. These include the location, shape, size, borders, internal echogenicity, and attenuation of the mass, as well as any associated findings such as skin thickening or architectural distortion. The location of a mass is usually described in either a quadrant or by a clockface ("o'clock") position. The shape of the mass may be round, oval, lobulated, or indeterminate. Each dimension of the breast mass should be measured accurately as there may be a disparity between the palpable and imaged abnormality. One should realize that compression of the breast mass by the transducer itself may alter the width of the lesion but not its volume. One should carefully examine the internal echogenicity of a mass, deciding if it is anechoic, hypoechoic, and whether the internal echoes are homogeneous or heterogeneous. Border delineation of a mass is important as carcinomas tend to have irregular borders whereas benign lesions such as cysts are smooth. The overall attenuation of the ultrasound beam by the mass is helpful in determining its internal matrix. Cysts typically demonstrate posterior acoustic enhancement, whereas many solid lesions do not. However, homogeneous benign and malignant solid masses occasionally have posterior enhancement. Associated findings may include thickening of Cooper's ligaments, skin retraction, and lymphadenopathy, and should be sought by the sonographer.[32] Thickened Cooper's ligaments appear as irregular thickening of the connective tissue septa that attach immediately beneath the skin. Skin retraction is best depicted on automated scanners that examine the patient in the prone position without compression. In general, only large abnormal auxillary lymph nodes are visible on ultrasound, and these will appear as oval or lobulated solid hypoechoic masses.

Cysts

Sonography is highly accurate in distinguishing cysts from solid masses in the breast. Cysts form from fluid-distended ductal and lobular systems, and their connection to the ducts may be found in occasional cases (Fig. 41–4.A,B). Cysts are typically round masses that demonstrate smooth walls, enhanced through transmission, lateral shadowing, and no internal echoes. Hemorrhagic or infected cysts may demonstrate low level internal echoes, but all simple cysts should have thin and smooth borders. Cysts must be examined thoroughly at very small intervals to evaluate for wall thickening and solid masses within the cyst. These findings may be seen in necrotic solid tumors as well as intracystic papillomas and carcinomas.[33] In addition, fluid-fluid layers may occur in intracystic tumors, necrotic tumors, or in cysts complicated by infection or hemorrhage (Fig. 41–4.C).

Cystic lesions may also exhibit a variety of complex configurations. Some may be benign histologically, such as those with one or more septa, but other cystic lesions may have a far more ominous significance. Between 1

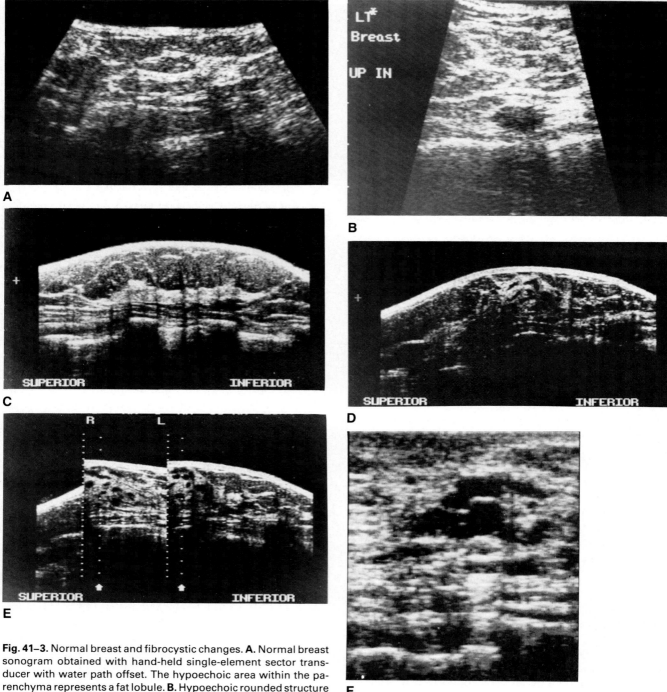

Fig. 41–3. Normal breast and fibrocystic changes. **A.** Normal breast sonogram obtained with hand-held single-element sector transducer with water path offset. The hypoechoic area within the parenchyma represents a fat lobule. **B.** Hypoechoic rounded structure posterior to pectoralis muscle represents costochondral junction portion of the thoracic rib. **C.** Sonotomogram of normal breast demonstrating echogenic parenchymal tissue surrounded by relatively hypoechoic subcutaneous fat. Cooper's ligaments are also identified as they course toward the under surface of the skin. **D.** Sonotomogram demonstrating slightly dilated lactiferous ducts. **E.** Same patient as **D** imaging dilated lactiferous ducts in short and long axis. **F.** Linear array hand-held sonogram of dilated lactiferous ducts. **G.** 25-year-old female who presented with cyclic pain and lumpiness in both breasts. The longitudinal 7.5 MHz sonograms show diffusely echogenic breast tissue with multiple "holes" and "channels" frequently seen in the microcystic type of fibrocystic disease. Some of the tubular-appearing structures are ducts.

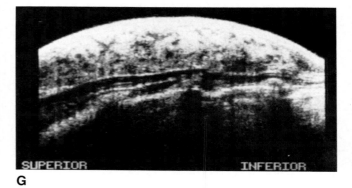

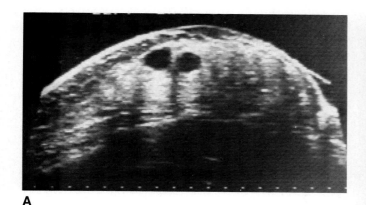

A

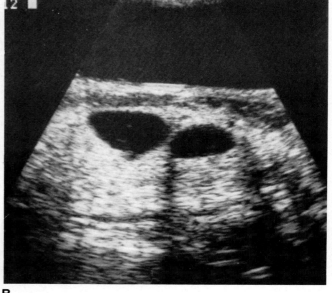

B

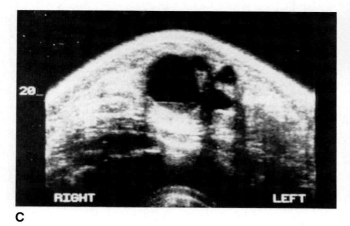

C

Fig. 41–4. Cysts. A. Automated sonogram demonstrating two well-defined cysts in the upper outer quadrant of the left breast. B. Hand-held breast sonogram demonstrating the same cyst. C. 35-year-old female who presented with palpable mass just inferior to the left nipple at 3 days. The transverse 7.5 MHz sonogram shows a cluster of cysts. The largest cyst has a fluid-fluid level within it. At biopsy, this was a cyst with hemorrhage into it. The anterior solid-appearing mass is actually "partial voluming" of another small cyst.

and 2% of carcinomas will mimic a cyst.[33–35] Some will be unilocular, but will have irregular borders, lack good through transmission, and have occasional scattered echoes within the lesion. Although not a specific finding for malignancy, some carcinomas present as cystic lesions exhibiting a fluid-fluid level, which results from the layering of two fluids of different specific gravities. They may also have definite tumor nodules seen within the cystic matrix.[33] It should be stressed that the most important and fundamental thought process in interpretation should be that either a lesion is a pure, simple cyst, or it is not.

Fibroadenomas

Fibroadenomas have been classically described as smooth-walled, round, or oval masses that have relatively uniform internal echo textures (Fig. 41–5). They may be evaluated and occasionally demonstrate posterior enhancement. However, many fibroadenomas do not have this "classic" appearance and they may exhibit irregular borders, heterogeneous internal echo texture, or posterior shadowing. Up to 20% of fibroadenomas were not visible on ultrasound in three reported series.[36–38]

Fibroadenomas are frequently located at the junction of subcutaneous fat and mammary parenchyma. They range in size from several millimeters up to more than 6 to 8 cm, beyond which they are classified as giant fibroadenomas. They may occur in any age group, but they are the most common palpable mass in women under age 35.

When fibroadenomas undergo degeneration and hyalinization, they frequently contain large, coarse calcifications that are large enough to see on ultrasound. Though most fibroadenomas, particularly in younger women, will not shadow with higher-resolution transducers, it has been our experience that some, particularly the hyalinized type, may exhibit acoustic shadowing. This phenomenon has also been documented by others.[38] Acoustic shadowing, therefore, is not specific for carcinoma.

Cystosarcoma phylloides is considered by some to be a variant of fibroadenomas. These lesions typically are very large solid masses and small internal cystic clefts or spaces are occasionally seen on ultrasound.[39] Up to 5% of cystosarcomas contain areas of malignancy but this, to date, has not been detected sonographically.

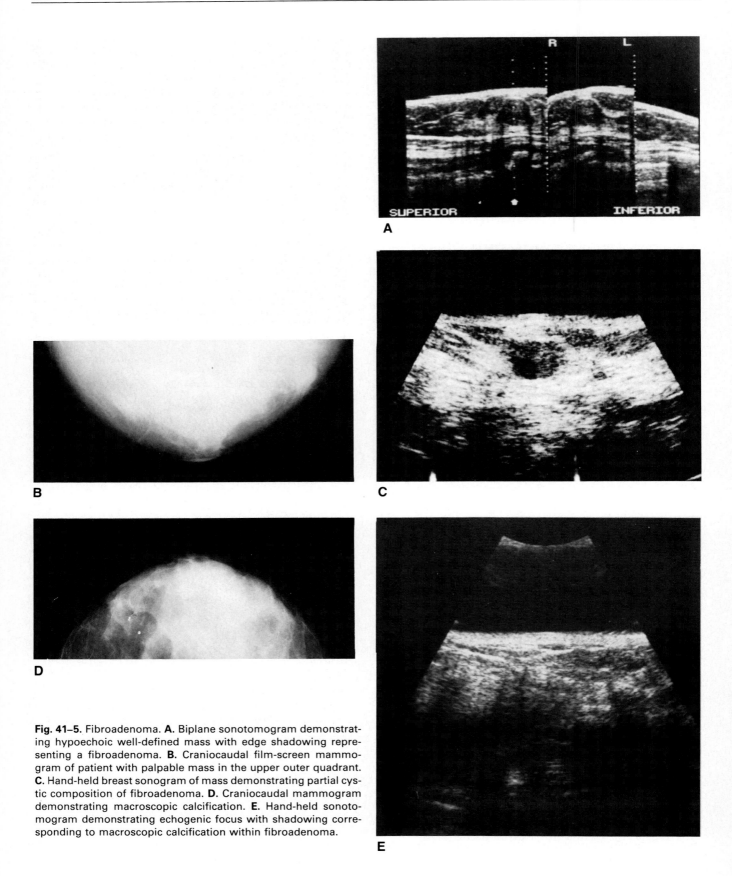

Fig. 41–5. Fibroadenoma. **A.** Biplane sonotomogram demonstrating hypoechoic well-defined mass with edge shadowing representing a fibroadenoma. **B.** Craniocaudal film-screen mammogram of patient with palpable mass in the upper outer quadrant. **C.** Hand-held breast sonogram of mass demonstrating partial cystic composition of fibroadenoma. **D.** Craniocaudal mammogram demonstrating macroscopic calcification. **E.** Hand-held sonotomogram demonstrating echogenic focus with shadowing corresponding to macroscopic calcification within fibroadenoma.

Fibrous Mastopathy

These masses usually represent a focal area of fibrous dysplasia.[40] They can either have poor or moderately well defined borders and can mimic in many cases the appearance of breast carcinoma (Fig. 41–6).

Galactocele

These are cystic lesions filled with a lipid material. On ultrasound, they are often anechoic, but show little or no posterior enhancement. They may contain low-level internal echoes arising from the proteinaceous milk contained within them (Fig. 41–7.B,C). They may be associated with a group of dilated ducts. While many occur in pregnant or lactating women, they may also be seen in older women.

Carcinoma

The sonographic findings in breast carcinomas depend in part on the histologic type of carcinoma.[32,41] The most common pattern, usually arising from infiltrating duct carcinomas, demonstrates a hypoechoic mass with ill-defined borders and posterior acoustic shadowing (Fig. 41–8). The irregular borders commonly correspond to the stellate appearance seen on mammography as the tumor infiltrates into the surrounding parenchyma by finger-like projections. There may be associated skin thickening and thickening of Cooper's ligaments (Fig. 41–8.G). Echogenic desmoplastic reaction may be seen surrounding the tumor (Fig. 41–8.H). Sonographic architectural distortion may also be present. Some malignancies, such as medullary and colloid carcinomas, may be cellular and well circumscribed and have an appearance similar to benign solid lesions such as fibroadenomas. The accuracy of ultrasound in detection of carcinomas depends largely on the size of the tumor and the type of underlying breast parenchyma. Small tumors may be difficult or impossible to see in fatty breasts. In addition, sonography is not accurate in the detection of microcalcifications associated with breast carcinoma, although they are occasionally seen within these masses. Isolated microcalcifications in the breast tissue are rarely visible. However, when associated with the early breast carcinoma, they can be depicted.[42]

Miscellaneous Conditions

Sonography has been found to be useful in evaluating the residual breast tissue in a patient who has a breast prosthesis (Fig. 41–7.D,E). Silicone prostheses are radiographically dense and may hide large areas of breast tissue. The remaining parenchyma can be examined sonographically for abnormalities.

Sonography of the breast after lumpectomy and ra-

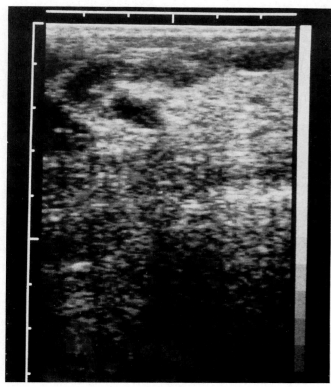

A

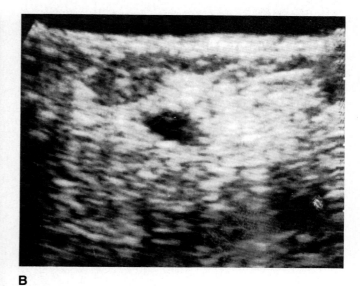

B

Fig. 41–6. Solid masses that can mimic carcinoma. **A.** Hypoechoic mass with irregular borders found in biopsy to represent fibrous mastopathy. **B.** Solid mass with irregular borders found to represent fibroadenoma.

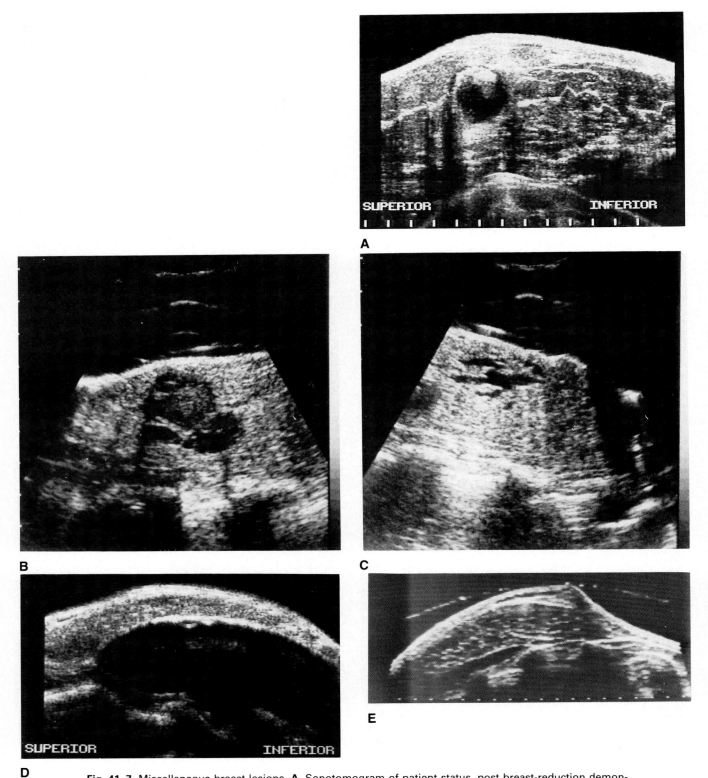

Fig. 41–7. Miscellaneous breast lesions. **A.** Sonotomogram of patient status, post breast-reduction demonstrating predominantly cystic mass with echogenic material layering anteriorly. At surgery, a breast abscess was found. **B.** Hypoechoic, lobulated, mass with good through transmission but internal echoes. **C.** Same patient as **B** demonstrating a cluster of dilated ducts. This patient had an infected galactocele. **D.** Sonotomogram of normal breast tissue anterior to silicone breast prostheses. **E.** Sonotomogram of male patient with gynecomastia.

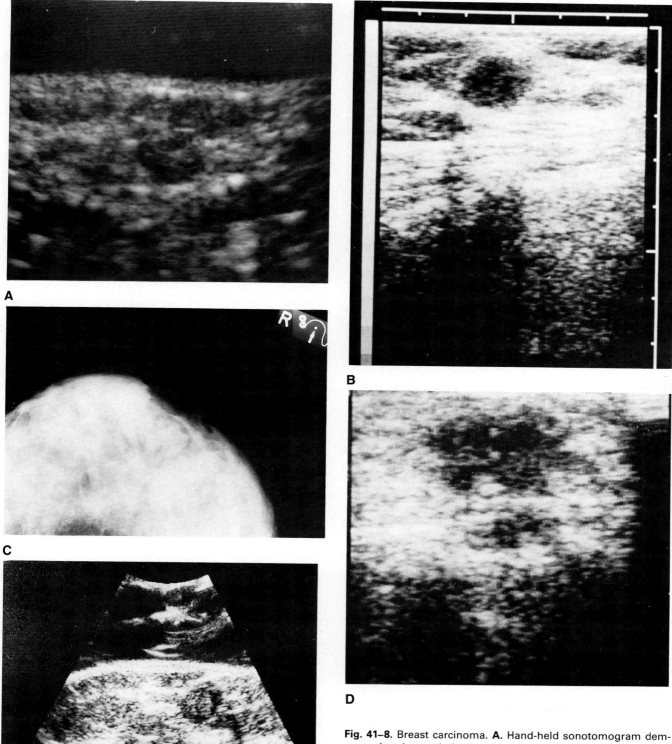

Fig. 41–8. Breast carcinoma. **A.** Hand-held sonotomogram demonstrating hypoechoic, moderately well-defined lesion representing infiltrating duct carcinoma. **B.** Sonotomogram obtained with hand-held linear array transducer demonstrating hypoechoic mass with irregular borders. Fine-needle aspiration showed malignant cells. **C.** Magnified craniocaudal mammogram demonstrating ill-defined lesion with stellate borders. **D.** Hand-held real-time sonogram of lesions in **C** representing infiltrating duct carcinoma. The stellate pattern corresponds to the finger-like projection of tumor throughout the parenchyma. **E.** Hypoechoic well-defined mass later found to represent a colloid carcinoma. (*Figure continued.*)

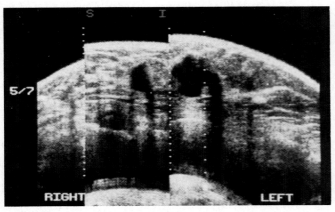

F–i

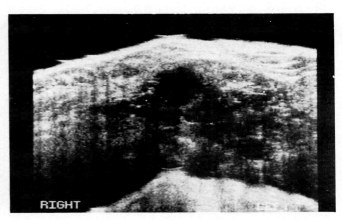

F–ii

Fig. 41–8. (continued). Breast carcinoma. **F.** 84-year-old female presented with a one month history of a right breast mass and palpable (R) axillary node. The mammograms showed an irregular mass corresponding to a carcinoma. Biplane 7.5 MHz ultrasound (i) of the breast mass shows an irregular hypoechoic mass with posterior enhancement. The internal echoes are very low level. At surgery this was a completely solid invasive ductal carcinoma. Ultrasound (ii) of the auxillary node shows the typical appearance of a smooth hypoechoic mass with low-level internal echoes. There is some posterior enhancement. At surgery this node was filled with metastatic breast cancer. **G.** 47-year-old female with (L) upper outside quadrant palpable mass. The XRM had shown a partly smooth mass suspicious for cancer. The transverse 7.5 MHz sonograms show a well-defined smooth solid mass. Cooper's ligaments appear to be "tethered" into the mass. At surgery this was a circumscribed invasive ductal cancer. (*Figure continued.*)

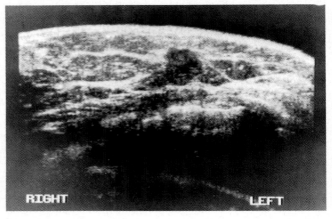

G

diation therapy is occasionally helpful in the patient with a difficult or equivocal XRM. The typical sonographic changes following radiation therapy include skin thickening, thickened Cooper's ligaments, increased echogenicity, and decreased compressibility of the breast.[43] Areas of focal fat necrosis may produce an irregular texture with an ill-defined border, similar to the sonographic appearance of carcinoma. Recurrent breast carcinoma has only rarely been seen on ultrasound. Lymphoma and metastases to the breast are often well-circumscribed, solid hypoechoic lesions, similar to the "classic" sonographic appearance of fibroadenomas. In other cases they may have irregular walls and posterior shadowing.[41]

NEW AND FUTURE DEVELOPMENTS

The ultimate goal still lies ahead. That is the detection and resolution of small masses within the breast, coupled with the ability to characterize these foci as either benign or malignant. Instruments with even better gray-scale

resolution will be available in order to address the first of these two objectives, detection. The ability to assess whether a focus is potentially malignant will most likely rely not only on the lesion characteristics outlined in this chapter, but will also be aided by two additional types of functional, quantitative information.

High-resolution, gray-scale ultrasound instruments with the ability to obtain simultaneous Doppler ultrasound information will be available. Thus detailed parenchymal images will be conveniently coupled with real-time blood flow data, allowing better assessment of either focal or diffuse breast pathology. In addition, information will also be available concerning tissue signature. It will most likely be obtained from the quantitative analysis of acoustic impedance information, derived from tissue interrogation with multiple frequencies. Phase shift and changes in velocity as the beam transverses the breast is also being investigated as a means for better tissue interrogation.[44]

Future development is also anticipated in the needle guides and slotted transducers required for guided biopsy (Fig. 41–9).[45] Sonography can be helpful in providing

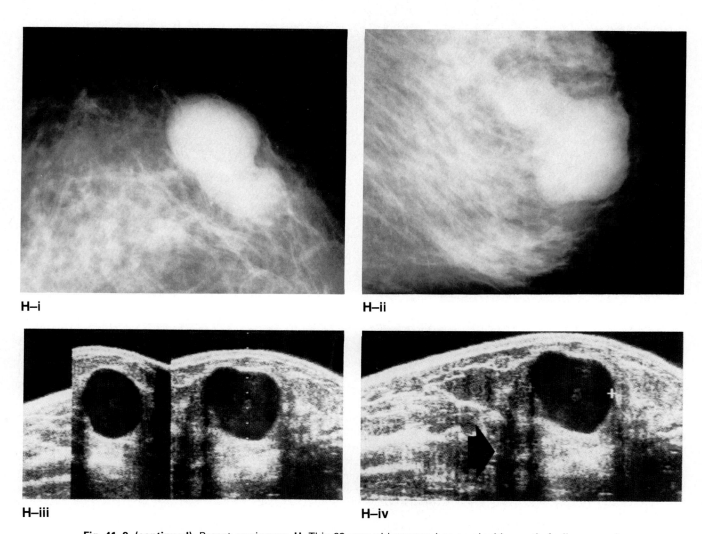

H–i

H–ii

H–iii

H–iv

Fig. 41–8. (continued). Breast carcinoma. **H.** This 63-year-old woman has a palpable, cystic-feeling mass in the medial aspect of the left breast. X-ray mammography (i = craniocaudal view; ii = magnified view) reveals a lobular, well-circumscribed mass measuring 4.5 cm. The biplane (iii) ultrasound shows through transmission indicating a lesion containing fluid, but it is not a pure, simple cyst. Rather, there is a triangular-shaped area of desmoplastic response along the superior aspect of the lesion, portions of which are dense enough to cast acoustical shadows (iv) (*arrow*). At excisional biopsy, this was found to be a ductal carcinoma. (*Figure continued.*)

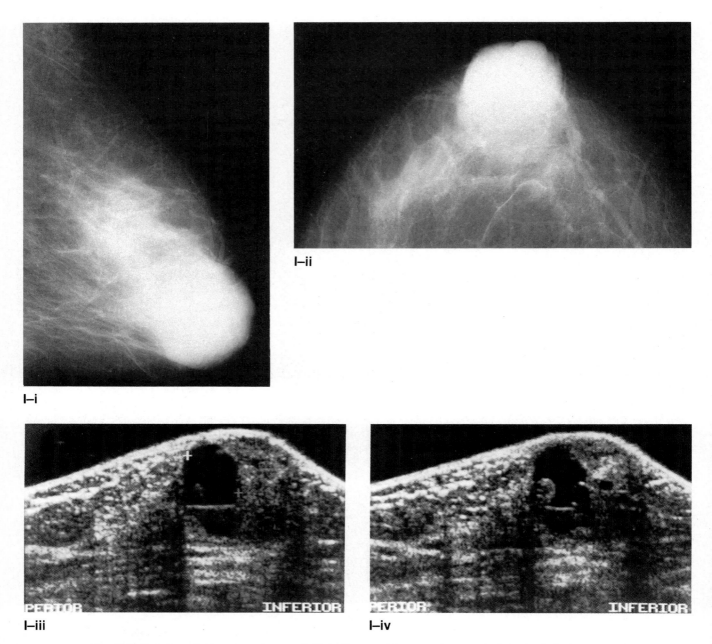

I–i

I–ii

I–iii

I–iv

Fig. 41–8. (continued). Breast carcinoma. **H.** This 63-year-old woman has a palpable, cystic-feeling mass in the medial aspect of the left breast. X-ray mammography (i = craniocaudal view; ii = magnified view) reveals a lobular, well-circumscribed mass measuring 4.5 cm. The biplane (iii) ultrasound shows through transmission indicating a lesion containing fluid, but it is not a pure, simple cyst. Rather, there is a triangular-shaped area of desmoplastic response along the superior aspect of the lesion, portions of which are dense enough to cast acoustical shadows (iv) (*arrow*). At excisional biopsy, this was found to be a ductal carcinoma. (*Figure continued.*)

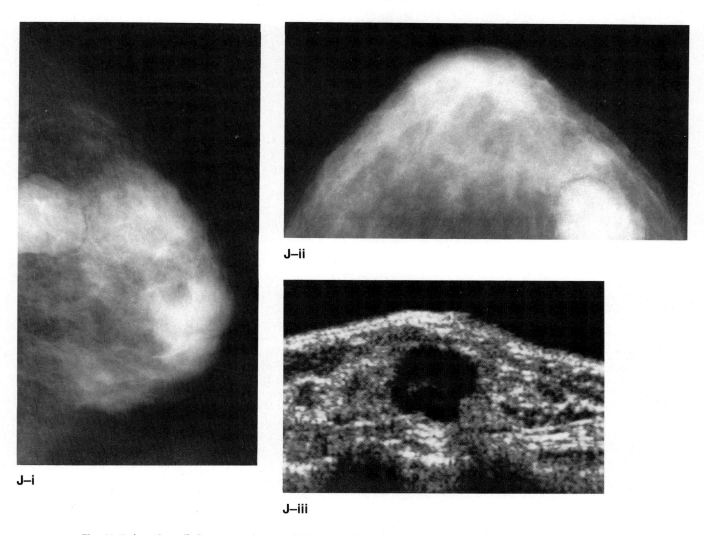

J–i

J–ii

J–iii

Fig. 41–8. (continued). Breast carcinoma. **J.** This is a 34-year-old woman presenting with a palpable, 3.5 cm lesion in the upper-inner quadrant of the left breast. On the XRM (i = mediolateral view; ii = craniocaudal view), the lesion appears well-circumscribed with an apparent "halo" sign along its perimeter. The ultrasound (iii) shows that although cystic in nature, it is not a pure, simple cyst. Instead, it has a thickened, irregular border and irregular internal echoes. At excisional biopsy, this was found to be an anaplastic medullary carcinoma.

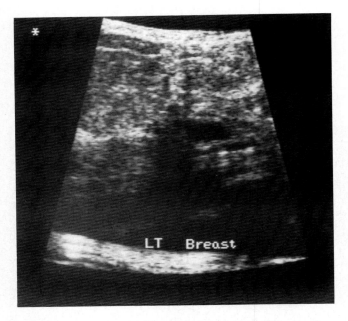

Fig. 41–9. Biopsy and fine-needle aspiration guidance. Fine-needle aspiration of mass suspected to be cystic. The needle is barely seen along the lateral aspect of the mass.

guided aspiration and fine needle biopsy of suspicious solid lesions.

SUMMARY

This chapter has discussed and illustrated the current clinical uses of sonography in the evaluation of breast disorders. Identification of cysts and guided biopsy are the two major clinical applications of this technique.

REFERENCES

1. Wild JJ, Neal D. Use of high-frequency ultrasonic waves for detecting changes of texture in living tissue. *Lancet.* 1951;1:655–657.
2. Wild JJ, Reid JH. Further pilot echographic studies on the histologic structures of tumors of the living intact breast. *Am J Pathol.* 1952;26:839–861.
3. Howry DH, Stott DA, Bliss WR. The ultrasonic visualization of carcinoma of the breast and other soft tissue structures. *Cancer.* 1954;7:354–358.
4. Kikuchi Y, Uchida R, Tanaka K, Wagai T. Early cancer diagnosis through ultrasonics. *J Acoust Soc Am.* 1957;29: 824–833.
5. Jellins J, Kossoff G, Buddee FW, Reeve TS. Ultrasonic visualization of the breast. *Med J Aust.* 1971;1:305–307.
6. Jellins J, Kossoff G, Reeve TS, Barraclough BH. Ultrasonic

gray scale visualization of breast disease. *Ultrasound Med Biol.* 1975;1:393–404.
7. Jellins J, Reeve TS, Croll J, Kossoff G. Results of breast echography examination in Sydney, Australia 1972–1979. *Semin Ultrasound.* 1982;3:58–62.
8. Kossoff G, Jellins J. The physics of breast echography. *Semin Ultrasound.* 1982;3:5–12.
9. Kelly-Fry, Kossoff G, Hindman HA. The potential of ultrasound visualization for detecting the presence of abnormal structures within the female breast. In: Proceedings of IEEE Ultrasonic Symposium. New York: IEEE Press. 1972:25–30.
10. Kelly-Fry E. Influences on the development of ultrasound pulse-echo breast instrumentation in the United States. In: Harper P, ed. *Ultrasound Mammography.* Baltimore: University Park Press. 1985:1–20.
11. Baum G. Ultrasound mammography. *Radiology.* 1977; 122:199–205.
12. Jackson VP, Kelly-Fry E, Rothschild PA, Holden RW, Clark SA. Automated breast sonography using a 7.5-MHz PVDF transducer: Preliminary clinical evaluation. *Radiology.* 1986;159:679–684.
13. Fleischer AC, Muhletaler CA, Reynolds VH, et al. Palpable breast masses: Evaluation by high frequency, hand-held real-time sonography and xeromammography. *Radiology.* 1983;148:813–817.
14. Rubin E, Miller VE, Berland LL, Han SY, Koehler RE, Stanley RJ. Hand-held real-time breast sonography. *AJR.* 1985;144:623–627.
15. Fleischer AC, Thieme GA, Winfield AC, et al. Breast sonotomography and high-frequency, hand-held real-time sonography: A clinical comparison. *J Ultrasound Med.* 1985; 4:577–581.
16. Hilton S, Leopold G, Olson L, et al. Real-time breast sonography: Application in 300 consecutive patients. *AJR.* 1986;147:479–486.
17. Seidman H, Gelb SK, Silverberg E, LaVerda N, Lubera JA. Survival experience in the breast cancer detection demonstration project. *CA.* 1987;37:258–290.
18. Tabar L, Fargerberg CJG, Gad A. Reduction in mortality from breast cancer after mass screening with mammography. *Lancet.* 1985;1:829–832.
19. Dupont WD, Page DL. Risk factors for breast cancer in women with proliferative breast disease. *N Engl J Med.* 1985;312:146–151.
20. Moskowitz M. Screening is not diagnosis. *Radiology.* 1979;133:265–268.
21. Dempsey PJ, Moskowitz M. Is there a role for breast sonography? *Clin Diag Ultrasound.* 1987;20:17–36.
22. Sickles E, Filly R, Callen P. Cancer detection with sonography and mammography: Comparison using state-of-the-art equipment. *AJR.* 1983;140:843–845.
23. Kalisher L. Factors influencing false negative rates in xeromammography. *Radiology.* 1979;133:297–301.
24. Martin J, Moskowitz M, Milbrath J. Breast cancers missed by mammography. *AJR.* 1979;132:737–739.
25. Egan RL, Egan KL. Detection of breast carcinoma: Comparison of automated water-path whole-breast sonog-

raphy, mammography, and physical examination. *AJR.* 1984;143:493–497.

26. Harper AP, Kelly-Fry E. Ultrasound visualization of the breast in symptomatic patients. *Radiology.* 1980;137:465–467.

27. Jellins J, Kossoff G, Reeve TS. Detection and classification of liquid-filled masses in the breast by gray scale echography. *Radiology.* 1977;125:205–212.

28. Texidor HS, Kazam E. Combined mammographic-sonographic examination of breast masses. *AJR.* 1977;128:409–417.

29. Cole-Beuglet C, Goldberg B, Kurtz A, et al. Ultrasound mammography: A comparision with radiographic mammography. *Radiology.* 1981;140:693–698.

30. Egan RL, Egan KL. Automated water-path full-breast sonography: Correlation with histology of 176 solid lesions. *AJR.* 1984;143:499–507.

31. van Dam PA, Van Goethem MLA, Kersschot E, et al. Palpable solid breast masses: Retrospective single- and multimodality evaluation of 201 lesions. *Radiology.* 1988;166:435–439.

32. Cole-Beuglet C, Sorino R, Kurtz A, et al. Ultrasound analysis of 104 primary breast carcinomas classified according to histopathologic type. *Radiology.* 1983;146:191–196.

33. Reuter K, d'Orsi CJ, Reale F. Intracystic carcinoma of the breast: The role of ultrasonography. *Radiology.* 1984;153:233–234.

34. Sadowsky N, Kopans DB. Breast cancer. *Radiol Clin North Am.* 1983;21:51–65.

35. Tabar L, Pentek Z, Dean PB. Diagnostic and therapeutic value of breast cyst puncture and pneumocystography. *Radiology.* 1981;141:659–663.

36. Heywang SH, Lipsit ER, Glassman LM, Thomas MA. Specificity of ultrasonography in the diagnosis of benign breast disease. *J Ultrasound Med.* 1984;3:453–461.

37. Jackson VP, Rothschild PA, Kreipke DL, Mail JT, Holden RW. The spectrum of sonographic findings of fibroadenoma of the breast. *Invest Radiol.* 1986;21:34–40.

38. Harper AP, Kelly-Fry E, Noe JS, Bies JR, Jackson VP. Ultrasound in the evaluation of solid breast masses. *Radiology.* 1983;146:731–736.

39. Cole-Beuglet C, Sorino R, Kurtz A, et al. Ultrasound, x-ray mammography, and histopathology of cystosarcoma phylloides. *Radiology.* 1983;146:481–486.

40. Herman G, Schwartz IS. Focal fibrous disease of the breast: Mammographic detection of an unappreciated condition. *AJR.* 1983;140:1245–1246.

41. Derchi LE, Rizzatto G, Giuseppetti GM, Dini G, Garaventa A. Metastatic tumors in the breast: Sonographic findings. *J Ultrasound Med.* 1985;4:69–74.

42. Lambie R, Hodgden D, Herman E, et al. Sonographic manifestations of mammographically detectable breast microcalcifications. *Ultrasound Med Biol.* 1983;2:509–514.

43. Meyer JE, Kopans DB. The appearance of the therapeutically irradiated breast on whole-breast water-path ultrasonography. *J Ultrasound Med.* 1983;2:211–213.

44. Chenevert TL, Bylski DI, Carson PL, et al. Ultrasonic computed tomography of the breast: Improvement of image quality by use of cross-correlation time-of-flight and phase-insensitive attenuation measurements. *Radiology.* 1984;152:155–159.

45. Rizzatto G, Solbiati L, Croce F, Derchi LE. Aspiration biopsy of superficial lesions: Ultrasonic guidance with a linear-array probe. *AJR.* 1987;148:623–625.

42 Legal Concerns in Diagnostic Ultrasound: An Overview

Albert L. Bundy

As in all other disciplines of medicine, the field of diagnostic ultrasound faces its own legal concerns. Rapidly growing sophistication of technology and users has caused this modality to assume a major role in health care, particularly in the areas of obstetrics and gynecology. Both sonographers and sonologists are confronting medicolegal issues that have not previously challenged the legal system. The lawyers and courts are not familiar with adapting the traditional doctrines of medical jurisprudence to this specialty. Besides the legal theory of negligent malpractice, other legal issues, such as agency relationships and informed consent, are likely to come into play. Those working in this field must familiarize themselves with these medicolegal concerns, because litigation in this area has continued to rise over the past several years.[1-9]

MEDICAL NEGLIGENCE LAW

The laws governing medical malpractice, or medical negligence, are largely a section of jurisprudence known as tort law. By definition, a tort is a civil (as opposed to criminal) wrong where a defendant breaches a duty he owes to the plaintiff. Tort law is further subdivided into intentional torts, such as assault, battery and trespass; strict torts which require neither intention to do harm nor negligence to render one liable; and negligence torts, which is the category into which medical malpractice cases fall.

There are four basic elements in a negligence action. They are duty, breach, proximate causation, and damages. To be successful, the plaintiff has the burden of proving each of these four elements. The plaintiff must establish that the defendant owed him a duty of care which he breached, and that this breach proximately resulted in the damages of which the plaintiff is complaining. At first glance, it seems that the plaintiff has a very difficult burden to prove but, in reality, some of these elements are easily dealt with by the court. For example, the duty of care is established by the physician-patient relationship. Even nonprimary care physicians, such as radiologists, establish legally binding physician-patient relationships daily with people they might never meet. The mere interpretation of a film that a patient willingly had taken is enough to establish a duty of care based on the physician-patient relationship.

The proximate causation element is also usually easily dealt with by the court as long as the alleged negligence was antecedent to the harm. The damages themselves do not have to be concrete or economically measurable. Complaints of noneconomic damages for pain and suffering give the courts leeway in determining just how much harm has been done.

The most difficult burden of proof for the plaintiff attorney is deviation from the standard of care. The standard which the courts rely on is called the "reasonable man standard": the defendant is expected to behave like a reasonable person under like circumstances, and the physicians and technologists must behave like reasonable physicians and technologists practicing ultrasound. To determine what this reasonable standard is, the court looks to publications, guidelines, and experts in the field.

While there is little legal precedent for many of the current problems facing diagnostic ultrasound, there is a large body of law on medical negligence in other specialties. Courts do recognize a status of "specialist" that encompasses many medical specialties and subspecialties. Routinely, the courts have held the specialist to a higher standard of care than the medical profession in general. Therefore, those claiming to be experts in diagnostic ultrasound will be held to the minimum standards of a specialist in this field.

Lack of proper training is certainly not a defense. A claim of "level I" versus "level II" practice would not hold legal relevance. Furthermore, the strict locality rule, where one must adhere to the standard of care of those in the same community, has been abandoned. Currently, adherence to a national standard of care is the order in most jurisdictions.

LEGAL ACTIONS INVOLVING DIAGNOSTIC ULTRASOUND

The statistics which follow were presented by Dr. Roger Sanders at the 1987 American Institute of Ultrasound in Medicine (AIUM) convention in New Orleans. Over the years, Dr. Sanders has surveyed various groups and memberships requesting any information regarding legal actions involving the use of ultrasound. These results were published twice in the *Journal of Ultrasound in Medicine* and have been presented by Dr. Sanders at the legal symposium during the AIUM meeting. The actual outcome in most of these instances is not known. Many cases may have been dropped or never became a real legal action. Some have proceeded to court at both trial and appellate levels. Nevertheless, the results of this survey are quite interesting. Regardless of the actual outcome, it is certain that complaints about ultrasound examinations are on the rise (Tables 42–1 to 42–3).

As can be seen from Table 42–1, the number of these legal actions more than tripled from 1983 through 1987. Also, as shown in Table 42–2, the vast majority of these actions involved the obstetric sonogram. This is not surprising when ultrasound is coupled with the already highly litigious field of obstetrics.

The alleged "missed diagnosis" has already proven to be of major legal concern to the general diagnostic radiologist. This continues to be the category into which most legal actions involving ultrasound seem to fall.

The most frequent offenders in the missed-diagnosis category are ectopic pregnancy, fetal anomalies, multiple gestations, and placenta previa. The "misreported" category includes those cases where the findings were not missed but were incorrectly interpreted or reported. These include misdating gestational age, calling a decidual cast a gestational sac, and interpreting adjacent bowel as a stone-filled gallbladder.

The "invented-lesion" category includes those instances where findings were made that, in fact, didn't exist at all. Examples include reporting IUDs when none were present, reporting fetal demise when the fetus was still alive, calling a normal gestation a molar pregnancy, and reporting a normal fetus as anencephalic.

The "failure-to-use category" is of more concern to the referring physician than the sonologist. Cases of failure to use ultrasound which have been cited include not using ultrasound when there are risk factors for intrauterine growth retardation, history of previous ectopic pregnancy, and elevated maternal alpha-fetoprotein.

TABLE 42–2. NUMBER OF LEGAL ACTIONS IN EACH EXAM TYPE

Exam Type	Number
Obstetrics	159
Gynecology	18
Abdominal	21
Neuro	1
Eye	4
Breast	2

From Sanders.[9]

Legal actions regarding procedure complications have arisen when there have been problems during an ultrasound-guided amniocentesis and when ultrasound guidance was not used for this. The issue of informed consent, which is discussed later, also comes into play here.

Sonographer-related problems have included alleged patient molestation, giving a diagnosis to the patient that differed from the final report, and deliveries occurring with the patient left unattended while running films.

In recent years, a few appellate court decisions have discussed the issue of failure to perform ultrasound. In the case of *Quellette v Subak* (379 NW2d 125 [Minn App 1985]), there was a medical malpractice action alleging negligence of care in pregnancy management with resultant injury to the newborn. The pregnancy was misdated clinically, which resulted in cesarian delivery of a postmature baby with signs of brain damage.

The trial court ruled in favor of the plaintiff, who claimed that a sonogram should have been performed to date the pregnancy. The appellate court reversed this decision, finding that the physician is not responsible for an honest error in judgment when choosing between alternative methods of diagnosis. In other words, the appellate court was of the belief that the failure to perform the sonogram did not constitute negligence but an error in judgment. It seems unlikely that today ultrasound

TABLE 42–1. TOTAL NUMBER OF LEGAL ACTIONS IN SURVEY

Year	Number
1983	64
1984	86
1985	134
1986	177
1987	205

From Sanders.[9]

TABLE 42–3. MAJOR CATEGORIES OF TYPES OF LEGAL ACTIONS

Category	Number
Missed Diagnosis	88
Invented Lesions	20
Misreported Cases	34
Failure to Use	32
Procedure Complications	15
Sonographer Related	4
Delayed Reports	2
Miscellaneous	10

From Sanders.[9]

involvement. Ultrasound physicians may be replaced in time-consuming diagnostic studies, such as pulsed Doppler real-time evaluation of the carotid circulation, because their time is too expensive.[14] The agency relationship will predictably achieve increasing importance in this particular situation.[3]

One of the outgrowths of DRGs and certificates-of-need has been the initiation of so-called "diagnostic imaging centers," which often include ultrasound. In this type of arrangement, physicians often form partnerships between their referring doctors (representing limited partners) and their parent imaging group (as general partners). The general partner acts in a fiduciary capacity for the limited partners. Several antitrust challenges can be anticipated, including unlawful tying arrangements, restraint of trade, and extension of liability for general partners acting as agents for the limited partner.[15] Legislation before the United States Congress could make these arrangements unlawful.

As imaging physicians expand their activities in the area of "interventive medicine," their malpractice exposure will increase. Intrauterine treatment of hydrocephalus, cardiac abnormalities, and urinary obstruction have been well described in the literature.[16] Intraoperative ultrasound procedures have placed imaging physicians at greater risk as well. It will be exceedingly difficult in some interventive procedures to legally determine when the sonologist is acting as a consultant (independent contractor) or as an agent of the surgical colleague. When summoned by the surgeon to perform imaging in the case of either an interventive or an intraoperative procedure, is the sonographer the agent of the surgeon, the sonologist, or both? To date, we are unaware of precedent decisions in this regard. These procedures are being performed increasingly and one can anticipate that a number of cases will soon be litigated.

Untoward events during medical procedures can have a variety of etiologies. Sonographers may act outside their scope of employment, physicians may not perform to the level of standard care, or the equipment may fail. If a patient is injured due to equipment failure, is the manufacturer liable, is the physician liable as insurer of a good result, or is the principal in whose behalf the sonographer, his agent, performed the study liable? In the United States, courts have ruled that the instrument manufacturer is the most responsible party to insure the appropriate technical performance of the machine itself and is, therefore, liable for harm to patients for faulty design or fabrication.[17] If the technology is inappropriately applied, then the physician is liable for any injury in which proximate cause can be established. The ultrasound physician is not an agent of the manufacturer.

Many areas of the law of agency in medical imaging are founded in common law theory. Circumstances in one country may result in the existence of precedent cases prior to litigation in another. These precedent decisions may be instructive by anticipating legal ramifications to continuing medical developments. Agency law is particularly appropriate to consider as health care delivery continues to increase in complexity and sophistication, necessitating a team approach.

Diagnostic sonography, because of the energy form employed and the previous lack of invasiveness, has been a discipline of medical imaging traditionally immune from concerted legal inquiry. The information it can now provide has recently placed sonography in the forefront of legal activity in the United States in cases of wrongful birth, wrongful life, and in questions regarding fetal viability. These will predictably extend the questions of agency relationships.

We hope that this chapter will provide some assistance in understanding certain of these problems, and recognize that new issues may have been introduced for which we can provide no solutions at present.

Acknowledgments

We wish to thank our colleagues in both medicine and law in our respective institutions. The manuscript was prepared in the editorial office of the Division of Radiological Sciences and the Vanderbilt Center for Medical Imaging Research. Tom Greeson, JD, Legal Counsel for the American College of Radiology, was particularly helpful, as were Ed Hollowell and Ward DeWitt.

REFERENCES

1. James AE Jr. Hickey lecture: Medical imaging technology in a societal context. *AJR*. 1985;144:1109–1116.
2. James AE Jr, ed. *Legal Medicine With Special Reference to Diagnostic Imaging*. Baltimore: Urban & Schwarzenberg; 1980.
3. James AE Jr, Sherrard TJ. The law of agency as applied to radiology. *Radiology*. 1978;128:257–260.
4. James AE Jr, Bundy AL, Fleischer AC, et al. Legal aspects of diagnostic sonography. *Semin in Ultrasound, CT and MR*. 1985;6:207–216.
5. James AE Jr, Bundy AL, Johnson BA, et al. Certain legal aspects of obstetrics and gynecology in ultrasound. In: Sanders RC, James AE Jr, eds. *Principles and Practice of Ultrasonography in Obstetrics and Gynecology*. 3rd ed. Norwalk, Conn: Appleton-Century-Crofts; 1985:617–624.
6. James AE Jr, Fleischer AC, Thieme G, et al. Diagnostic ultrasonography: Certain legal considerations. *J Ultrasound Med*. 1985;4:427–431.
7. James AE Jr, Hall DJ, Johnson BA. Some applications of the law of evidence to the specialty of radiology. *Radiology*. 1977;124:845–848.

8. James AE Jr, Waddill WB III, Feazell GL, et al. The new medical imaging technologies as evidence. *Journal of Contemporary Law* (University of Utah College of Law). 1984;2:105–130.

9. Certificate of need in an antitrust context. *J Health Polit Policy Law.* 1983;8:314–319.

10. James AE Jr, Winfield AC, Rollo FD, et al. An analysis of the combined effects of certificate-of-need legislation (CON) and changes in the granting of hospital privileges. *Radiology.* 1982;145:229–231.

11. James AE Jr, Sloan FA, Hamilton RJ, et al. Antitrust aspects of exclusive contracts in medical imaging. *Radiology.* 1985;156:237–241.

12. James AE Jr, Sherrard TJ. Agency. In: James AE Jr, ed. *Legal Medicine with Special Reference to Diagnostic Imaging.* Baltimore: Urban & Schwarzenberg; 1980;135–146.

13. James AE Jr, Sloan FA, Pendergrass HP, et al. Hospital cost regulation: Certificate-of-need and diagnosis related groups. *Noninvasive Medical Imaging.* 1984;4:259–263.

14. Johnson AC, Price RR, Erickson JJ, et al. Medical imaging in the 1980s: Certain perspectives. *Indian J Radiol Imaging.* 1984;37:287–294.

15. James AE Jr, ed. *Medical/Legal Issues for Radiologists.* Chicago: Precept Press; 1987.

16. Reece EA, Hobbins JC. Ultrasonography and diabetes mellitus in pregnancy. In: Sanders RC, James AE Jr, eds. *Principles and Practice of Ultrasonography in Obstetrics and Gynecology.* 3rd ed. Norwalk, Conn: Appleton-Century-Crofts; 1985;297–320.

17. *Dubin v Michael Reese Hospital* 83 Ill2d 277 (1980).

44 The Concepts of Wrongful Life and Wrongful Birth and Their Relation to Diagnostic Sonography

*A. Everette James, Jr. • Arthur C. Fleischer •
Everette James III • Albert L. Bundy •
Jeannette C. James • Frank H. Boehm*

The recent focus on fetal and infant rights has involved the ultrasound physician in a number of cases of great importance. To date, legal precedents in this area have not been established. Thus, our roles have not been clearly defined and the societal issues involved are exceedingly complex. One might suggest that if these issues were better understood by physicians, and could be placed in an appropriate intellectual perspective by policy makers, the response to perceived societal demands would be more appropriate. We hope that this chapter will provide some assistance in that regard.

The concepts of wrongful birth and wrongful life are often confused, and unfortunately, as medical terms they are often used interchangeably. Wrongful birth cases are based on the legal theory of breach of duty by a physician to practice or impart medical information about potential fetal defects with due care. To be actionable, the parents must establish that inadequate warnings of potential anomalies had been given or inadequate or inappropriate testing had been performed. The damages recovered by the parents in such a case include the expense of the child's medical treatment as well as custodial and educational care. The compensated damages should be attributable to the infant's or child's defective condition. Medical and educational expenses, as well as mental anguish and emotional stress, have been found to merit compensation in certain cases of wrongful birth.[1]

A wrongful life action, in contrast, is brought by the child to recover extraordinary life expenses. These expenses are those anticipated during the individual's life as a result of being born with a defect that was either not discovered by the physician or, on discovery, was not properly acted on. Although the plaintiffs in these two forms of action are different, usually the parents in wrongful birth and the child in wrongful life, legal theory and analysis of circumstances in these cases have a number of similarities. Wrongful birth cases have generally been more successful than wrongful life actions, but the material risk of liability to the physician is much the same in both.

WRONGFUL BIRTH

It may be more instructive to consider wrongful birth in some depth before commenting on the concept of wrongful life. The action of wrongful birth conforms to the traditional structure of tort principles. The most crucial element to be established in a successful case is the concept of duty. Do physicians have a duty correlative to a parent's responsibility to prevent the birth of a defective child?[2,3] This was formerly a moot point, but medical science now has standardized investigative or diagnostic methods to predict and, after conception, detect the birth of a defective child.

Is the responsibility to detect a fetal deformity after conception greater than the responsibility to determine before conceiving, whether or not the parents' genetic traits significantly increase the risk of an infant being born less than whole? Thus, is the ultrasonographer as responsible as, or more responsible than, the geneticist?

Advances in biomedical imaging technology in detecting intrauterine defects have been well documented.[4-6] The dissemination of this information has both raised public awareness and raised expectations from patients and society in general. Communication regarding the virtues of ultrasound in terms of spatial and contrast resolution and the promise of magnetic resonance have created a favorable public climate for their introduction and routine use.[5,7] The professional and lay literature has also fostered the idea that these modalities should be widely distributed and almost universally applied. These data and communications have created the belief, as well, that diagnostic tests performed with these marvels of technology approach infallibility, thereby greatly increasing the physician's responsibility and liability because of a change in expectations.

Our legal system, hopefully with the advice of organized medicine, as well as the public, must decide whether or not new modalities such as pulsed Doppler real-time ultrasound, x-ray computed tomography, digital radiology, and magnetic resonance imaging confer upon parents the right to prevent the birth of a defective child. Do these medical advances provide to society the means of avoiding the extraordinary economic and emotional expense of defective children? Some courts have decided that in recognition of the benefits afforded by these medical advances, parents have the right to prevent defective births, and physicians have a responsibility correlating to that right. This responsibility includes communicating to the parents material information that could alter the decision of whether or not to abort a conception.[8]

In wrongful birth claims, the injury to the child is not the cause of the parents' injury. Rather, the birth of the child is the cause of the injury to the parents. Compensation can be recovered as a result of financial damages due to medical expense, loss of child's love and injury to the parent-child relationship, and deprivation of a child's services to the parent. Damages for emotional injury should be weighed against the benefits due to the birth of a child even in an impaired state. When one is considering injury from the viewpoint of parents, the standard of reference in that case would be a whole or unimpaired child.

WRONGFUL LIFE

Wrongful life has been considered by some to be the child's equivalent to wrongful birth by the parent. As previously noted, wrongful life actions have not historically been as successful in court because the traditional tort concepts are often difficult to substantiate.[9,10] Duty can only be established if the court admits that the fetus possesses rights and that the physician had a responsibility to that particular fetus. The establishment of this is, at best, problematical.

Employing the concept of "for suability," the duty of a physician could potentially extend or be projected as far back into the medical history as preconception.[11] It also follows that, if a person could be foreseeably endangered by a physician's conduct, then the physician may be accorded retroactive liability. In wrongful life cases, a very difficult determination for sonologists is whether or not the fetus would have been born had the parents known about an intrauterine abnormality based on ultrasound studies. Even more problematic is the circumstance when the sonographic study is inconclusive. This gives rise to the determination of whether or not the study was of diagnostic quality to meet the community standard.

Another difficulty in assessing the importance of wrongful life cases is in determining whether or not an impaired life is preferable to nonexistence.[12] Some courts have felt that to award damages to impaired infants due to being born less than whole would represent a disavowal of the sanctity of human life. Other courts have held that a less-than-whole child is entitled to redress in the form of financial compensation just as are other members of society who have been injured through no fault of their own. By equating a physician's duty to a child to that of the parents', some courts have expressed the belief that this standard would discourage incompetent medical practices and would foster proper genetic counseling and ultrasound testing.[11]

As noted, the settling of damages has been problematic in cases of wrongful life. The quantification of damages is difficult because courts simply cannot measure the difference in the value of a life in an impaired condition to compare it to the absence of life or even to a normal life. However, most courts, while recognizing that this quantification represents a substantial dilemma, do not agree that this should preclude bringing the action of wrongful life. Certain elements of this situation can be accounted; the expenses for medical care and special training for children with congenital defects are certainly calculable. Other areas do not lend themselves to ready computation.

The major difficulty for the medical profession in accepting the validity of wrongful life actions is the legal inability to establish proximate cause. Can the claim be established that, except for the physician's negligence, the parents would have aborted that particular pregnancy? Usually this is a retrospective analysis by the court, based on testimony by plaintiffs that is inherently biased and self-serving. The issue of fairness is difficult for physicians to accept but does not appear as difficult for the legal system.

IMPLICATIONS OF TECHNOLOGIC ADVANCES

The legal concepts of wrongful birth and wrongful life are of particular importance to diagnostic sonography. The application of biomedical engineering advances has made it possible to detect many intrauterine congenital defects that would predictably result in an impaired child. With the advent of gray scale ultrasound, the resolution of textural soft tissue characteristics allowed improved evaluation of the placenta, adnexal region, and details of the fetus itself. Real-time ultrasound with simultaneous Doppler capability has permitted a much-improved determination of fetal viability. Evaluation of the physiologic abnormalities associated with structural derangements that had previously escaped detection by conventional imaging methods is now possible. The portability of real-time ultrasound units and the ability to image continuously from many different angles have greatly increased our diagnostic capacities.

The improvements in diagnostic sonography have also created in the mind of the public and among many physicians the belief that ultrasound approaches an ideal imaging method. Thus, if an ultrasound study has been performed and an intrauterine defect not detected when one was, indeed, present, this may be regarded as prima-facie evidence for the existence of negligence and malpractice.[13] Additionally, if sonography represents a "perfect" test, then should it not be employed in every pregnancy? In this instance, what is standard of care?

The limits of spatial and contrast resolution for ultrasound instrumentation mean that certain intrauterine lesions may not be of sufficient size to be detected with present technology.[14] Thus, in wrongful life cases, a plausible defense might be that the fetal defect was too small to be seen on a "state of the art" ultrasound study. The limits of resolution are difficult to establish because they vary with the patient's size, the fetal age, the amniotic fluid volume, and fetal lie.[15]

In some cases of wrongful life, plaintiff's attorneys have claimed that standard of practice would dictate that an ultrasound study be performed in every pregnancy. This, however, is not the case. Several years ago, the NIH consensus panel on ultrasound in obstetric care recommended that an ultrasound study be obtained only when "medically" indicated, leaving the decision to the physician's perception of the clinical condition of the mother and fetus.[16] Groups at high risk for congenital defects were included in the population for which a diagnostic sonogram was recommended. In wrongful life cases, it appears to be an adequate defense, at present, to allege that the medical circumstances did not meet the criteria for which an imaging study would be mandatory.[17]

The sensitivity and specificity of ultrasound in detecting the presence of an intrauterine abnormality is further complicated by the concept of level I and level II studies. Level I evaluation by ultrasound is described as a study only to screen for fetal viability and cursory examination to detect only gross anatomic derangements. It is implied that the liability for a level I ultrasound examination is not as great as in a level II study. This at best provides for two levels of patient care. It permits a tacit compromise in basic quality control and in procedure performance. We suggest that this is a flawed concept, and does not appear to serve any useful purpose. In fact, it implies that a physician can elect to perform a study with less than standard of care or due care and raises yet another issue of who should properly perform and interpret the study. Could they be persons of lesser training

and competence than those performing a level II study?

Because there is no legal impediment to any licensed physician acquiring and employing ultrasound, it is difficult to assess the conditions and expertise that constitute community standard of care in performing diagnostic sonography studies and interpretation. Wording in the transcript of *Turpin v Sortini*,[11] for example, suggests that ultrasound testing should be encouraged, and the partial relief of awards for damage might have further use as a positive benefit for ultrasound. The proceedings from this trial do not appear to offer suggestions as to which health care provider should perform and interpret these ultrasound studies. How will the "turf" of obstetric ultrasound be decided? Our discussion in the overview chapter of the case of *White v Rockingham Radiologists* (see Chapter 43) may provide some insight.[18]

At present, there is no standardized examination or board to provide a determination of professional competence in ultrasound. Some ad hoc testing and guidelines are present, but no subspecialty examination exists as a regular procedure.[19] Several specialty boards offer examinations of special competence in diagnostic sonography, but no separate board or board equivalent exists at present. Although fellowship and preceptorship programs in ultrasound are available, these also are not standardized, and no established methods to evaluate these programs exist.[20] They may be evaluated as part of residency programs' review in radiology and in obstetrics and gynecology, but only in a general context.

As noted, the legal implications of wrongful life cases are significant for our discipline. With the magnitude of awards and the percentage of successful cases increasing, potential litigants will continue to increase. As the "addictive" nature of diagnostic testing through imaging becomes more widespread, it will become much more routine to obtain ultrasound studies in normal pregnancies. Nonfeasance may well become an actionable legal theory in instances of children born with an abnormality making them less-than-whole. Failure to perform an ultrasound study, considered as malpractice, might well be a result of the technologic evolution as improvements in equipment and examination techniques continue.

The sonographer predictably will become involved in subsequent wrongful life suits. As in any trial, certain elements of proof and legal activities will be required to establish a certain line of reasoning. Expert testimony will be necessary to establish certain facts, such as whether a study should have been obtained, whether the lesion should have been resolved by the capabilities of the instrumentation, whether the study was performed with due care, whether the sonographer's interpretations were sufficient and specific to constitute community standard of care, and whether the results of the study were communicated adequately and in a timely fashion.

To address the first issue, at present an ultrasound

study should be obtained only if medically indicated. The instrumentation should meet the community standard if not the ideal state-of-the-art. A quality assurance program should be in place and functioning as routine "conduct of the shop." These may very well obviate the questions of resolution as there is little agreed-upon scientific data regarding instrument capabilities in vivo.

Complete ultrasound studies of the pelvic region, adnexa, and appropriate other areas should be obtained. In our judgment, no level I examinations should be performed. Timely and accurate communication to the referring physician or, when appropriate, the patient is standard practice and a universally agreed-on desirable activity. Still, difficulties may arise as to the content of the consultative report to the referring physician. In cases where abortion of the fetus is being considered, this may be a major issue in assessing liability. Thus, the responsibility of the sonographer in cases of wrongful life and wrongful birth appears to be an ever-increasing one.

SUMMARY

We hope this chapter will further the understanding of the concepts involved in wrongful life and wrongful birth, and will assist the conduct of medical practice in such a way as to minimize risks to patients and with regard to the liability of physicians, technicians, and hospitals. If sonographers are involved in wrongful life cases, we trust the data presented will assist them in understanding the legal and societal environment in which they are suddenly thrust. As a secondary benefit, we hope this communication may assist the defense attorney to effectively argue against the plaintiff's legal theory. Knowledge should provide understanding, if not relief.

Acknowledgments

We are appreciative of the use of the resources of the Vanderbilt School of Medicine, the Institute of Public Policy Studies, and the Center for Medical Imaging Research (CMIR). Legal colleagues Tom Greeson, James Blumstein, James Neal, and Melvin Belli provided editorial assistance. Lonnie Burnett and Ann Wentz gave us insight from the obstetric perspective. Philippe Jeanty was most helpful in furthering our knowledge of ultrasound in genetic disorders.

REFERENCES

1. *Harbeson v Parke-Davis*, 98 Wash2d 460, 656 P2d 483 (1983).

2. *Phillips v United States*, 508 F Supp 544,545 n.1 (DSC 1981).

3. Rogers TD. Wrongful life and wrongful birth: Medical malpractice in genetic counseling and prenatal testing. *SC Law Rev.* 1982;33:739–741.

4. Jeanty P. *Obstetrical Ultrasound.* New York: McGraw-Hill; 1984.

5. Fleischer AC, James AE Jr. *Real-Time Sonography.* Norwalk, Conn: Appleton-Century-Crofts; 1984.

6. Sanders RC, James AE Jr, eds: *The Principles and Practice of Ultrasonography in Obstetrics and Gynecology.* 3rd ed. Norwalk, Conn: Appleton-Century-Crofts; 1985.

7. Partain CL, James AE, Rollo FD, Price RR. *Nuclear Magnetic Resonance Imaging.* Philadelphia: WB Saunders; 1983.

8. James AE Jr, Bundy AL, Fleischer AC, Gore J, Sanders RC, Hobbins JC. Legal aspects of diagnostic sonography. *Semin in Ultrasound, CT, MR.* 1985;6:207–216.

9. *Curlender v Bio-Science Labs*, 106 Cal App3d 811, 165 CalRprtr 477 (1980).

10. *Becker v Schwartz*, 46 NY2d 401, 386 NE2d 807, 413 NYS2d 895 (1978).

11. *Turpin v Sortini*, 31 Cal3d 220, 643 P2d 954 182 Cal Rptr 337 (1982).

12. *Berman v Allan*, 80 NJ 430, 404 A2d 8 (1979).

13. James AE Jr, Fleischer AC, Thieme G, et al. Diagnostic ultrasonography: Certain legal considerations. *J Ultrasound Med.* 1985;4:427–431.

14. Thieme GA, Price RR, James AE Jr. Ultrasound instrumentation and its practical applications. In: Sanders RC, James AE Jr, eds. *The Principles and Practice of Ultrasonography in Obstetrics and Gynecology.* 3rd ed. Norwalk, Conn: Appleton-Century-Crofts; 1985.

15. Gibbs SJ, Price RR, James AE Jr. Image perception. In: Coulam CM, Erickson JJ, et al, eds. *The Physical Basis of Medical Imaging.* New York: Appleton-Century-Crofts; 1981.

16. NIH: Diagnostic Ultrasound Imaging in Pregnancy Report of Consensus Conference, Washington. United States Department of Health and Human Services, 1984.

17. James AE Jr, Bundy AL, Johnson BA, et al. Certain legal aspects of obstetric and gynecologic ultrasound. In: Sanders RC, James AE Jr, eds. *The Principles and Practice of Ultrasonography in Obstetrics and Gynecology.* 3rd ed. Norwalk, Conn: Appleton-Century-Crofts; 1985.

18. *White v Rockingham Radiologists, Ltd.*, 820 F2d 98, 4th Cir, 1987.

19. James AE Jr, Chapman JE, Carroll F, et al. Ethical choices in high technology medicine: Current dilemmas in diagnostic imaging. *Health Care Instrumentation.* 1986;1:158–167.

20. James AE Jr, Garrett WJ, Bundy A, Fleischer AC, Vallentine JR. The commonality and contrasts of agency law and relationships in sonography. *Journal of Australasian Radiology.* 1986;30:298–301.

Index

Page numbers followed by f refer to illustrations.
Page numbers followed by t refer to tables.

Page numbers followed by *f* refer to
illustrations.
Page numbers followed by *t* refer to tables.

Page numbers followed by *f* refer to
illustrations.
Page numbers followed by *t* refer to tables.

Page numbers followed by *f* refer to
illustrations.
Page numbers followed by *t* refer to tables.

Page numbers followed by *f* refer to
illustrations.
Page numbers followed by *t* refer to tables.